Community health

Community health

Lawrence W. Green, B.S., M.P.H., Dr.P.H.

Professor and Director, Center for Health Promotion Research
and Development, University of Texas Health Science Center at Houston;
Visiting Lecturer, Division of Health Policy Research and Education,
Harvard Medical School and Harvard School of Public Health,
Boston, Massachusetts

C.L. Anderson, B.S., M.S.P.H., Dr.P.H.

Former Professor and Head, Hygiene and Environmental Sanitation,
Oregon State University, Corvallis, Oregon

FOURTH EDITION

with **135** *illustrations*

The C. V. Mosby Company

ST. LOUIS • TORONTO • LONDON   1982

MOSBY

A TRADITION OF PUBLISHING EXCELLENCE

Editor: Charles K. Hirsch
Assistant editor: Michelle Turenne
Manuscript editor: Elizabeth O'Brien, Selena V. Bussen
Book design: Susan Trail
Cover design: Suzanne Oberholtzer
Production: Barbara Merritt, Ginny Douglas

FOURTH EDITION

Previous editions copyrighted 1969, 1973, 1978

Printed in the United States of America

The C.V. Mosby Company
11830 Westline Industrial Drive, St. Louis, Missouri 63141

Library of Congress Cataloging in Publication Data

Green, Lawrence W.
    Community health.

    Rev. ed. of: Community health/C.L. Anderson,
Richard F. Morton, Lawrence W. Green. 3rd ed.
1978.
    Includes bibliographies and index.
    1. Public health.   2. Public health—United
States.   I. Anderson, C.L. (Carl Leonard),
1901–   .   II. Title.   [DNLM: 1. Community health
services.   2. Public health. WA 546.1 G796c]
RA425.G74   1982   362.1   81-18785
ISBN 0-8016-0187-8   AACR2

C/VH/VH   9   8   7   6   5   4   3   2   1   01/B/075

PREFACE

This book is about community health rather than about personal hygiene. Personal health practices are the essential building blocks of community health, but the promotion of such practices through the planning and delivery of programs for *populations* distinguishes community health programs from medicine and self-care. Community health encompasses many medical and self-care activities, but its concern is with the coordination and integration of these activities with the needs, goals, and resources of whole communities.

Community health is more concerned with the availability and accessibility of adequate health resources for the care of all rather than for the special care of a few. This book, therefore, addresses questions of distribution, participation, and organization more than biomedical processes and techniques; prevention more than cure; the dissemination and application of health knowledge more than its source or its control; and communities more than individual patients.

Just as the individual faces health problems, the community also faces or anticipates health problems that must be solved or prevented. In the solutions to community health problems some new promotional approaches are emerging. In the United States, federal funding to state and local health departments and for medical and hospital facilities and services has had a catalytic effect, but other resources and efforts have also been important in community health advances in the past decade. Much of

this edition is directed to a discussion of these recent advances.

Ironically, with all of the investments in medical facilities and technology of the Western nations, they appear to have reached a plateau in their contributions to reductions in death rates. Certainly, to break away from these plateaus will require ingenuity and concerted effort in dealing with human health on all levels and in all aspects. Prevention or correction of such risk factors as smoking, alcoholism, other drug misuse, injuries, and malnutrition presents the best opportunities for extending life expectancy. This applies to community action as well as to individual life-style.

An aging population and the possibility of a population exceeding the supply of energy arouse concern. Zero population growth is still some distance in the future, but great strides have been made in extending family planning to all segments of communities.

Legislation such as the Traffic and Motor Safety Act in the United States and mandatory seat belt laws in Australia has given impetus to renewed efforts to reduce motor vehicle injuries. Most nations have not truly come to grips with this destructive force. Congressional indifference and languid resignation of the public must be replaced with a vigorous, scientifically based program to deal effectively with this ubiquitous threat.

Fitness programs to promote mental, social, and physical health are given emphasis in both Western society and Communist Asia. Recognition is given to the role of recreation in the correction of disabilities and in rehabilitation. With each passing year the role of the community becomes more important in providing a recreational program to meet the needs of most of the community's citizenry. Recreation and fitness as an investment in health is not a new concept, but the resurgence of interest in fitness is a societal change of major significance for health.

Alcoholism and the prevention of alcohol and other drug addictions are of interest and concern to most communities. Like many other health problems, drug misuse has long been with us, and, like some other health problems, it has multiplied in gravity at a geometric rate. As with most such problems, community action can make a contribution to the solution of alcohol and drug misuse.

The major changes to be found throughout this edition include updated concepts, facts, and figures, including charts, flow diagrams, and models that replace outdated illustrations. Chapter 4 on human behavior and community health education is a new chapter that introduces a model of health promotion planning. Also new to this edition are sections on objectives for 1990 in disease prevention and health promotion and model standards tables for community health, which are both presented in a form to allow students to fill in their own community needs.

In preparing this revision we have increased the emphasis and use of administrative, educational, and epidemiological concepts and methods. A problem-solving approach is now used to complement the more purely descriptive character of previous editions. Information on adult health has been expanded so as to feature adolescent and adult coverage more equally. New sections on mental health, community organizations, and communication and transportation problems and solutions have been added to the community geriatrics chapter, Chapter

7. Discussions of hospital facilities in the community mental health chapter, Chapter 8, have been reduced in light of recent de-institutionalization of psychiatric care. Greater emphasis is now given to health and economic aspects in the community recreation and fitness chapter, Chapter 9, especially to fitness programs in work settings.

Reorganization of the communicable disease control chapter, Chapter 10, reflects the recent eradication of smallpox and new epidemiological principles of disease control. Expansion of Chapter 11 on community safety and injury control includes additional coverage of motor vehicle and burn injuries, falls, and violent deaths proportionate to their occurrences in the community. The chapter on life-style and community health promotion, Chapter 12, (formerly the compulsive behaviors chapter) applies the new model of health promotion planning introduced in the new Chapter 4. Also included is a major expansion of nutrition and world hunger issues.

The environmental health chapters, Chapters 13 to 17, reflect recent concerns with toxic agents, chemical and nuclear wastes, air and noise pollution, and energy and conservation issues. The health services chapters, Chapters 18 to 21, offer a more comparative view of current U.S. systems and those of other English-speaking countries (Canada, Australia, and New Zealand) and European countries.

This revision was completed as one of us (L.W.G.) returned to teaching after 2 years of directing the U.S. Office of Health Information, Health Promotion and Physical Fitness and Sports Medicine in the Office of the Assistant Secretary for Health.* We are indebted to Virginia Li Wang and David Levine at The Johns Hopkins University, Judith Ottoson and

---

*No official support or endorsement of this edition by the U.S. Department of Health and Human Services is intended nor should be inferred.

Beatrice Hamburg at Harvard University, Ruby Isom, Beverly Wright, and Kay Andreoli at the University of Texas, Donald Iverson at the Connecticutt State Department of Health, and Charles K. Hirsch and Michelle Turenne at The C.V. Mosby Company for their encouragement and support at various points in this revision. We also thank the publisher's reviewers—Ruth Ann Althaus, Ph.D., George Williams College, Downer's Grove, Illinois; Mark Dignan, Ph.D., The University of North Carolina at Greensboro; Dan D. Gowings, Associate Professor, Ball State University, Muncie, Indiana; Bryan J. Gray, D.Ed., North Texas State University, Denton, Texas; and Richard H. Needle, Ph.D., The University of Minnesota at Minneapolis—and the many college and university instructors whose reviews and comments have helped shape this revision.

Lawrence W. Green
C.L. Anderson

CONTENTS

9 Community recreation and fitness, 221

10 Communicable disease control, 253

PART ONE

Overview

1

THROUGH THE CENTURIES

The history of public health might well be written
as a record of successive redefinings of the unacceptable.

Sir Godfrey Vickers

Community health promotion has been interwoven with the philosophy, religion, economic conditions, form of government, education, science, aspirations, and folklore of any given period. The history of community health therefore reflects the advances and declines of societies and human conditions.

Civilization depends on the quality and distribution of health in the general population. Health in turn is dependent on human advancement in various spheres. Cast in the historical framework of a time, community health is not something apart from the life of the time—it is a result of life-styles as well as a barometer of that period. Community health promotion is an attitude constantly evolving in its acceptance of conditions and in its aspiration to change those conditions.

Community health practice today is not isolated from the past; it is built on and retains the best of the past. A new discovery may lead to the abandonment of a well-accepted practice, or it may lead to a new method of applying what has been an accepted health principle. Vestiges of health advances of the past are a legacy of scientists and other pioneers whose continual quest for better health led to the periodic redefinition of unacceptable conditions by the people they served.

CONCEPT OF COMMUNITY HEALTH PROMOTION

One of the leading figures in the history of public health, C.-E. A. Winslow, characterized public health practice as the science and art of preventing disease, prolonging life, and promoting health and well-being through organized community effort for the sanitation of the environment, the control of communicable infections, the organization of medical and nursing services for the early diagnosis and prevention of disease, the education of the individual in personal health, and the development of the social machinery to assure everyone a standard of living adequate for the maintenance or improvement of health.

The definition of *community health promotion* that will be used in this book is *any combination of educational, social, and environmental supports for behavior conducive to health*. The educational interventions may be directed at high-risk individuals, families, or groups or at whole communities through mass media, schools, worksites, and organizations. Social interventions may include economic, political, legal, and organizational changes designed to support actions conducive to health. Environmental supports include the structure and distribution of physical, chemical, and bi-

3

ological resources, facilities, and substances required for people to protect their health. The health behavior of a community includes the actions of the people whose health is in question and the actions of community decision makers, professionals, peers, teachers, employers, parents, and others who may influence health behaviors, resources, or services in the community.

Organized community effort is the key to community health. There are some things the individual can do entirely alone, but many health benefits can be obtained only through united community effort. Community health promotion is necessary to make the fruits of health science available to all citizens.

HISTORY OF COMMUNITY HEALTH
Egyptian and Babylonian health practices

The ancient papyrus discovered by Edwin Smith indicates the early use in Egypt of prescriptions, particularly of opium, minerals, and root drugs. ℞ was the astrological sign of Jupiter, under whose protection medicine was placed. The association of moon and lunatic arose from the relationship of religion and astrology. Alcoholic intoxication was thought to be due to the spirits of the fruit that was used in making the beverage. Pharmaceutical preparations played an important role in attempts to treat disease, although most of the successes are attributed to placebo effects. Medication was not universally available or acceptable.

Excavations have revealed that the Egyptians had community systems for collecting rain water and for disposing sewage. Herodotus, in the fifth century BC, described the hygienic customs of the Egyptians. Personal cleanliness, frequent baths, and simple dress were emphasized. Earth closets were in general use.

Hammurabi, a great king of Babylon who lived around 2000 BC, formulated a set of laws called the Code of Hammurabi that governed the conduct of physicians and provided for

health practices. The code also regulated and defined unacceptable conduct in general.

Yet from the standpoint of community health practice, the Egyptians and Babylonians went backward as the centuries advanced. Hebrew and Greek health practices went far beyond those of Egypt and Babylon.

Hebrew Mosaic Law

Early Hebrew society extended Egyptian concepts of disease and the community promotion of health through the regulation of human conduct by the Mosaic Law or Code. Human conduct is fundamental in all health—community as well as personal. With the Hebrews, a weekly day of rest was a health as well as a religious measure. Family relations and sexual conduct were directed to the best interests of personal, family, and community health. While the Hebrews had rather crude concepts of the spread of disease, they did make concerted efforts to prevent disease spread. The first practice of preventive medicine was the segregation of lepers, as recorded in Leviticus. Recognition that eating pork at times resulted in illness led the Hebrews to regard pork as unclean and to forbid it in the diet.

The Mosaic Law or Code provided for (1) personal and community responsibility for health, (2) maternal health, (3) communicable disease control, (4) segregation of lepers, (5) fumigation, (6) decontamination of buildings, (7) protection of water supplies, (8) disposal of wastes, (9) protection of food, and (10) sanitation of campsites. Without the aid of fundamental knowledge of the nature of infectious disease, the health efforts of the Hebrews were not highly effective. Nevertheless, they defined unacceptable conditions and mobilized community forces against them.

The glory of Greece

The Greek era in history extends over many centuries, but the Classic Period was the years

460 to 136 BC. The Greeks excelled in physical aspects of personal health. Games, gymnastics, and other exercises were directed toward their definition of physical strength, endurance, dexterity, and grace. Harmonious development of all faculties was the guiding philosophy. Exercise was supplemented by measures in personal cleanliness and dietetics. The Classic Period of Greece is characterized by its emphasis on the individual. As a consequence, very little attention was given to environmental sanitation. Yet Hippocrates wrote the definitive treatise on environment and health with his trilogy *Air, Waters, and Places* (Dubos, 1968, p. 114).

The Greeks did not borrow from other nations. The Hindus of ancient India had practiced surgery for at least a century, but there is no evidence that the Greeks used the Hindu methods of surgery, despite Alexander's conquests on the Indian subcontinent.

The Roman empire

With the destruction of Corinth in 146 BC, the health knowledge and health practices of the Greeks migrated to Rome and were welcomed by the rising Roman empire. In the philosophy of the Romans, however, the state and not the individual was of primary importance. To the Romans, the individual existed merely to serve the state. With this extreme emphasis on the state, it is not surprising that the influence of Greek hygiene should soon fade through neglect.

The Romans had a special talent for military science, and their administrative and engineering attainments were reflected in their many community health projects. At all times the welfare of the state was primary and that of the individual was subservient. The registration of citizens and slaves and the taking of a periodic census served to help in planning community health measures, although their primary purpose was doubtlessly mercenary. Regulation of building construction, the prevention of nui-

sances, and the destruction of decaying goods and buildings were measures that are still practiced in the modern state. Building regulations provided for ventilation and even for central heating. Town planning was directed toward sanitation measures as well as toward other needs. Public sanitation was promoted through the construction of paved streets with gutters. Street cleaning and repair were standard procedures in the interest of sanitation, although modern health officials regard these measures as being of esthetic rather than of direct health importance. Drainage networks carried off rain and other water, all of which was of some health significance. Removal of garbage and rubbish, although desirable in any society, was not of as great health significance as the Romans contended. Public baths were promoted as community health measures. Although street cleaning, garbage removal, and public baths were of minor health value, several other measures promoted by the Romans were of significant importance to health.

Roman officials had sufficient understanding of health to provide a protected water supply for their cities. Water was brought to Rome from great distances via aqueducts, some of which are still incorporated into the water system of Rome. City sewerage systems were built, and some of these drains are still part of the sewerage system of the city. This ability of the Romans to design and construct public water and sewerage systems enabled Rome to grow to a city of 800,000 during the reign of Julius Caesar. The Greeks, who depended on family wells and private refuse disposal, were more limited in the size to which their cities could grow. Corinth at the pinnacle of its greatness had a population of only 35,000.

The downfall of the Western empire was related to social degeneration. The term *Byzantine*, which refers to the Eastern Roman empire, connotes luxury and sloth. Even in this atmosphere, Galen (AD 130-201) did some experimentation relating to health, but his extreme dogmatism limited the value of his work. Contrasted to the attempt of Galen to understand disease is the statement of Saint Augustine (AD 353-430): "All diseases are to be ascribed to demons."

Dark Ages

The early years (AD 476-1000) of the medieval period of history are usually referred to as the Dark Ages. Western civilization was in a chaotic, almost formless state. The only existing science was fostered by the state and was but a trifle. Virtually the entire emphasis of the time was on the spiritual aspects of life because the clergy were the only educated class. Rejection of the body and glorification of the spirit became the accepted pattern of behavior. It was regarded as immoral to see one's body. People seldom bathed, and they used dirty garments. The use of perfumes appears to have stemmed from the attempt to conceal body and other unpleasant odors about the person. The more one could neglect and abuse one's body, the more esteemed one was. A legendary example of body neglect is of Saint Stylites, who sat on top of a pole for 16 years to expose his body to the abuse of the elements. It was as though health itself had been defined as unacceptable. The poor diets of the time resulted in the use of spices to overcome the bad odor and the foul taste of the food.

During the sixth and seventh centuries, Mohammedanism arose. After the death of Mohammed, a series of pilgrimages to Mecca began. Each pilgrimage was followed by a cholera epidemic. All through history migrations have been a vehicle of disease spread.

The spread of leprosy was from Egypt to Asia Minor and then to Europe. Most nations decreed lepers unacceptable and civilly dead. Lepers were required to wear identifying clothing and to warn of their presence by a bell or a horn. This isolation, however, together with the early death of lepers, virtually eliminated leprosy in Europe.

Medieval pandemics

The later medieval period, from AD 1000 to about 1453, is of special interest because of the severe pandemics of the time and the attempts to deal with the spread of disease. (*Pandemics* are widespread epidemics, usually affecting more than one country. *Epidemics* are outbreaks of disease that have spread through a population.) Between the years 1096 and 1248, the six great crusades to the holy lands were of health significance. To provide crusaders who were fit for the long journey, attention was given to building up the best possible level of health. While the approach was somewhat that of the ancient Greeks in building up physical prowess, the general result was that of building up a better condition of well-being in that one segment of the population. However, in their journeys the crusaders picked up cholera, and the death rate among them was high.

In 1348 bubonic plague, or the Black Death, followed a devastating path from Asia to Africa, Crimea, Turkey, Greece, Italy, and up through Europe. Some idea of the devastation of the disease can be gathered by referring to the deaths in several of the large cities in Europe: Paris, 50,000; Seine, 70,000; Marseilles, 16,000 in 1 month; Vienna, 1,200 daily; Florence, 60,000; and Venice, 100,000. Boccaccio reported that in the terrible outbreak of plague in Florence in this year, feelings, pity, and humanity were forgotten. Families deserted their sick. In Venice the government appointed three guardians of public health and in 1374 denied entry to the city of infected or suspected travelers, ships, or freight. In 1403 a quarantine of 40 days was imposed on anyone suspected of having the disease. In England 2 million died, representing approximately half the total population of the country. London had 100,000 deaths. Over a number of years

London's deaths exceeded its births. If it were not for the influx of people from the rural areas, London's population would have declined steadily. Estimates that approximately 25 million people died of the Black Death in Europe attest to the virulence of the bubonic plague.

Control measures. Pandemics were attributed to storms, comets, famines, drought, crop failures, insects, and poisoning of wells by the Jews. However, discerning officials of various communities recognized the possible relationship of crowding, poor sanitation, and migrations to the outbreak and spread of disease, and some communities took steps to establish control measures. In 1377 at Rogusa it was ruled that travelers from plague areas should stop at designated places and remain there free of disease for 2 months before being allowed to enter the city. Technically, this is the first official quarantine method on record. In 1383 Marseilles passed the first quarantine law and erected the first official quarantine station.

Measures to control disease spread were not highly effective. The need was for a scientific understanding of the cause and nature of disease and its spread. Scholars of the time who turned toward the scientific approach to pestilence were open to surveillance and public persecution. As a consequence of such resistance, there could be little progress in the understanding of disease.

Renaissance

The beginning of the Renaissance is associated with a revival of learning that was germinating in Italy, stimulated by the fall of Constantinople in 1453. For many historians, the Renaissance as applied to western and northern Europe encompasses the period from AD 1453 to 1600.

From the standpoint of community health, the Renaissance was particularly important because of its movement away from scholasticism and toward realities. It was an age of individual scientific endeavor, and it ushered in a spirit of inquiry that would lead to the understanding of the cause and nature of infectious disease. The fifteenth and sixteenth centuries produced such distinguished figures as Copernicus, da Vinci, Vesalius, Galileo, and Gilbert. By the middle of the sixteenth century, scholars had differentiated influenza, smallpox, tuberculosis, bubonic plague, leprosy, impetigo, scabies, erysipelas, anthrax, and trachoma. Diphtheria and scarlet fever were not recognized as separate diseases but were recognized as being different from all other diseases. Fracastorius (1478-1553), a physician of Verona, recognized that syphilis was transmitted from person to person during sexual relations. Learning was advancing, but the resulting social concentration, expanding trade, and movement of populations tended to spread disease. Knowledge of communicable disease control lagged behind disease spread, and great plagues still harassed Europe.

Colonial period

During the colonial period from 1600 to 1800, community health in North America, Australia, Africa, Asia, and South America was dependent on developments in Europe. No account of this period would be complete without some mention of health problems in Europe and the contributions that European scholars made to health.

Community health in Europe. Between 1600 and 1665 Europe suffered three severe pandemics of bubonic plague. The plight of London indicates the severity of the outbreaks. In 1603 a sixth of London's population died of the plague. In 1625 another sixth was destroyed by the plague, and in 1665 one out of five of London's residents died from the same disease.

This same era produced Descartes (1598-1650), Voltaire (1694-1778), and Boyle (1627-1691). This last named scholar, a distinguished

Englishman, made a prophetic pronouncement: "He that totally understands the nature of ferments and the fermentation shall probably be much better able than he who ignores them to give a fair account of certain diseases (fevers as well as others) which will perhaps be never properly understood without an insight into the doctrine of fermentation." William Harvey (1578-1657) fairly accurately described the circulation of human blood. In 1658 an English investigator, Sydenham (1624-1689), made a differential diagnosis of scarlet fever, malaria, dysentery, and cholera. Some historians contend that most of Sydenham's discoveries were accidental, but it should be acknowledged that chance favors the disciplined mind. Sydenham is generally regarded as the first distinguished epidemiologist.

Athanasius Kircher (1602-1680) examined the blood of victims of plague, using a microscope of 33 diameters, and thereby instituted a new method of study. In 1676 a Dutch draper and city hall janitor, Anton van Leeuwenhoek (1632-1723), using a microscope with magnification of 200 diameters, succeeded in seeing bacteria, protozoa, red corpuscles, and spermatozoa. Robert Hooke (1635-1703) also worked with the microscope, as did Marcello Malpighi (1628-1694) who studied the microscopic structure of tissues and laid some of the early foundations for histology.

In 1693 an astronomer, Edmund Halley (1656-1742), compiled the Breslau Table of births and funerals. This represented a contribution to the growth of vital statistics. In 1762 M.A. Plenciz, a physician of Vienna, studied scarlet fever and other infectious diseases and concluded that each infectious disease was caused by a specific kind of thing. While he did not identify "thing" factually, his theory predated the discoveries of Pasteur and Koch by a century.

Edward Jenner (1749-1823), a British physician and son of a Gloucestershire clergyman, scientifically demonstrated the effectiveness of smallpox vaccination. In 1796, using matter from pustules on the arm of a milkmaid who had contracted cowpox, Dr. Jenner vaccinated a young boy. Six weeks later he inoculated the boy with smallpox virus and demonstrated that the boy was immune to smallpox. Dr. Jenner demonstrated scientifically that inoculation with cowpox virus can produce immunity to the smallpox virus. He received his idea of inoculating with cowpox vaccine to prevent smallpox from the practice of English peasants of allowing themselves to contract cowpox in the knowledge that they would then be safe from smallpox. Reports indicate that some form of smallpox vaccination had been practiced in Turkey previous to Dr. Jenner's time, but he generally is credited with the first scientific vaccination against smallpox.

Health in the colonies. There was little interest in community health in the British, French, Dutch, and Spanish colonies on the other continents. Community health action was taken only during epidemics and consisted essentially of isolation and quarantine. Sanitation consisted of community tidiness or general housecleaning.

Smallpox ironically aided the European settlers of America. Introduced to the east coast by the Cabot and Gosnold expeditions, the disease eliminated so many of the Indians that the new settlers were able to colonize with little or no opposition. Yet smallpox took its toll among the whites as well and obliterated some of the early settlements. Some notable pandemics were those of Massachusetts Bay colonies in 1633, New Netherlands (New York) in 1663, and Boston in 1752. Of Boston's 1752 population of 15,684, only 174 completely escaped the smallpox pandemic. During the life of George Washington, 90% of the people who attained the age of 21 had had smallpox, and 25% of those infected by smallpox died. The significance of public health in history is reflected by these statistics in the context of the 1980 announcement of the World Health Organization

(WHO) that smallpox had been totally eradicated from the earth.

Yellow fever became a bigger scourge than smallpox during the eighteenth and nineteenth centuries. In 1793 Philadelphia had the greatest single epidemic in America. Of a population of about 37,000, more than 23,000 had the disease and over 4,000 of these died. A citizen's committee appointed to deal with the problem drew up the following set of regulations:

1. Avoid contact with a case.
2. Placard all infected houses.
3. Clean and air the sickroom.
4. Provide hospital accommodations for the poor.
5. Keep streets and wharves clean.
6. Encourage general hygienic measures such as quick private burials, avoidance of fatigue of mind and body, avoidance of intemperance, and adaptation of clothing to the weather.

Vinegar and camphor were used on handkerchiefs to prevent infection. Gunpowder was burned in the streets to combat the disease. Simple and perhaps as ineffective as these measures may have been, they represented a sincere attempt of communities to combat the disease based on the fragmentary knowledge people had of yellow fever. Frosty nights on October 17 and 18 ended the epidemic. Citizens of Philadelphia did not understand the "miracle," but from the vantage point of today we know that the frost killed the *Aedes aegypti* mosquito, the temporary host or vector for yellow fever. Modern health authorities are indebted to Dr. Benjamin Rush for a magnificent report of the Philadelphia epidemic published in 1815.

Health advances during the colonial period were made mostly during the eighteenth century. Occupational hygiene and the safety and well-being of the worker were given specific attention. Infant hygiene was not founded on any scientific basis but was represented in a humane attempt to give better care to the child.

Mental hygiene was limited to a sympathetic understanding and care of the mentally disordered.

In 1639 the Massachusetts colony passed an act stating that each birth and death must be recorded, and the Plymouth colony did likewise. In 1647 Massachusetts Bay colonies passed regulations to prevent the pollution of Boston Harbor. Between the years 1692 and 1708 Boston, Salem, and Jamestown passed laws dealing with nuisances and offensive trades. In 1701 Massachusetts enacted legislation providing for isolation of smallpox cases and for ship quarantine.

Superstitions expressed in witchcraft and other practices of the time indicate that the colonial period in history was hardly one in which to expect any great advances in health science. In America during George Washington's time the average duration of life was about 29 years. Measured by today's standards, the men who wrote the American Declaration of Independence and drew up the Federal Constitution were extremely young. Decidedly few of them were over the age of 40.

Boards of health were established in New York and Massachusetts in 1797 as a result of the yellow fever outbreaks. Local boards of health were established in Petersburg, Virginia (1780), in Baltimore (1793), in Philadelphia (1794), in New York (1796), and in Boston (1799). Paul Revere served as chairman of the Boston Board of Health. While all these were formally organized health boards, none of them functioned as boards of health function today.

Early nineteenth century

From 1800 to 1850 North America experienced rapid industrial expansion. As remarkable as this was, public health activities were stymied, and many epidemics occurred. The rapid growth of cities out-stripped other developments. Community health could hardly flourish under such conditions, and organized health measures were almost nonexistent.

Community health promotion in England. Developments in England in the first half of the nineteenth century were important for several reasons. Public health was officially recognized in England in 1837 when legislation relating to community sanitation was enacted. This indication of an awakening interest in community health led to the appointment of a factory commission to study the health conditions of the laboring population of the nation. Particular emphasis was placed on the study of child employment conditions. Edwin Chadwick, a civilian who had a special interest in social problems, was made secretary of the Factory Commission. In 1842 his "Report on the Inquiry Into the Sanitary Condition of the Laboring Population of Great Britain" appeared. Chadwick's colorful descriptions of the deplorable conditions of the time had more than just a popular appeal. They aroused the determination of well-meaning people to improve the conditions of the laboring class, particularly the child employment conditions. Chadwick's report pointed out that half the children of the working classes died before their fifth birthday. While the death rate and infant mortality do not indicate the complete picture of a nation or community, the length of life and the infant death rates reported by Chadwick indicate health conditions in which mere survival could be the sole health goal (Table 1-1).

The impact of such appalling health conditions is reflected in the loss at an early age of some of England's outstanding literary figures of the time. Shelley died at the age of 30, Keats at 25, Byron at 36, Robert Burns at 37, Charlotte Brontë at 39, Emily Brontë at 30, and Ann Brontë at 29. On the continent, Chopin died at 40, Felix Mendelssohn at 38, and Franz Schubert at 31. One might speculate on what these master artists might have produced for humankind if today's knowledge of health could have been applied during their lives.

Chadwick's report led to the establishment of a board of health in 1848. John Simon was appointed first medical health officer of London. England was not yet ready for the reforms that Chadwick's report pointed out, for the general board of health lasted but 4 years. Perhaps his enthusiasm led to overpromotion. Nevertheless, his report stands as a landmark in the history of public health.

Health developments in the United States. Not until the close of the first half of the nineteenth century was there a significant American development in community health promotion. Lemuel Shattuck (1793-1859) drew up a health report that was to serve as a guide in the field of health for the next century. Shattuck successively was a teacher, historian, sociologist, statistician, and state legislator. From the health standpoint he was a layman, but with an intense and intelligent interest in sanitation. He was appointed chairman of a legis-

TABLE 1-1. Mean age of death and infant death rates, England, 1842*

Class	Mean age of death		Infant deaths per 1,000 births (England)
	London	England	
Gentry, professional persons, and their families	44	35	100
Tradesmen, shopkeepers, and their families	23	22	167
Wage classes, artisans, laborers, and their families	22	15	250

*Based on Chadwick. See Richardson, B.W.: The health of nations. A review of the works of Edwin Chadwick, vol. 2, London, 1887, Longmans Green & Co.

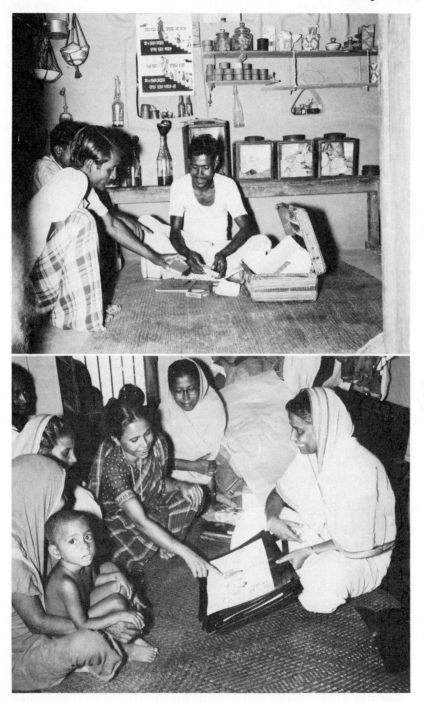

FIG. 1-1. Modern community health and contraceptive technology is delivered today in many developing countries through ancient channels of communication and distribution similar to those of the eighteenth and nineteenth centuries in Europe and America.

Courtesy Public Health Education Research Project, University of California, Berkeley.

lative committee to study sanitation and health problems in the Commonwealth of Massachusetts. The report was written by Shattuck and published in 1850. This report revealed Shattuck's insight and foresight. It charted health pathways for generations to come, and many of its provisions have not yet been fully attained. The importance of this remarkable document can be appreciated by reviewing its various recommendations:

1. Establishment of state and local boards of health
2. Collection and analysis of vital statistics
3. Systematic exchange of health information
4. Sanitation programs for towns and buildings
5. System of sanitary inspections
6. Studies on the health of school children
7. Studies of tuberculosis
8. Study and supervision of health conditions of immigrants
9. Supervision of mental disease
10. Control of alcoholism
11. Control of food adulteration
12. Exposure of nostrums
13. Control of smoke nuisances
14. Construction of model tenements
15. Construction of standard public bathing and wash houses
16. Preaching of health from pulpits
17. Teaching the science of sanitation in medical schools
18. Prevention as a phase of all medical practice
19. Routine health examinations

Shattuck was considerably in advance of his time. In addition, he did not have the flair for writing that Chadwick possessed. He did not depend on vivid descriptions of appalling conditions. The report produced no results until 1869, when a Massachusetts state board of health was established. Its membership included both laymen and physicians. The Shattuck report served as the guide for the board in its early years of activity. The wisdom of Shattuck's report stands as a valued guidepost in the history of public health in America.

Modern era of health

The modern era of health is dated from 1850 to the present. It represents an organized, disciplined attack on problems of health and disease, growing out of a general recognition of the importance of a united public approach to health protection, initially in Western societies and later in the Third World. In America interest in community health became a necessity with the rapid expansion in the latter half of the nineteenth century and continuing on into the twentieth century.

The modern era of health can be divided into five phases. The first phase (1850-1880) was the *miasma* phase; the second phase (1880-1920), the *disease control* phase or health protection era; the third phase (1920-1960), the *health resources* or medical phase; and the fourth phase (1960-1975), the *social engineering* phase. The fifth phase came in the late 1970s with the *health promotion* phase, sometimes referred to as the "second revolution in public health," in which the behavior and life-style of individuals and communities were recognized as the major causes of illness, disability, and death.

Miasma phase (1850-1880). The term *miasma* literally means noxious air or vapor. During this period the approach to disease control was based on the misconception that disease was caused by noxious odors, dirt, and general lack of cleanliness. Diphtheria was thought to be caused by gases associated with putrefaction. The term *malaria* literally means "bad air." Because it was observed even as early as Hippocrates that people who ventured about at dusk were those who invariably contracted malaria, the common belief persisted into the late nineteenth century that the disease was a result of the particular air existing at dusk. Here was an illustrious example of interpreting mere coincidence as a cause-and-effect relationship.

Disease control efforts were directed entirely toward general cleanliness. Garbage and refuse collection became important to communities. Street cleaning was pursued relentlessly. These general cleanliness measures were not directed at the specific causes of disease and consequently were of little value in control.

Quarantine conventions were held in a number of cities. The first of these was a 3-day convention held in Philadelphia in 1857. The topics discussed at the first convention indicate the interests of the 54 people who were in attendance: prevention of typhus, cholera, and yellow fever; port quarantine; stagnant and putrid bilge waters, droppings, or drainage from putrescible matter; and filthy bedding, baggage, and clothing of immigrant passengers where they had been confined. The convention recommended the vaccination of all incoming immigrants.

The first state health department was organized in Massachusetts in 1869, with Dr. Henry I. Bowdich as the first head. The department's program was directed to the following six areas:

1. Professional and public education in hygiene
2. Housing
3. Investigation of some diseases
4. Slaughtering
5. Sale of poisons
6. Conditions of the poor

Measured in terms of present standards in public health, the program of the first state health department would rate rather poorly.

The American Public Health Association was founded in 1872 at Long Beach, New Jersey. Dr. Stephen Smith was the first president. The new association proposed to go considerably beyond the thinking of the quarantine conventions as well as to deal with sanitation, prevention and transmission of disease, and longevity, hospital hygiene, and all other health problems that arose that would be of interest and of concern to the public.

Public health teaching had its inception during this period. An English manual of hygiene by E.A. Parkes, professor of military hygiene in the army medical school of England, was published in 1859. The first as well as subsequent editions were in use in America. In 1879 A.H. Buck edited his pioneering text, *Hygiene and Public Health*. This volume deals with environmental sanitation, housing, personal hygiene, child hygiene, school hygiene, industrial hygiene, food sanitation, communicable disease control, disinfection, quarantine, infant mortality, and vital statistics. Several distinguished men contributed to the volume. Dr. J.S. Billings wrote the introduction with foresight in the jurisprudence of hygiene. His concepts, such as the following, are also enunciated by present leaders in public health:

1. County lines are not natural boundaries and have no relation to causes of disease.
2. Administrative health areas should be large enough and populous enough to require full-time sanitary and executive forces.
3. There should be nonpracticing full-time health officers with medical education.
4. The health officer should be specially trained for his job.
5. If a municipal board of health is properly constituted so that its relationship to the medical profession is harmonious, it should be charged with the supervision of all medical charities such as hospitals and dispensaries.

Schools of public health were not founded until a later time, but the seeds of professional public health preparation were being planted before the disease control phase of the modern health era was reached.

Disease control phase (1880-1920). This phase might be properly termed the *bacteriology phase* because it was initiated by the work of Louis Pasteur, Robert Koch, and other bacteriologists who demonstrated that a specific organism causes a specific disease. With the knowledge that an organism causes a certain disease, it was now possible to change from general measures in attempting to control diseases to specific measures in protecting health by blocking the routes over which the causative agents would travel. As it became apparent that certain vehicles served as the means for the transmission of disease-producing organisms, attention was directed to such specific measures as the protection of water supplies, milk, and other foods, the elimination of insects, and the proper disposal of sewage. A natural further advance was the development of laboratory procedures.

The scientific productivity of the bacteriologists of this period is legendary. The French bacteriologist Louis Pasteur (1822-1895), in addition to demonstrating that a specific organism causes a specific disease, also made other outstanding contributions to bacteriology. He disproved the theory of spontaneous generation, discovered the fowl cholera bacillus and the cause of silkworm disease, and developed a method of inoculation against rabies. Robert Koch (1843-1910) discovered the tubercle bacillus and the streptococcus. He also discovered the cholera vibrio, which he demonstrated was transmitted by water, food, and clothing. In 1893 Theobald Smith of the U.S. Department of Agriculture showed that Texas fever in cattle was transmitted by ticks; thus the concept of an intermediate host, or vector, was established. In 1896 Dr. Bruce, a British army surgeon, demonstrated that African sleeping sickness was transmitted by the tsetse fly. In 1898 Sir Ronald Ross in India and Battista Grassi in Italy demonstrated that malaria was transmitted by the *Anopheles* mosquito. In 1900 Walter Reed, Jesse W. Lazier, James Carroll, and Aristides Agramonte demonstrated that yellow fever was transmitted by the *Aedes* mosquito.

Although Pasteur's work in the treatment of rabies was developed in 1883, it was not until 1894 that Emil von Behring (1854-1917) developed his procedure for use of diphtheria anti-toxin for the successful treatment of diphtheria. In 1904 Sir Almroth Edward Wright developed the use of dead organisms for inoculation against typhoid fever. During this same period Lord Joseph Lister (1827-1912) developed the practical use of phenol (carbolic acid) as an effective antiseptic.

Official public health departments were staffed with bacteriologists, laboratory technicians, sanitarians, sanitation inspectors, sanitary engineers, quarantine officers, and others who specialized in disease control measures. With the extreme emphasis placed on isolation and quarantine during the first 2 decades of the twentieth century, one might with justification refer to these 20 years as the "tackhammer" period in public health history. To the public of that time, ubiquitous quarantine officers with their hideous placards were the identifying symbol of public health.

Limited as the health protection programs of this period were, they had an apparent effect in reducing the death rate. A comparison of the death rate for 1930 with the average death rate for the years 1881 to 1885 indicated a pronounced reduction in deaths in western Europe and in the United States.

Health resources phase (1920-1960). Medical examination of the men being inducted into the U.S. Armed Services during World War I was the first broad-scale barometer of the health status of the people of the United States. With health standards for induction lower than previously had prevailed, the Armed Services still found it necessary to reject 34% of the men examined because of physical and mental disabilities. The nation was appalled to learn that one third of its youth were unfit for military service. Professional health personnel analyzed the data obtained in the medical examination of draftees and arrived at a conclusion that was to change the course of public health in America.

Public health experts learned from the data that while communicable diseases had been controlled quite well, other health hazards and problems had been neglected. Many of the defects reported could have been prevented, and most of the defects could have been corrected. It was clear that the public health program had neglected the citizen as an individual and that future efforts of public health programs must be directed to individual citizens. It became apparent that it was necessary to build up and maintain the highest possible level of health resources for each individual citizen. The prevention of communicable disease was not enough.

State health departments began expanding their programs and directing their efforts toward personal health services as well as toward community disease control. This required administrative reorganization within the state health departments and the inclusion of many new specialties in the health services.

In 1911 Guilford County, North Carolina, and Yakima County, Washington, organized the first full-time county health departments. The organization of official health departments on a county basis was slow in developing until the second decade of the positive phase of health resources. Then, under the stimulus of financial support from such organizations as the Rockefeller Foundation, the Children's Fund of Michigan, the Kellogg Foundation, and the U.S. Public Health Service, county health departments became recognized as the desirable health unit in the age of modern transportation. County health departments with full-time professional personnel gradually displaced the city health departments with part-time health officers and nonprofessional personnel. Only a few large cities with full-time professionally prepared personnel still continue to function apart from the 3,102 counties in the United States.

The largest investments during this era, however, were not in public health services or even in personal health services for mothers, infants, and children, but rather in three other resources: hospitals, health manpower, and biomedical knowledge from research. The Hill-Burton Act passed in 1946 provided for the construction of massive facilities for medical care. Medical, nursing, and dental schools proliferated to train the personnel required to staff the new hospitals. The National Institutes of Health was established to generate the research and strengthen the knowledge resource from which scientific medicine and public health could draw new methods, drugs, vaccines, and diagnostic tests.

Voluntary health agencies had been established in the United States previous to 1920, but following this date these voluntary organizations played an increasingly important role in the promotion of health in the United States, particularly through health education. Voluntary health organizations are somewhat uniquely an American creation. Their major contribution was in bringing to public attention the importance of certain health problems. At the same time, some of them oversold the importance of relatively rare diseases, causing the public to contribute unnecessary services or resources at the expense of more urgent or pervasive problems. The burden of being solicited for contributions repeatedly by too many voluntary agencies led many communities to establish joint fund raising under "community chests" and "united campaigns." The voluntary agencies also tended to be drawn into the aura of medical research and medical services, usually at the expense of their public health education function. Thus even in the private sector the resources for community health during this era were concentrated in medical rather than health activities.

Social engineering phase (1960-1975). By 1960 it had become apparent that technical health advances and personal health resources were not available to all people. Indeed, large segments of the world and of each community were completely isolated from developments in health. The husbanding of human resources required that the products of technological developments be made available to every world citizen. The social aspects of health were given a new priority.

To make the advances of health science available to all people posed a pyramid of problems because of the various individuals and groups unable to acquire the benefits of health knowledge and health services. The poor—economically, educationally, and socially—often missed the benefits of community health programs. The economic barriers were considered the most urgent, so medicare and medicaid legislation was passed in the United States to put purchasing power in the hands of the poor and medically indigent to enable them to acquire needed health services.

The other problems of educational and social isolation of the poor required carrying health resources and services to those who apparently were not receiving the benefits of health programs. The "outreach" services of public health nurses and indigenous community health workers thus became a mainstay of local health departments.

Migrant workers are an example of a group requiring health services adapted to their needs. Other groups who also need special community health services are mothers, infants, children, adolescents, and the chronically ill and elderly. For all of these groups, more than health services is necessary. These groups need assistance in other aspects of living. Opportunities must be provided that enable these people to enrich their lives; limited though that enrichment may appear to be. This also calls for the enlistment of many community resources, voluntary and official agencies, in many different categories of human services besides health.

Creating a favorable environment and favorable living conditions for these people means creating opportunities for self-improvement, calling for a form of social engineering not previously used for the betterment of the underpriviledged. This approach has been criticized as being paternalistic. Yet to offer people more

healthful channels of living and to help them develop the ability to guide their own mode of life is no more paternalistic than to award people state scholarships for a college education.

The modern community health program covers all citizens of all ages, but of necessity it must give a proportionately higher degree of attention to the people at greatest risk who are usually the least knowledgeable and of the lower social, economic, and educational strata. The human ecology involved is apparent. The health of these people affects the health and economy of the entire community. Abandoned to their own resources, many people would decline in health and consequently in their social condition.

Community health programs must give highest priority to the allocation of resources to those least able to provide for their own health needs. These people are entitled to a better quality of health, an extended productive life, and a greater life expectancy—the objectives of community health programs.

The trend in community health programs during the late 1960s was the funneling of federal funds through state and county agencies to provide for medical and hospital services for certain medically deprived groups in the community. Certain guidelines were laid down by the federal agencies, but within these stipulations health departments had considerable leeway in the use of these funds. Most of the funds go to practicing physicians for professional services rendered to citizens who otherwise would not have the medical care they need. This tendency to channel some of the funds for medical services through the county health departments cast an additional burden on the staffs of these local health departments because seldom was provision made for additional personnel.

By the early 1970s the resources of health facilities, manpower, and research developed in earlier decades had been more equitably distributed to the poor and the medically indigent. This had occurred in the United States as a result of the "New Society" legislation of the Kennedy years and the "War on Poverty" legislation of the Johnson years. In Europe, Canada, Australia, Asia, and Africa even more sweeping social and medical reforms were made. In the United States citizens in most communities had a greater voice in allocating health resources at the local level as a result of the "maximum feasible participation" provision in most of the legislative acts requiring policy and planning bodies for neighborhood health centers and other new entities to include 51% lay membership. The 1960s had achieved a closing of much of the gap between high-income and low-income people in their use of medical services.

These accomplishments, however, were not universally reflected in the mortality and morbidity statistics. The differences between the death and disease rates of rich and poor, black and white, urban and rural populations persisted. Indeed, the increasing expenditures on health care (mostly medical care) were not yielding proportionate improvements in the health of nations in general. The rapidly escalating costs of medical care were attributed to the high medical technology and facilities created by the earlier investments in medical resources, now made more universally accessible by new health insurance coverage and related programs of distribution. The 1970s, then, were devoted heavily to the search for ways to contain the costs of medical care.

The search for cost-containment strategies in the United States led first to the "health planning" acts of the late 1960s and early 1970s; then to "peer review" requirements to encourage medical practitioners to restrain themselves in the use of unnecessary medical procedures; then to new forms of delivery, such as "health maintenance organizations," designed to encourage physicians to keep their patients out of hospitals rather than to admit them unnecessarily. During this period of concentrated

tinkering with the *medical* care system, the *health* care system was almost forgotten. State and local health departments lost much of their financial base to medical institutions and much of their political force to health planning agencies.

Health promotion phase (1975-present). By the mid-1970s there was a renewed interest in disease prevention and health promotion. This occurred almost simultaneously in several English-speaking countries. The United States began the decade with the report of *The President's Committee on Health Education,* but the Canadians followed soon after with a more comprehensive and influential report by the Minister of National Health and Welfare, *A New Perspective on the Health of Canadians* (Lalonde, 1974). In Great Britain the famous "red book" was issued by the government with the title *Prevention and Health: Everybody's Business, 1976,* and a three-volume House of Commons report from the Expenditure Committee on Preventive Medicine was issued as well. The Scottish Health Education Unit published *Effectiveness and Efficiency in Health Education* (Tones, 1978). The prolific Americans continued their refocusing with a series of official documents and legislative acts, including the *Forward Plan for Health* issued by the Public Health Service in 1976; the National Health Information and Health Promotion Act of 1976; the task force report, *Preventive Medicine USA* (1976); the two-volume Surgeon General's report on health promotion and disease prevention, *Healthy People* (1979); and *Promoting Health, Preventing Disease: Objectives for the Nation* (1980). The Australian Commonwealth Department of Health published *Health Promotion in Australia 1978-79* (Davidson, Chapman, and Hull, 1979).

• • •

This edition of *Community Health* has been revised in the chapters that follow largely on the basis of recent historical landmarks. The foregoing historical background can be understood as a repeated redefining of the primary or prevalent causes of illness and death, from supernatural causes in the earliest Egyptian through Medieval times, to natural causes in the Greco-Roman and modern eras, to social causes in the midtwentieth century, to personal or behavioral causes in the present health promotion period. The personal or behavioral causes of the current health concerns, however, must be understood and addressed in their historical, cultural, social, economic, and community contexts. This chapter has addressed the historical context of community health, including some of the social, cultural, and economic forces that shape history and health simultaneously. Later chapters will draw on history to help one understand more clearly how social, behavioral, environmental, and technological forces can be harnessed and directed in the planning and development of community health. Finally, it is helpful for one in understanding and applying these several forces to draw back from the provincial perspective of his or her own community and cast the historical, social, behavioral, environmental, technological, and health trends in national and international perspective.

Health promotion will gain momentum in the 1980s as more professionals and decision makers recognize the growing importance of behavior as the key to preventing or controlling the leading causes of death and disability. Heart disease, cancer, stroke, and accidents make up the majority of deaths in Western countries today. All of these have as their primary causes one or more behavioral or lifestyle problems. The voluntary adaptation of behavior conducive to health is the goal of health education. Combined with social and environmental supports for such behavior, health education becomes health promotion. This edition of *Community Health* will emphasize health promotion.

SOME COMMUNITY HEALTH MILESTONES OF THE PAST 2 CENTURIES

1780 Petersburg, Virginia, board of health created
1789 French Revolution results in the granting of every citizen a right to public support for health and other services
1790 First U.S. census
1796 Scientific smallpox vaccination from cowpox by Jenner
1798 First city health department, Baltimore
1831 New York City water supply provided
1832 England's Health and Morals Act passed
1842 Massachusetts registration of births and deaths
1844 Dorothea Dix crusade for humane treatment of mentally ill
1848 England's General Health Board created
1850 Shattuck's Massachusetts sanitary report
1851 European health conference
Paris sewer system installed
1852 Founding of the American Pharmaceutical Association in Philadelphia
1854 First fireproof building in United States
1857 First electric fire alarm system
1859 First milk inspectors required by law in Massachusetts
1860 Red Cross founded in Geneva, Switzerland
1862 Internal revenue taxes on tobacco and alcohol go into effect
1866 Bathhouses operated by a municipality opened in Boston
1868 Clinical thermometer comes into general use
1869 Royal Sanitary Commission established in England
Massachusetts State Board of Health created
1872 Founding of the American Public Health Association
1873 Germ theory of disease advanced
1879 Gonococcus identified
1880 Typhoid bacillus discovered
Pneumococcus identified
Malaria plasmodium discovered
1882 Tubercle bacillus discovered
1883 Rabies treatment successful
Cholera vibrio discovered

1884	Diphtheria bacillus identified
1889	Massachusetts Public Health laboratory and Johns Hopkins Hospital opened with new patterns of scientific health care
1893	Lawrence, Massachusetts, water treatment plant completed
1894	Diphtheria antitoxin successfully demonstrated
	Pasteurella pestis, cause of plague, discovered
1895	Discovery of the x-ray
	Cause of hookworm discovered
	Relation of *Anopheles* mosquito to malaria established
1899	International Sanitary Bureau organized
1901	Infectious nature of yellow fever established
1902	U.S. Public Health Service established
	Relation of *Aedes aegypti* mosquito to yellow fever demonstrated
1904	Typhoid fever immunization successful
1905	Spirochete of syphilis identified
1906	Pure Food and Drug Act passed
	Standard methods of water analysis adopted
1908	Chlorination of Jersey City water supply
1909	Successful treatment of syphilis using arsphenamine
	Hemophilus pertussis identified
1910	International Board of Health, Rockefeller Foundation, created
1911	Chemical nature of vitamin D (calciferol) discovered
	Milk pasteurization proved effective
1913	Harvard School of Public Health established
	Pellagra demonstrated to be a deficiency disease
1914	National Safety Council established
1916	First birth control clinic opened in Brooklyn, and School of Hygiene and Public Health established at Johns Hopkins University, Baltimore
1918	U.S. Department of Agriculture booklet published, which apportioned food into five groups
1920	Prohibition enacted by Eighteenth Amendment to U.S. Constitution
1922	Insulin treatment of diabetes mellitus demonstrated
1923	Health Section of League of Nations founded

1925	Diphtheria toxoid used successfully
1930	National Institutes of Health established
1933	Influenza virus A identified
	Prohibition repealed
1935	Social Security Act passed
1938	Venereal Disease Control Act
1941	Penicillin demonstrated
	Papanicolaou develops cervical smear for cancer detection
1942	Seven food groups defined by National Wartime Nutrition Guide
1943	Streptomycin antibiotic effects demonstrated
1948	World Health Organization (WHO) founded
1949	Cultivation of poliomyelitis virus
1952	Poliomyelitis vaccine successful field test
1953	Public Health Service joined with new Department of Health, Education, and Welfare
1954	Rubeola virus identified
1956	Poliomyelitis attenuated virus vaccine field test
1961	Peace Corps established
1963	Measles vaccine demonstrated successfully
1964	Mumps vaccine developed
	Economic Opportunity Act launches the "War on Poverty"
	Surgeon General's Report on Smoking and Health
1966	Rubella vaccine trial tested
	Fair Packaging and Labelling Act
1967	Medicare and Medicaid begin coverage
1969	Rubella vaccine introduced
1970	National high blood pressure education and screening programs initiated
	Family Planning and Population Research Act signed
	Occupational Health and Safety Act signed
1971	White House Conference on Aging
	Sickle Cell Disease Program initiated
1973	Health Maintenance Organization Assistance Act
1974	National Institute on Aging established
	A New Perspective on the Health of Canadians published
	National Health Planning and Resources Development Act replaces Comprehensive Health Planning and Regional Medical Programs

1975 National Center for Health Education established

U.S. Supplemental Food Program for Women, Infants, and Children

1976 Health Information and Health Promotion Act signed

1977 WHO announces the eradication of smallpox in Asia

1978 National initiatives in childhood immunization, adolescent pregnancy, smoking, and nutrition announced

1979 American and Australian national reports on health promotion

1980 Smallpox officially declared eradicated worldwide

Department of Education created, leaving Public Health Service and Health Care Finance Administration in Department of Health and Human Services

QUESTIONS AND EXERCISES

1. Why and how does a knowledge of the past in any field of human endeavor benefit those who now work in that field?
2. Illustrate how disease has altered the course of history.
3. Why should people in the parahealth professions have a broad knowledge of community health?
4. Why was the Mosaic Law or Code of special importance to the advancement of the community health movement?
5. Using examples, explain how the political philosophy of a nation affects its health program.
6. What specific lesson in health can the present generation gain from a study of health conditions during the Dark Ages?
7. To what extent did the Renaissance influence the direction of community health?
8. What, in your judgment, was the most important health discovery in Europe during the period of American colonization between 1600 and 1800?
9. Evaluate this statement: "Colorful reporting can get more public action than scientific fact."
10. Evaluate this assertion: "Lowering the death rate among laborers and their families does not improve their lot because it results in a surplus of laborers."
11. Appalling health conditions had an adverse effect on literary and musical productivity during the golden age of arts and letters in Europe. What factors in America today have a deterrent effect on productivity in the field of arts and letters?
12. In 1850 Lemuel Shattuck listed a considerable number of health recommendations that were carried out in the next century. What health recommendations would you make for future America?
13. What questionable health practices in the miasma phase of health are still regarded by the general public as important to health?
14. What is the basis for the contention that scientific public health should be dated from 1880?
15. Why did the application of scientific methods have such a profound effect on the death rate in Europe and the United States?
16. Why is the postponement of death not sufficient as the objective of a community health program?
17. Explain what is meant by the expression, "Public health is social engineering."
18. In what respects is the development of local health departments of more importance than the development of state or provincial health departments or the national health agencies?
19. What single health discovery has been of greatest value to you?
20. What determines who benefits most from present community health programs?

BIBLIOGRAPHY

Bartsocas, C.S.: Two fourteenth century descriptions of the "Black Plague," J. Hist. Med. **21**:394, 1966.

Blake, J.B.: Public health in the town of Boston, 1630-1823, Cambridge, Mass., 1959, Harvard University Press.

Buck, A.H.: Hygiene and public health, Philadelphia, 1879, William Wood and Co.

Calder, R.: The lamp is lit, the story of WHO, Geneva, 1951, WHO Division of Public Information.

Chapin, C.V.: A report on state public health work based on a survey of state boards of health, Chicago, 1916, American Medical Association.

Chapin, C.V.: The papers of C.V. Chapin, New York, 1934, The Commonwealth Fund.

Davidson, L., Chapman, S., and Hull, C.: Health promotion in Australia 1978-79, Canberra, Australia, 1979, Commonwealth of Australia.

Dubos, R.: Man, medicine and environment, New York, Praeger Publishers, Inc., 1968.

Duffy, J.: History of public health in New York City, 1625-1866, New York, 1968, Russell Sage Foundation.

Great Britain Expenditures Committee: First report from the Expenditures Committee, Session 1976-77, Preventive Medicine, London, 1977, HMSO.

Green, L.W.: Research and demonstration issues in self-care: measuring the decline in medicocentrism, Health Educ. Monogr. **5**:161, 1977.

Health in America: 1776-1976, Rockville, Md., 1976, Health Resources Administration.

Healthy people: the Surgeon General's report on health promotion and disease prevention, 2 vols., Washington, D.C., 1979, DHEW (PAS) Pub. No. 79-55071A.

Henschen, F.: History and geography of disease, translated by Joan Tate, New York, 1966, The Delacorte Press.

History and American public health, Am. J. Public Health **55:**1, 1965.

Hobson, W.: World health and history, Baltimore, 1963, The Williams & Wilkins Co.

Kargon, R.H.: Science in Victorian Manchester: enterprise and expertise, Baltimore, 1977, The Johns Hopkins University Press.

Knowles, J.H., editor: Doing better and feeling worse: health in the United States, New York, 1977, W.W. Norton & Co., Inc.

Lalonde, M.: A new perspective on the health of Canadians, a working document, Ottawa, 1974, Government of Canada.

Leff, S., and Leff, V.: From witchcraft to world health, New York, 1957, Macmillan Publishing Co., Inc.

Leff, S., and Leff, V.: Health and humanity, New York, 1962, International Publishers Co., Inc.

Lerner, M., and Anderson, O.W.: Health progress in the United States, 1900-1960, Chicago, 1963, University of Chicago Press.

Lewis, R.A.: Edwin Chadwick and the public health movement, 1823-1854, Clifton, N.J., 1970, Augustus M. Kelley, Publishers.

Means, R.K.: A history of health education in the United States, Philadelphia, 1963, Lea & Febiger.

Miller, G.: Bibliography of the history of medicine in the United States and Canada 1939-1960, Baltimore, 1964, The Johns Hopkins University Press.

O'Brien, H.R.: Fifty years in public health, Camp Hill, Pa., 1967, Henry R. O'Brien.

Preventive medicine USA: A task force report, New York, 1976, Prodist.

Promoting health, preventing disease: objectives for the nation, Washington, D.C., 1980, Public Health Service.

Public Health Service: Forward plan for health, FY 1978-82, Washington, D.C., 1976.

Ravenel, M.P., editor: Half century of public health, New York, 1970, Arno Press, Inc.

Richardson, B.W.: The health of nations. A review of the works of Edwin Chadwick, vol. 2, London, 1887, Longmans Green & Co.

Rogers, D.E., and Blendon, R.J.: The changing American health scene: sometimes things get better, J.A.M.A. **237:**1710, 1977.

Rogers, F.B.: Man and his changing environment: historical perspective, Am. J. Public Health **51:**1637, 1961.

Rosen, G.: A history of public health, New York, 1958, MD Publications, Inc.

Rosen, G.: Preventive medicine in the United States, 1900-1975, New York, 1975, Science History Publication.

Rush, B.: Medical inquiries and observances, ed. 4, Philadelphia, 1815, University of Pennsylvania Press.

Schwartz, J.L.: Early histories of selected neighborhood health centers, Inquiry **7:**3, 1970.

Shattuck, L., et al.: Report of the Sanitary Commission of Massachusetts, 1850, New York, 1948, Cambridge University Press.

Shryock, R.H.: Medicine and society in America, 1660-1860, New York, 1960, New York University Press.

Sigerist, H.E.: Landmarks in the history of hygiene, London, 1956, Oxford University Press.

Sigerist, H.E.: History of medicine, 2 vols., London, 1951, 1961, Oxford University Press.

Tones, B.K.: Effectiveness and efficiency in health education, Edinburgh, 1978, Scottish Health Education Unit.

Wain, H.: A history of preventive medicine, Springfield, Ill., 1970, Charles C Thomas, Publisher.

Wilcox, C.: Medical advance, public health and social evolution, New York, 1965, Pergamon Press, Inc.

Winslow, C.-E. A.: The untilled fields of public health, Science **51:**23, 1920.

2

THE COMMUNITY AND ITS HEALTH

Social influences exert their power, either good or bad, upon all who come within their reach.

E.H. Janes (1876)

A MODEL OF COMMUNITY HEALTH

The modern community health program must combine the elements of environmental, social, and behavioral interventions, because both health and community are made up of all three elements. The environmental elements of the community interact with human biology to produce the natural history of health in which the members of the community adapt to a changing environment, learn from their adaptation, adjust their behavior, and protect or enhance their health (Fig. 2-1).

The history of community health, as described in the preceding chapter, is a social history in which people have organized themselves into families, institutions, communities, and societies to exercise more control over the environment and over the behavior of each other. Rules of behavior become community norms that are transmitted from one generation to another as culture. Culture defines acceptable social organization (family interaction patterns, roles and responsibilities of institutions and leaders, and the functions of government) as well as individual behavior. The influence of all these cultural, economic, organizational, and institutional forces on the environment, on individual behavior, and on health may be referred to as the social history of health. Social

history is imposed on the natural history of health, positively or negatively, at the junctures of environment and behavior, as shown in Fig. 2-2. Community organization for health promotion specifically attempts to channel these social forces in ways that will support behavior that is more conducive to health.

The social history of health is also an economic history of communities. Behavior is expressed at the community level as a social norm, which means that it becomes widely expected. A widely expected behavior in relation to goods and services is expressed in economic terms as *demand*. For example, people who shift their purchasing behavior in large numbers from butter to margarine establish a norm and create a demand for more margarine. Demand, in turn, influences *supply* of the goods and services in the same way that norms influence culture with respect to nonconsumable goods such as family roles and responsibilities. Supply of highly demanded consumable goods in a community determines price or value of those goods and services, just as culture defines the value individuals place on noncommensurable (abstract) goods such as loyalty, faith, love, responsibility to care for children, and specific health goals or values.

Individuals allow these social and natural

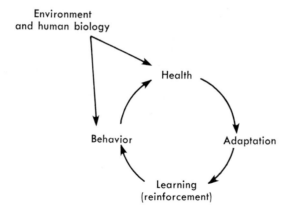

FIG. 2-1. The natural history of health.

From Green, L.W.: Natural, social and personal histories of health. In Whither health education? Proceedings of the Second National Conference, Dublin, 1980, Bureau of Health Education.

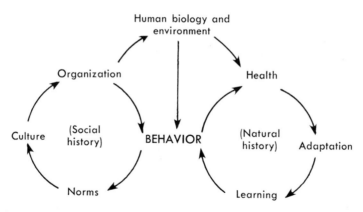

FIG. 2-2. The social history of health imposes positive and negative influence on health through the organization of behavior and the environment.

From Green, L.W.: Natural, social and personal histories of health. In Whither health education? Proceedings of the Second National Conference, Dublin, 1980, Bureau of Health Education.

forces to dictate their behavior and life-styles to a greater or lesser degree, depending on their economic and geographical circumstances, their personal experience, and their beliefs, values, and attitudes. Motivation is a combination of these forces converging on behavior through personal histories, as shown at the bottom of Fig. 2-3. Before these concepts

and the community model of the natural, social, and personal determinants of health are discussed further, some features of their connections should be noted.

The first feature to be noted in the three cycles in Fig. 2-3 is that they are continuous rather than static. This was the lesson of Chapter 1 in which the history of community health

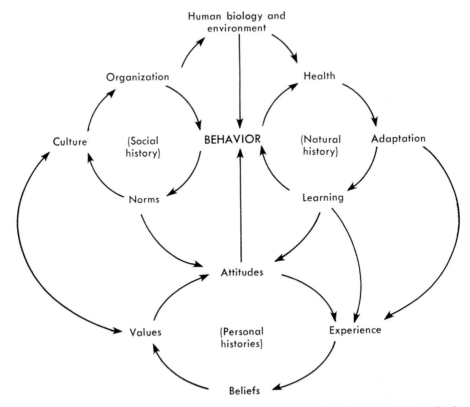

FIG. 2-3. The place of personal histories and motivation in the development of life-style (behavior) and health shows the interaction of environmental, social, and individual determinants in community health.

From Green, L.W.: Natural, social and personal histories of health. In Whither health education? Proceedings of the Second National Conference, Dublin, 1980, Bureau of Health Education.

was characterized as a continuous redefining of unacceptable conditions. Redefinition of acceptable or unacceptable conditions is partly a social process in the cultural and organizational response to changing conditions, partly a natural process in the connection between learning and behavior, and partly a personal response to both the social and natural conditions imposed on the individual.

The second feature of the three cycles is that they connect with each other in such a way that everything influences and is influenced by everything else, however indirectly or remotely. This is the lesson of Chapter 3 on hu-

man ecology and epidemiology. The concept of community implies an interdependence of the many elements on each other. As one element changes in nature (the environment or human biology) it sets up a series of adaptations in the natural history of health that in turn require some adjustments in society, altering the course of the social history of community health. These changes influence the personal histories of some, if not all, individuals in the community, altering their health-related experiences, beliefs, values, and attitudes in varying degrees.

The third feature of the three cycles is that

behavior is the pivotal factor linking personal and social history to health. According to the arrows representing causation, personal history can influence health only through behavior. The behavior may be individual action (self-care, life-style, or preventive action), or it may be collective action (community organization, family decision, group petition, neighborhood action, voter recruitment, or other social process). Collective action results in some change in the organization of health resources or the environment to influence health. Chapter 4 will address the central role of behavior as a mediator of personal and community forces that might influence health.

Finally, Fig. 2-3 shows only two arrows impinging directly on health, one representing the direct influence of behavior on health, and the other representing the direct influence of human biology and environment on health. All other elements of the three cycles influence health indirectly through one of these three direct determinants of health. Community organization of health resources can influence all three.

Diffusion of community health problems or innovations

An example of how the health history cycles operate in the community will help illustrate the use of these concepts in analyzing a community health innovation or problem. The initial stimulus to community action could be a positive alteration in the environment, such as the introduction of a beneficial, new medical technology, or a negative alteration, such as a new industrial technology that is hazardous to the health of workers employed to operate it. The new technology in the environment could thus influence both health and behavior (follow the arrows in Fig. 2-3). The impact on health, positive or negative, would result in some physiological adaptation in the people affected. They would learn, consciously or unconsciously, from the adaptive response of their bodies, which would reinforce subsequent behavior related to the health sign or symptom.

If a number of people adjust their behavior at the same time, a social process of developing new norms of behavior in the community is set into motion. For example, if the people who benefited from a public health or medical innovation, such as a new vaccine, all felt better during a subsequent epidemic, they would learn that vaccines are good, and they would respond enthusiastically to the next vaccination campaign. The enthusiastic behavior of the early adopters of the vaccine would create a norm or social model for the majority of their friends and acquaintances who would gradually adopt the behavior of seeking vaccination themselves, until the practice would be so widespread and accepted that it would become a part of the community's culture. Once acculturated, the innovation would become organized or incorporated into existing organizations and institutions. This organizational response then would have the power to influence the environment and behavior with regard to the availability of the vaccine in the environment, mass communication about the advantages of the vaccine, legal requirements for vaccination before admission to schools, and other community effects. The natural history and the social history of response to the introduced vaccine would influence individual experience, attitudes, beliefs, and values concerning the vaccine in numerous ways. These personal perceptions or adjustments to the new vaccine would make the behavior of accepting the vaccine more or less likely to occur in different individuals, depending on their personal histories.

Hence this model of community health provides a sequential placement of the numerous elements and phenomena that make up the full spectrum of responses to a health threat or health innovation. It could be made more complex by elaborating on the biomedical process of natural history in greater detail and the sociological and psychological processes of social and personal histories more fully, but the additions would be elements that could be subsumed under those contained in Fig. 2-3. Let us now focus on the four most immediate determinants of community health shown at the top of Fig. 2-3: human biology, environment, behavior, and organization.

HEALTH FIELD CONCEPT

The health field concept was used to formulate strategies for improving Canadian health (Lalonde, 1974). The original concept (Laframboise, 1973) classed the determinants of health into four categories: biology, environment, lifestyle, and health care organization.

Human biology encompasses the health outcomes that directly derive from the biology of humans. The genetics of the individual, growth, and aging are examples. This component is a necessary substrate for the remaining three categories, but there is little that individuals or communities can do to alter it except through genetic counseling and attention to the special health problems and requirements of various stages in the life cycle.

Environment includes all those factors related to health that are external to the human body and over which the individual has little control, yet over which the community may have a larger degree of control. Examples include safe, uncontaminated food, air, water, and drugs; control of air, water, and noise pollution; effective garbage and sewage disposal; and prevention of spread of communicable diseases. Providing a safe social environment by accident and fire prevention, gun control, and television programs that do not glorify and exploit violence are further examples. Urbanization, with resultant crowding and poor housing, is an environmental influence on community health.

Rapid social change with disintegration of established community values and their replacement by newer, untested mores may cause alienation and stress. Pursuit of private pleasure at the cost of common good may result in deterioration of community health, both physical and mental.

Life-style, the third category, covers decisions by individuals that affect their health, including self-imposed risks such as cigarette smoking, overeating, drug misuse, alcoholism, promiscuity, careless driving, and failure to wear seat belts. Lack of exercise, recreation, or relief from pressure of work or other stressors are further examples of self-imposed risks that are health hazards.

The fourth category in the health field concept is the one that has received the most attention and money and from which an unrealistic expectation of health improvement has developed. Health care organization is the category reserved for provision of medical services. Elements are medical practice, nursing, hospitals, nursing homes, dental services, drugs, mental health, and other community health services. An array of interventional methods, usually applied late in the natural history of disease, when little in the way of cure can be expected but much in the way of effort and cost can be expended, are elements of this category. Society has developed a dependence on this fourth category while overlooking the benefits to be derived from health-related changes in environment and life-style.

CONCEPT OF COMMUNITY

A community may be considered a social unit in which there is a transaction of a common life among the people making up the unit. As a social group, functioning with norms of behavior and organization of resources, it regulates both the environment and behavior.

A community may exist in a fairly limited territory, but more and more the community is characterized by a constantly enlarging geographical expanse. Our concept of community has changed from the limited view that a city in its boundary constitutes a community to a consideration of the interaction of social norms and organizations. A few decades ago a single large city was regarded as an independent community. Today we speak of a metropolitan area, implying that the entire area functions as a unified community. The Standard Metropolitan Statistical Area (SMSA) is a county or group of contiguous counties containing at least one city of 50,000 inhabitants or more.

In the promotion of health it is necessary to think of the areas outside the legal limits of a city as being an integral part of the total community. Erecting hospitals, establishing clinics, and providing other medical services today require planning based on the use of modern transportation and require an estimate of the health needs of the population served. Such planning is best accomplished by elected bodies including consumers as well as health providers. By so doing, it is possible to organize more efficiently for all people living within the area and having a common interest in health resources and facilities. It is interesting to observe that long-established industrial communities are adult-centered and suburbs are child-centered. To the suburbanites the needs of the children seem to command first priority. This is significant in health promotion.

Concisely stated, a community is a group of inhabitants living in a somewhat localized area under the same general regulations and having common norms, cultures, and organizations.

COMMUNITY ENVIRONMENTAL FACTORS

The number of people living in a community is a significant factor in dealing with community health problems, yet a large city can be thought of as a group of villages. Varying economic and other environmental influences can identify communities within the community. Environmental factors to be recognized in diagnosing community health problems include the physical environment; geography, topography, and climate; neighborhood organization; and industrial conditions.

Physical environment. The overall physical conditions of a community sometimes account for the general health of the community. Perhaps more important, the physical environment sometimes reflects the community's general health status. This applies to the mental, emotional, and social health of a community as well as to the physical health. The community that possesses a degree of orderliness usually reflects an awareness and a pride in the well-being of its citizens. Clean air and water, however, are the critical environmental factors in health.

Geography, topography, and climate. Geography refers to the surface of the earth. Topography indicates the features of a region or locality. Together with climate, these two phenomena relate to special community health problems. Lowlands, marshy areas, and hot climates give rise to health problems not of particular concern elsewhere. Tropical diseases are limited in most instances to such areas. Dry, dusty areas may create health conditions differing from those of more humid regions. The minerals of an area, the types of soil, and the functions of the rivers, canals, waterways, and harbors can be significant factors in determining the general health of the locality, depending on how the people use these natural resources.

Neighborhood organization. A neighborhood generally has been thought of as an area that houses a population for which one elementary school is ordinarily required. A neighborhood ranges in size from 1,000 to 3,000 families. This usually means an entire population of about 5,000. Areas deviating from this general pattern are common and can be designated as true neighborhood units, especially as the birthrate declines.

The compactness and uniformity of neighborhoods vary. Some of the older, longer established neighborhoods have an amazing unity and rapport. Some of the newer neighborhoods, particularly in the suburban areas, frequently are neighborhoods in area only. Speculative building in the suburbs, combined with a mobile population, tends to produce communities of individuals who are almost transients, with scant allegiance to a common health standard. Time is needed before the influence of schools, churches, and community groups becomes established. Social unity in such neighborhoods is loose. The degree of neighborhood unity, past practices, leadership, and established standards all contribute to existing health conditions. More important, however, is the nature of the neighborhood unity that exists when a particular health problem arises and must be dealt with on a cooperative basis. Where a long-established neighborhood cohesiveness already exists, the necessary leadership and united support will be mobilized quickly, and a program to solve the health problem will be initiated summarily. In a neighborhood where very little cohesiveness has been developed, valuable time will be consumed in the effort to mobilize the neighborhood's resources in dealing with the health problem requiring attention. Such a neighborhood may require several years to deal with a health problem that a more cohesive neighborhood will have well in hand in a matter of days.

A common health problem can be a highly important catalyst in unifying a neighborhood. A common concern about a situation that threatens health or is important in the promotion of health can bring people together, promote mutual respect, and provide a common purpose that will provide a sense of neighborhood unity that will prevail for years to come.

Solving neighborhood problems through collective action builds pride and cohesiveness. Only when reasonably diligent effort on the part of the neighborhood has failed and the health problem is critical should the neighborhood resort to legal means. Political action can usually avert the necessity of litigation.

Very few health problems arise that must be dealt with summarily. Sufficient time is usually available for working out a satisfactory solution. It is a fortunate neighborhood that has united to deal with problems in the past because of the unity such common purposes engender. It is a wise neighborhood that anticipates public health problems lying ahead and that has developed some form of organization and collective action.

Industrial conditions. Health problems can be identified sometimes with particular industrial conditions that prevail either within the community or that indirectly affect the community. A "garden city" or a residential community will not have some of the health problems that citizens in a highly industrialized community will encounter. An industry that causes a great deal of noise may create special problems of an emotional as well as of a physical nature. The social health of the community can be affected by chemical plants creating obnoxious odors. A mining community or a logging community living in the shadow of extreme occupational hazards is a community different from one in which industrial accidents are rare.

A particular industry will have direct effects on the health of a community, in addition to secondary effects in the type of people an industry attracts to a city. Certain industries engage workers who have a high regard for health and who live under conditions conducive to the promotion of a high level of health. Other industries seem to attract workers whose attitudes toward health tend to result in a community life in which health is not highly valued or pursued.

SOCIAL AND CULTURAL FACTORS

The difference between communities does not lie simply in the observable physical characteristics of the buildings, industries, and topography. Communities are identified by certain social and cultural factors that distinguish them. The traditions of the long-established community, social stratification in a community, the religious influences, the tenure of residence, and other social and cultural processes operate in giving a distinctive personality to a community. These same factors both directly and indirectly influence the health of the community. The recognition of health problems, the promotion of community health, and the ability to deal with health emergencies will be affected by the cultural and organizational influences that have evolved over the years.

Traditions and prejudices. New health problems, new aspects of old health problems, different health requirements, and new discoveries call for new approaches to health. In some communities long-established conventions, unwritten but generally understood, prove to be a barrier to attempts to deal with evolving health needs. In some instances these orally transmitted notions are not readily identifiable but appear as norms of resistance in the form of "We have always done it this way." Perhaps an even greater obstacle to health advances in the community are certain preconceived judgments or values relating to health matters or health procedures. A health bias can be as deeply ingrained as a religious bias. Sometimes they are the same.

Socioeconomic status (SES). The population may be classified into strata on the basis of income, residence, occupation, or education. According to which of these four criteria are used, the resulting hierarchy is graduated into any number of upper, middle, and lower SES levels. SES influences life-style, which in turn governs environmental exposures, customs, and habits that affect health status. There is considerable overlap between income and residence as well as between occupation and education. The latter is the most powerful determinant of the four criteria with regard to influence on health-related behavior. Persons of high educational attainment often enjoy the best health status, and they respond to appeals from health professionals and modify their behavior in a positive, health-related manner, for example, smoking cessation, weight control, exercise programs, dental care, and immunization status. In contrast, persons of a low educational level often suffer the worst health and are more difficult to reach with persuasive health messages. There frequently exists a cultural barrier between the efforts of health professionals to educate and the perceptions of people with less education.

Communicable diseases cut across all strata

of society, although generally the lower strata are more affected than those higher up on the pyramid. Prevention and control of communicable diseases among the less privileged groups indirectly protect and thus benefit the entire population. In general, public health activities are most needed by members of low-income groups and individuals of less educational attainment, but all people in a community will benefit from an overall community health program.

Social norms. Customs and norms imbued with ethical significance can have the force of laws. Usually the social norms of a community can serve as an asset in the promotion of community health. It is sometimes necessary to change established customs in a community to obtain the necessary gains that modern health procedures can contribute. Modification of customs in a community usually represents a compromise. Attempts to eliminate or reverse a custom often generate hostile resistance to a health program. When norms are transmitted from one generation to the next, they become embedded in the culture of the community.

The inertia of norms and custom is a conservative force in the modern community. Communities with broad social-mindedness and a concept of intercommunity and intracommunity action provide the necessary tenable basis for dealing with health problems on the broad scale that modern living requires.

Religious influences. Communities composed of citizens of diverse religious faiths living in harmony permit no particular denomination or group of churches to dominate the community. The total effect is to enrich the community life and provide a cooperative spirit in which community health promotion can flourish. This effect is achieved if those who provide the community's health leadership properly seek the support of the many church groups in the community. Health leadership must be sensitive to possible conflicts, religious or otherwise, that may exist in a community.

Political influences. Not all community health

programs or factors are official or political in nature. Law enforcement is not a highly significant factor in modern community health promotion, yet the caliber of officials a community has and the extent of social-mindedness in its officialdom both directly and indirectly affect community health standards. The willingness of community officials to raise taxes for health promotion and their interest in giving a high priority to matters of health are significant in the final determination of the kind of health people of a community will have. Even when official support of community health is inadequate, however, it is possible through other avenues, through other agencies, and through other means to promote community health action.

Economy. The size of a trade area, the importance of farm people in a trade area, the diversity of industry, the fluctuations in the economy, and the extremes of rich and poor are of significance to community health. Different economic conditions mean differences in the money available for food, clothing, housing, and other basic needs. They also mean differences in money available for health facilities, health services, schools, sanitary facilities, leisure time activities, and general health promotion programs.

The family income that an economy provides appears to be directly related to the level of health enjoyed by the people in a community. Surveys indicate that people in prosperous cities live longer than people who reside in low-income cities. It must be recognized that the factor of income may conceal several factors or variables. It may mask the general educational level of a people, and it may conceal groups that would tend to live longer under most circumstances. Prosperous communities usually provide more and better medical facilities than impoverished communities, a factor of overrated importance in community health.

Tenure of residence. Growth in population is a sign of a prosperous community and usually of a healthy community. Population growth may cause certain temporary displacements within a community that may be adverse to health promotion. Additional schools may be required, and additional community services may be necessary. There may be some disorganization during the time between the occurrence of these new needs and their fulfillment. This is the experience of suburban communities adjacent to large metropolitan areas, especially during periods of heavy immigration and most dramatically with refugee settlements. In such communities the tenure of residence of a good many of the families is relatively short. Usually the newcomers are young couples with families of small children. In other communities where families are moving in and out constantly, an unfavorable health situation usually exists. A high number of transient families tends to lower the stability and social networks that support the health of a community.

In many of the smaller villages of a nation there is a tendency for the younger people to move away, so that today most of the small rural and even nonrural villages are populated by older people. With a proportionately high percentage of their citizens over 65 years of age, these small communities find themselves faced with low birthrates, high death rates, and the special health problems of the elderly. Many of these communities are unable to provide the necessary health facilities and services for the health needs of their older citizens. Some communities are fortunate in being near to or part of a large community in which complete health services are available. Health Systems Agencies are attempting to plan for the needs of these outlying communities by linking them with urban facilities and resources.

ORGANIZATIONAL FACTORS

In any community there will be a diversity of agencies and individuals providing services of direct and indirect health significance. Too frequently there is little coordination or integration of services, and considerable overlapping of functions frequently exists. Despite the lack of efficient coordination, the fact that both tax-supported and non-tax-supported health services are available is important to the health-conscious citizen who knows how to use health services to the best advantage of self, family, neighborhood, and community.

Tax-supported services. The official agencies that contribute to the health of a community usually touch the individual citizen directly. Some of the services given by these tax-supported agencies may be of an indirect nature, but the majority of their services directly affects individual citizens in their everyday living. Obviously, the most important of these tax-supported agencies is the county, city, or district health department. Other official agencies also providing health services include the department of welfare, public hospitals, special boards and commissions, department of public works, public schools, local housing authority, agricultural agency, recreation agency, and the police department. Each of these, individually and cooperatively, has an important role in community health promotion.

Non-tax-supported services. Certain health services are available to citizens of most communities through voluntary agencies or organizations present in the typical community. Civic clubs, church groups, parent-teacher associations, Red Cross, visiting nurse associations, and the community hospital are classic examples. Special clinical services, as well as medical care and hospital service plans, may also be available.

National voluntary health organizations may have an indirect effect on the health of any given community and in some instances may play a direct role in the health of individual citizens. These national voluntary health organizations serve several functions, such as education, demonstrations, supplementing official activities, supporting official health activities, and

coordinating community health efforts. Some of these organizations are concerned with specific diseases. In the United States this group would include chapters of organizations such as the American Cancer Society, American Heart Association, American Lung Association, and March of Dimes.

A prevalent nontax-supported service in most communities is the private practitioner. The practicing physician, the dentist, the nurse, and other health specialists provide indispensable services to the community. The medical society, the dental society, and medical service plans must be included in any appraisal of community health services.

Model standards for community health. As one means of assessing one's own community and applying the principles and methods of community health promotion, the user of this textbook is encouraged to examine the status of health, health organization, and health services in a specific community in comparison with national objectives and model standards. In each chapter of this book objectives will be suggested based on national and international consensus as to the levels of health possible in the present or near future and the types of organization and services that should be in progress to accomplish the expected health outcomes. The student or practitioner using these objectives and standards is encouraged to adapt them to local conditions by inserting an appropriate target date and to identify indicators of their achievement or implementation, as in the table on p. 32.

QUALITY OF HEALTH

Many people not incapacitated nevertheless do not have the quality of health that would enable them to live effectively and enjoyably. Many people regarded as being well actually do not possess a high quality of health. They may be free from disabilities and overt symptoms and yet not possess an adequate level of well-being.

Text continued on p. 39.

Administration and supporting services in community health*

Goal: Administration and supporting services of the official health agency or any other agency will ensure that the agency plans, organizes, manages, and coordinates services within its jurisdiction to meet the collective health needs of the population in an effective and efficient manner.

NOTE: This standard, unlike many others in later chapters, has been developed principally for the official health agency as the lead health agency of the community. Most elements of this standard do, however, have direct application to any entity administering a community health program and should be considered as appropriate objectives of each subsequent standard.

Focus	Objectives	Indicators	Population in need
	Process (actions and services)		
General administration	1. By 19 ___ an administrative apparatus for coordination of all official health agency activities will be established.	a. An agency goal statement defining its philosophy, beliefs, and purposes b. An agency organizational chart delineating lines of authority and functional relationships c. Administrative files documenting internal agency communication channels, e.g., (1) Regularly scheduled staff conferences with minutes (2) Provision for conferences with individuals, as necessary (3) Written, dated, signed, and cataloged directives, guidelines, memoranda, etc. d. Administrative files documenting external agency communication channels, i.e., agency staff participation in (1) Health councils (2) Interagency committees (3) Community and area-wide planning groups	The community
Federal, state, local legislation and guidelines	2. By 19 ___ the official health agency will be cognizant of and responsive to all relevant federal, state, and local statutes and regulations. NOTE: *This objective recognizes the imperfection of statutes and regulations and the need for their periodic review and update. This need is especially*	a. Current file of all relevant federal, state, and local statutes and regulations b. Inventory of applicable laws, rules, and regulations compared with official health agency records and reports c. Agency involvement in review and updating of applicable codes	The community

important for agencies promulgating regulations.

			The community
Manpower	3. By 19 — sound personnel management practices for the agency or program will be established.	a. Current written personnel policies and procedures manual b. Maintenance of personnel records system c. Existence of staff development system	
	3a. By 19 — the staffing patterns and qualifications necessary for agency operations will be identified and established.	a. Inventory of staff qualifications and minimum requirements b. Personnel roster and statements of qualification	
	3b. By 19 — the agency will develop or have access to intramural and extramural performance-based training programs relative to the needs of the agency, the programs and employees for which the agency has responsibility.	a. Existence of an educational needs assessment system b. Existence of performance-based in-service training programs and continuing education c. Availability and use of work-related training courses and meetings	
Fiscal management	4. By 19 — sound fiscal management practices for the agency will be established.	a. Maintenance of a fiscal record system consistent with a written fiscal policies and procedures manual (1) Appropriate books, ledgers, registers, and fiscal reports b. Compliance with acceptable accounting and auditing practices c. Detailed annual program budget d. Detailed, written fee collection schedules, as appropriate	The community
Office management practices	5. By 19 — communications systems appropriate for conducting agency business will be established and reviewed periodically.	a. Provision for reception, telephone answering and channeling, and word processing during regular business hours and during other hours for health emergencies b. Provision for prompt issuance of licenses and permits and other documents during regular business hours	The community

*Based on Model standards for community preventive health services, Washington, D.C., 1979, Public Health Service, U.S. Department of Health and Human Services.

Continued.

Administration and supporting services in community health—cont'd

Focus	Objectives	Indicators	Population in need
Office management practices—cont'd		c. Provision for files of records and correspondence, readily available to appropriate agency personnel d. Availability of standardized records and forms for uniform reporting by agency personnel e. Record maintenance practices in conformity with the required record retention schedules and procedures established to protect individual confidentiality and rights	
Legal services	6. By 19 ___ the official health agency will have adequate legal services to support its operations.	a. Documentation of agency access to legal review and consultation for its various administrative practices, program operations, staff duties and responsibilities, and authorities relating to enforcement powers b. Access to legal services to draft necessary legislation and maintain liaison with legislative branch of government	The community
Facilities and equipment	7. By 19 ___ the agency will be assured that facilities and supplies necessary to carry out its objectives are available and maintained.	Maintenance of perpetual inventory of facilities equipment and supplies	
Physical plant technical requirements	8. By 19 ___ the agency will be cognizant of and responsive to relevant federal-state-local health facility codes and ordinances.	Documentation that all agency facilities conform to relevant federal-state-local health facility codes and ordinances, e.g., periodic facility inspection reports	The community
	9. By 19 ___ the agency will ensure that its facilities and services are distributed and arranged to minimize barriers to access, with special attention to the mobility disadvantaged and the physically handicapped.	a. Accessibility of facilities b. Distribution of facilities	The community

NOTE: *Time and distance factors are important considerations in the use of many personal health services (e.g., perinatal care, family planning, general primary care). Individual program standards may articulate some arbitrary limits, recognizing that deviations from these may be justified for special circumstances. These circumstances deserve close attention.*

Program management process	10. By 19 — agency-wide management practices and procedures for the various program components of the agency will be established.	a. Identification of professional management responsibility for each agency program area b. Maintenance of a management system designed to accomplish the following: (1) Periodic comprehensive review of agency programs (2) Identification and resolution of operational problems	The community
Program management (planning)	11. By 19 — an agency-wide planning and evaluation system will be established.	a. Identification of professional responsibility for planning and evaluation b. Inventory of community and agency programs and capacities c. Existence of systematic internal and external review processes	
	11a. By 19 — a system of monitoring existing agency operations to determine progress and need for continuation, refinement, redirection or expansion of agency operations will be established and maintained.	a. Existence of system b. Periodic reports with analysis that provide current information in the following areas: (1) Program administration and funding (2) Program description (3) Program delivery activity (4) Program recipient characteristics	
Program management (consumer awareness)	11b. By 19 — the agency will establish and maintain a system to review its programs periodically for their sensitivity to consumers' (individual, family, and community) unique needs, values, experiences, awarenesses, understanding, language and cultural differences, rights, and dignity.	a. Existence of system b. By-laws that contain language defining the term *consumer* and provide for such representation in the agency decision-making process c. Documentation of consumer representation on agency boards, councils, committees, commissions, and task forces	The community

Administration and supporting services in community health—cont'd

Focus	Objectives	Indicators	Population in need
Program management (consumer awareness—cont'd)		d. Written guidelines for and documentation of solicitation of public participation in health care programs e. Existence of consumer education programs f. A stated policy of free public access to program information of a nonindividually identifiable nature g. Agency publications that reflect sensitivity to the ethnic, cultural, and linguistic differences that may be barriers to the understanding of its consuming public h. Agency personnel composition compared to the community it serves in terms of ethnicity, cultural differences, and principal languages spoken in the community i. Existence of a written consumer grievance policy and procedures manual	
Health planning and development	11c. By 19 ___ determine and define, based on analyses and interpretation of health statistics and other pertinent information, the health needs and priorities of the community.	a. Existence of systematic agency planning process b. Existence of a written comprehensive health master plan or plans containing priorities and objectives based on needs, supply of resources, and local demands c. Evidence of periodic updating of plan d. Evidence of agency participation in community and area-wide health planning e. Compatibility of agency plan and those of planning agencies relating to the agency f. Maintenance of file of agency planning documents	The community
Research policy	12. By 19 ___ the agency will have an established policy concerning its participation in and support of research and demonstration activities.	a. Existence of policy	The community

Program area	Objective	Indicator	
	12a. By 19 ___ where technical capabilities and necessary resources are available the agency will have a mechanism for conducting research concerning major causes of death and disability and experimental testing of methods that appear to provide means for preventing death and disabling disease.	Existence of mechanism	The community
	13. The agency will publish and make available periodically to agencies and individuals health statistics and publications of general interest.	a. Availability of materials b. Publications	
Program evaluation	14. By 19 ___ the agency will establish a mechanism for evaluation and assessment of existing programs and the determination of factors that interfere with the effectiveness or reduce the efficiency of established agency programs.	Evaluation and assessment mechanism	
	14a. By 19 ___ the agency will have available to it an inventory of community health programs.	Inventory	
	14b. By 19 ___ the agency will have a systematic internal and external periodic program review process.	Program review mechanism	
	14c. By 19 ___ the agency will periodically report to the community on its objectives, activities, and accomplishments.	Reports to governing bodies, legislative bodies, elected officials, and the public	
Vital records	15. By 19 ___ the official health agency will cooperate with the established program for the collection, tabulation, and analysis of vital records, or in its absence, shall maintain such a program.	Vital records administration program	The community

Continued.

Administration and supporting services in community health—cont'd

Focus	Objectives	Indicators	Population in need
Vital records—cont'd	15a. By 19 — the community will have a designated registrar and, as needed, a deputy registrar or subregistrars with the authority and accountability to protect the integrity and accountability of vital records and to ensure the efficient and proper administration of the system of vital statistics.	Designated registrars	
	15b. By 19 — the registrar will establish mechanisms to ensure that each birth, death, marriage, and divorce that occurs in its jurisdiction is reported, recorded, and registered, and of which authorized copies are authenticated; and the registrar will make vital records available to authorized members of the public in a timely fashion.	a. Existence of mechanisms b. Provision for prompt issuance of public documents during regular business hours	
	15c. By 19 — the agency will maintain a file of and be familiar with vital statistics laws, rules, regulations, and instructions issued by the state registrar and other appropriate official agencies.	File	The community
	15d. By 19 — the registrar will provide fire protection and security systems to preserve vital records.	Existence of fire protection and security systems	
	15e. By 19 — the agency will participate in a mechanism for the analysis and publication of vital statistics data for this area.	Evidence of participation	

The health goal that the community health program seeks for every citizen is not only an absence of disabling defects and disorders, but also a vitality, buoyancy, and abundance of energy that enables the people of the community to do the things they reasonably expect to do, with a corresponding enjoyment and gratification in living. Not perfect health, but a high level of well-being in which an individual finds life stimulating, is a realistic goal for citizens of every community.

Despite the advances that have been made in longevity and communicable disease control during this century, poor health, with its attendant human suffering and soaring social and economic costs, remains all too prevalent in every segment of most communities. Of significance in Western societies today is the fact that most of the serious diseases and disabilities people can control are related to personal habits: drinking, smoking, drug misuse, overeating, poor nutrition, lack of exercise, and careless behavior. If people can be helped to change these habits, both individual health and the quality of life can be greatly improved.

Not all solutions will be behavioral. Indeed, in the last years of the twentieth century, as in the first years, the results of basic research, technological development, and environmental modification may offer further control of health problems. Currently, however, knowledge to prevent or minimize many health problems is not being used to a satisfactory degree. After-the-fact medical care, unfortunately, still takes precedence over programs of disease prevention and health promotion.

The challenge, then, is for innovative and creative community programs to support better health practices and health protection. Given the ever-increasing social and economic burden of health care costs resulting from negative community conditions and individual behaviors, what are the areas in which improved preventive health services can have the greatest effect, and what are the communications techniques and the substantive messages that should be given priority?

PROBLEMS AND POTENTIALS

Consistent with the reports of the governments of Australia, Canada, Great Britain, and the United States, Tables 2-1 through 2-8 outline examples of some health problems that seem to offer the best opportunity for amelioration through a more creative approach to health education, preventive services, and community environmental control. The eight problems selected as being most susceptible to change have been divided into the four health field areas of human biology (life cycle), human behavior (life-style), organization (life supports), and environment (life threats). Within these broad categories, examples of priority health problems are outlined in the following manner:

1. A brief statement of the scope of the problem
2. The prevailing misconceptions and attitudes that underlie individual and community behaviors that are injurious to health
3. The negative behaviors themselves
4. The range of health problems resulting from such behaviors
5. The affirmative goals and benefits to individuals and communities that might accrue from a successful program of health

In all socioeconomic groups there are too many mothers and fathers who are unaware of the principles of child health and successful parenting. The relationships among these problems are shown in Table 2-1.

While the birthrate in America is declining overall, the number of school-age girls who become pregnant each year is rising. Of all girls in the United States, 10% will give birth before age 18. Largely owing to prenatal ignorance and neglect, the prematurity rate at this age is over 20%, greatly increasing the chances of mental retardation and other birth defects. The incidence of poverty is twice as high among women who become mothers when they are under 17, and 60% of all teenagers who carry their children to term are on welfare. These are but a few of the statistical measures of a health program that are largely a result of ignorance, fear, and lack of access to proper care.

The goal for a program of community health promotion in this area is the attainment of fewer mental, physical, emotional, and social problems for individuals, their children, and society, also, the birth of healthier infants to mothers and fathers who understand the principles of child health and successful parenting. The result for society is stronger families with reduced dependence on publicly financed social supports such as welfare, medical assistance, mental health services, and institutionalized care.

TABLE 2-1. Community health problems related to the human biology of the life cycle—prenatal and postnatal care and parenting*

Misapprehensions, beliefs, attitudes	Behaviors	Resulting health problems

Lack of knowledge of early signs of pregnancy and prenatal diagnosis
Lack of knowledge of prenatal care resources
Lack of recognition of seriousness of fetal damage possible through careless or heedless behavior, such as smoking or taking drugs and alcohol during pregnancy
Lack of knowledge of adequate nutrition
Lack of knowledge of and proper preparation for childbirth
Failure to recognize postnatal symptoms
Lack of awareness of proper principles of child development and practices of good child care
Lack of awareness of needs for communication and stimulation between mother and child
Inability to recognize the dangers to the child of health abuses and emotional disorders of the parents
	Failure to seek early pregnancy diagnosis and care
	Poor maternal nutrition, use of drugs and alcohol during pregnancy, and lack of prenatal care leading to prematurity
	Failure to make careful physical and emotional preparations for childbirth, including proper preparation for caesarian section, which runs from 10%-20% in young mothers
	Failure to take advantage of available community-based postnatal and well-baby health services
	Failure to give infant adequate attention and stimulation of various stages of development
	Failure to practice parenting skills and attitudes needed for successful child raising
	Inability to control emotional tendencies in self, which may lead to neglect and child abuse
		Damage to fetus and infant
		  a. Prematurity
		  b. Low birth weight
		  c. Birth damage
		  d. Risk of high infant mortality
		  e. Risk of mental retardation and other infant health and developmental problems
		  f. Congenital problems
		  g. Risk of disease and untreated anomalies due to lack of prenatal and postnatal care
		Damage to mother
		  a. Psychological and emotional unpreparedness for child birth and parenting
		  b. Maternal and perinatal mortality due to lack of adequate care
		  c. Emotional, psychological, and physical problems continuing and worsening as child grows older
		  d. Danger to mother in second trimester abortion
		Damage to infant and child
		  a. High incidence of infant and child health problems and anomalies because of lack of timely medical care
		  b. Infant at increased risk as to mental retardation and other developmental disabilities
		  c. Child neglect, child abuse, and consequent mental, physical, and social problems for the parents and their children

*From Green, L.W., et al.: The Johns Hopkins University and Medical Institutions, Baltimore, 1979; Harvard University Division of Health Policy Research and Education, Boston, 1981; and The University of Texas Center for Health Promotion Research and Development, Houston, 1982.

While the issue of sexual responsibility extends to all age groups, the effects of sexual irresponsibility, whether through ignorance or peer group pressure, have an impact with particular severity on the teenage population, the results of whose sexual behavior pose one of the nation's most rapidly growing health problems (Table 2-2). Venereal disease among this population has reached epidemic proportions; the number of recorded teenage abortions has increased 50% over the past 5 years; congenital anomalies are more frequent in children born to this age group; illegitimate births are now around 15% of all births, and this rate is rising.

The goal of education for greater sexual responsibility is healthier children born to more mature mothers and fathers into stronger, more stable families with greater economic security. The result for society is girls able to complete education, avoid welfare, and get better jobs. Education should also reduce prematurity, retardation, and child abuse and neglect, with attendant social and economic benefits.

TABLE 2-2. Community health problems in the life cycle—sexually transmitted diseases*

Misapprehensions, beliefs, attitudes	Behaviors	Resulting health problems
Lack of knowledge or misunderstanding of individual sexual vulnerability and its consequences	Sex without contraception	Teenage pregnancies (age 10 to 14 birthrate up 30% in the past 10 years).
Ignorance of contraception: myths and misinformation	Failure to obtain early medical care in response to venereal disease and symptoms	Venereal disease
Ignorance of signs, symptoms, and treatment resources for venereal diseases	Reporting pregnancy too late and not following through with prenatal care	Second trimester abortion
Ignorance of signs and symptoms of early pregnancy and of need for early professional diagnosis and care in the event of pregnancy, disease, and other consequences of sexual activity	Inability to cope with decision making relative to a pregnancy, i.e., abortion, marriage, carrying child to term, adoption, etc.	Excessive stress leading to a. Mental health problems b. Psychosomatic illnesses, such as peptic ulcers; gastrointestinal symptoms c. Alcoholism, drug misuse
Fear of censure, peer group rejection, family anger leading to denial of pregnancy (or disease), and failure to seek timely care	Failure to obtain family support and adequate counseling within community to reinforce values and make necessary life adjustments	Poor life adjustment
Inability to withstand peer pressure to engage in sexual activity before either readiness or desire is present		Problems of prematurity, low birth weight, etc., in infants
Ignorance of existence of prevention, support, and clinical care in community facilities and how to avail self of their services		Problems of infant care and child abuse arising from unwanted or unplanned births
Ignorance of emotional and sociological causes of sexual activity; lack of commitment to sexual responsibility		Mental, emotional, and physical disabilities resulting from inability to cope with sexual activity before emotional or physical readiness
		High-risk pregnancies; infants and children suffering a variety of mental and physical developmental disabilities

*From Green, L.W., et al.: The Johns Hopkins University and Medical Institutions, Baltimore, 1979; Harvard University Division of Health Policy Research and Education, Boston, 1981; and The University of Texas Center for Health Promotion Research and Development, Houston, 1982.

Although the aging process is common to all, there is at present a general lack of knowledge, awareness, and understanding of its nature and consequences (Table 2-3). The elderly are increasing in absolute numbers as well as proportionately in Western nations. One in ten Americans is now 65 or over, and by the year 2030 this will increase to one in six. With the fertility rate declining, the absolute number of babies born diminishing, and the death rate falling to under 9 per 1,000 people, the growing number of older Americans poses complex social, economic, and health problems. Even as their health care needs continue to rise in overall amount and cost, the major social and economic institutions contribute to their health problems through rejection, loss of usefulness, and unavailability of appropriate support facilities.

The goal of education in human development and aging is to create greater understanding of the emotional and physical processes at every stage of development, to create greater acceptance and use of those in the oldest age group, and to motivate people to assume more responsibility in caring for their own well-being. The result for society is increased and prolonged productivity; reduced delinquency and welfare dependency; improved mental, emotional, and physical well-being of older citizens in particular; and reduced dependency on publicly funded social support systems.

TABLE 2-3. Community health problems from the human biology of the life cycle—human development and aging*

Misapprehensions, beliefs, attitudes	Behaviors	Resulting health problems
Lack of recognition among all individuals of the various stages of the maturation and aging process	Treatment of the aging by society based on false stereotypes: helplessness, deteriorating learning processes, loss of function and control, etc.	Stress resulting from lack of understanding of the aging process
Negative, unrealistic attitudes toward the process of senescence and old age	Unresponsiveness of individuals and social institutions to the specific physical and emotional needs of the aging	Emotional, mental, and social disfunctions
Lack of recognition of the symptoms of chronic and functional illnesses and ignorance of coping mechanisms	Rejection of the aging process in the individual, resulting in unrealistic and often bizarre attempts to retain youth	Psychosomatic and functional illnesses: peptic ulcers, bowel malfunctions, insomnia, skin rashes, etc.
Lack of acceptance of the ultimate fact of dying and death as a universal experience	Neglect early warnings of illnesses common to the older citizen	Lack of preparation for dying and death
Lack of knowledge of community-based health and social services and how to gain access to them	Delay of appropriate diagnosis and treatment of health problems associated with or incidental to the aging process	Uncontrolled chronic diseases leading to premature disability and death
Lack of knowledge of nutritional needs of the aging	Inadequate diet and failure to eat sufficient amounts of healthful foods	Unattended disabilities leading to restrictions of activity, isolation, underemployment, and ultimate hastening of onset of serious illness, dying, and death
Lack of awareness on the part of society of the value of the aged in terms of their wisdom and experience in dealing with life's problems, their relative physical and mental soundness, and their potential in fulfilling needed social roles (i.e., advising, counseling, helping to care for the very young, etc.)	Disfunction of the social system, creating particular problems for the aged by denying them work, a useful social role, adequate economic opportunity, and a voice in influencing social and political institutions	Serious nutritional deficiencies
		Mental, emotional, and physical incapacity resulting from loss of "role" in life and useful function in society

*From Green, L.W., et al.: The Johns Hopkins University and Medical Institutions, Baltimore, 1979; Harvard University Division of Health Policy Research and Education, Boston, 1981; and The University of Texas Center for Health Promotion Research and Development, Houston, 1982.

For a nation that has the capacity of using up almost 30% of the world's resources to support the life-style and standard of living of 6% of the world's population, Americans are singularly inept in their dietary practices (Table 2-4). With almost 20% of all Americans at least 10 pounds (4.5 kg) overweight, poor health is courted in both nutritional intake and in the lack of exercise needed to burn off fat-producing calories. There is some evidence that behavioral changes are taking place as a result of campaigns to reduce consumption of eggs and animal products and to create awareness that poor dietary habits, fats, cholesterol, and sedentary living are hazardous to health. There is still, however, excessive intake of saturated fats and lack of sufficient and vigorous exercise among all segments of society.

The desired goal of a community health promotion program on behalf of improved diet and exercise is healthier, more productive individuals at every stage of the life cycle. Results of such an outcome will be a substantial reduction of social and economic costs to the individual, family, insurance group, employer, and society from chronic, diet-related disease and disabilities resulting from lack of exercise.

TABLE 2-4. Community health problems: behavior and life-style—nutrition and exercise*

Misapprehensions, beliefs, attitudes	Behaviors	Resulting health problems
Lack of specific, continuous concern for nutrition and exercise as necessary concomitants to a healthy life-style	Poor food selection, bad dietary habits, inappropriate timing of food intake (poor breakfast habits, especially)	Obesity and nutritional imbalance are prime risk factors for
Prevalence of food fads, conflicting diets, use of vitamins and certain health foods	a. Excessive calorie intake b. Excessive intake of sodium, sugar, and fats, especially among children who are most vulnerable to advertising	a. Cardiovascular disease b. Diabetes c. Pulmonary misfunction d. Arthritis e. Mental and emotional disorders
Confusion as to proper nutrition instilled by advertising messages on behalf of packaged and processed foods, snacking items, and desserts	c. Fad crash diets for personal treatment of obesity Failure to burn up calories through regular, vigorous exercise	Crash treatment of obesity may introduce the use of and dependency on amphetamines or restrict diet dangerously to nonnutritive foods over an extended period of time
Confusion as to necessary requirements for appropriate weight loss regimen due to prevalence of popular nostrums and "cures" for obesity	Prevalence of sedentary leisure time activity: nonwalking, nonexercise, spectator sports, driving short distances, short-term exercise, fads and quickie substitutes for regular physical activity	Excessive weight, physical weakness, and cardiovascular disease due to lack of sufficient, regular exercise
Lack of awareness of the meaning, duration, and intensity of exercise needed for fitness and good health		

*From Green, L.W., et al.: The Johns Hopkins University and Medical Institutions, Baltimore, 1979; Harvard University Division of Health Policy Research and Education, Boston, 1981; and The University of Texas Center for Health Promotion Research and Development, Houston, 1982.

While some studies indicate a slackening in the use of some hard drugs, the use of alcohol has become almost epidemic, especially among younger Americans (Table 2-5). It is estimated that there are almost 6 million alcoholics in the United States whose cost to themselves and society runs into the billions of dollars. The use of amphetamines, marijuana, and other mood-changing drugs, such as hallucinogens, remains high. According to government statistics, more than half of all Americans aged 22 to 25 have used marijuana; 10% of all adults have used hashish; almost 8% of all Americans between 12 and 17 have used psychotherapeutic drugs.

The goal of a community health promotion program in this area is healthier, more productive individuals who are able to use their own emotional resources to cope with life. The result of a successful program would be a substantial reduction in social and economic costs of chronic absenteeism and poor job performance, crime, violence, accidents, family dislocation and disintegration, health care, and dependence on publicly financed social supports.

TABLE 2-5. Community health problems: behavior and life-style—alcohol and drug misuse*

Misapprehensions, beliefs, attitudes	Behaviors	Resulting health problems
Lack of recognition that excessive alcohol or mood-altering drug usage reflects a chronic disorder and can have serious effects on social, mental, economic, physical, and emotional aspects of the individual's life Failure to recognize causes of pressures and tensions that lead to hazardous coping such as "pill popping" and drinking Failure of parents and surrogates to recognize and provide substitutes for drugs (especially those who start their children on drug habituation through availability of aspirin, sleeping tablets, tranquilizers, etc.) Failure to recognize that individuals can exercise judgment and maturation in the use of alcohol Lack of recognition or understanding of physical, mental, behavioral indicators of alcoholism and drug misuse	Lack of moderation in the use of substances having an effect or influence on mental state, emotion, and behavior Failure to seek professional counseling and therapy before symptoms become chronic Failure to adjust habitual use early enough when pathological symptoms appear Dogmatic, absolute prescription of any use of alcohol or drugs that leads adolescents, especially, to illicit experimentation and immoderate use Failure to seek out or provide alternative modes of support, expression, relief, or therapy as coping mechanisms in place of behavior or emotion-modifying substances	Alcohol a. Liver disease b. Acute hepatitis c. Chronic cirrhosis d. Liver cell cancer e. Gastritis f. Trauma while drunk (falls, auto accidents, irrational acts of bravado, etc.) g. Aspiration pneumonia h. Seizures i. DT's j. Anemia k. Malnutrition l. Fetal alcohol syndrome Drugs a. Hepatitis b. Death from overdose c. Emotional, mental, societal, and economic impacts resulting from drug dependency. (Crime associated with drugs alone costs the United States $10 billion per year.)

*From Green, L.W., et al.: The Johns Hopkins University and Medical Institutions, Baltimore, 1979; Harvard University Division of Health Policy Research and Education, Boston, 1981; and The University of Texas Center for Health Promotion Research and Development, Houston, 1982.

While cigarette smoking by adult Americans is less common than before the release of the Surgeon General's report in 1964, the number of cigarettes smoked each year has risen appreciably, and smoking has actually increased among certain high-risk segments of the population, such as teenagers and young women (Table 2-6). Statistics indicate that the heaviest smoking now takes place among male youth aged 15 to 24, followed closely by males under age 15 and females between ages 17 and 24, the group at greatest risk during pregnancy.

The goal of limiting the smoking of cigarettes is to produce healthier, more productive individuals with increased life span, not habituated to such a harmful, even lethal, activity. The desired outcomes are reduction of damage to the fetus with attendant long-term health costs, as well as reduction of chronic, smoking-related disease with parallel reduction in health costs to society.

TABLE 2-6. Community health problems: behavior and life-style—smoking*

Misapprehensions, beliefs, attitudes	Behaviors	Resulting health problems
Belief that cigarette smoking is glamorous or a symbol of sexual maturity, rather than a habit harmful to health with lethal possibilities, especially for women during pregnancy	Excessive cigarette smoking beginning in early adolescence. (Growth of smoking among younger women multiplies the chance of immoderate smoking during pregnancy.)	Coronary heart disease, peripheral vascular disease, cancer Increased fetal and neonatal deaths due to smoking during pregnancy Deaths and injury from fires caused by smokers
Belief among teenagers, especially, that smoking is necessary for social acceptbility among peers	Peer pressure to smoke, resulting in early experimentation and habituation	
Lack of awareness of differences among smoking materials (pipes, cigars, filter and low nicotine and tar cigarettes) that can mitigate the health dangers of smoking	Failure to choose least dangerous forms of smoking material if habituated and unable to cut down or stop smoking readily	
Lack of knowledge of programs and agencies available on a community basis to help individuals stop smoking	Failure to use available sources of assistance in cutting down or stopping smoking	
Lack of understanding among parents that their smoking behavior will have a significant influence on their child's attitudes and actions	Parental smoking behavior coupled with usual prescription against smoking on the part of their children generally leads to resistance and rebellion against parents' dictum	
Lack of an awareness that smoking is used at times as a coping mechanism substituting for more creative and effective solutions to problems	Failure to deal directly with the problem of smoking habituation through alternative coping mechanisms or to seek more appropriate therapeutic resources to resolve need to smoke	

*From Green, L.W., et al.: The Johns Hopkins University and Medical Institutions, Baltimore, 1979; Harvard University Division of Health Policy Research and Education, Boston, 1981; and The University of Texas Center for Health Promotion Research and Development, Houston, 1982.

Many significant health problems can be prevented if there is a greater and more timely use of formal health services and facilities and a recognition of the supportive role of families, friends, and other community members in the prevention and health care process, including self-care (Table 2-7).

The goal of education in the better use of health services is to stimulate active involvement of each individual in personal health care, thereby increasing knowledgeable choices and appropriate care-seeking behaviors. This would result in diminishing cost, improved morbidity and mortality, increased accessibility or professional services when needed, together with a more rational pattern of self-help and use of facilities.

TABLE 2-7. Community health problems: organization of life supports—use of health services and family or community supports*

Misapprehensions, beliefs, attitudes	Behaviors	Resulting health problems
The individual Lack of awareness of the potential of each individual for personal decision making regarding health (especially in disease and accident prevention due to faulty or incomplete health education) Suppression of recognition or ignorance of signs and symptoms of poor health; fear of involvement in the health services system Quasi-religious attitude toward the role of the physician in society Reliance on institutional health care to provide total prevention and treatment process **The community** Lack of recognition of need to improve emergency services for entire population Lack of recognition of or apathy toward the need to improve health care services in both economically deprived urban areas and remote and inaccessible rural areas Lack of concurrence on appropriate care-seeking behavior among and between providers and patients	**The individual** Failure to make knowledgeable choices in personal decisions regarding both prevention and treatment aspects of health behavior Delay in seeking diagnosis of and treatment for suspicious physical, mental, or emotional symptoms Acquiescence in apparently unnecessary procedures, operations, etc., through overreliance on a single source of diagnosis or medical opinion **The community** Failure to develop self-help, self-service facilities in communities in which the individual himself can perform significant diagnostic procedures at regular intervals or at onset of symptoms, i.e., blood pressure, blood sample, urinalysis, etc. Failure to develop an emergency care system in which individuals can provide helping services, i.e., cardiopulmonary resuscitation, etc. Failure to remove geographic and economic barriers to care through inadequate or disproportionately distributed health care resources	Serious illnesses due to failure to seek care in timely fashion Financial barriers to health care Geographic barriers to health care; inadequate distribution of health care resources

*From Green, L.W., et al.: The Johns Hopkins University and Medical Institutions, Baltimore, 1979; Harvard University Division of Health Policy Research and Education, Boston, 1981; and The University of Texas Center for Health Promotion Research and Development, Houston, 1982.

Sickness, injury, and death from accidents and exposure to environmental hazards have increased greatly since 1960. Accidents are now the fourth leading cause of death in America, ranking just behind heart, malignant, and vascular diseases. While some exposure to accidental hazard is inescapable in society, a high proportion of these threats to life is the result of specific and general environmental factors that are capable of amelioration, as well as lack of awareness of dangers that can be corrected through education (Table 2-8).

TABLE 2-8. Community health problems: life threats—injury control and environmental exposure*

Misapprehensions, beliefs, attitudes	Behaviors	Resulting health problems
The individual	**The individual**	Pulmonary disease, acute toxicities, heart diseases, cancer, accidents
Lack of knowledge of environmental pollutants, toxicants, dangers at work, play, home, travel; occupational hazards; sociocultural factors leading to health hazards and accidents (tv violence, automobile driving habits, etc.)	Careless or heedless behavior at home, at work, on the streets, and elsewhere that endangers self and others	Specific work-related chronic diseases, i.e., black lung, etc.
Unawareness of proximity to self of dangers and unawareness of degree of susceptibility	Failure to attempt to change conditions recognized as, or suspected to be, hazardous	Sociobehavioral and emotional disorders
Misinformation about environmental hazards (i.e., presence of carcinogens in water, harmful substances in working environment such as asbestos.)	**The community**	a. Excessive risk taking
	Institutional violations of health and safety codes and standards. Failure of appropriate agencies to mandate compliance with proper environmental safeguards; failure of industries or unions to make a safe work environment a significant factor in labor-management relations	b. Criminal behavior
Ignorance of mechanisms available to change unsafe conditions and eliminate most environmental hazards		c. Violence
		Injuries, trauma, disabilities among all age groups
The community	Acquiescence in, or apathy toward, social, economic, or institutional factors in health and safety, (i.e., crowding, poor housing, violation of laws and codes, etc.)	
Lack of identification of high-risk populations	Failure to concentrate prevention education on individuals and groups at high risk of injury or environmental exposure	
Ignorance of appropriate techniques and appeals effective in changing behavior or minimizing risks	Insistence on unworkable and impractical absolutist solutions. (e.g., "pure water," "clean air," "risk-free environment")	

*From Green, L.W., et al.: The Johns Hopkins University and Medical Institutions, Baltimore, 1979; Harvard University Division of Health Policy Research and Education, Boston, 1981; and The University of Texas Center for Health Promotion Research and Development, Houston, 1982.

Reduction in the social and economic impact of death and disability of individuals in their most productive years is the major goal of injury control. Higher morale among workers through reduction of accidents and improvements in health through safer working conditions, better employee relations, greater productivity and job effectiveness, and reduction in chronic disease and costs of compensation and long-term health care all represent the potential benefits of a community health program in injury control. The ecological and epidemiological context of these and other problems and potentials for community health are the subjects of the following chapters.

QUESTIONS AND EXERCISES

1. What are the advantages and disadvantages of a high degree of mobility in a population?
2. What constitutes the community in which you live?
3. What favorable characteristics would you look for in a community?
4. Make an analysis of the neighborhood in which you live.
5. Explain how one dramatic incident can unite a community in a common health cause.
6. Explain how one citizen can provide the spark necessary to deal with a long-existing, unresolved health problem.
7. Using an example, show how a particular industry attracts a particular type of people with particular health problems.
8. What are some obstacles to community health progress?
9. Analyze this statement: "It is impossible to eliminate community customs but not difficult to modify them."
10. Why should churches have an interest in community health?
11. To what extent does economics enter into community health promotion?
12. Evaluate this statement: "Transient families are community health liabilities."
13. Apply one or more of the model standards for administration and supporting services in community health to a community by investigating the indicators to determine when the community did, or will be able to, accomplish the objectives.

BIBLIOGRAPHY

American Public Health Association: Health is a community affair, New York, 1970, The Association.

Conant, R.W.: Politics of community health, National Commission on Community Health Services, Washington, D.C., 1968, Public Affairs Press.

Engel, A.: Perspectives in health planning, New York, 1968, Oxford University Press, Inc.

Fox, J.G., and Zatkin, S.R.: Innovations in family and community health practice and the law, Fam. Commun. Health 1:19, 1978.

Ginzberg, E.: Urban health services: the case of New York, New York, 1970, Columbia University Press.

Green, L.W.: Status identity and preventive health behavior, Pacific Health Education Reports, No. 1, 1970, University of California School of Public Health, Berkeley.

Green, L.W.: Natural, social and personal histories of health. In Whither health education? Proceedings of the Second National Conference, Dublin, 1980, Bureau of Health Education.

Hanlon, J.J., and Pickett, G.: Public health: administration and practice, ed. 7, St. Louis, 1979, The C.V. Mosby Co.

Henkle, O.B.M.: Introduction to community health, Boston, 1970, Allyn & Bacon, Inc.

Jones, B., editor: The health of Americans, Englewood Cliffs, N.J., 1970, Prentice-Hall, Inc.

Kosa, J., et al.: Poverty and health: a sociological analysis, Cambridge, Mass., 1969, Harvard University Press.

Laframboise, H.L.: Health policy: breaking it down into more manageable segments, J. Can. Med. Assoc. 108:388, Feb. 3, 1973.

Lalonde, M.: A new perspective on the health of Canadians, Ottawa, April, 1974, Canadian Department of Health and Welfare.

Larimore, G.: Health planning, Arch. Environ. Health 20:128, 1970.

Meadows, P.: Public health in a new community, Am. J. Public Health, 60:1980, 1970.

Michael, J.: A basic information system for health planning, Public Health Rep. 83:21, 1968.

Morgan, L.S.: Community development: observation around the world, Am. J. Public Health 55:607, 1967.

Paul, B.D.: Health, culture and community. New York, 1967, Russell Sage Foundation.

Prohansky, H., et al.: Environmental psychology: people and their physical settings, ed. 2, New York, 1976, Holt, Rinehart and Winston, Inc.

Sarason, S.B., and Lorentz, E.: The challenge of the resource exchange network, San Francisco, 1979, Jossey-Bass Publishers.

Smith, B.C.: Community health, an epidemiological approach, New York, 1979, Macmillan Publishing Co., Inc.

Taugenhaus, L.J.: A division of community health services, Arch. Environ. Health 20:732, 1970.

Watkin, D.M.: Personal responsibility: key to effective and cost-effective health, Fam. Commun. Health 1:1, 1978.

Wing, K.R.: The law and the public's health, St. Louis, 1976, The C.V. Mosby Co.

3

HUMAN ECOLOGY AND EPIDEMIOLOGY

Each of us is responsible for everything,
and to every human being.

Dostoevski

The natural history of health described in Chapter 2 reflects a cycle of adaptation to the environment as a biological phenomenon. Inherent in the individual is a psychophysiological pattern expressing the need and desire for survival. This biological pattern gives force and direction to the means the individual employs to promote his or her own well-being as well as to postpone death. The individual alone can do much to enhance his or her survival, but the community and society, through collective action, can aid the individual to survive. Society itself is benefited, because society's greatest resource is its members. For its own survival, society must organize measures for the conservation of human resources.

But in striving to organize resources, control behavior, and regulate the environment to meet its survival needs, society creates new problems, some of them harmful to health. The production of nuclear energy produces a Three-Mile Island incident; coal mining strips mountains of protective foliage, causing erosion and flooding; importing oil by tanker ships from abroad pollutes the ocean when an accident occurs. Each of the past methods of meeting society's energy needs, for example, has produced other problems. The *social history* of

health, then, is imposed on the *natural history* as a help and a hazard. The help can be great when organized at the societal level, because resources and authority of the greatest magnitudes can be pooled and deployed at that national level. Yet the hazards are greater when authorities who make highly centralized decisions fail to take into account the special needs and delicate balance of human resources at the local level. It is for this reason that community health planning and community-based health services are essential to an ecologically sound, culturally sensitive, socially responsive health system.

The human species is widely dispersed over the face of the earth. Of all forms of life, humans possess the greatest degree of adaptability, being able to adjust to a greater variety of conditions than any other living form. In the arctic region as well as in the tropics, humans have the great ability to bend nature to will and to solve problems of survival created by environmental conditions. In solving one problem relating to survival, however, society frequently creates another problem. Survival and health are constant challenges in which humans look for other problems as soon as they have solved one. Good public health is good ecology based on sound epidemiology. Community health planners must keep this principle constantly before them as they redefine unacceptable conditions and strive for higher levels of wellness.

HUMAN ECOLOGY

Human ecology is the study of the relations between human beings and their environment. Society deals with an environment that is physical, chemical, biological, social, and behavioral. Society lives in an organic relationship with the environment. Most of the time society alters the environment to its advantage, but at times alteration of the environment reacts to the disadvantage of specific communities, populations, or individuals.

Some problems of environmental control cut across several disciplines, indicating that the field of human ecology is a collective discipline. A listing of environmental factors and academic disciplines that are the concern of human ecology would be somewhat arbitrary. However, the physical-chemical factors of human ecology could include the following:

Climate
Food production
Air pollution
Radiation
Noise
Debris
Soil
Fuel

The biological factors of human ecology could include

Food production
Food conservation
Growth and development
Nutrition
Physiological effects
Poisons, toxic agents
Pathogens
Other parasites
Vectors
Water pollution

The social and behavioral factors of human ecology could include

Social structure
Communication
Learning
Economics
Mobility
Leisure
Stress
Population imbalance
Culture

This chapter will deal with those factors relating to the conservation of human resources and will leave discussions of other factors to subsequent chapters.

ADAPTATION AND CONSERVATION

Society has not conquered nature and doubtless never will, for biological laws are always at work, and ignoring these laws will not alter their certain, inevitable course. Society can modify the course of nature and alter conditions to aid in survival. Society even makes it possible for the biologically weak to survive. A common misconception is that this "artificial selection" is dysgenic in that it enables the "poorest" segments of our species to survive. However, biologists contend that there is no such thing as artificial selection, that it is just as much natural selection when the brain is used to aid survival as when legs and wings are used.

The natural cycle of health in Chapter 2 featured adaptation as a product of health. Any challenge to health results in adaptation. Successful adaptation is learned and incorporated in subsequent behavior, and such behavior contributes to health.

There is little evidence that the human species today is biologically inferior to ancestors of previous centuries or biologically better. Civilization recognizes values other than biological endowment. Why should not people wih diabetes have the right to life? By making it possible for these people to survive, society in return has received the intellectual, artistic, and other benefits that the special gifts of many of these people have made possible.

Conservation is not the hoarding of resources but the wise use of them. Conservation of human resources means the husbanding and most effective use of the environmental factors most essential to survival, quality of well-being, and the extension of the prime of life. Conservation entails balancing future needs as well as present requirements. Conservation of human resources means giving consideration to climatic conditions, food supply, use of land, fuel, and water, the birthrate, other living forms, technological developments, and other factors fundamental to the existence of the human species.

CLIMATIC AND SEASONAL EFFECTS ON HEALTH

People living in the temperate zones have a longer life expectancy than people living in the tropics. This holds true also for people who normally live in temperate zones but who migrate to the tropics and live there. In conditions of excessive heat, physical and mental activity decline, bodily functioning tends to become reduced, and resistance to infection is apparently less than under cooler temperatures. Standard aptitude and intelligence tests administered to college students reveal lower performances in the heat of summer than in the cool days of the winter months. Experiments with rats indicate reduced performance when the ambient temperature is increased.

With animal husbandry it has been observed in the United States that twice as much time is required to grow a steer to a 1,000-pound weight in Louisiana as is required in the northern states. The animal's maximum weight in Louisiana is considerably less than that of the animal raised in the northern states.

Temperature cycles of the world have had a significant influence not only on the health of the human species but also on the economy and general culture of nations. During the glory of Greece and the height of Rome, Europe was in the throes of a cold cycle that provided ideal temperatures for agriculture in the Mediterranean area. Culture flourished in those nations that enjoyed a thriving agriculture, but those nations in northern Europe that had prevailing temperatures too low for growing crops declined culturally as well as in other respects. During the period of low temperatures, the population of Ireland consisted of sheep, goat, and cattle herders and their families. Vegetable crops were almost nonexistent. Ireland's general culture declined with its economy.

During the Dark Ages, the thermometer had swung to the other extreme and reached its peak about AD 850. Grapes and other crops usually associated with the Mediterranean area grew abundantly in England. This was the period when the Norsemen were making their explorations ot the North American continent and elsewhere. During this hot era, Greece experienced a steady decline as her agriculture and general economy faded. Ireland flourished and probably was the most cultured nation in Europe. This hot period was followed by a cooling period. Ice that formed in some of the northern nations during the year AD 1000 did not begin to melt until the onset of the present upward trend of temperature.

The most recent rising phase of the temperature cycle appears to have begun around 1880, but the rise in temperature was not appreciable until the period beginning in 1930. Since that time there appears to have been a gradual, somewhat irregular, but nonetheless measurable increase in the world's temperature. Glaciers are receding and objects and forms of life frozen in ice 1,000 years ago are being exposed. How long this upward cycle will continue no one can predict accurately. Whether a predicted constant temperature rise during the next 200 years will materialize, no one knows, but the rising increase in carbon dioxide is providing an atmospheric layer that holds heat next to the earth.

Seasonal variations in health and vital rates are partly a consequence of climate and partly a consequence of cultural and social traditions associated with seasons and holidays. In the United States the highest death rates tend to occur in the winter months, as shown in Fig. 3-1. The holiday season surrounding Christmas and New Year's is known to contribute a large share of the increase through automobile acci-

dents, suicides, and heart attacks. The relatively higher incidence of respiratory conditions and associated deaths in the winter attests to some climatic effect, but how much of this is attributable to exposure to cold temperatures and how much is attributable to being more exposed to the transmission of communicable diseases among people enclosed together in warm but confined spaces is still contested. The latter explanation is preferred by most epidemiologists, suggesting that social norms of adaptation

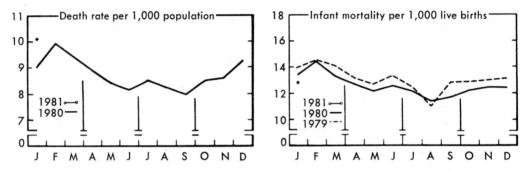

FIG. 3-1. Seasonal variations in mortality in the United States.

From National Center for Health Statistics, Public Health Service, U.S. Department of Health and Human Services: Monthly Vital Statistics Report 30(1):2-3, April 20, 1981.

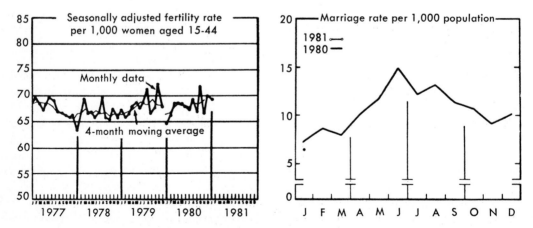

FIG. 3-2. Seasonal variations in fertility and marriage rates in the United States.

From National Center for Health Statistics, Public Health Service, U.S. Department of Health and Human Services: Monthly Vital Statistics Report 30(1):1-2, April 20, 1981.

to climatic conditions are important both in providing protection and in exposing the individual to additional risks.

Seasonal adjustments on vital rates are made by averaging monthly rates for several consecutive months, as shown in Fig. 3-2. Although American marriage rates follow a predictable pattern of seasonal and monthly variation, fertility rates are much less predictable and less associated with marriage rates than one might expect in some primitive and traditional societies where cultural and social restrictions on birth control are operating differently. Society imposes both positive and negative influences on natural cycles and conditions.

Society does not now possess technological knowledge to alter the world's temperature. Society must, however, adapt to any climate that may occur if it is to prosper and even survive. Certainly air conditioning, refrigeration, and other technical developments indicate that society has already attacked the problem of excessive heat. Changes in agricultural crops and procedures will be inevitable if the rising temperatures continue. New problems in parasitism and in human physiology will appear.

Some nations may benefit from the warm centuries ahead and rise to positions of dominance in the world, whereas other nations may decline in relative importance in the world. This equation is compounded today, however, by the availability and location of fuel and other natural resources.

WORLD POPULATION

From 1910 to 1980 the world population increased from 1.5 to 4.3 billion (Fig. 3-3). The rate of increase is such that, if maintained, the population will double in 40 years. However, the world birthrate declined from 34 per 1,000 in 1965 to below 30 per 1,000 in recent years for the first time in recorded demography. The United Nations and the World Bank predict that it will not stabilize until it reaches 10 or 11 billion people within the next 150 years. Long-term predictions of population growth are very speculative, because many factors, including technological, legislative, climatic, and cultural factors influence population growth.

At the present time, two thirds of the people of the world do not have sufficient food. There are over 450 million severely malnourished

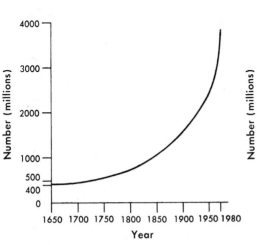

FIG. 3-3. World population, 1650-1980.

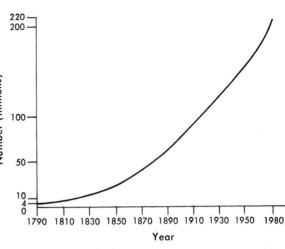

FIG. 3-4. Resident population, United States, 1790-1980.

people in the world, and the number is increasing. In 1976 increases in food production reached only 3.1%, and only 1.2% in the neediest countries. Where starvation exists, disease flourishes. The malnourished are more susceptible to infection than the well-nourished. Famines cause people to migrate and, by so doing, to spread infectious disease. Only if there are sufficient technological developments in the fields of agriculture and health, and only if these advances are made available to all nations, can the present rate of population increase be expected to continue during the present century.

BIOTIC POTENTIAL

Perhaps human population changes can best be understood by a consideration of the biotic potential of a nation as related to environmental resistance. Environmental resistance is expressed in parasitism, food supply, accidents, cold, heat, fuel supply, and other factors that may affect life adversely. The biotic potential of the human is generally thought of as a birthrate of 50 per 1,000 per year. This rate has been attained in the Ukraine over a 5-year period and in Bengal over a 10-year period. During the 10-year period from 1930 to 1940, the Warm Springs Indians of Oregon had an average birthrate of 50 per 1,000 per year. Scientific advances in the prevention and correction of human infertility and sterility could raise the present acknowledged maximum human birthrate, but this maximum is currently accepted.

Government policy

Government policy directly affects birthrates. A pronatal policy embodies inducements and rewards for large families, and the reverse is true of antinatal policy. U.S. policy has been generally inconsistent in this regard. Both the birthrate per 1,000 population and the absolute number of births have been falling since 1957 (4,300,000) to 1976 (3,128,000)—a 27% de-

cline. A more recent increase to 3.5 million was noted in 1980.

To a certain extent, society can bend nature and control the environment. The extent to which societies will be able to control the factors of environmental resistance will be the important element in determining the direction of human population growth in the world in the immediate future as well as over the coming centuries. For an individual nation to survive, it must have a positive vital index. The vital index is the difference between births per 1,000 and deaths per 1,000 population (Fig. 3-5). If the United States has a birthrate of 15.8 per 1,000 and a death rate of 8.7 per 1,000, it has a vital index of 7.1. When a nation's vital index begins to approach 2, that nation's population is becoming stable. If deaths exceed births in a nation, that nation will have a negative vital index symptomatic of national decline.

Food limits

Poverty and hunger. Poverty is the primary cause of hunger. Nearly 40% of the people in the nonsocialist developing world live in such dire poverty that they cannot provide themselves with a minimally adequate diet. This impoverished one fifth of humanity lacks the land to grow its own food or the money to buy it— even in years when local crops are good, world production is high, and storage bins are filled to overflowing. This massive poverty means that even doubling food production on present patterns would not materially change the status of the great majority who are hungry and malnourished today.

Sharp extremes of wealth and poverty persist between and within nations. Three major national factors, acting within the environment defined by international economic constraints, give rise to most developing world poverty: inequitable distribution of resources and income, low productivity and slow economic

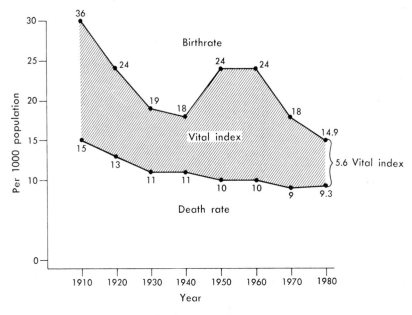

FIG. 3-5. Vital index, United States, 1910-1980.

growth, and excessive population increases. These major factors interact with one another and a number of subsidiary factors to perpetuate world poverty, and thus hunger.

Measures for overcoming world hunger. Lasting solutions to world hunger can result only from rapid, equitable, and self-reliant economic growth. The industrialized nations can do their part by providing various forms of development assistance. The effort, however, to assure equitable economic growth cannot end with developmental assistance, no matter how generous and effective. Because hunger and poverty are deeply rooted in political and economic relations among nations, fundamental changes in global patterns of food production, trade, and finance are needed to improve the conditions within which the developing countries themselves must break the cycle of stagnant agricultural productivity, hunger, poverty, high birthrates, unemployment, and disease.

The economic prospects of poor nations and poor people depend heavily on the evolution of the international economy as a whole. A number of related factors will govern the general direction of the world economy and the performance of individual communities and developing nations. In addition to the economic health of the industrialized nations, these factors include developments in world trade, private and public capital flows, and energy issues, among others. The rate at which the world economy grows during the next 20 years will make the major difference between the possibility of better conditions of life or continuing misery for millions of people. It is imperative that policymakers in every nation search for all possible ways to further economic growth as the most self-sustaining means of overcoming hunger.

Food production worldwide has been steadily increasing over the past 20 years, although there are wide regional variations. In the 1960s and 1970s food production increased at a faster pace in the developing countries than in the developed countries, yet because of much higher population growth rates in the developing countries, per capita food supplies are growing smaller where the need is greatest. In Africa, in particular, food production per capita has declined dramatically in recent years. If present trends continue, substantial portions of the developing world will encounter rapidly increasing food grain shortages and increasing hunger and malnutrition as domestic demand outstrips the ability of nations to grow or purchase their own food.

The necessary increase in agricultural productivity in the developing world will not occur without substantially greater investments of financial and human resources in Third World agriculture. Actions to alleviate hunger must be taken in an international environment that complements and supports the goal of balanced, self-reliant development. This environment consists of many elements of which the most important are the trade flows that link the developing and industrialized nations and the tariffs and other government policies that shape the composition of that trade.

Despite the wealth and abundance of food in the developed nations, there are pockets of poor, hungry people within their national borders. Readily identifiable groups with high incidence of hunger in the United States are migrant and seasonal farm workers, native Alaskans, American Indians, the elderly, and those with incomes below the poverty level. Although federal programs have made great progress in reducing domestic hunger and malnutrition over the past 10 years, much more needs to be done.

The U.S. Food Stamp, Elderly Feeding, and Women-Infants-Children (WIC) programs have made large improvements in the nutrition of the poor. The persistence of hunger and malnutrition in the United States can be attributed in part to the fact that only about 60% of the eligible poor persons participate. Significant improvements in nutrition can be achieved by increasing participation in these programs *without instituting any new programs*. The cost of existing programs, however, would certainly increase with fuller participation.

At present, the nutritional status of the U.S. population is still largely unknown, despite many useful studies. Nor is there any single office, agency, or department that fully coordinates and analyzes information or identifies the major gaps in the current body of knowledge. There is widespread agreement on the genuine need for such information.

Finally, to be consistent with supporting self-reliant growth in the developing world, the developed nations must focus on the same goal for their own poor and malnourished. The President's Commission on World Hunger (1980) recommends that

The United States Government undertake a systematic effort to assess the nutritional status of American citizens through a National Nutrition Surveillance Program.

The Congress act to remove the expenditure limit on Federal funding for the Food Stamp program and to increase resources for all domestic feeding programs with a demonstrated record of success.

The United States adopt a national policy of economic development, designed to foster balanced growth and full employment, which supports the objective of self-reliance for all Americans.

In the United States the population increased at a rate of 0.7% per year in 1980. In terms of food supply there is no threat of a "population explosion." The United States can produce sufficient food for a population at least 10% greater than its current population without being hard pressed. Distribution of food still poses a problem, but production is not likely to be a concern for some years to come. The critical domestic problems created by the present population increase are prices and inflation, waste disposal, and transportation. Satisfactory disposal of both solid and liquid wastes challenges the nation's economic means and technological know-how. The inadequacy of transportation systems, particularly around metropolitan areas, is now further complicated by the fuel crisis.

Zero population growth in the United States would mean reducing the birthrate to the level of about 10 per 1,000 people. This could be a deciding factor in solving the problems of waste disposal and transportation; however, there could be an adverse effect on the nation's economy. Throughout the history of the United States the nation's economy has been based on an anticipated increase in the number of consumers. Zero population growth would cause some problems, but the long-range benefits of a reduced population growth outweigh the difficulties.

Fuel limits

The Western world faced a major fuel crisis some 400 years ago when Europe ran out of wood. Since time immemorial wood had provided heat and shelter. The dense forests that covered the continent and the British Isles seemed inexhaustible, so much so that no thought was given to conservation or management. And as long as the population remained relatively sparse and stable, the consequences were not serious. But in the sixteenth century prices for firewood and lumber suddenly began to skyrocket.

The shortage was particularly acute in England and Wales whose collective population had doubled within a century and a half—from about 3 million in 1550 to twice that figure by 1690. At the same time the mass movement from country to city got under way, creating excessive demands for building material. London alone grew from 60,000 inhabitants in 1534 to some 530,000 in 1696, making it the largest city in Europe and perhaps in the world.

Similar trends marked the population explosion throughout much of Europe, but other pressures contributed to depleting its forest reserves: the shipbuilding boom in the age of exploration, the soaring production of metal ore mines with their wood-burning smelteries, and the rising consumption of wood pulp—used in the manufacture of paper—following the invention of printing.

Eventually coal came to the rescue. A massive shift from wood to coal, along with the discovery of vast new forest reserves in the New World, helped to overcome that particular crisis. Coal, however, turned out to be much more than a mere substitute; compact and efficient as a fuel, it made possible a whole new technology that led to the industrial revolution and ultimately to our current worldwide difficulties.

One lesson of this earlier near disaster is that there are few final answers. But if each solution engenders new problems, facing up to them is what led society out of the Stone Age—reason enough to hope that the latest challenge will again be met.

Facing up to new problems, however, may be difficult. In 1980 a majority (83%) of Americans believed the energy problem was a hoax perpetrated by the oil companies. Nearly half now believe that we do not have an immediate problem, and one third believe that we will not have a fuel problem even in the next 5 years. Clearly, an educational problem for the 1980s, comparable to the need for population education in the 1970s, is energy education. Only half of the Americans in the 25- to 36-age range could answer correctly 50 key energy questions in 1980.

EPIDEMIOLOGY

The companion science to ecology in community health is epidemiology. Both represent perspectives on health that go beyond the individual. Whereas ecology views the individual in the context of environment, epidemiology views the individual in the context of a population. Epidemiology is the science of the causes, frequencies, and distribution of diseases in a population.

The methods of epidemiology allow the community health worker to collect, tabulate, analyze, and interpret statistical facts about the occurrence of health problems, risk factors, and deaths in a community. Physicians, nurses, and others trained in clinical sciences sometimes have difficulty standing far enough away from the individual patient to see the larger patterns of disease occurrence in their population of patients. The epidemiological method and perspective on health enables clinical workers and public health officials to specify, describe, and understand such patterns so that they can see the common characteristics of those who have the problem in contrast to the characteristics of those who do not have the problem. The comparison may reveal the cause or the source of a disease of unknown origin. Most of the breakthroughs in medicine, especially preventive medicine, that emerged from the laboratory of an immunologist or a physiologist had their first leads from an epidemiologist or other investigator applying the epidemiological method.

The early focus of epidemiology was on epidemics, as the name implies. The transmission of communicable diseases in populations, when traced systematically, provided clues to the mode of transmission. Some proved to be air-

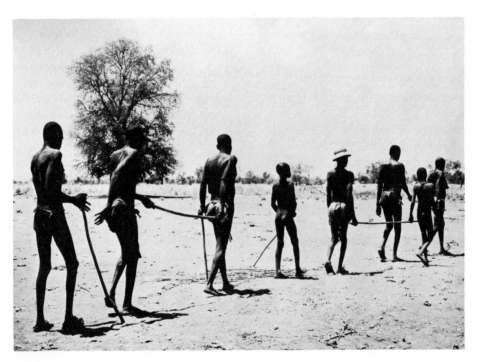

FIG. 3-6. Onchocerciasis, or river blindness, is widespread in Central America and in large stretches of central Africa. The disease is caused by a minute worm transmitted to humans by the bite of infected flies. A multitude of these worms invading the eye causes ocular disturbances and sometimes blindness. In many communities blind adults must be led by the children. A World Health Organization (WHO) expert committee on onchocerciasis reported infection rates of 80% to 100% in various countries of Africa and South America.
Courtesy WHO.

borne, some waterborne, some foodborne, and some transmitted by an intermediate host such as a rat, mosquito, fly, tick, or bird. Such clues enabled community health workers to interrupt the transmission of some diseases through quarantine, pest control, water purification, food protection, immunization, or solid waste disposal.

As communicable diseases have come increasingly under control, the methods of epidemiology have been turned to analyzing the comparative frequencies and distribution of chronic diseases, degenerative diseases, and even injuries, addictions, and risk factors such as smoking, hypertension, obesity, and health habits or behavioral patterns. These studies, again, have provided the clues and hypotheses on which advice to the public and further research have been based in developing national campaigns against smoking, alcohol and drug misuse, malnutrition, blood pressure, dental caries, and childhood accidents.

The frequencies and distribution of diseases are compared by measures of incidence and prevalence. *Incidence* refers to the number of new cases of the disease or condition that occur within a given time period (week, month, or year). *Prevalence* refers to the number of cases that exist at one point in time. Thus incidence is influenced entirely by how rapidly a disease is spreading. As such, it is the most sensitive measure of an outbreak or epidemic of a communicable or acute infectious or toxic agent disease. Prevalence is influenced both by incidence and by the duration of the disease or condition, hence its wider use in measuring chronic diseases and disabilities. It is difficult to measure the incidence of chronic degenerative diseases because they are usually undetected until they reach an acute stage. Incidence rates are derived usually from health department reporting systems that require hospitals, clinics, and even private physicians to report every new case of a communicable or infectious disease they encounter. Prevalence

rates usually come from screening and detection programs and special surveys of populations.

Pandemics

The term *pandemic* literally means "all people" and is used to denote a disease conflagration over a considerable area. A statewide outbreak of a disease may be regarded as a pandemic, but generally the term is used to denote a nationwide, continentwide, or worldwide outbreak. The past has seen devastating pandemics of bubonic plague, yellow fever, cholera, smallpox, typhus fever, and syphilis. The 1918-1919 influenza-pneumonia pandemic caused 400,000 deaths in the United States, 10 million deaths in India alone, and more than 20 million deaths throughout the world. In some of the underdeveloped nations of the world during the past decade pandemics of acute infectious diseases such as cholera have occurred. These outbreaks have usually been confined to a single nation or to a small group of nations. Even in the underdeveloped nations there is not likely to be a devastating pandemic of an acute infectious disease such as occurred in the past, but moderately severe outbreaks can be expected for decades to come. In the more developed nations scientific advances in the field of epidemiology make even a moderate pandemic of an acute infectious disease highly unlikely.

Chronic infections still plague vast segments of the population in many nations of the world. At the present time there are more than 200 million malaria cases in the world, 260 million hookworm cases, 650 million people with ascarids (a roundworm), and 5 million cases of leprosy, of which 3 million are in Asia. Asia has 335 million people who harbor the parasitic ascarid. Each of these Asians will harbor between six and nine adult ascarids. The total weight of the worms thus carried by these 335 million Asians will be in the neighborhood of 37,500 tons and will consume as much food each day

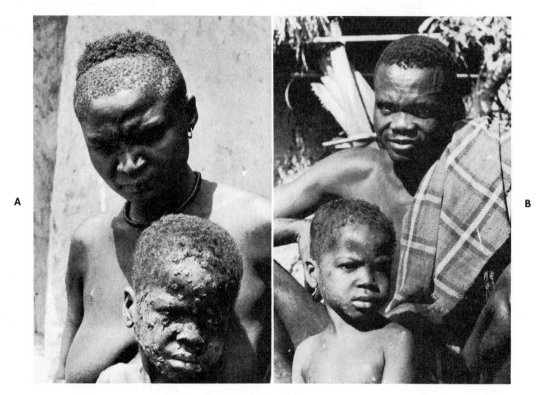

FIG. 3-7. A, Yaws: the affliction of this 5-year-old African boy. Yaws is a widespread disfiguring treponemal disease causing deep-seated infirmity if untreated. It can be cured by a single injection of long-acting penicillin. **B,** Yaws conquered: the same 5-year-old African boy, 10 days after receiving a single injection of penicillin.

Courtesy WHO.

as a population of more than 40,000 people.

Indonesia had 15 million cases of yaws before a staff of Indonesians trained by United Nations technologists and supplied with penicillin from the United Nations proceeded to wipe out the disease. One injection of penicillin usually cures yaws, so that virtually the entire Indonesian population is now free of the disease.

In Australia, Europe, and North America diphtheria, influenza, meningitis, encephalitis, poliomyelitis, and other infectious diseases that conceivably could break out in pandemic form can be controlled effectively with the means at our command. A mutant pathogen of humans may arise and challenge society's ability to control the spread of disease. Our ability to solve disease control problems that might arise will depend on advances in our knowledge of infection and its control.

AGRICULTURE, TECHNOLOGY, AND HEALTH

The relationship between the vitality of a nation's agriculture and the nation's health is readily recognized. The food supply of a nation not only determines the health of the people, but also the nature of its population growth. America's farm situation is undergoing some changes that are of interest in terms of the nation's health and its population. According to

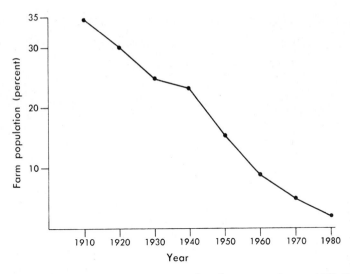

FIG. 3-8. Farm population as percentage of total U.S. population, 1910-1980.

the records of the U.S. Bureau of the Census, the farm population declined from 35% of the total in 1910 to less than 4% of the total in 1980.

The number of farms in the United States also declined, but the average acreage of each increased from 138 to 390 acres. The total farmed acreage also increased to 1,121 million in 1970 from 879 million in 1910. Agricultural specialists report that it is desirable to shift 40 million acres of cropland acreage into other uses. They also report that 216 million acres could be shifted from grassland and woodland to cropland. About 280 million acres of productive land have been destroyed by neglect. However, at least 33 million acres of land not now in production could be reclaimed with adequate irrigation. Whenever we see topsoil washed away, we should remind ourselves that it takes from 2,000 to 5,000 years to build 1 inch of topsoil and that the average depth of topsoil in the United States is only about 8 inches.

Every year thousands of acres of farmland are taken out of production for highways, air-

fields, golf courses, industrial plants, housing developments, and other purposes. The productivity of agriculture not only is basic to a society's health and the extent of its population growth but is the key to its general cultural advancement. In a nation where less than 20% of the employed can supply its people with food, it is possible to have other workers available for industry, transportation, construction, education, music, painting, writing, entertainment, and the multitude of other pursuits that make possible a more fruitful and complete mode of living through the diversity of experiences and services that are made available.

The development of DDT, BHC, and other insecticides has been a milestone in society's battle with insects. The battle against weeds is yielding to technological developments. The use of 2,4-D, DNBP, and 2,45-T has reduced the amount of cultivation necessary on farms. Experimentation yielding better seeds, better strains of plants and animals, and the addition of antibiotics to animal feeds has increased the productivity of farms. Improved methods of food processing, better refrigeration, improved

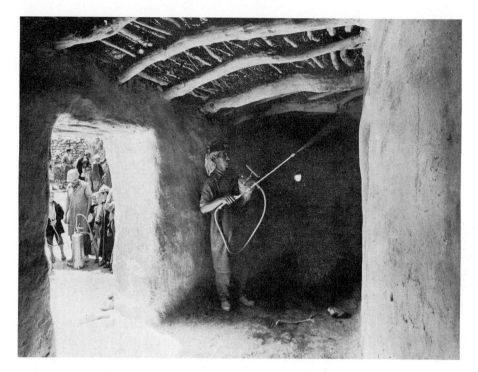

FIG. 3-9. Malaria eradication in a Moroccan village by spraying DDT. WHO started a malaria eradication program in 1955, and today the disease has been controlled in large parts of Southeast Asia, Europe, and the Americas.

Courtesy WHO.

packaging, and better methods of food preservation have reduced food wastes and thus contributed tangibly to the total food supply available.

But such technologies also bear less wholesome fruits. Fertilizers and chemicals used against weeds, insects, and fungus have accumulated in the soil, water, and in some food products to the point that new hazards to health have been introduced. Where environmental health was once concerned primarily with microorganisms, today environmental health and occupational health are concerned chiefly with toxic agents of the chemical variety.

LIFE SPAN AND LIFE EXPECTANCY

Life span and life expectancy are two different phenomena, one biological and the other epidemiological. Life span is the recognized biological limit of life. Based on present knowledge, biologists tend to set the human life span at 120 years. They recognize that with an increase in our knowledge of human biology, this figure may be projected upward, perhaps by even more than 30 years. The figure is generally set at 120 years because scientists do not possess reliable data of human beings living beyond this age. The usual report of people living beyond 120 years emanates from primitive areas where unreliable records or no records at

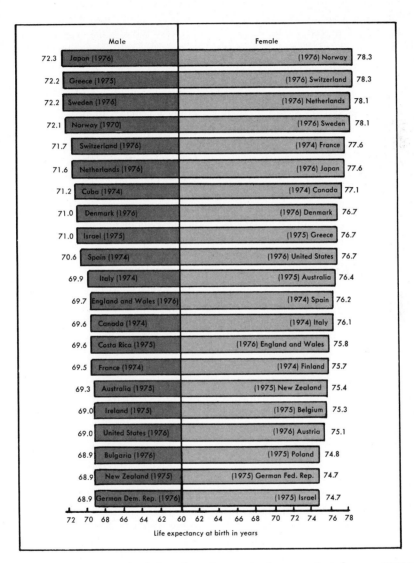

FIG. 3-10. Life expectancy at birth for selected countries by sex: selected years, 1974-1976.

all exist. Biologists acknowledge that in all probability even the person who lives to age 115 years has shortened his or her life by adverse health practices. Scientists recognize that improper dietary practices, infections, excessive fatigue, prolonged exposure, inadequate rest, and other factors may well have shortened the life of the person who lives to age 115. Obviously, not all people have a life span of 120 years. Some people likely have a life span considerably below 100 years. This is indicated by failure of any member in some lineages to reach the age of 60 years. Life span is an inherited characteristic that is determined at the time of the fertilization of the ovum by the sperm. The person can do nothing to extend the span but inadvertently or unwisely does many things to prevent realization of his or her life span.

Life expectancy is an epidemiological concept that refers to the average duration of time that individuals of a given age can expect to live, based on the longevity experience of the population. Expectancy is expressed as the average number of years an individual of a given age can expect to live. These averages are based on the assumption that the longevity experience of the immediately preceding years will prevail in the future, even though future developments likely will be favorable to an extension of longevity beyond what the immediate past years indicate.

All averages on expectancy apply to the age group. Obviously, individuals within a group will vary, some experiencing an expectancy considerably above the average and some below the average.

Americans have been prone to assume that they possess the greatest life expectancy of any people in the world. Data from the World Health Organization (WHO), as shown in Fig. 3-10, has caused Americans to reflect on their relative world position in terms of life expectancy. With all of America's medical, hospital, and other health facilities, along with her favorable economic position, it was embarrassing to find that life expectancy in the United States does not compare favorably with that in many other industrialized countries. Of 21 countries with the highest life expectancies for males, and for which recent data were available, 16 had higher life expectancies at birth for males than the United States. Japan, Greece, Sweden, and Norway had the longest life expectancies for males (more than 72 years). Life expectancy for males in the United States was 69.3 years in 1977, 70.0 in 1980.

For females, however, only 6 of the 21 countries with the highest life expectancies had higher life expectancies at birth for females than the United States. Norway, Switzerland, the Netherlands, and Sweden had the longest life expectancies for females (more than 78 years). Life expectancy for females in the United States was 77.1 years in 1977, 77.6 years in 1980.

In every country, life expectancy was greater for females than for males. France and the United States had the greatest differentials between sexes—8.1 and 7.6 years in 1980, respectively—while Israel and Greece had the smallest—3.7 and 4.5 years, respectively.

The expectation of life at birth attained a record of 73.2 years in 1977 for the total American population. This continues the general upward trend in this measure over the past several decades as shown in Fig. 3-11.

Under the mortality conditions prevailing in 1948, an infant born in that year could expect to live an average of 67.2 years. Between 1948 and 1968, 3 years were added to life expectancy, and an additional 3 years were added between 1968 and 1977. Thus the gain in the 20-year period was the same as the gain during the last 9 years. This expectation of life at birth represents the average number of years that a group of infants would live if they were to experience throughout life the age-specific death rates prevailing in 1977.

Females have gained more years than males,

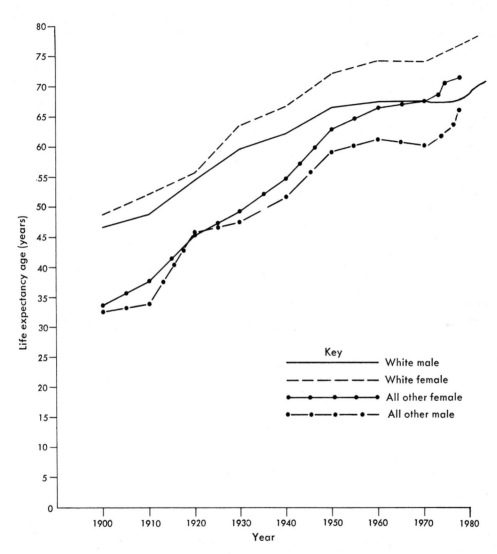

FIG. 3-11. Estimated average length of life in years at birth, United States, 1900-1980.
From reports of the National Center for Health Statistics.

especially nonwhite females who now have a longer life expectancy than white males. From 1950 to 1977 white females had a 5.5-year increase, and all other females had a 10-year increase over males. In contrast, white males had only a 3.5-year increase, and all other males had a 5.5-year increase during the same period. Since females historically have had longer life expectancies than males, a greater differential existed between male and female life expectancy in 1977 than it did in 1950.

While the difference between life expectancy for males and females has increased, the difference between life expectancy for white people and people of all other races has been reduced substantially. In 1950 white people could expect to live about 8 years longer than people of all other races. By 1977 this differential had decreased to 5 years.

The greatest gain in life expectancy during the first half of the twentieth century can be attributed to the prevention of deaths in infancy and childhood. However, in recent years progress has been made in extending the length of life by the postponement of death in the later age brackets so that in 1976 life expectation of a person of 40 was nearly 8 years greater than the life expectation of a person of 40 in the year 1900.

Data on life expectation at birth are important, but equally significant are data on life expectancy at various ages. Studies indicate that college graduates have a greater life expectancy than that of the general population. Even noncollege graduates, by the application of sound health principles and the use of available medical and health facilities and services, can extend their life expectation considerably beyond the average if they possess a basic biological endowment or life span of over 100 years.

A phenomenon of interest but without a complete explanation is that the people of seven U.S. Midwestern states consistently have a greater life expectancy than that of the people of most other states in the nation. Iowa, Kansas, Minnesota, Nebraska, North Dakota, Oklahoma, and South Dakota regularly exceed the national life expectation figures by at least 2 years and occasionally 3 years for both the male and the female. No acceptable explanation of this phenomenon has been made. The national origin of the population, economic means, climate, vocations, living practices, and other factors have been analyzed, but nothing has been discovered that distinguishes the population of these states from the population of other states.

Two neighboring states, Utah and Nevada, have similar climates and geography but extreme differences of life expectancy, reflecting their differences in life-style. A study in Alameda County, California, demonstrated the importance of life-style by tracing an increase of 11 years in life expectancy for 45-year-old males who followed simple and basic living habits associated with smoking, weight control, moderate alcohol consumption, hours of sleep, regularity in meals, good nutrition, and physical activity. An additional dimension of life-style that has emerged from secondary analyses of the Alameda study as a major determinant of increased life expectancy is social supports. Those males who had more friends, more memberships, or more family available to them lived longer.

FACTORS DETERMINING LIFE EXPECTANCY

Longevity is a general term that incorporates a vast number of factors significant to individuals who are interested in appraising their own life expectancy. Fortunately, no one knows precisely when he or she will die, but it is possible to establish the approximate probable lifetime by a statistical procedure called health hazard appraisal or health risk appraisal, which weights various characteristics of the individual according to the known correlation of those characteristics with mortality. This procedure allows the individual to identify how many years he or she could add to his or her life, with some statistical probability, by changing specific health practices, circumstances, or conditions throughout life. Some of these factors, however, are not changeable.

Race. Fig. 3-11 indicates that the racial factor is important in longevity. At the time of birth, the white male has a life expectancy greater than the nonwhite male, and the white female has an expectancy greater than the nonwhite female. These data doubtless conceal some economic factors that are adverse to the nonwhite individual.

After age 74 years, however, there is a crossover in the white-nonwhite rates in both sexes. Whites enjoy lower mortality rates until age 74 years, when nonwhite mortality becomes lower and remains so. Nonwhites who have surmounted the economic barriers and environmental hazards to health may represent a hardier group of survivors compared with their white counterparts of similar age.

Inheritance. Long-lived parents tend to have long-lived offspring. What actually is transmitted is not the abstraction, long life, but rather the adequate body structure, the efficiently functioning organs and systems, resistance to diseases, the ability to recover from injury or disease, the capacity to produce the necessary body enzymes, and the various other attributes necessary for long life. Studies in England on the nobility and upper-class families, conducted by Karl Pearson and M. Beaton, demonstrated a marked consistency between the length of life of parents and their offspring. In a comparable study, S.J. Holmes obtained the same findings.

Dr. Raymond Pearl, the American biometrist, used a different approach to avoid errors common in studies based on geneologies. Dr. Pearl devised the method of "Total Immediate Ancestral Longevity" (TIAL), which is the sum of the ages at death of both parents and all four grandparents of a given individual. There is little likelihood that the TIAL will fall below 100 or will exceed 600. Dr. Pearl found that for all of his subjects 90 years of age or over (longevous group), 46% had two long-lived parents, while in the unselected subjects (control group), only 12% had two long-lived parents. The significant difference in the two percentages doubtless represents inherited endowment. The possibility remains that biased factors exist. A study was made by Dr. L.I. Dublin and H.H. Marks of 118,000 white males, ages 20 to 64 years, granted life insurance between 1899 and 1939. At every age the lowest death rate occurred for those men who had both parents living when the insurance was granted. At the other end of the scale, the death rate was highest among those men whose parents were both dead at the time the insurance was issued.

In considering the influence of inheritance on the length of life, one should not overlook the fact that living in a long-lived family usually means certain environmental advantages that could be favorable to longevity. Having both parents living to look after his welfare should be an aid to an individual in obtaining the highest possible portion of his potential, both in quality of health and length of life. Certainly gains in the longevity of the general population must be attributed to environmental gains rather than genetic changes. Inherited longevity still has its advantages in determining one's length of life, but with modern advances perhaps these advantages are not as great as they were at the turn of the century.

Gender. At birth, the American white female has an expectancy greater than the male, as seen in Fig. 3-11. Although the differential between the life expectancy of the female and the male declines during the ensuing years, she tends to have an advantage all through life. A female appears to inherit a better constitution in terms of long-wearing qualities. She has less bulky musculature and more flexible soft tissues. She is less prone to heart disorders and arteriosclerosis. She has lower blood pressure and a higher white cell count, both of which are to her advantage. She has an advantage in not being called on to do as much heavy manual labor. She engages in less hazardous occupations, and her accidental death rate is much lower than that of the male. Perhaps as important as any factor is that she has worked under less daily tension. The American male seems to shorten his life by the intensity of his daily living and the tension that he experiences in his vocational pursuits. Females seem to possess both the means and the social encouragement to give release to their emotions, a practice the male could emulate to his benefit.

With emancipation of the female, however, her advantage in longevity may decrease. Adolescent groups now contain the same proportion of female cigarette smokers as males, although females smoke fewer cigarettes and inhale less. Unfortunately, they find it more difficult to stop smoking than males, and recidivism is higher in females. The habit of cigarette smoking is equated with freedom and social advancement in the advertisements directed at females. Obesity is more prevalent in females than in males, particularly in the lower socioeconomic groups. As females seek more employment and achieve economic parity with males, the differential in mortality may decline.

Occupation. The general designation of occupation as a factor in longevity incorporates a number of variables such as the types of individuals who go into the different occupations, the hazards in the occupations, the economic position of different occupations, and the educational background of men in the various occupations. Longest lived are clergymen, lawyers, engineers, teachers, doctors, and farmers, essentially in this order. Next longest lived are business executives, white collar workers,

and skilled tradesmen. Shortest lived are the unskilled workers, miners, quarrymen, and granite workers.

Income. Favorable living conditions, associated with income, have a definite influence on longevity. Families with a favorable income are able to avail themselves of the best medical care, proper nutrition, good housing, and other advantages that make a longer life possible. People living in cities with a high level of income live longer than those living in cities of low income. The advantage conferred by high income is no longer effective, however, in very old age groups, that is, those over 85 years. After this age, genetic endowment is totally dominant, and socioeconomic status is of no influence on further life expectancy.

Marital status. Married men live longer than single men. Many men in poor health prefer to remain single, which partially accounts for the shorter life expectancy of the single men. Doubtless the orderly life of the married man operates to his advantage in preserving his life. Among women, the picture of longevity varies. Up to the age of 40, married women have a greater life expectation than single women, but thereafter married women and unmarried women have the same life expectancy.

Body build. An individual inherits a particular type of body build that can be modified but little through nutrition or other means. While people of certain body builds live longer than those of other body types, no one is doomed to a short life expectation merely on the basis of his body build. People who are of average height and weight tend to live longest. As a group, people of very large stature do not live as long as those who are smaller than average in height and weight. Being extremely underweight during young adulthood has an adverse effect on length of life. Those who are somewhat underweight in later years tend to have a favorable life expectancy. Obesity, particularly in the later years of life, has an adverse effect on longevity. People more than 25% overweight have a 75% higher death rate than those in the average weight category.

Temperament and habits. Easygoing people outlive fast-paced and excitable individuals. Tension, overstrain, overeating, and general excessiveness associated with high-tension living tend to shorten life. Cigarette smoking and heavy drinking both reduce life expectancy. Manual labor, even heavy manual labor, before the age of 40 does not appear to affect the length of life, but hard manual labor continued after the age of 40 years does appear to shorten life. Generally, people of a temperament that leads to a pattern of moderation in living reap benefits from their modes of life in terms of more years added to their lives.

Blood pressure. Low blood pressure, unless extremely low, favors longevity. The higher the blood pressure, the shorter the life, partially resulting from the relationship of blood pressure to heart and kidney disorders and stroke. An unusually rapid or irregular pulse is usually associated with short life expectancy. Individuals with high blood pressure or with rapid pulse need not assume the fatalistic attitude that they are doomed to a short life and can do nothing to extend their expectation. Modern medical treatment and their own efforts can have a significant effect on reducing pulse rate and blood pressure, and on postponing death.

INDIVIDUAL APPLICATIONS

Both the individual and the community can take effective measures to extend life expectancy, starting with study of the most likely causes of death. More than 76% of all deaths this year in the United States will result from three causes: cardiovascular diseases, cancer, and accidents. Breaking these data down on the basis of age groups, we can be more specific in concentrating our attention on the most likely cause of our death. In addition, if the citizens of a community were informed on what they can do to promote their own quality of health and postpone death, life expectancy

could be extended appreciably in that community. Seven of the ten leading causes of death are subject to reduction chiefly through informed individual actions.

A community can contribute to life expectancy through an effective program of health education that gives citizens a knowledge of what they as individuals can do to promote their present health. Individuals should be concerned about the condition of their heart, arteries, kidneys, lungs, and other vital structures. Periodic health appraisals and examinations would give them an assessment of the condition of these structures and warn them against the development of the various chronic disorders of adulthood. People need to adopt a positive health-oriented mode of behavior, emphasizing proper diet and rest, regular exercise, avoidance of tobacco and moderate use of alcohol. A life-style of moderation with a value system consistent with health can result in zestful living and longevity. A community program of adult health promotion that includes periodic tests or examination with a suitable follow-up should yield tangible results in extending life expectancy and reducing disease and disability.

Any community with adequate and accessible health services and facilities is contributing to the life expectancy of its citizens. The extent to which these services and facilities actually contribute to the postponement of death and the quality of life will depend on the understanding that citizens have of these services and facilities and the extent to which they avail themselves of the health services as well as other nonmedical resources and opportunities for health promotion in their community.

Research and the understanding, prevention, and control of heart disease, cancer, and other principal causes of death will largely determine the future extension of life expectancy. A single breakthrough on the problem of cancer may well have a marked influence on life expectancy. New methods and techniques in heart surgery could increase life expectancy at age 50 by a few years. Inroads on the accidental death rate could have a profound effect on life expectancy.

MEASURING PROGRESS

The U.S. Surgeon General's 1979 report on Health Promotion and Disease Prevention presented a set of broad goals for the nation for each of five age groups:

- To continue to improve infant health, and by 1990 to reduce infant mortality by at least 35% to fewer than 9 deaths per 1,000 live births
- To improve child health, foster optimum childhood development, and by 1990 reduce deaths among children ages 1 to 14 by at least 20% to fewer than 34 per 100,000
- To improve the health and health habits of adolescents and young adults, and by 1990 to reduce deaths among people ages 15 to 24 by at least 20% to fewer than 93 per 100,000
- To improve the health of adults, and by 1990 to reduce deaths among people ages 25 to 64 by at least 25% to fewer than 400 per 100,000
- To improve the health and quality of life for older adults, and by 1990 to reduce the average annual number of days of restricted activity due to acute and chronic conditions by 20% to fewer than 30 days per year for people aged 65 and older

Advances toward most of these health goals for different age groups are readily tracked through death statistics. The long-term goal of a health promotion and disease prevention strategy, however, must not only be to achieve further increases in longevity, but also to allow people to find an independent and rewarding life, free of constraints of at least those health problems that are within their capacity to control. Success in such a large endeavor is not easily measured. The average number of days of restricted activity that people experience each year, ascertained through household interview surveys, is an example of one available indicator of health status.

Progress toward the broad goal of reducing the heavy human and economic costs imposed on populations by avoidable disease and disability demands action on many fronts. Specific objectives have been formulated in 15 priority action areas, including five aspects of environmental protection, five changes in peoples' daily habits of living, and five areas of preventive health services concerned with the degree of attention that health professionals and health institutions devote to helping their patients stay well. Employers, school systems, product designers and manufacturers, food distributors, the insurance industry, and many other important groups of a society outside its health system often play crucial roles in preventing unnecessary injury and death and in promoting healthier life-styles. Such a multitude of groups enormously complicates the task of constructing a tracking and surveillance system to measure the quality of actual efforts and the amount of progress in disease prevention and health promotion.

Collecting the necessary data to construct a relevant profile of health risks, public and professional awareness, and available services constitutes another major constraint on the measurement of progress toward objectives. By definition, progress toward preventing disease or reducing risks can only be followed over time when good baseline data exist and where such data are likely to be available in the future. Unfortunately, there is no necessary congruence between the importance of any particular objective and the availability of data to make it measureable. For example, no data currently exist to show how many communities and how many people in the United States are likely to be exposed to contaminated groundwater during the 1980s from toxic wastes introduced into their immediate environments during the 1950s, 1960s, and 1970s. Nor is it known how many children each year suffer injuries and death from abusing parents. Regardless of the importance that society may attach to prevention in such areas, the absence of data prevents the formulation of measurable objectives. Thus they cannot be included in the surveillance system.

Such imbalance in the elements included in a community health profile can only be remedied by improving the community's capabilities for securing reliable, continuing information of special or emerging importance to the community's health. To improve the relevance of the surveillance system to the major challenges community health faces today requires epidemiological data systems that can be used as follows:

- To determine the incidence of hypertension, heart diseases, and stroke
- To assess the status of hypertension control
- To determine the impact of a range of prenatal preventive measures on the physical and psychological development of infants and children over time
- To monitor the extent to which children are currently immunized against childhood diseases
- To determine the occurrence of a variety of sexually transmitted diseases to provide a basis for preventive strategies in local areas
- To measure environmental hazards, both those of a continuing nature and those resulting from isolated incidents
- To provide information on concentrations of hazardous agents in air, food, and water
- To correlate occupational, life-style behavior and health and illness records and use them to assess the extent and distribution of cancer and other possibly occupationally related illnesses, including heart disease, and of occupational injuries

- To monitor trends of common infectious agents not now subject to public health surveillance and measure their impact on health care cost and productivity
- To review the actuarial experience on differential life expectancy and hospital use of smokers and nonsmokers
- To monitor and evaluate the impact of misuse of alcohol and drugs on health status, accidental injuries, interpersonal aggression and violence, outcomes of pregnancy, and the emotional and physical development of infants and children
- To detect nutritional problems among especially vulnerable population groups and provide a basis for decisions on national nutrition policies
- To evaluate the effects of participation in programs of physical fitness on job performance and health care cost
- To enlarge the knowledge about stress as a risk factor in mental and physical health and the impact of stress management in reducing risks

Future surveillance systems will need to track changes in the public's knowledge of risk factors for particular diseases and conditions, the extent to which people are making changes in their behavior in efforts to reduce their risks, and their success in maintaining the changes they make. Surveys conducted during the 1970s by the National Center for Health Statistics and by private survey organizations have already accumulated a good deal of the necessary baseline data for the United States. Smaller countries have more uniform and consistent systems for the collection of data on a national scale.

The first elements of a system to track measurable prevention objectives at the community level are outlined in the table on pp. 78 and 79. Additional objectives for monitoring and surveillance in relation to special population groups and specific health problems will

Objectives and measures to assure that communities have the capacity to provide epidemiological surveillance*

Goal: The community will be served by a surveillance and epidemiology system that (1) detects, monitors, and investigates conditions contributing to morbidity and mortality in the community and (2) provides the necessary data for analysis appropriate to the development of prevention and control measures and research strategies.

Focus	Objectives	Indicators	Population in need
System establishment maintenance	1. By 19 ___ the community will be served by a surveillance system for acute and chronic conditions of public health significance.	a. The presence of a system of routine reporting of specified conditions of public health significance b. The presence of additional systems of surveillance, including one or more of the following: (1) sentinel physicians, (2) statistically representative hospital-based reporting, (3) laboratory reporting, (4) disease registers, (5) special surveys, (6) supplemental systems to corroborate routine surveillance methods, (7) supplemental surveillance system to detect unusual conditions of public health significance in the community c. Presence of a system for data analysis and use of analyses	The community
Investigation and control	2. By 19 ___ the community will have available competent medical, statistical, and epidemiological consultation and other services necessary (a) to carry out investigations, special studies, and data analyses, (b) to institute appropriate control measures against conditions of public health significance in the community, and (c) to evaluate the impact of control measures.	A demonstrable system to provide immediate telephone consultaton as well as on-site assistance for investigaton, control, and evaluation processes within 24 hours	The community

Laboratory support	3. By 19 —— the community will have access to laboratory facilities necessary for the timely diagnosis confirmation of diseases and conditions of public health significance.	A demonstrable system of timely access to laboratory services	
Information sharing	4. By 19 —— the surveillance program will have an appropriate and timely system of communicating surveillance and epidemiological data to public health officials, practicing physicians, and the community as a whole.	a. One or several of the following: (1) a regular newsletter (2) a regular channel of communicating to practicing physicians, (3) a reliable means of rapid communication through the public media (e.g., for emergency notification) b. A measure of reader acceptance and use of established system	The community, particularly health care providers

*Based on Model standards for community preventive health services, Washington, D.C., 1979, Public Health Service, U.S. Department of Health and Human Services.

appear in corresponding tables in later chapters.

Promoting community health in virtually all spheres will have some influence on life expectancy. Maternal, infant, and child health programs, adult health programs, prevention of disorders, communicable disease control measures, safety promotion, industrial hygiene programs, reduction of alcoholism, improved sanitation, programs to deal with disasters, and the extension of community health services, directly and indirectly, influence the length of life that people of the community will enjoy. Because we know the specific leading causes of death, we have specific targets toward which to direct our efforts. Programs can be directed into channels leading to likely dividends. This holds true for a community program, and it is equally true for the individual. Knowing statistically what the causes of death most likely might be, using health education and methods such as health risk appraisal, the wise person can use all of the measures, devices, and services available to aid in postponing his or her death.

QUESTIONS AND EXERCISES

1. Explain this statement: "Man is born a biological being, he has to become a social being."
2. What evidence is there that the human being possesses an inherent drive to survive?
3. What evidence is there that the advances in health sciences have had a dysgenic effect on America's population?
4. What is meant by the conservation of human resources?
5. Analyze this statement: "People in the tropics of the southern hemisphere do not live as long as those in the northern hemisphere because of the south's excessive heat."
6. For the past 30 years the Alaskan glaciers have been reducing rapidly. What interpretation do you make of this, and what is the significance of the phenomenon?
7. Speculate as to what effect a constantly rising world temperature would have on life expectancy, health, the economy, and the general culture of Canada, Russia, the Scandinavian nations, and the Mediterranean nations.
8. In what type of nation does hunger pose the greatest threat?

9. Predict the world population for the year 2000, and present the factors that were considered in arriving at your estimate.
10. One county with a vital index of 16 has a neighboring county with a vital index of 4. What differences would you expect to find in the two counties?
11. What has been the effect of the discovery of DDT on the health and culture of the world?
12. What has been the effect of advances in agricultural technology on the health and culture of the world?
13. Analyze this statement: "Clear up disease and you promote starvation because there will be more mouths to feed."
14. Why does Sweden have a greater life expectancy than the United States?
15. What factors probably account for the poor life expectancy of the American male at age 50?
16. Why do females in the United States live longer than males?
17. Explain the paradox that a child born in the United States can expect to live a greater number of years after his first birthday anniversary than after the day on which he was born.
18. Why do college graduates have a greater life expectancy at age 30 than people of the same age who have not attended college?
19. What is the role of economics in life expectancy?
20. What are the social and the economic consequences of the American wife outliving her husband by an average of 8 years?
21. What factors are favorable for a long life for clergymen?
22. Cigarette smoking markedly increases the risk for certain major diseases. List four.
23. Appraise your own present health status in terms of life expectancy
24. Study the established health practices of five of your acquaintances who are more than 70 years of age. What did you learn of value to you?
25. How would you proceed to make this knowledge available to the citizens of your community?
26. Consider the program to educate teenagers not to smoke. How could this program be extended to include all factors that most threaten a long life?
27. To what degree is the extension of life expectancy a matter of community education?
28. Which is most important, a long life, an enjoyable life, or a productive life, and are the three incompatible for one individual?

BIBLIOGRAPHY

Abel-Smith, B: Poverty, development, and health policy, Geneva, 1978, Public Health Papers, No. 69, World Health Organization.

Belloc, N.B., and Breslow, L.: Relationship of physical health and health practices, Prev. Med. 1:409, 1972.

Berg, A.: Nutrition, development, and population growth, Popul. Bull. 29:1, 1973.

Borgstrom, G.: World food problems, New York, 1973, Intext Educational Publishers.

Bureau of the Census, U.S. Department of Commerce: Statistical abstract of the United States, Washington, D.C., Bureau of the Census. (Current.)

Cheney, E.S.: U.S. energy resources: limits and future outlook, Am. Sci. 62:14, 1974.

Clark, W.: Energy for survival; the alternative to extinction, New York, 1974, Anchor/Doubleday.

Conference on Records and Statistics, Washington, D.C., 1980, National Center for Health Statistics, DHHS Pub. No. (PHS) 81-1214.

Darnell, R.: Ecology, Dubuque, Iowa, 1972, William C. Brown Co., Publishers.

Fuchs, V.: Who shall live? New York, 1975, Basic Books, Inc., Publishers.

Green, L., Wilson, R., and Bauer, K.: Objectives for the nation in disease prevention and health promotion and requirements to measure our progress, Proceedings of the 18th National Meeting of the Public Health Conference on Records and Statistics, Washington, D.C., 1980, National Center for Health Statistics, DHHS Pub. No. (PHS) 81-1214.

Lockley, R.M.: Man against nature, New York, 1971, International Publishers Co., Inc.

McNerney, W., editor: Working toward a healthier America, Cambridge, Mass., 1980, Ballinger Publishing Co.

Miller, G.T., Jr.: Living in the environment: concepts, problems, and alternatives, Belmont, Calif., 1975, Wadsworth Publishing Co. Inc.

National Vital Statistics Division: Vital statistics of the United States, Washington, D.C., Government Printing Office. (Annual.)

Odum, H.T.: Environment, power and society, New York, 1971, John Wiley & Sons, Inc.

Office of the Assistant Secretary for Health: Facts of life and death, Washington, D.C., 1978, National Center for Health Statistics, DHEW Pub. No. (PHS) 79-1222.

Office of Health Information and Health Promotion: Health highlights 1976-1977, Washington, D.C., 1978, Public Health Service.

Office of Health Research, Statistics, and Technology: Health United States 1980, Washington, D.C., National Center for Health Statistics. (Annual.)

President's Commission on World Hunger: Report of the President's Commission on World Hunger, Washington, D.C., 1980, The Commission.

Prohansky, H., et al.: Environmental psychology: people and their physical settings, ed. 2, New York, 1976, Holt, Rinehart and Winston, Inc.

Ridgeway, J.: Politics of ecology, New York, 1971, E.P. Dutton & Co., Inc.

Shimkins, D.B.: Man, ecology, and health, Arch. Environ. Health **20**:111, 1970.

Shottenfeld, D., and Fraumeni, J., Jr., editors: Cancer epidemiology and prevention, Philadelphia, 1981, W.B. Saunders Co.

Stevens, K.M.: Ecology and etiology of human disease, Springfield, Ill., 1967, Charles C Thomas, Publisher.

Wade, N.: World food situation: pessimism comes back into vogue, Science **181**:634, 1973.

World Health Organization: Demographic yearbook, Geneva, The Organization. (Annual.)

World population growth and response, 1965-1975, Washington, D.C., April, 1976, Population Reference Bureau, Inc.

4

HUMAN BEHAVIOR AND COMMUNITY HEALTH EDUCATION

Health is the ability to perform certain valued social roles.

Talcott Parsons

The fourth scientific cornerstone of community health, in addition to biomedical sciences, ecology, and epidemiology, is the behavioral and social sciences. These are not independent of the first three because the relevance of human behavior to community health is chiefly a matter of how human behavior influences biological, ecological, and epidemiological processes. The behaviors of individuals (as shown in Fig. 2-2) become the life-style norms of populations, which in turn influence the modeling and transmission of attitudes, culture, and values, as well as diseases. In the social history of health, normative behavior becomes organized, and organized behavior has a cumulative effect on the environment and therefore on the ecology of health. Finally, the environment, especially the social environment, influences individual behavior.

These interactions have given rise to subspecialties among the four scientific disciplines, such as environmental epidemiology, behavioral ecology, behavioral medicine, social medicine, medical sociology, and social epidemiology. The application and delivery of the scientific products of these disciplines fall heavily on community health workers, especially health educators. Community health education is the combination of methods designed to facilitate voluntary adaptations of behavior conducive to health. The broader efforts of community health promotion, to be described in subsequent chapters, may go beyond voluntary changes in behavior to include certain regulatory and environmental control strategies designed to channel and support behavior conducive to health.

HEALTH BEHAVIOR AND LIFE-STYLE

Human behavior relates to health in both direct and indirect ways. The *direct* effect on health of personal or social behavior is that which exposes an individual, group, or population to excessive risks that may cause sudden injury, disease, or death or to repeated doses of normal risk that may become addictive or cumulative in their effect. Eating a poisonous or infected food, for example, would be a behavior that exposes the individual or a population to an immediate and excessive risk. Such acute risks in food production, distribution, advertising, and consumption have been minimized in the social history of health by the environmental and regulatory controls administered by our public health agencies. Today the risks are more often taken or imposed in smaller doses, as with chemicals and less lethal or virulent substances or actions, but with a cumulative effect that is nearly imperceptible until they reveal themselves in chronic conditions such as obesity, elevated blood pressure or serum cholesterol levels, reduced lung function or physical conditioning, or drug dependency.

Direct behavioral risks and benefits to health also have been referred to in previous chapters (see Fig. 2-1) as part of the natural cycle of health. In the natural cycle of health self-protective behavior is a response to prior adaptive experience and environmental influence. The direct ways that behavior influences health, then, include preventive behavior and self-care behavior, including diet and physical fitness actions (see Tables 2-4 through 2-6).

As part of the social history of health, previous chapters have featured behavior as having additional *indirect* influence on health through social norms, culture, organization, and environment (see Fig. 2-2 and Tables 2-7 and 2-8). The organizational and environmental routes to health are additional but not unre-

lated to behavior as determinants in the health field concept. They usually require social action and planning at a community level.

The relative importance of behavior among the four factors in the health field concept is illustrated in Fig. 4-1. In addition to the direct influence of behavior on health, much of what can be accomplished in the environment and in the organization of health services depends on human behavior. Behavior can influence health indirectly through the environment to the degree that people will plan individual or community actions to bring about changes in the environment (see Table 2-8). Examples of behavior in community environmental concerns include participating in waste disposal, rat control, or lead paint removal efforts in the neighborhood, or voting on referenda or for elected officials in support of community water fluoridation, automobile safety provisions, food and drug labeling, air and water pollution controls, and regulation of the production, distribution, and advertising of harmful substances.

In addition to the direct effects of behavior on

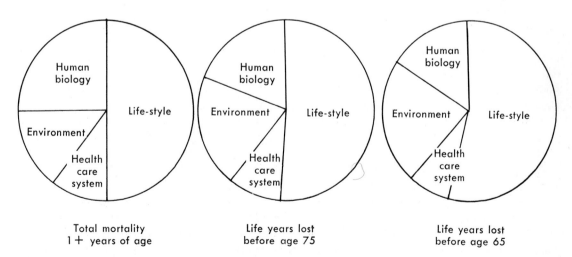

FIG. 4-1. Human behavior is paramount in the direct control of health through personal hygiene, life-style, and other preventive or self-care actions. Life-style behavior also influences the health care system, the environment, and human biology.

From Centers for Disease Control, U.S. Department of Health and Human Services, 1979.

health and the indirect effects of behavior through environmental exposures or control, behavior can influence health indirectly through health services in three ways: (1) the public creates and distributes services through individual and community action in the legislative and health planning process, (2) the public uses available services in a timely and appropriate way, and (3) the public follows the medical or preventive regimens prescribed by its health service providers (see Table 2-7).

COMMUNITY HEALTH EDUCATION

The aim of health education in the community is to elicit, facilitate, and maintain positive health practices by assuring that people are competent and supported in the voluntary adoption of activities conducive to their health. Health education planning is concerned not only with initial preventive actions, appropriate use of health services, health supervision of children from birth to adolescence, and adherence by adults and children to appropriate medical and nutritional regimens, but also with the development in children and youth of a foundation for future health. Within their families and with peers at school, children form predispositions—knowledge, attitudes, and values—that can prevent or promote many of the health problems of later adult life. Planning is required to assure that these several channels of influence on health are appropriately combined and designed to support voluntary adaptations of behavior conducive to health.

Health education planning in the community is based on the systematic application of theories and methods from the behavioral sciences, epidemiology, ecology, administrative science, and communications. Community health education assumes that beneficial health behavior in both children and adults will result from a combination of planned, consistent, integrated learning opportunities. This assumption or proposition is based partly on direct scientific evidence from the evaluation of health education programs in schools, at worksites, in medical settings, and in the mass media. It is based also on indirect evidence borrowed from experiences outside the fields of health and education. Community development, cooperative extension, social work, and other enterprises in human service and behavior change all have contributed to the understanding of planning for change at the community level.

Planned activities to influence voluntary changes in behavior, as opposed to casual, incidental learning experiences distinguish the educational approach to community health; other change strategies that may be excessively permissive, legal, or coercive must also be distinguished. Behavioral changes resulting from education are by definition voluntary and freely adopted by people, with their knowledge of alternatives and probable consequences. Some behavioral change strategies may have unethical components. Behavior modification techniques, for example, qualify as appropriate health education methods so long as the patient or consumer has freely requested or consented to apply the techniques to achieve a behavioral result, such as controlling eating or smoking habits, that he or she desires. Principles of community health education planning call for the participation of consumers, patients, or citizens in the planning process.

Use of the mass media qualifies as an educational channel for community health up to the point that the media are controlled exclusively by commercial or political interests whose use of the media is strictly for profit or propaganda. The regulation of advertisers and the media may be necessary as a more coercive, economic, or legal strategy to protect consumers from, for example, deceptive advertising claims concerning the health value of food products. Community health promotion, then, is the combination of health education with related organizational, environmental, and economic supports for behavior conducive to health.

PRINCIPLES OF HEALTH EDUCATION

A health education plan should derive from an acknowledged health problem or risk in the community and the corresponding program objectives to prevent the problem or reduce the risk. Insofar as it is an integral part of a total community health program, and the achievement of the behavioral goals is but an interim step toward the achievement of health objectives, why should one devote the time and effort required to plan the educational component separately? Focused planning of the educational component of a community health program allows one to increase the potential for successful change by applying behavioral science theory and methods in assessing the behavioral requirements of the program and the corresponding knowledge, attitudes, values, beliefs, norms, skills, and supports required for those behaviors. From these assessments a wiser choice of the messages and experiences required to produce voluntary changes in these causes of health-related behavior can be made. Then the educational methods and resources to be deployed can be more carefully planned and budgeted. Evaluation of the program can also be based on the educational diagnosis by measuring the changes in each of the causes diagnosed as responsible for the health behavior in the community.

The principle of cumulative learning. A large portion of the health status of a population is determined by behavior, as seen in Fig. 4-1. Behavior is the sum of a long-term, complex synthesis of personal and cultural experience and social, economic, and other environmental circumstances and genetic inheritance. Therefore to effect behavioral change, health education in any setting requires a planned sequence of experiences and activities over time, tailored as closely as resources will allow to the circumstances and prior experiences of specific groups.

The principle of multiple targets. Health education objectives such as knowledge, attitudes, and behavior are intermediate to the final health objectives of a community health program. To achieve the ultimate health objectives, several causes of health problems must be addressed by the health education program. This means that not only the characteristics and predispositions of the target population must be taken into account, but also the social systems that enable its behavior and the motivation and ability of providers, parents, teachers, employers, and peers to communicate and reinforce the preferred behaviors.

The principle of aggregating educational targets. The difference between developing teaching programs based on the classroom model and developing health education programs based on the community model is similar to the difference between the clinical-medical model and the community-epidemiological model. Prescribing for a patient based on the history and symptoms of that one person is less complex than determining the right balance in treating a community or population in which many histories and symptoms vary. A health education program must accommodate many varied personal histories, because an educational diagnosis cannot be carried out on each patient or consumer. Community health education and most patient education plans must be designed to modify the educational strategies for various subpopulations on the basis of visible or easily identified characteristics, because it is seldom possible to analyze each individual's educational needs in community programs.

The principle of participation. The prospects for success of programs requiring citizen, consumer, or patient cooperation are greatly increased when members of the community as well as staff and health service–provider organizations are included early in the program genesis. The early involvement of both consumers and providers in identifying problems, assessing their causes, and anticipating barriers to change provides greater assurance that the health education effort will pursue relevant and realistic goals, will employ acceptable methods, and will proceed with the commitment of those involved to the program activities and goals.

The principle of situational specificity. Health education activities vary so widely that it is sometimes difficult for health workers to discern their similarities. Methods used in the accomplishment of educational objectives range from instructional methods, such as group discussion, individual counseling, behavior modification, educational technology, and staff development, to community methods, such as the use of mass media, political actions, and community organization. There is nothing inherently superior or inferior about any of these methods. Their appropriate application depends on the situation. Regardless of the visible activity—whether it is a group of mothers discussing infant nutrition, the PTA president advocating an appropriation before the city council, or an in-service training session with outreach workers—there are theories and principles based on previous research and evaluation to guide the selection and coordination of the methods with the overall educational component of the community program. The selection of methods, then, should be based on an explicit educational diagnosis of the situation.

The principle of intermediate targets. Health education seldom has an immediate, direct impact on behavior. It predisposes behavior primarily through changes in knowledge, attitudes, beliefs, values, and perceptions. It also reinforces behavior by strengthening the social supports of relatives and significant others. It can enable or support behavior through changes in community resources, skill development, and referrals. These represent the full range of intervening variables through which health education should be expected to influence health behavior and which therefore should be considered in the selection and co-

ordination of educational experiences.

The principle of multiple methods. Because there are multiple targets for health education, no single educational input by itself should be expected to have significant, lasting impact on health behavior unless it is supported by other educational input. Health education strategies must be cumulative and mutually supportive of the several factors facilitating a behavior conducive to health.

The principle of diversity. The best combination of educational methods, media, and messages for some people is not necessarily the best combination for others or for the same people in other situations. Therefore educational methods within programs should vary according to the audience characteristics and circumstances, and this means that a variety of learning opportunities or experiences must be provided to assure that different people are exposed to the methods most likely to facilitate their decisions relating to health.

The principle of health promotion. Health education cannot claim and should not be expected to accomplish more than voluntary behavior change. Unless the additional organizational, economic, and environmental supports for the behavior also change, health education might only frustrate the learner. Health education may succeed, for example, in changing the dietary knowledge, motivation, and skills of a population of pregnant women, but unless the diet prescribed is economically accessible and culturally compatible in that population, the effectiveness of the health education methods may be limited. Similarly, if the knowledge, skills, and social supports imparted by a community health program are not applied in behavior, the success of the health education component may be limited by organizational, legal, or economic factors that must be addressed with health promotion interventions beyond health education.

The principle of administration. The educational component of community health programs should have (1) the education plan written not separately or independently but within the context of the larger health program plan, (2) the responsibility for coordination of the educational component fixed on a designated person, (3) the responsibility for each educational intervention assigned to specific people, and (4) a budget for personnel, materials, and other costs. The process of health education may then be defined as any combination of learning opportunities designed to facilitate voluntary adaptations in behavior conducive to health. The principles of administration are implied by the terms *combination* and *designed*.

DIAGNOSTIC STAGE OF EDUCATIONAL PLANNING FOR COMMUNITY HEALTH*

A community health plan begins with an analysis of a social problem or quality of life concern and the incidence, prevalence, and cause of the health problems associated with the social problem in a given population (Fig. 4-2). The first step, then, is a social diagnosis of the quality of life concerns of the community. Step 2 is an epidemiological diagnosis. Step 3 is a behavioral analysis of the priority health problem to determine specific behaviors causing the problem. For each behavior implicated in the cause of each health problem, a further analysis of the factors influencing the behavior is needed in step 4 before educational methods are selected. Health education based more on traditional or favorite techniques than on systematic analysis of behavior and of the learning problems influencing the behavior will tend to be inefficient if not ineffective. Indeed, the selection of appropriate behavioral objectives and adequate methods and materials that make up an educational intervention (step 5)

---

*Based on Green, L.W., Krenter, M.W., Deeds, S., and Partridge, K.: Health education planning: a diagnostic approach, Palo Alto, Calif., 1980, Mayfield Publishing Co.

depend to a considerable extent on the accuracy of the preceding steps in problem diagnosis. While political and legislative decisions often determine some of the priorities and direction of community health programs, local health planners will have to develop, from the best epidemiological evidence available, a sound and rational basis for setting the objectives of their own priority health problems before planning the health education components of the program.

1. Social diagnosis. The starting point should be some assessment of the social concerns of the community to ensure that the health planning is cast in the proper context of the social problems or quality of life concerns paramount in the community. This step requires an understanding of the subjective concerns and values of the community, as well as objective data on social indicators such as unemployment, housing problems, teenage pregnancy, violence, and poverty.

2. Epidemiological diagnosis. The educational components of community health programs are developed within the context of a social concern or quality of life issue in the community that has been analyzed and redefined as a health problem and that becomes the ultimate target of an overall program goal. The sponsoring agency should use the most recent available demographic, vital, and sociocultural information to define the characteristics of the subpopulations experiencing the health problem. The problem should be further analyzed on the basis of the experience of related agencies and a review of previously published reports. To gain perspective on the experience of the community with the health problem, similar data from other cities, states, or regions should be compared. Particular attention should be paid to the rates in subpopulations (age, sex, race, and income groups) within the community relative to comparable rates in other communities or in national statistics.

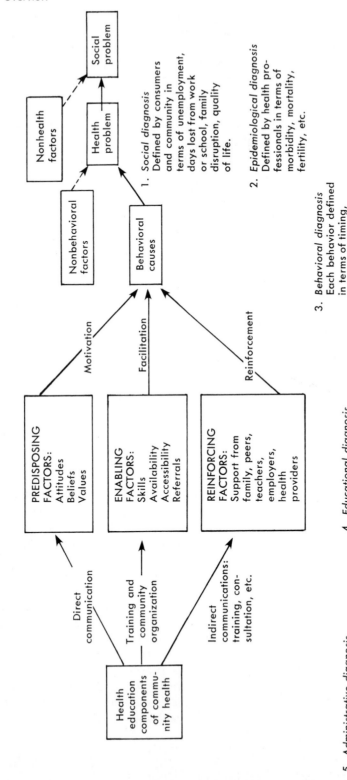

FIG. 4-2. Relationships among factors considered in the assessment of health education needs.

Adapted from Green, L.W., Kreuter, M.W., Deeds, S., and Partridge, K.: Health education planning: a diagnostic approach, Palo Alto, Calif., 1980, Mayfield Publishing Co.

1. *Social diagnosis*
   Defined by consumers and community in terms of unemployment, days lost from work or school, family disruption, quality of life.

2. *Epidemiological diagnosis*
   Defined by health professionals in terms of morbidity, mortality, fertility, etc.

3. *Behavioral diagnosis*
   Each behavior defined in terms of timing, frequency, quality, range, duration.

4. *Educational diagnosis*
   These factors need to be analyzed for each behavior.

5. *Administrative diagnosis*
   Interventions are matched with educational and behavioral objectives from steps 3 and 4, budgeted, sequenced, and coordinated.

An example* of health statistics to be reviewed in the epidemiological diagnosis of a community might include rates, such as the following, of maternal and child health in a rural area that is populated mainly by a low-income minority agricultural group:

The community maternal death rate of 65.5 per 100,000 births compared to the state rate of 18.4.

The community infant death rate of 34.5 per 1,000 compared to the state rate of 21.0.

The community fetal death ratio remains at 24.9 in spite of an overall decline in the state to 14.6.

The health problems that might be identified from these statistics are the high incidence of prematurity, low infant birth weights, a pattern of fetal distress and respiratory distress at delivery, and observed failure of infants to thrive. A visiting nurse service also might report data such as the prevalence of anemia and the incidence of gastrointestinal infections and respiratory diseases.

At this stage difficult decisions must be made to place greater priority on some problems than on others. Patients, consumers, parents, and various health service providers within the community may perceive the problems of mothers and children differently than the sponsoring health agency. The two groups may differ also in ranking the priority or urgency of various health problems.

Consideration of varying community perceptions should take place early in program development. Health programs are not likely to be successful without community support and par-

ticipation in the planning process. Consumer participation in the planning process not only generates support for program activities, but also helps identify population subgroups within the community, such as adolescent mothers and preschool youth who may have special problems and educational needs. Information on these subpopulations should be assembled, information that includes geographical distribution; occupational, economic, and educational status; age and sex composition; ethnicity; health indicators, including age-specific morbidity; and service utilization patterns. Representatives of the consumers or target groups indicated should then be recruited to assist in step 3.

3. Behavioral diagnosis. The foregoing information and definition of the health problem, the program goal, and the high-risk subpopulations should identify the task of specifying the behavioral problems or barriers to the community solution of the health problem. The following guidelines should be considered in the behavioral diagnosis.

- The behaviors presumably contributing to the health problem should be specified as concretely as possible. An inventory of as many possible behavioral causes as one can imagine should be made.
- The nonbehavioral factors (environmental, human biology, and technological factors) contributing to the problem should be identified so that they may be recognized as determinants for which strategies other than health education must be developed.
- There should be a review of evidence that the behaviors identified as possible causes are amenable to change through educational interventions and that such change will improve the health problem in question.
- For each health problem, one or more of the following relevant dimensions of health behavior should be identified:

*From Green, L.W., Wang, V.L., Deeds, S., et al.: Guidelines for health education in maternal and child health, Int. J. Health Educ. Suppl. **21**(3):1, 1978. The maternal and child health examples refer to Chapter 5, but the same approach to health education planning can be applied to the problems described in subsequent chapters. A full application of this diagnosis and planning framework is illustrated in Chapter 12 in relation to drug misuse.

Dimension	Example
Time or promptness of the behavior	Prenatal care begins with the first trimester of pregnancy
Frequency of the behavior	Prenatal visits are every sixth week in the second trimester
Quality of the behavior	Foods with low fat or low sugar content are selected in preference over those high in these substances
Range taken of health behaviors	Prenatal care is obtained, plus diet control regimen followed, plus smoking reduced or stopped
Persistence or follow-through with health behavior	All booster shots are obtained following initial immunization, or medical care is continued through prenatal, delivery, and postnatal periods

- The reasons for selecting specific behaviors as the priority focus of the educational interventions should be justified. An assessment should lead to the selection of specific behaviors that will be the target of the educational interventions. Rarely, if ever, does an agency have the resources necessary to influence all the behaviors contributing to a health problem or set of problems. An initial selection of some of the behaviors should be made. The selection often must be influenced by policies governing required services of the agency, legal and economic factors affecting the desired behaviors, agency resources and expertise available, political viability of the educational interventions, the possibility of continued funding, and the probability of quick program success.

The two most important objective criteria for selection of priority behavioral targets for health education are (1) the evidence that the behavioral change will make a difference in the reduction of the health problem and (2) the evidence that the behavior is amenable to voluntary change.

Examples of nonbehavioral factors influencing the previously defined health problems include

- Genetic factors
- Economic base
- Occupation
- Environmental isolation

Examples of behavioral causes of the previously defined health problems include

- Consumption of proper nutritional diet
- Acceptance of medical supervision at each stage from prenatal to postnatal year for mother and child
- Postponement of pregnancy to age 18 and avoidance after age 40
- Spacing of pregnancies over 24 to 30 months
- Reduction in total number of pregnancies
- Avoidance of physical and emotional stress during pregnancy
- Avoidance of fetal insult (reduction in smoking and alcohol, aspirin, and other drug ingestion)

4. Educational diagnosis. The behaviors selected should be subjected to further analysis for assessment of their causes. The following sets of factors should be considered as causes of each behavior:

Predisposing factors: Knowledge, attitudes, beliefs, and values that motivate people to take appropriate health actions.

Enabling factors: Skills and the availability and accessibility of resources that make it possible for a motivated person to take action.

Reinforcing factors: The attitudes and climate of support from providers of services, families, community groups, and so on, that reinforce the health behavior of an individual who is motivated and able to adopt the behavior but who will discontinue the behavior if it is not rewarded.

Representatives of the various segments within the agency and community who will be affected by the program should be consulted in these analyses. By assessing the predisposing, enabling, and reinforcing factors influencing the health behaviors in the earlier example, the most useful interventions on which to concentrate health education can be decided. By consulting with the target women themselves, one could adapt the health advice to fit the circumstances of these women more appropriately. Examples of the factors identified in an educational diagnosis of maternal and child health follow:

Predisposing factors: Attitudes toward pregnancy as a way of fulfilling needs other than reproduction; belief that pregnancy and childbearing are the only acceptable roles for young women.

Enabling factors: Scarcity and cost of recommended foods; inaccessibility of emergency care, transportation problems in getting to clinics for prenatal and well child care; clinic hours preclude attendance by working women.

Reinforcing factors: Husbands do not support contraceptive behavior; loss of income from inability to work in fields may be an incentive for family planning for some, but exemption from work may reward pregnancy for others; crowded clinic and waiting time does not reward clinic attendance.

Failure to assess some of these factors and to develop a community health education program addressed to all three sets would seriously limit the impact of the program. Fig. 4-2 summarizes the relationships among the factors that were considered in the foregoing procedures. The analysis proceeds from right to left, with methods of health education decided last in the administrative diagnosis.

5. Administrative diagnosis. Selecting the health educational methods for a community health program follows almost automatically from a thorough identification and ranking of predisposing, enabling, and reinforcing factors influencing the health behaviors. Administrative diagnosis then includes the assessment of available resources to support preferred methods, the coordination and budgeting of these methods into a timetable that corresponds to the community health program, and the constructive participation by staff and area residents who, in addition to understanding and defining the program's intent, also contribute to the setting of priorities, the determination of acceptable approaches, the informational content and phraseology, the suggestion of barriers and facilitators to the achievement of program objectives, the identification of indigenous resources, and the review (pretesting) of educational media and materials. By including community members in the planning, one obtains their personal commitment to realizing program success. Most importantly, their participation enables program planners to incorporate consumer interests, perspectives, and values into the educational activities of the program. The principle of consumer participation applies equally well to representatives of related agencies, institutions, and organizations in the community and to the agency staff who will implement the program activities.

Resources in the community may already be channeling funds and efforts into areas related to the proposed educational program. Others may have been active in previous years. It is important to survey the activities, organizations, and individuals behind these resources to avoid overlap and to integrate services.

The program plan is based on survey information obtained from organizations and agencies at national, state or provincial, and local levels (e.g., schools, citizens' groups, industry, labor organizations, religious groups, colleges, advertising agencies, drama groups, drug stores); local facilities (e.g., libraries, health centers, training centers, town halls, gathering places); personnel (e.g., volunteers, agency staff, social workers) whose functions relate to health education, training, experience, and supervision; community events (e.g., fairs, festivals, conventions, public and private meetings); communications resources (e.g., numbers of telephones, use of radios, billboards, local television and radio stations, newspapers, newsletters, organization bulletins); and funding sources available for the educational program through the health service agency itself and related organizations. This identification and assessment of available resources should lead to the further refinement of objectives, strategies, and methods. Some previously written objectives may be accomplished earlier or more extensively if more resources are obtained. Additional intermediate objectives may be needed for the development of resources that are inadequate.

PLANNING FOR THE DELIVERY OF COMMUNITY HEALTH EDUCATION

The planning steps outlined in this section are not entirely sequential. They begin during the preceding diagnostic stages and continue through the organizational, implementation, and evaluation stages.

Priority target populations for specific educational components

The people at risk, or those who are affected by the health problem, are easily identified once the health problem has been defined. They are the target for most of the educational interventions and thus the beneficiaries, or target group, who the planners should consult. Education must also be directed toward groups not affected by the health problem but who are in a direct position to influence those who are. These "gatekeepers" and social reinforcers (parents, spouses, teachers, peers, employers, and "opinion leaders") are often an intermediate or additional target population for educational interventions.

As implied in Fig. 4-2, the primary target group will receive direct communication designed to influence their predisposition to accept the recommended health practices. One intermediate target group for community organization efforts would be directors of other agencies who control resources that would enable or facilitate the health behavior to be practiced. Another intermediate target group would receive training, consultation, or supervision in reinforcing the recommended health behavior. In relation to the predisposing factors, the primary target population should be described in terms of geographical, occupational, economic, educational, age, sex, and ethnicity distributions. The characteristics that provide the basic analysis for the specification of community health programs are also the basis for the development of educational interventions. Representative persons from the described population should be included in the further development of the educational plans. In relation to the enabling and reinforcing factors, intermediate target groups—controllers of needed resources for the health behavior—and those who can reinforce the behavior—transmitters of information—should be contacted and their participation in planning solicited.

If behavioral data are not available on the target population, descriptive information may be obtained by a "diagnostic-baseline sample survey" or estimated from survey statistics obtained elsewhere and applied to local census data on the demographic characteristics of the target population in question.

Behavioral objectives

The behavioral objectives stage overlaps with the previous planning stage. It is at this point of specifying behavioral objectives and the consequent educational objectives, however, that the educational component of the community health program should begin to emerge as an entity distinct from other technologies and services.

The objectives derive from the findings of the behavioral and educational diagnoses. The proper statement of the objectives should lend purpose to the program plan and direction to its implementation. The test of objectives is their ability to communicate expected results. Lucidity and precision in their formation should (1) provide limits to expenditure of time and effort on specific educational interventions, (2) identify criteria for measurement of program achievement, (3) lead to task anaylses for selection, training, and supervision of staff, and (4) provide orientation to cooperating agencies and to the general community.

Time spent on the formulation of objectives in educational planning is sometimes more important than in the planning of some administrative and service components because education appears to be more abstract and difficult to define or measure than some of the more familiar activities of community health programs.

Objectives should be expressed in terms of outcomes. They may apply to providers and to the system as well as to the consumers. Each objective should answer the question, *Who* is expected to achieve or become *how much* of *what* by *when* and *where*?

Who—Target groups or individuals expected to change

How much—The extent of the condition to be obtained

What—The action, change in behavior, or health practice to be obtained

When—The time in which the desired condition is to be obtained

Where—The place in which change will be observed, usually implied within the specification of who

The desired behaviors (what) should derive from the behavioral diagnosis and should describe what the participants will (be able to) do or not do as a result of the program that they could not or did not do (as much) before the program. The conditions of the action should be stated in the following way:

Who—Derived from some logical portion (percentage) of the target group

How much—Or to what extent will partially be a function of available resources

Where—Geographical, political, or institutional boundaries derived in part from the original description of the health problem

When—Or how soon, or within what time period, will be determined by the urgency of the health problem in the community and by the rate of change that can be expected from the amount and type of effort devoted to the program

The objectives should be so explicated as to lead to assessment criteria. They should be stated in concrete terms with at least an implied if not stated scale of measurement that can be used to evaluate their accomplishment. Given the stated program goal for the earlier example—To raise the survival rate of mothers, infants, and children through raising the quality of prenatal care and promoting the optimum growth and development of children.—the following health objectives for the community health program might apply:

• To reduce maternal mortality within Counties A and B by 10% within the first 2 years and an additional 15% the next 3 years, continuing until the state average rate is reached.

• To reduce infant mortality to the state average within 10 years.

Behavioral objectives then could take the following form:

• In the county 1,850 women under 40 who are at high risk of problem pregnancy will receive two general health checkups the first year of the program.

• In this group 80% of pregnancies will be detected within the first trimester.

• Of the pregnant women 95% will be delivered by qualified medical personnel in obstetric facilities during the first year of the program.

In the first behavioral objective, the following apply:

Who—Women in the county who are under

40 and have selected characteristics (e.g., age, socioeconomic status) associated with high-risk pregnancies

How much—1,850

What—Receiving two general health checkups

When—During the first year of the program

Note that in most public health or population-based programs, "how much" refers to the number of people or percentage of the population, whereas for individuals "how much" would refer to the level of accomplishment (e.g., two checkup visits).

Educational objectives

Educational objectives are the intermediate or subobjectives to the behavioral objectives (Fig. 4-3). These must be accomplished before it is possible to achieve a change or development in behavior. These intermediate changes are defined by an analysis of the predisposing, enabling, and reinforcing factors referred to in the behavioral diagnosis, along with the assessment of the barriers and facilitators, which is indicated in the following section. To avoid a shotgun approach to communications, the planners should consider the knowledge, attitudes, skills, organizaton, and training required of people to move toward stated objectives. The various types of educatonal objectives that flow

from these causes of behavior can be described as follows.

Informational objectives. Informational or cognitive objectives relate to the knowledge and beliefs necessary on the part of individuals or groups to address or cope with the health problem, services, and activities. In other words, who will comprehend how much of what information?

Attitudinal objectives. Attitudinal or affective objectives relate to the predispositions or feelings people hold toward certain health problems or practices or toward means to be employed in certain health measures (e.g., contraceptives or immunizations)—what will sufficiently motivate people to take appropriate health action?

Skills. Persons may have to learn certain skills, such as reading thermometers, recording observations, and judging symptoms, to be able to use services or self-care procedures effectively.

Community organization objectives. Making services accessible through community organization may require the reordering of community priorities or the redistribution of resources.

Training objectives. Training to bring about specified changes in staff knowledge, behavior, and attitudes can encourage and reinforce de-

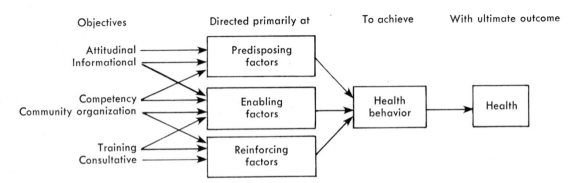

FIG. 4-3. Types of educational objectives and their relationship to behavioral objectives and health status objectives as the ultimate outcome of community health programs.

sired behavior. Similar objectives may be written for parents, employers, spouses, peers, and community opinion leaders. Training may take various forms such as consultation, group work, supervision, or continuing education.

Assessment of barriers and facilitators to implementation

A realistic view of implementing the educational plan requires an assessment of factors that may impede carrying out program activities. At the same time, certain existing characteristics of the community may facilitate program success. Both the barriers and supports to the program should be considered.

Barriers to the achievement of educational objectives can assume several forms: social, psychological, and cultural barriers (e.g., citizen and staff bias, prejudice, misunderstanding, taboos, unfavorable past experiences, values, norms, social relationships, official disapproval, rumors); communication obstacles (e.g., illiteracy, local vernacular); economic and physical barriers (e.g., low income and inability to pay for prescribed drugs or the means of transportation to medical services, long distances over difficult terrain to medical facilities); and legal and administrative barriers (e.g., residence requirements to be eligible for services, legal requirements that the program operate within defined geographical boundaries).

Facilitators to the achievement of program objectives go beyond the mere absence of barriers. The knowledge, predispositions, and skills of area residents favorable to the implementation of the program may include past and favorable experience with similar programs, high credibility of the program sponsoring agency, high education levels of consumers, dynamic and favorable local leaders and organizations, skilled staff with experience, open channels of communication with consumers, and support from other agencies. In addition, some geographical and physical enabling factors may serve as program assets (e.g., population distribution and density, access to facilities).

In considering factors that may impede or support the program, it should be emphasized that the introduction of new or unfamiliar schemes for promoting awareness and health behavior has its greatest opportunity for success when integrated into existing systems of knowledge transfer and influence within the community. Schools, local media, clubs, churches, neighborhoods, and ethnic associations are the most effective channels of communication. Also, the identification of barriers should be included in additional objectives that indicate how much and when each of the barriers is to be surmounted in the program.

THE ORGANIZING STAGE

Organization of the educational components of the community health program follows the development and refinement of the planning operations. At this stage, if involvement of concerned persons has been obtained and planning is detailed and thorough, staff, volunteers, and cooperating agencies will be in agreement over the program's aims and general strategies. At this stage they should be committed to assuming their roles in the educational efforts. To initiate the program will require more specific planning and resource identification, equipment and materials assembly, design of procedures, and training and orientation of personnel.

Many health workers and allied personnel may be uninformed of the methods of health education, while others may feel that educational efforts are too slow, complex, and of dubious efficacy. Therefore a flexible training plan that allows people time to discuss their concerns and that provides encouragement and support is indicated. The health education training should be differentiated from technical training related to health and medical content. Health education training underscores the attitudinal and behavioral factors essential to long-term health maintenance, the cultural perceptions of the clients, and the neccessity of well-planned and properly sustained action to achieve the health behavior changes required by the objectives of the community health program.

Priority

Resources can always be considered scarce in relation to the great needs in community health. To ensure the most economical use of the resources available, priorities among alternative educational activities must be considered. Related to this pressing need for efficiency is the need for effectiveness. This requires the selection of the most effective combination of educational interventions and activities available. The first step is to determine which procedures are feasible, given limited staff, services, money, and time, and then to combine these resources to achieve the best support of program objectives. The latter should be done in light of the educational diagnosis, not as an isolated step in planning.

The following considerations should help set priorities: obtain opinions from community members on priorities for educational services; delineate the areas that will provide the greatest benefits to the most recipients; and phase program activities with a gradual beginning, limiting number and range of activities, with initial emphasis on areas most amenable to quick and easy success and activities requiring minimum staff training. Most of these decisions should be guided by reviewing the most recent scientific literature on the evaluation of health education methods and programs.

There should be a contingency plan to aid program survival in the event of future reduction of resources. Beyond these general principles, the selection of educational efforts in strategic patterns or combinations is subject to the particular circumstances of each site.

Development of educational methods and media

Having set priorities and selected strategies, the planners can proceed to develop and schedule the use of educational tools and methods. Methods, media, and materials may be classified according to visual, audio, interpersonal, and multimedia attributes and can be preassessed in terms of their acceptability to the particular group, convenience (time demands, manpower requirements, situational concerns—light, sound), efficiency (fixed costs, continuing costs, space and maintenance requirements, staff and time needs to convey a message), and effectiveness (in communicating messages, arousing attention and interest, promoting interaction, using suitable repetition and message retention techniques, encouraging desired attitudes and adoption of principles).

Every experience the client has with services and with staff in clinic situations entails some learning that may be helpful, detrimental, or neutral to the achievement of the program's objectives. It is recognized that communication involving interpersonal or two-way processes provides the most favorable environment for learning, and it generally has greater long-term behavioral effects. Pamphlets of mass media are often appropriate in the early phases of a program or when other methods with more lasting outcomes are not feasible. It must be acknowledged that a single educational intervention isolated in time be relied on to have a significant, lasting impact on an individual's health behavior. Only through repeated educational inputs, including reinforcement by health staff, aides, community leaders, friends, and family, can health education affect human behavior related to contemporary community health problems.

Orientation and training

In the orientation and training aspect of the organizing stage, the staff (including volunteers, teachers, employers, parents, peers, agricultural agents, and other community leaders) should accept the fact that the objectives of health programs are achieved primarily by the actions of consumers, namely, the target population. Accordingly, the staff must be instructed in how they can affect client behavior, both positively and negatively.

Staff training may include orientation aimed at sensitizing the staff members to their educational function and to the general objectives of the education program, preparation in recognizing educational opportunities, communication skills and reinforcement techniques, training priorities for those staff members in contact with consumers and continuing education.

As the primary link between the health service and the consumers, community aides and volunteers must be aware of their special role in the health education process. Their potential influence through interaction with community residents should be emphasized in the planning of the program.

Volunteers are not free of cost. Proper use of volunteers requires continuous, careful supervision and training, which should be budgeted in the educational plan. A thorough plan for training volunteers might include a content designed to foster their interest in health education and in the program's need for their insight into the attitudes, reactions, and daily lives of the service group; training in communications skills and teamwork roles; and educational responsibilities and limits of volunteers.

Data collection and records

Statistics are used for educational planning and replanning; for continuous monitoring of program impact; for supervision, training, and staff development; and for evaluation of program process and outcome. Information collection requiring additional paperwork must always be weighed against other demands for time. Small additions and checklists may be integrated into existing records with little effort and consequent staff acceptance. For more intensive narrative reporting and recording, special efforts during limited time period may be acceptable and provide sufficient data without generating staff resistance and unmanageable amounts of paperwork. The educational plan should clearly identify the use and purpose of new forms and records.

Scheduling

Timing is crucial to the success of the educational plan of action and requires an analysis of when, where, and who is responsible for implementation. This analysis will provide the lead time estimated and the completion date required for each activity in relation to the total program and with consideration given to the training required, production schedules for material, and staff loads.

A task analysis and time sequence of activities should integrate the educational implementation with the total program plan. External events should be considered in the scheduling for coordination with community happenings, school openings, holidays, and related community schedules.

THE IMPLEMENTING STAGE

The implementing stage is a logical progression from the previous stage of diagnosis, planning, and organizing. Very little can be stated in a program plan about implementation that is not already covered in preceding sections of the plan. Lines of authority and communication (supervision and feedback) should be detailed. Good records and documentation, quality control, and other process evaluation can provide immediate feedback on whether everything is working satisfactorily. Peer review among health professionals helps to maintain quality control, but it must be based on standards and documentation of practice. Feedback on pa-

Health education objectives for communities.*

GOAL: Community residents will have the necessary knowledge, skills, capacity, and opportunity to improve and maintain individual, family, and community health; use preventive health services, practices, and facilities appropriately; understand and participate, where feasible, in decision making concerning their health care; understand and carry out prescribed medical instructions; and participate in community health decision making.

Focus	Objectives	Indicators	Population in need
	Process		
Integration of health education services	1. By 19 ___ all community prevention programs will have an identifiable strategy for the use of health education, including, at a minimum, the following: a. A statement of educational objectives b. Specification of target groups c. Educational methods to be employed d. Periodic evaluation of educational effectiveness	Existence and use of strategy Percent of programs having identifiable strategy	The community
Promotion of individual health maintenance	2. By 19 ___ the health education component of all community prevention programs will be conducted to provide the necessary knowledge, skills, and capacity to assure that individuals a. Assume greater personal responsibility for improving and maintaining optimum health for themselves, their families, and their community (e.g., smoking cessation) b. Use preventive services, practices, and facilities appropriately (e.g., well baby care) c. Participate in community health decision making	Percent of prevention programs where (as relevant) there is an emphasis on increased individual responsibility for health Evidence of citizen participation in community health decision making	

Appropriate use of health services and resources	3. By 19 — the community will be served by an information and referral system concerning available health facilities, resources, and services.	Existence of information and referral system Evidence of continuing cooperation from relevant agencies in providing information to the system Use of system by community Level of public media involvement	The community
Patient education	4. By 19 — all patients able to do so will participate in educational experiences designed to help them a. Understand their current health status b. Understand prescribed personal preventive services, procedures, or practices, their relative benefits and risks (e.g., vaccine reactions, chronic disease treatment), and alternatives to prescribed treatments c. Participate in the development of their preventive health care plan if they choose to do so	Documentation in patient record of Patients' following prescribed instructions Patients' accepting or rejecting preventive service, practice, or procedure Presentation of benefits and risks	Patients receiving preventive care
Citizen involvement in community health decisions	5. By 19 — a mechanism will exist in the community to ensure that a. Health-related boards and committees obtain advice and guidance from consumers b. Orientation and training is provided for members of boards, committees, task forces, etc. c. Citizen participation in health-related decision making is assured	Presence of formal and informal means of obtaining such input Documentation of action taken as a result of such input Documentation of programs presented Documentation of outreach activities and responses	The community

*Based on Model standards for community preventive health services, Washington, D.C., 1979, Public Health Service, U.S. Department of Health and Human Services.

tients' or clients' utilization and satisfaction should provide data for program adjustment and replanning. Community surveillance will aid in continuous health education planning.

EVALUATION

Evaluation is the comparison of an object of interest against a standard of acceptability. It is, at the very least, an assessment of the worth of a program, a method, or some other object of interest. It may provide an estimate of the degree to which spent resources result in specified activity and the degree to which performed activities attain goals. The determination of whether goals have been met is based on criteria indicated by precise statements of objectives along with subjective impressions and reporting. Hard data are sometimes available and can be used to maintain continuous evaluative research efforts. Evaluation can suggest which of several alternative educational strategies is the most efficient and which steps have an effect on the behavior specified. Evaluation provides accountability for time spent. Results usually offer a sense of accomplishment to staff and consumers or sponsors of the program.

Process evaluation

Process evaluation or formative evaluation refers to continuous observation and checking to see whether program activities are taking place with the quality and at the time and rate necessary to achieve the stated objective. Sources of data for continuous process evaluation often include budget reports on monthly expenditures in specific categories where rate of expenditures would indicate amount of program activity relevant to achievement of objectives. The standards of acceptability in process evaluation usually are based on professional consensus, as in the table on pp. 98-99. Process evaluation also may be based on statistics or observations from daily encounters with consumers, patients, or clients, such as clinic attendance records that are tabulated weekly,

monthly, or quarterly for total numbers of new and old patients attending specific clinic sessions. Systematic samples of the records can be tabulated to obtain more detailed estimates of progress or status on variables such as broken appointment rates, sources of referral for specific clinics or problems, and trimester of first visit for pregnant women. A third type of data available for process evaluation is administrative records. Personnel records on the number of home visits attempted, the number completed, the number of group sessions conducted, and the time allotted for various educational functions can be tabulated periodically.

Feedback mechanisms should be set up so that the information that is collected can be used by supervisors and peers in reviewing performance. Time should be allowed in staff meetings and community meetings for consideration of strengths, weaknesses, and readaptation of ongoing programs. There should be a plan for charting records over time or comparing progress statistics with other programs or standards.

Outcome evaluation

Outcome evaluation, sometimes referred to as summative evaluation, is when the achievement of objectives is assessed by evaluation of expected outcomes. The precision with which objectives are stated determines the usefulness of this assessment. Information and data should be determined in advance. Baseline information should be obtained on a period prior to the program's inception for comparison with similarly gathered data from the period of the program or the period following the program. Statistical procedures to assess differences in outcomes should be selected in advance of data collection.

The basic questions addressed by outcome evaluation of health education are the following: What are the measurable results of program efforts in the promotion of health behavior? Has there been any change in the attitudes of the clients toward the recommended actions or change in their ability to carry out the recommended actions or change in the resources and social support for such actions in the community?

Ideally, the evaluation of a specific educational component (e.g., a pamphlet or a group discussion) should not depend on the comparison of a group of patients who receive only that method with a group of patients who receive nothing. The comparison should be made between a group who receive a comprehensive health education program and another group who receive everything *except* the component to be evaluated. Thus there should be overall outcome statistics (knowledge, attitude, and behavioral outcomes) for the entire program and separate statistics on subgroups who were exposed to the entire program except for specific methods or materials of interest. The finding of no significant difference would indicate methods or materials that could be eliminated from the program to reduce costs (increase efficiency).

Reporting on progress or outcomes of health education and community health programs is a continuous process and should occur at any stage of developing or conducting the educational program in which important or unusual observations or decisions are made. Program developments and results need to be made available to the affiliated organizations, agencies, and institutions participating in the program and to the clients and general public. Their continued participation can be encouraged by addressing their contribution to, or influence on, the program development. Case histories and reports should be published in professional journals and newsletters for use by other departments, programs, or projects and to contribute to the advancement of professional knowledge and practice.

QUALIFICATIONS FOR THE EDUCATIONAL SPECIALIST

Desirable qualifications for the person assigned the responsibility for planning and im-

plementing the community health education program include training in public health or community health education and experience in a community health agency or institution. Competencies in health education include the following:

1. Planning at the community level (as distinct from formal classroom and individual instruction level), including epidemiological and sociological methods, community organization, and health services administration
2. Assessment and adaptation of communications to attitudinal, cultural, economic, and ethnic determinants of health behaviors
3. Educational evaluation within the context of community health (as distinct from formal curriculum evaluation), including biostatistics and behavioral research methods

When these skills are not available within the staff of a community health agency, consultation for the planning and preparation stages of health education programs may be obtained from other organizations in the same way that specialized medical, nursing, statistical, engineering, or administrative consultation is used to supplement the expertise of the agency.

SUMMARY

Human behavior accounts for approximately half of the years of an average person's life lost prematurely in Western societies. Behavior is developed and modified through learning processes that can be designed in health education to empower people to make their own voluntary adaptations of behavior conducive to health. In addition, health promotion can build further supports for health behavior through organizational, economic, and environmental adaptations in the community. The planning and implementation steps outlined in this chapter apply to most of the following chapters.

QUESTIONS AND EXERCISES

1. What trends have you noticed in recent years in your community or among your friends in health behavior and health concerns? Can you find objective data to support your observations? If not, how would you go about verifying your subjective view of these trends in health behavior?
2. Identify one or two national or international health campaigns or programs spanning a number of years. How do you account for the public concern with these different health problems at different times? What were the major features of the health education component of these programs? Why have different programs or problems at different times required different health education methods?
3. Identify and describe the demographic characteristics (geographic location, size, age, and sex distribution, etc.) of a population (students, patients, workers, residents) whose quality of life you would like to improve. You will follow the population you choose through most of the remaining exercises below. Look ahead at these exercises to be sure the population is appropriate for the diagnostic and planning steps required.
4. How did (or would)* you involve the members of the population you selected in exercise 3 in identifying their quality of life concerns? Justify your methods in terms of their feasibility and appropriateness for the population you are helping.
5. How did (or would) you verify the subjective data gathered in exercise 1 with objective data on social problems or quality of life concerns?
6. Display and discuss your real or hypothetical data* as a quality of life diagnosis, justifying your selection of social, economic, or health problems for priority attention on the basis of their perceived and objective importance in the lives of your population.
7. List the health problems related to the quality of life concerns identified in your population in exercise 6.
8. Rate (low, medium, high) each health problem in the inventory according to (a) its relative importance in affecting the quality of life concerns and (b) its potential for change.
9. Discuss the reasons for your ratings of health problems as having high priority in exercise 8a in terms of their

*It is recommended that these exercises be carried out with a real population accessible to the student or practitioner. But if this is impractical, the exercises can best be followed with a well-described hypothetical population by using actual census data and health information from similar populations. For a more complete explanation of procedures to carry out these exercises, see Green, L.W., Kreuter, M.W., Deeds, S., and Partridge, K. (1980).

prevalence, incidence, cost, virulence, intensity, or other relevant dimensions. Extrapolate from national, state, provincial, or regional data when local data are not available.
10. Cite the evidence supporting your ratings of health problems in exercise 8b. Refer to the success of other programs or to the availability of medical or other technology to control or reduce the high-priority health problems you have selected.
11. Write a program objective for the highest priority health problem, indicating who will show how much of what improvement by when.
12. In relation to the highest priority health problem identified in your program objective in exercise 11, list the specific behaviors in your population that might be causally related to the achievement of that objective.
13. Rate (low, medium, high) each behavior in your inventory according to its (a) prevalence, (b) epidemiological or causal importance, and (c) changeability.
14. Provide or cite objective evidence supporting your ratings in exercise 13. Extrapolate or interpolate from national, state, provincial, or regional data when local data are not available or cite data from similar populations or studies elsewhere.
15. Write a behavioral objective for your population (who) showing what percentage (how much) will exhibit the behavior or change the behavior (what) by a given date or amount of time from the beginning of a program (by when).
16. For one of the high-priority behaviors you selected in the previous exercises, make an inventory of all the predisposing, enabling, and reinforcing factors you can identify.
17. Rate each factor believed to cause the health behavior according to each of two criteria: importance and changeability. Give each factor a rating of low, medium, or high on each criterion.
18. Write educational objectives for the three highest priority determinants of the health behavior: one objective for a predisposing factor, one for an enabling factor, and one for a reinforcing factor.
19. For the population and health problem you have analyzed, identify three educational methods that would appear to be most appropriate.
20. Analyze how your program would affect and be affected by other programs and units within a health agency or educational institution.
21. Describe the interorganizational coordination that would be required to achieve the objectives of your program.

BIBLIOGRAPHY

American Hospital Association: Media handbook: a guide to selecting, producing, and using media for patient education programs, Chicago, 1978, The Association.

American Hospital Association: Medication teaching manual: a guide for patient counseling, Chicago, 1978, The Association.

American Hospital Association: Implementing patient education in the hospital, Chicago, 1979, The Association.

American Hospital Association: Staff manual for teaching patients about chronic obstructive pulmonary diseases, Chicago, 1979, The Association.

American Hospital Association: Staff manual for teaching patients about diabetes mellitus, Chicago, 1979, The Association.

American Hospital Association: Staff manual for teaching patients about hypertension, Chicago, 1979, The Association.

American Hospital Association: Staff manual for teaching patients about rheumatoid arthritis, Chicago, 1979, The Association.

Barofsky, I., editor: Medication compliance: a behavioral management approach, Thorofare, N.J., 1977, Charles B. Slack, Inc.

Bernstein, L., Bernstein, R.S., and Dana, R.H.: Interviewing: a guide for health professionals, ed. 2, New York, 1974, Appleton-Century-Crofts.

Bertera, R., and Green, L.W.: Cost-effectiveness of a home visiting triage program for family planning in Turkey, AM. J. Public Health **69:**950, 1979.

Biehler, R.F.: Psychology applied to teaching, ed. 2, Boston, 1974, Houghton Mifflin Co.

Bowden, C.L., and Burstein, A.G.: Psychosocial basis of medical practice, Baltimore, 1974, The Williams & Wilkins Co.

Brieger, W.R.: A behavioral guide for evaluating patient educators, Int. J. Health Educ. **23:**55, 1980.

Bugelski, B.R.: The psychology of learning applied to teaching, ed. 2, Indianapolis, 1971, The Bobbs-Merrill Co., Inc.

Campbell, A., Converse, E., and Rodgers, W.L.: The quality of American life: perceptions, evaluations and satisfaction, New York, 1976, Russell Sage Foundation.

Casey, P.H., and Whitt, J.K.: Effect of the pediatrician on the mother-infant relationship, Pediatrics **65:**815, 1980.

Cohen, M.M.: Instructions for parents, New York, 1980, Appleton-Century-Crofts.

Cohen, S., editor: Compliance: the behavioral dimensions, Lexington, Mass., 1978, Lexington Books.

Dalis, G.T., and Strasser, B.B.: Teaching strategies for values awareness and decision making in health education, Thorofare, N.J., 1977, Charles B. Slack, Inc.

Danaher, B.G.: Smoking cessation programs in occupational settings, Public Health Rep. **95:**149, 1980.

Deeds, S.G., Hebert, B.J., and Wolle, J.M.: A model for patient education programming, Washington, D.C., 1979, American Public Health Association.

Education manual for a health education program, Bowie, Md., 1978, Robert J. Brady Co.

The John E. Fogarty International Center for Advanced Study in the Health Sciences: Preventive medicine, U.S.A.: health promotion and consumer health education, New York, 1976, Prodist.

Freedman, C.R.: Teaching patients, San Diego, 1978, Courseware, Inc.

Freedman, C.R., and O'Neal, H.: Teaching your patients to take better care of themselves, San Diego, 1979, Courseware, Inc.

Green, L.W., and Kansler, C.: The scientific and professional literature on patient education, Detroit, 1980, Gale Research Co.

Green, L.W., Kreuter, M.W., Deeds, S., and Partridge, K.: Health education planning: a diagnostic approach, Palo Alto, Calif., 1980, Mayfield Publishing Co.

Green, L.W., Lewis, F.M., and Levine D.M.: Balancing statistical data and clinical judgments in the diagnosis of health education needs, J. Community Health **6:**79, 1980.

Green, L.W., Wang, V.L., Deeds, S., et al.: Guidelines for health education in maternal and child health, Int. J. Health Educ. Suppl. **31**(3): 1978.

Griffith, H.W.: Instructions for patients, ed. 2, Philadelphia, 1975, W.B. Saunders Co.

Griffith, H.W.: Drug information for patients, Philadelphia, 1978, W.B. Saunders Co.

Haynes, R.B., Taylor, D.W., and Sackett, D.L.: Compliance in health care, Baltimore, 1979, The Johns Hopkins University Press.

Insel, P.M., and Roth, W.T.: Core concepts in health, ed. 2, Palo Alto, Calif., 1979, Mayfield Publishing Co.

Kidd, J.R.: How adults learn, New York, 1973, Association Press.

Knowles, M.S.: The modern practice of adult education, rev. ed., Chicago, 1980, Association Press.

Knowles, M.S.: The adult learner: a neglected species, ed. 2, Houston, 1978, Gulf Publishing Co., Book Division.

Lazes, P., editor: The handbook of health education, Germantown, Md., 1979, Aspen Systems Corp.

Leventhal, H., et al.: Cardiovascular risk modification by community-based programs for lifestyle change, J. Consult. Clin. Psychol. **48:**150, 1980.

Levin, L.S., Katz, A.H., and Holst, E.: Self-care: lay initiatives in health, New York, 1976, Prodist.

Litwack, L., Litwack, J.M., and Ballou, M.B.: Health counseling, New York, 1980, Appleton-Century-Crofts.

Mager, R.F.: Preparing instructional objectives, ed., Belmont, Calif., 1975, Fearon Publishers.

Mahoney, M.J.: Cognition and behavior modification, Cambridge, Mass., 1974, Ballinger Publishing Co.

Mahoney, M.J., and Thoresen, C.E.: Self-control: power to the person, Monterey, Calif., 1974, Brooks/Cole Publishing Co.

Maslow, A.: Motivation and personality, ed. 2, New York, 1970, Harper & Row, Publishers.

Mico, P.R., and Ross, H.S.: Health education and behavioral science, Oakland, Calif., 1975, Third Party Associates.

Nierenberg, J., and Janovic, F.: The hospital experience, Indianapolis, 1978, The Bobbs-Merrill Co., Inc.

O'Connor, A.B.: Nursing: patient education, New York, 1979, American Journal of Nursing Co.

Pohl, M.L.: The teaching function of the nursing practitioner, Palo Alto, Calif., 1979, William C. Brown Co., Publishers.

Redman, B.K.: The process of patient teaching in nursing, ed. 4, St. Louis, 1980, The C.V. Mosby Co.

Reilly, D.E.: Behavioral objectives in nursing: evaluation of learner attainment, New York, 1975, Appleton-Century-Crofts.

Rogers, E.N., and Shoemaker, F.F.: Communication of innovations: a cross-cultural approach, New York, 1971, The Free Press.

Ross, H.S., and Mico, P.R.: Theory and practice in health education, Palo Alto, Calif, 1980, Mayfield Publishing Co.

Sommers, A.R., editor: Promoting health: consumer education and national policy, Aspen Systems, Inc., 1976.

Squyres, W., editor: Patient education: an inquiry into the state of the art, New York, 1980, Springer Publishing Co., Inc.

Von Haden, H.I., and King, J.M.: Educational innovators' guide, Worthington, Mass., 1974, Charles A. James Publishing Co.

Wang, V.L., Terry, P., Flynn, B.S., et al.: Multiple indicators of continuing medical education priorities for chronic lung diseases in Appalachia, J. Med. Educ. **54**:803, 1979.

Weiss, C.H.: Evaluation research: methods of assessing program effectiveness, Englewood Cliffs, N.J., 1972, Prentice-Hall, Inc.

Windsor, R.A., Green, L.W., and Roseman, J.M.: Health promotion and maintenance for patients with chronic obstructive pulmonary disease: a review, J. Chronic Dis. **33**:5, 1980.

Zander, K.S., et al.: A practical manual for patient teaching, St. Louis, 1978, The C.V. Mosby Co.

PART TWO

Promoting community health

5

MATERNAL, INFANT, AND CHILD HEALTH

Their mother hearts beset with fears,
Their lives bound up in tender years.
Christina Rossetti

Promoting the health of a community means addressing the special health needs and the different health problems of the various segments within the population. Health problems of expectant mothers, infants, children, adults, and the aging have many things in common, but each category has special aspects of these common problems as well as unique problems. Community measures to promote the health of one group frequently will be applicable to the needs of other groups, but directing the community's attention to the specific needs of a particular population segment will assure the necessary measures to protect and promote the health and general well-being of that specific group.

Maternal, infant, and child health encompasses community preventive care issues for the potential mother and her condition before and after the delivery of the infant, the care of the infant and child, and the education of the public in immunization, dental care, nutrition, substance misuse, physical fitness, and stress in these maternal, infant, and child states. Special attention is given in this chapter to preventive health services and health promotion approaches that should be incorporated into prenatal care, such as proper nutrition and the avoidance of alcohol and drug consumption and smoking. Included in the discussion is a de-

scription of certain health care service programs and how their services relate to prenatal, infant, and child health needs. This chapter and subsequent ones also propose the establishment of specific high priority populations and problems for prevention and health promotion by setting forth a number of assumptions and objectives, together with research and data needs, that should increase the impact of community health promotion activities on problems in pregnancy, infant, and child care.

PROGRESS IN MATERNAL HEALTH PROMOTION

At the turn of the century, when the population in the United States was about 76 million, more than 20,000 women died in childbirth each year. Some 80 years later, with a population of more than 220 million, the yearly number of deaths of women resulting from complications of childbirth has been reduced to less than 400. The chances of a woman's surviving childbirth in the United States today are about 8,999 out of 9,000. This improvement in survival should continue.

Maternal mortality

Maternal deaths are those associated with deliveries and complications of pregnancy, childbirth, and puerperium. Rates are on a ba-

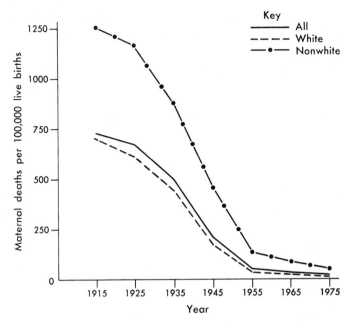

FIG. 5-1. Maternal mortality by race, United States, 1915-1975.

Data from Vital Statistics of the United States, vol. 2, 1976.

sis of 100,000 live births occurring in a given year to mothers of each age and racial group. The causes of maternal mortality have altered, reflecting the relative decline of hemorrhage, infection, and toxemia. Anesthetic misadventures are relatively more common now as other causes have decreased and as the number of patients receiving anesthesia for childbirth has increased. Paradoxically, advances in medicine have provided challenges in obstetrics. Patients with congenital heart disease as well as juvenile diabetics are now able to become pregnant, and their safe delivery demands skill. The contributions of abortion to maternal mortality have dramatically decreased with safe, legalized abortions in contrast to criminal, septic abortions.

Widespread availability of effective contraceptive techniques has reduced the number of unwanted pregnancies, which in turn has reduced maternal mortality. The radical changes in abortion laws and contraceptive use are the result of societal pressures to which public, ed-

ucation, and medicine have responded.

In 1977 in the United States there were fewer babies born to teenage women, partly because there are fewer teenage women. On the other hand, the actual birthrate among teenagers rose for the first time since 1970. The fertility rate rise was for the 18- to 19-year-old age group only. Fertility rates for teenagers under 18 fell.

Despite the fact that more teenagers in the United States used contraceptives in 1976 than in 1971, the number of pregnancies had increased in 1976, presumably because more teenage women were having sexual intercourse. It is estimated that 70% of teenage conceptions were unplanned, and 46% of teenage births were unplanned.

For teenagers 14 and under, the fertility rate was 2.0 per 1,000, and the abortion rate was 2.2 per 1,000 in the United States. For those 15 to 17, the fertility rate was 34.5 per 1,000, and the abortion rate was 21.9 per 1,000. For those 18 to 19, the fertility rate was

82.2 per 1,000, and the abortion rate was 45.0 per 1,000. Rates of repeat pregnancies in teenagers who have had a first out-of-wedlock conception decreased by 40% between 1971 and 1976. For teenagers whose first pregnancies ended in abortion, the percentage of those who became pregnant again in 2 years fell from 67% to 24%.

DES daughters are those women who were exposed to the drug diethylstilbestrol when their mothers took the drug before their birth. DES was prescribed from the 1940s into the 1970s for women with pregnancy complications. In addition to being at increased risk of cancer of the vagina and cervix, DES daughters are also more likely to have problems in their pregnancies. The rate of unfavorable birth outcomes for a group of women exposed to DES was about one and three quarters that of a control group of women, where *unfavorable birth outcome* was defined as a miscarriage, a stillbirth, or an ectopic pregnancy. Out of groups of 220 exposed women and 224 unexposed women, 83 (38%) of the DES-exposed women had unfavorable outcomes, two thirds of which were miscarriages.

Pregnancy is no longer the leading cause of school dropouts, which it was prior to 1975. Women now have choices available in planning for children by means of contraception, terminating unwanted pregnancies by abortion, continuation of schooling during and following pregnancy, and antenatal services for safe delivery. The community role lies in making potential users of these options aware of them and counseling as to appropriate choice. Early and reliable pregnancy testing is now available. This is important, because antenatal care should be sought early in pregnancy, preferably during the first 3 months.

Legal abortions

Safety of abortions is closely correlated with the stage of pregnancy; abortion performed at less than 12 weeks of gestation, when suction curettage is used, is very safe, with a mortality of only one tenth of the low rate prevailing at term delivery.

Of the 3,105 counties in the United States, only 718 have physicians or medical facilities providing abortions, according to a study released in 1980 from the Alan Guttmacher Institute. Over 1 million women nationally who needed abortions in 1977 were unable to get them in the counties they lived in, and about half of these women were unable to get them at all.

Even in counties that provide abortions, more than half of the women in need of abortion cannot get one in those counties. This is because in underserved areas the providers are often private physicians who do a few abortions for their own patients and are unwilling to do abortions for women they do not know.

Similar problems exist between countries in Europe and Latin America. For example, over 3,000 women from Ireland cross the Irish Sea each year to receive abortions in England because they cannot obtain them in Ireland.

The women least adequately served in the United States are those living in rural areas and those who are Medicaid-eligible women whose states no longer fund Medicaid abortions. Public and private hospitals do only 30% of abortions. Freestanding clinics handle most of the case load. Strategies to provide abortion services could include starting freestanding clinics in more populous regions, encouraging physicians in hospitals to provide the services, and establishing clinics in county hospitals, with satellite clinics providing services in smaller communities out from the main facility.

Direct means for promoting maternal health

Antenatal care emphasizes early detection of abnormalities and identification of the high-risk mother and infant. At the first visit a complete medical, surgical, and obstetrical history is obtained, and a physical examination is performed. Routine laboratory data are obtained, including blood type and rhesus factor determination; urinalysis; complete blood count; rubella titer; tests for syphilis, gonorrhea, and abnormalities of hemoglobin synthesis (sickle cell); and cervical smear. A social worker may interview the couple and discuss the community resources that are available. The antenatal visits provide an opportunity for education in health-related behavior, including dental care, avoidance or reduction of cigarette smoking, balanced exercise, and rest. A supportive, nonjudgmental, warm, sympathetic climate is maintained so that communication and cooperation is enhanced between patient and provider, and responsibility is shared. Precautions in the early stages of pregnancy include avoidance of infection, avoidance of exposure to irradiation, and avoidance of ingestion of drugs. These three factors contribute to congenital defects. Nutrition in pregnancy is most important, and the diet must contain adequate protein. Nutrition maintenance should be a continuum, with infancy, childhood, pregnancy, lactation, and geriatrics being special points along it. Women should be prepared for safe childbearing by adequate nutrition before pregnancy, rather than merely during it. Height of the mother is important, for taller women have larger pelvic bones, and as height falls below 5 feet the percentage of mothers experiencing difficulty in delivery resulting from pelvic problems increases sharply. Height is related to nutrition during the growth period, before the epiphyses close and bone growth ceases. Also important is nutrition in adolescence, after growth ceases but before pregnancy occurs, or preconception nutrition. Mothers who are normal or overweight have a better pregnancy outcome than those who are underweight.

High-risk pregnancies can be identified so that they can be given special care. Predictors are age, particularly under 15 or over 35 years; previous obstetrical difficulty such as unexplained stillbirths, premature deliveries, and abortions; and mothers who are under 60 inches in height or those who smoke a pack of cigarettes daily. Education for childbirth should start at school in human biology studies. During pregnancy the most effective education is in peer group sessions, when experienced mothers can lead others. The removal of fear is of greatest benefit, and attendance of fathers is of value in sharing. Visits to the delivery and newborn suites and meeting the staff are beneficial. Various professional and lay groups endorse different plans of preparation and practices during childbirth, but the common thread is of open discussion, question and answer, and removal of fear. Couples in such programs will enjoy the emotional experience of pregnancy and delivery. Recent studies have shown reductions in the amount of analgesia and anesthesia used by women who participated in childbirth classes, as well as shortened labor.

Perinatal mortality is the number of fetal deaths (stillbirths) from the twenty-eighth week of pregnancy plus the number of deaths in the first week of life per 1,000 live births (Fig. 5-2). This reproductive index makes up both intrauterine and extrauterine deaths and is a measure of the quality and efficiency of the obstetrical and neonatal services. Deaths that occur during this time span (currently, 15.4 per 1,000 live births) may be ascribed to hazards of the birth process. Perinatal mortality is most heavily influenced by the prematurity rate, which is the percentage of all babies born who weigh 2,500 grams or less (5 1/2 pounds). The survival of such infants is naturally lower than that of term-sized infants, mainly because the respiratory system of premature infants is not sufficiently mature to adapt to extrauterine life. Advances in neonatology, through the use of intensive care nurseries or prematurity centers, have been tremendous so that survival is improving for all birthweight ranges. Perinatal mortality is falling, but its decline is limited by the prematurity rate, which has remained constant since 1950 in the United States. It was thought that the prematurity rate would fall in response to improved social conditions, but a

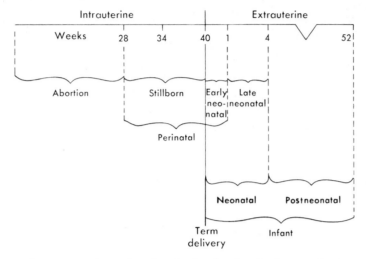

FIG. 5-2. Reproductive mortality is based on fetal and infant deaths in each of eight periods, some overlapping with others.

complex interaction of factors has been operating. A high proportion of births now derive from adolescent mothers and those in lower socioeconomic strata, and both these groups have increased prematurity rates. Mothers aged less than 15 years had a prematurity rate twice that of other mothers in 1977, and black babies were twice as likely as white babies to be born prematurely (16.1% and 7.4%, respectively). Risk factors for prematurity include (1) previous history of premature delivery, (2) age less than 15 years, (3) lower socioeconomic group, (4) height under 60 inches, (5) more than 15% underweight, and (6) a history of cigarette smoking. These factors are interrelated and are amenable to community influence in nutrition, in family planning, and in health education.

PROMOTING INFANT HEALTH

Infant mortality is the number of deaths occurring under 1 year of age per 1,000 live births. Deaths in the first week of life contribute both to perinatal and infant mortalities.

At the beginning of this century, about 100 of every 1,000 infants (10%) born in the United States died in the first year of life. This figure has progressively declined to reach 29.0 per 1,000 infants in 1950, 20.0 per 1,000 in 1970, 16.1 per 1,000 in 1975, and 13.0 per 1,000 in 1979. However, there remain large differences in infant death rates among subgroups of the population and between geographic areas. A black child is almost twice as likely to die before reaching 1 year of age than a white infant. Between 1975 and 1977, in Mississippi, the rate of infant deaths was 20.6 per 1,000 births, while in Maine the rate was 11.2 per 1,000.

Infant mortality can be divided into two components: (1) neonatal mortality, occurring in the first 28 days after birth, which largely reflects prenatal and perinatal circumstances and events and (2) postneonatal mortality, occurring between 28 days and 365 days of age, which is dependent on parenting and other aspects of the infant's environment (Fig. 5-2). Problems and intervention strategies differ between these two components. Pregnancy prevention, prenatal care with risk assessment and management, and newborn intensive care represent our major weapons to combat neonatal deaths. Parenting instruction, especially for

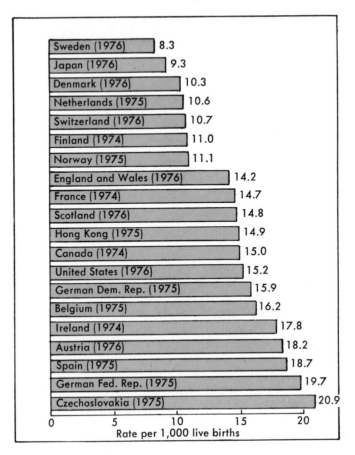

FIG. 5-3. Infant mortality, selected countries.

From World Health Organization: Demographic yearbook, Geneva, 1977; and National Center for Health Statistics, U.S. Department of Health and Human Services, 1980.

new mothers, including care and feeding of infants, illness surveillance and care, and use of pediatric services, is one technique to reduce postneonatal infant deaths. Neonatal mortality accounts for more than two thirds of infant death, and it is in this component that the largest gains are being made today. However, postneonatal problems will increase in priority if the currently successful trends in reducing neonatal mortality continue throughout the 1980s.

International comparisons of infant mortalities are often made (Fig. 5-3); however, it must be kept in mind that infant mortality in advanced countries is much influenced by deaths in the first month of life, which make up 80% of the deaths in the first year. This high proportion results from the reduction in deaths caused by infectious causes, which earlier in this century contributed to the high infant mortality (Fig. 5-4). Reduction of infant mortality depends now on reducing deaths immediately following birth. This in turn means reducing the prematurity rate. Countries that have low infant mortalities, for example, Norway and Sweden, have prematurity rates of

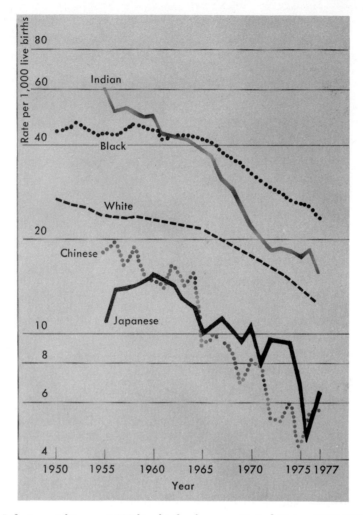

FIG. 5-4. Infant mortality per 1,000 live births, by race, United States, 1950-1977.

From National Center for Health Statistics, U.S. Department of Health and Human Services, 1980.

about 3% compared with 7.6% in the United States (6.1% for whites, 13.3% for blacks). Weight for weight, babies have a higher survival rate in the United States than in any other country because of advanced neonatology. But the United States must contend with relatively more low birth weight babies, which adversely affects reproductive indexes. Improvements will also stem from reduction in the needless waste of infant lives caused by ac-

cidents and by infectious diseases. Community action is effective here in providing a safe environment by legislation; immunization programs; reduction of burns, traffic accidents, alcoholism, and child abuse; and education of mothers to bring their children to a physician early in illness when infectious disease may be successfully treated. Adequate provision of community resources to provide alternate child care facilities for working mothers is imperative.

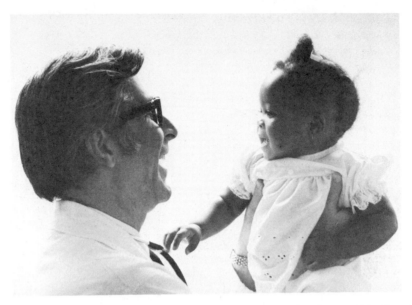

FIG. 5-5. Child health promotion. The health department medical and nursing staff conducts routine and special examinations of well children in ambulatory clinics.

Courtesy Johns Hopkins Medical Institutions.

COMMUNITY HEALTH PROGRAMS FOR CHILDREN

Basic health services for the prevention of disease and the early identification of illness or disability should be available to all children. Well-child clinics providing assessment of growth and development, nutrition, nurturing and anticipatory guidance, and immunization for all children should be available. Well-child care at regular intervals may be performed by allied health personnel other than physicians. Competent pediatric nurse practitioners, experienced public health nurses, and all physician's assistants working in tandem with psychologists and educators can assess the progress of a child, interpreting these steps and the next to be expected for the person caring for the child.

Fostering the mother-infant bonding and using anticipatory guidance to prevent problems will enable the child to grow up in a healthy and well-structured atmosphere. Early recognition of social and psychological components will permit early and simple correction of adverse circumstances.

Basic health services with well-child clinics should also include an immunization program.

Immunization programs and procedures

Many infectious diseases stimulate the production of protective antibodies that usually confer long-lasting, even lifelong, protection against reinfection. Vaccines and toxoids stimulate production of these antibodies without disease. At present there are eight diseases for which routine vaccination is widely recommended in the United States: seven (diphtheria, measles, mumps, pertussis, polio, rubella, and tetanus) through vaccination of all children in the first years of life (annual birth cohort, approximately 3 million), and one (influenza) through routine annual vaccination of individuals at high risk of complication or death from influenza infection (approximately 40 million people, mostly over 65 years of age).

Decisions to recommend routine use of immunizing agents are typically based on the risk of acquiring the disease, the severity of the disease or its consequences, the efficacy of the vaccine, the safety of the vaccine, and the number of doses required for initial immunization or boosters.

From the 1950s through the mid-1970s remarkable progress was made in the reduction of vaccine-preventable diseases throughout the world. Immunization programs historically focused primarily on the protection of children against the childhood diseases, which only 30 years ago produced extensive mortality and residual disability even in the most advanced countries. In the United States the 1955 Poliomyelitis Vaccine Assistance Act, later expanded by the Vaccine Assistance Act of 1962, supported extensive growth in state-level programs, providing all children with immunizations against the major childhood vaccine-preventable diseases. As more vaccines were developed, the list of diseases to be combated was expanded, and the number of reported cases fell as the vaccines came into wide use. As the disease incidence fell, however, efforts to immunize all children did not receive the priority they warranted, and levels of immunity to many of these diseases among children crested and, in some places, declined.

A nationwide immunization campaign in the United States was announced in 1977 with the goal of raising the immunization level of children fully protected against these diseases from an estimated 60% to 90% by the fall of 1979. Particular attention was paid to the gap between immunization levels in affluent communities and those in low-income areas and to the differences in levels between school-age and preschool children.

To remedy these problems and achieve this goal, the U.S. Department of Health, Education, and Welfare (now the Department of Health and Human Services) contracted with various organizations, stepped up the emphasis on improved immunization levels for users of grant-supported primary care facilities serving low-income populations, and launched a national outreach and education effort to encourage immunization. Organized professional groups, such as the American Academy of Pediatrics, the American Academy of Family Practice, the National Medical Association, the National League of Nursing, and the American Hospital Association all made substantial contributions to this effort. Local chapters of such voluntary groups as the National Council of Negro Women, the General Federation of Women's Clubs, the Parent-Teacher Association, and the American Red Cross participated extensively at the local chapter level. Organized sports provided publicity, with the National Basketball Association, the National Football League, and Major League Baseball donating time for immunization messages during broadcasts of games. Business helped also. McDonald's Restaurants, for example, took on childhood immunization as a special project. The AFL-CIO launched an education campaign among its membership, and school systems in many states have stepped up enforcement of school entry immunization laws and have expanded the requirements to include more diseases. For example, the number of states requiring immunity from mumps increased from 2 in 1977 to 18 in 1979, and 5 states enacted school immunization laws for the first time during the same period. Today all 50 states have school immunization statutes that will help ensure that all U.S. children are protected against vaccine-preventable childhood diseases.

The support of all of these groups has produced progress. Of the 24 million children in kindergarten through eighth grade in the United States, 91% are immunized. Of those newly entering school in the fall of 1980, 92% had been immunized against measles, 89% against rubella, 81% against mumps, 95% against polio, and 96% against diptheria, pertussis, tetanus (DPT), versus immunization levels ranging from 66% to 75% in 1977. Cases of these diseases have also declined in number. The Surgeon General of the U.S. Public

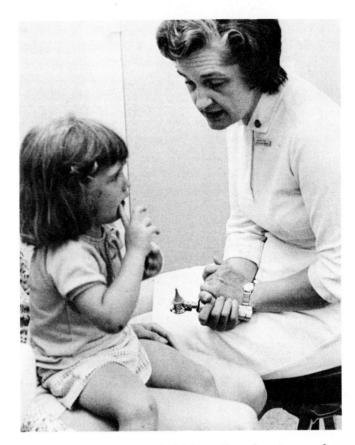

FIG. 5-6. Health education for parents and children. Clinical settings tend to maximize the quality but minimize the quantity of information effectively transmitted.

Courtesy Johns Hopkins Medical Institutions.

TABLE 5-1. Recommended schedule of active immunizations for normal infants and children

Age	Diphtheria, pertussis, tetanus*	Polio	Measles†	Rubella†	Mumps†
2 months	X	X			
4 months	X	X			
6 months	X	X (optional)			
15 months			X	X	X
18 months	X	X			
4-6 years	X	X			

*Children should receive a sixth tetanus-diphtheria injection (booster) at age 14 to 16 years and every 10 years thereafter.
†Measles, rubella, and mumps vaccines can be given in a combined form at about 15 months of age with a single injection.

Health Service has set forth the following objectives for 1990:

- To have 90% of all children complete the basic set of recommended immunizations.
- To have 95% of all children in all grades of schools or licensed preschool settings immunized.
- To improve the reporting of childhood diseases to better track the incidence of outbreaks.

The generally recommended age to begin routine immunizations is 2 months. The first vaccines given are diphtheria and tetanus toxoids combined with pertussis vaccine, or DTP, in addition to trivalent oral poliovirus vaccine, TOPV. Measles vaccine for rubeola is most effective when given after 1 year of age because all maternal transplacental antibody has been catabolized by then. In some populations where natural measles occurs frequently in the first year of life, it is indicated to administer the rubeola vaccine as early as 6 months of age. If this is necessary in this community, a repeat dose of measles vaccine should then be given after the age of 1 year to immunize any infants whose earlier vaccine response had been blocked by passive immunity (Table 5-1).

Selected screening programs

Screening for tuberculosis prior to rubeola vaccine should be performed routinely. In addition, a hematocrit for anemia during the first 6 months of life should be done on all children. This is particularly important in the small birth weight infant who has grown quickly.

Other diseases to be screened for depend on the community and the population at risk. Thus screening for sickle cell anemia, Tay-Sachs disease, thalassemia, and other genetic diseases should be done if the population is of the appropriate ethnic origin.

Screening should be carefully performed for illness prior to placement in day-care centers or prenursery school situations. It should be repeated again for the preschool physical examination, and hearing, speech, and eye examinations should be performed. Routine screening for these conditions can be performed by trained paramedical personnel. Dental evaluation and fluoride therapy for the prevention of caries are also necessary.

School health education programs

Education programs within the school setting aimed at preparing children for parenthood as well as their personal hygiene, nutrition, and sexuality should be instituted on a community-wide basis. The cooperation of the schools should be sought, since children are a captive audience during their school hours. Furthermore, attendance of parents at school functions enables an extension of health education to the family.

Children and youth are healthier today than ever before, certainly as measured by the usual morbidity and mortality indicators. Today, however, there are different threats to the health of children and youth, often characterized as the "new morbidity," for which environmental (social, physical, familial, and economic) and behavioral factors have been identified as causative or contributive. Some special childhood problems of concern to those who will work with these age groups are learning disorders, inadequate school functioning, behavioral problems, speech and vision difficulties, mental retardation, child abuse and neglect, and accidents and injuries. For youth, the principal threats to health are violent death and injury, abuse and neglect, alcohol and drug misuse, unwanted pregnancies, sexually transmissible diseases, and the environment. Adolescents experience unique health problems, and our traditional indexes do not represent well the nature of their problems. Limited attention has been given by the health care sector to this age group, as will be seen in the next chapter.

Characteristics developed during childhood can lead to adult diseases and disability. As many as 40% of youth ages 11 to 14 are now estimated to have already present one or more of the risk factors associated with heart disease (U.S. Department of Health, Education, and Welfare, Public Health Service, 1979b). Most of these were developing at earlier ages in the home and through health habits.

It is the family that has profound effects on the health and educational status of its members. The national goals to improve the health of children and youth and to prevent consequences of the "new morbidity" are highly dependent for their achievement on the familial environment. But the family is no longer seen as the sole agent of children's socialization; the emerging understanding is that both the child and the family are affected by every institution of society. With the focus now on children in context, living in a complex world of family interactions and societal forces, attention to the impact of families and school on children's health will make children targeted units for delivery of health and educational services.

The Surgeon General's report (U.S. Department of Health, Education, and Welfare, Public Health Service, 1979a), identifying strategies for better health for children and youth, recognized the potential and relatively untapped role of families and schools. More than 40 million U.S. children and youth spend most of the day in school, and "No group is more able than schoolteachers to provide information and instruction that can help young people make decisions that promote good health and prevent disease." In regard to the family, the Surgeon General's report viewed the role of parents as "critical." Parents enhance the opportunities for their children's health by fostering healthy personal habits and by ensuring availability and use of appropriate childhood health services.

The dramatic shift in child and youth health priorities suggests the need for the reassessment of health strategies—services and policies organized around the enhancement of health and the prevention of disease. The chal-

lenge for schools to participate in future programs in child health has been eloquently stated (U.S. Department of Health, Education, and Welfare, Public Health Service, 1979a).

Health services for chronic disease and disorders

Special health services for chronic disease and disorders such as cerebral palsy, epilepsy, and congenital malformations require careful planning within the community. Different health professionals need to be involved, and continuity as well as comprehensiveness of care are essential to prepare the child for the best quality of life possible. Much of the care may be provided by nonmedical providers, particularly in the school setting and in other areas in the community. Unfortunately, because of the large number of programs that provide services for problems, obtaining care may reveal a frustrating maze. Many programs provide only parts of the full care needs for each child, and each program may have different eligibility rules as well as a separate point of entry that is often difficult to locate.

In complicated congenital deformities, such as meningomyelocele, children frequently require the services of more than one program or need a service that is not provided within the community in which they live. There is no greater deterrent to the effective and efficient care of children with chronic disease than the fragmentation of services as a result of the isolation of categorical programs.

Clinics that are aimed at the physically handicapped, with all the related physiotherapy and educational needs provided for in that particular child, may not be adaptable for children with straightforward educational problems lacking the physical components.

Habilitation programs for an orthopedic deformity may not be available for children damaged by trauma. Again, the fusing eligibility and elimination rules may result in children slipping between the cracks of programs that are narrowly categorical.

Organization

During the past 40 years in the United States many programs have been developed by the federal government and by the states to provide some health services for children. These programs have had a major role in improving the health of the nation's children. There is general agreement that for a number of reasons some of them are now less effective. The federal Maternal and Child Health (MCH) and Crippled Children's Services (CCS) programs of Title V of the Social Security Act were created in 1935 to provide national leadership in the field of maternal health and child health and to direct the state Maternal and Child Health and state Crippled Children's programs. Thus the state Maternal and Child Health programs remain the major providers of basic health services for mothers and children, and the state Crippled Children's programs remain the major public system for providing services for children who require special health services for chronic diseases and disorders. The legislation that created these programs did not relate them to community health programs as needed to provide a direct patient service. Other categorical programs created by Congress have independent organizational structure at the federal, state, and community level, that is, Title I programs, the Developmental Disabilities program, and the Early and Periodic Screening, Diagnosis and Treatment (EPSDT) program. Some of these function at the national, state, and community level parallel to, or even in open competition with, each other and with the MCH and CCS programs. The result is a duplication of services, inefficiencies in administration, and increased costs. More importantly, the fragmentation of service results in some children receiving suboptimum care or not receiving needed services.

Mental retardation and mental health programs

Different states and different communities have tried to approach the mental retardation programs with special units for the identification and care of such children. Mental health programs frequently dovetail into the adult services and may function through the schools.

Health-related services

Psychological services may be obtained through mental health programs or the school system. It is the responsibility of each community to determine the organization of its community child center. The services offered in such a center should be strongly influenced by national and state or provincial goals, but services offered should be determined by the community after careful study of that community's needs. The organization of the community child center should be the responsibility of the community itself. Thus the number and type of health services provided in such centers will vary a great deal. Services, for example, for the protection of the juvenile, the management of teenage pregnancy and abortion counseling, and sexually transmitted disease programs should be available for all children who need them.

U.S. OBJECTIVES FOR CHILD HEALTH BY 1990

Death rates of children (Fig. 5-7) do not tell the entire story of child health in the United States, but certainly a knowledge of what causes deaths at the various ages of childhood should be of benefit in any community health program. Specific death rates point out where specific emphasis must be placed if we are to save the lives of our children. Comparisons between selected countries (Fig. 5-3 and Fig. 5-8) indicate the potential for improvement. Tables for one particular year do not necessarily represent the exact picture for all years, yet the 1976 experience of the United States is fairly typical of the years from 1950 to the present for most English-speaking countries. While the rates from year to year shift slightly, the general relative positions of the various causes of

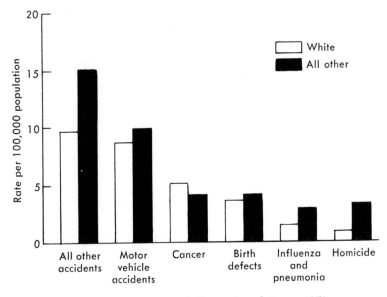

FIG. 5-7. Six leading causes of mortality for children, United States, 1976.

Based on data from the National Center for Health Statistics, Division of Vital Statistics, U.S. Department of Health and Human Services.

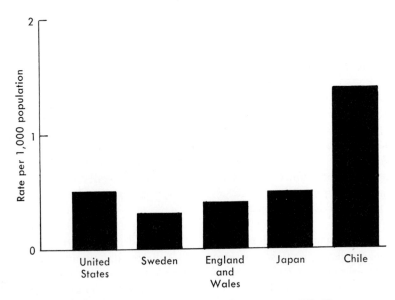

FIG. 5-8. Death rates for ages 1 to 14 years, selected countries, 1975. The most recent year of data for Chile is 1971.

Data from National Center for Health Statistics, Division of Vital Statistics, U.S. Department of Health and Human Services; and the United Nations.

death have remained quite constant during this period.

To say that all of these deaths could have been prevented would be unrealistic, but to say that at least half of them could have been prevented with our present knowledge and means would be a reasonable appraisal. Certainly accidental deaths, which loom so prominently in the statistics of childhood, can be reduced materially. Deaths from infectious diseases can be controlled better than is indicated in the statistics. The health of mothers and children in all countries can be further improved, and the death rates for this group should be reduced as follows.

Improved health status

- By 1990 infant mortality (deaths for all babies up to 1 year of age) should be reduced to no more than 9.0 deaths per 1,000 live births. (In 1978 infant mortality in the United States was 13.8 per 1,000 live births.)
- By 1990 no racial or ethnic group should have infant mortality in excess of 12.0 deaths per 1,000 live births. (In 1978 infant mortality in the United States for blacks was 23.1 per 1,000 live births and for American Indians, 13.7 per 1,000 live births. The rates for Hispanics are not yet separately available.)
- By 1990 the neonatal death rate (deaths for all babies up to 28 days old) should be reduced to no more than 6.5 deaths per 1,000 live births. (In 1978 the neonatal death rate was 9.5 per 1,000 live births in the United States.)
- By 1990 the perinatal death rate (late fetal deaths plus infant deaths up to 7 days old) should be reduced to no more than 5.5 per 1,000.* (In 1977 the perinatal death rate was 15.4 per 1,000 in the United States.)

*The perinatal death rate is expressed in terms of late fetal deaths plus live births.

- By 1990 maternal mortality should not exceed 5.0 per 1,000 live births for any ethnic group (black and Hispanic) and any community. (In 1978 the overall rate in the United States was 9.6; the rate for blacks was 25.0, more than three times the rate for whites, which was 6.4; the rate for American Indians was 12.1; the rate for Hispanics is not yet separately available.)
- By 1985 the incidence of neural tube defects should be reduced to 1.0 per 1,000 live births (In 1979 the rate was 1.7 per 1,000 in the United States.)
- By 1990 rhesus hemolytic disease of the newborn should be reduced to below a level of 1.3 per 1,000 live births (In 1977 there were 1.8 per 1,000 in the United States.)
- By 1990 the proportion of pregnant women with iron deficiency (low hemoglobin) should be reduced to 3.5%. (In 1978 the proportion was 7.7% in the United States.)
- By 1990 low birth weight babies (2,500 grams and under) should constitute no more than 5.0% of all live births. (In 1977 in the United States they constituted 7.1% of all births—12.8% of black births and 5.9% of white births.)
- By 1990 growth retardation of infants and children caused by restricted access to food should have been eliminated. (In 1972 to 1978 it was estimated that 10% to 15% of infants and children in the United States suffered growth retardation due to diet inadequacies.)

Reduced risk factors

- By 1990 no ethnic group of the population (black and Hispanic) and no county should have a rate of low birth weight infants (prematurely born and small-for-age infants weighing less than 2,500 grams) that exceeds 9.0% of all live births. (In 1978 in the United States the rate for whites was about 5.9%, and for blacks about 12.9%;

the rate for American Indians was 6.7%; the rate for Hispanics is not yet separately available from national data. The rate for some other nations is 5.0% and less.)

- By 1990 the proportion of women who breast-feed their babies at hospital discharge should be increased to 75%. (In 1975 in the United States the proportion was 35%.)
- By 1990 the majority of infants should leave hospitals in car safety carriers (Baseline data are unavailable. See also objectives for communicable disease control [Chapter 10], community safety and injury control [Chapter 11], and life-style and community health promotion [Chapter 12]).

Increased public-professional awareness

- By 1990 85% of women of childbearing age should be able to choose foods wisely (state special nutritional needs of pregnancy) and understand the hazards of smoking, alcohol, pharmaceutical products, and other drugs during pregnancy and lactation. (Baseline data are unavailable. See also Chapters 10 and 12.)

Improved services-protection

- By 1990 virtually all women and infants should be served by a regionalized system of primary, secondary, and tertiary care for prenatal, maternal, and perinatal health services. (In 1979 in the United States approximately 400,000 (12%) births occurred in geographical areas served by such a system.)
- By 1990 90% of women in ethnic groups (black and Hispanic) and in any community should obtain prenatal care during the first trimester of pregnancy. (In 1978 in the United States 40% of black mothers and 50% of American Indian mothers received prenatal care during the first trimester. The percent of Hispanics is unknown.)

- By 1990 virtually all pregnant women aged 35 and older and others at high risk of congenital fetal damage should have access to information on amniocentesis and prenatal chromosomal diagnosis, as well as therapy, as indicated. (In 1978 about 10% of women aged 35 and over underwent amniocentesis in the United States.)
- By 1990 all pregnant women at high risk of having a fetus with a condition diagnosable in utero should have access to information on amniocentesis and prenatal chromosomal diagnosis, as well as therapy as indicated. (Baseline data are unavailable.)
- By 1990 all women who give birth should have appropriately attended safe care, provided in ways acceptable to them and their families. (In 1977 less than 0.3% of births in the United States were unattended by a physician or midwife.)
- By 1990 all newborns should be provided neonatal screening for metabolic disorders for which effective and efficient tests and treatments are available (e.g., phenylketonuria [PKU] and congenital hypothyroidism). (In 1978 about 75% of newborns in the United States were screened for PKU; about 3% were screened for hypothyroidism in the early 1970s, with the rate now rapidly increasing.)
- By 1990 virtually all infants and their families should be able to participate in primary health care that includes well-child care, screening, diagnosis, and treatment for conditions requiring special services; counseling to families in parenting and child development; nutrition; immunization; automobile safety; and other accident prevention, including poisoning. (Baseline data are unavailable.)
- By 1990 all states or provinces should require comprehensive school health education at elementary and secondary levels, including nutrition education. (In 1979 in the United States only five states required

comprehensive school health education, with course content determined by grade level. Only 10 states mandate nutrition as a core content area. See also Chapters 10 and 12.)

Improved surveillance-evaluation systems

- By 1990 a system should exist for comprehensive and longitudinal assessment of the impact of a range of prenatal factors on infant and child physical and psychological development (e.g., maternal exposure to radiation, ultrasound, dramatic changes in temperature, toxic agents, smoking, alcohol, exercise, drugs, and stress).
- By 1990 a comprehensive, national nutrition status monitoring system should be operative to provide yearly detection of nutritional problems for certain population groups, as well as baseline data for decisions on national nutrition policies.

• • •

At the community level, these national objectives must be adapted to local circumstances. Model standards for community objectives and actions in maternal and child health are suggested in the following standards tables (pp. 124-135). Dates for their accomplishment are left open to be adjusted according to priorities and resources available in a given community.

Text continued on p. 136.

MATERNAL AND CHILD HEALTH (MCH) OBJECTIVES AND ACTIONS FOR COMMUNITIES*

GOALS:
1. The MCH-related morbidity and mortality statistics for any community will not exceed those for the nation by more than 10%.
2. Every expectant mother will maintain good health, learn the art of child care, and bear a normal infant.
3. All women capable of bearing children will participate in a comprehensive health program that emphasizes preventive care for themselves and their families.
4. All infants, children, and youth will participate in a comprehensive health program that emphasizes preventive care.
5. Child abuse and neglect will be eliminated.
6. The incidence of preventable injuries and deaths occurring among children will be reduced.
7. All children, including those with chronic handicaps, will function at their optimum level.

Focus	Objectives	Indicators	Population in need
	Outcomes in health status		
MCH general	1. By 19___ MCH mortality and morbidity statistics for ethnic, socioeconomic, or geographic subgroups within the community will not exceed those of the entire community by more than 20%.	MCH morbidity and mortality statistics both for the community and for ethnic, cultural, and racial subgroups within the community	All infants, children and youth, and women capable of bearing children (from the time of menstruation)
Maternal and perinatal health	2. By 19___ the number of unplanned pregnancies will represent less than ___% of all pregnancies. (See table on pp. 134 and 135 for further detail on family planning.)	a. Total births by age, race, and marital status of mother b. Unwanted births by age, race, and marital status of mother c. Children put up for adoption within 12 months of birth d. Elective abortions by age, race, and marital status of mother e. Women practicing contraception (childbearing age, exposed to pregnancy)	All pregnant women
Maternal and perinatal health	3. By 19___ pregnant women with toxemia will not exceed 2% of all pregnant women in the community.	Toxemia of pregnancy rate for the community	All pregnant women
	3a. By 19___ there will be 0 septic abortions occurring in the community.	Number of septic abortions	
	3b. By 19___ the number of infants born weighing less than 2500 grams will not exceed 7% of the total.	Rate of low birth weight	All neonates

Infant and child health	4. By 19___ infant mortality will not exceed 10 per 1,000 live births.	Number of live births and number of deaths in first year	All infants
	4a. By 19___ all groups of children will grow according to established norms. NOTE: *Percentile growth curves on populations of children are one of the best readily available measures of their health. In a population that conforms to a standard distribution of height, short children are not necessarily less healthy than tall ones. But a population that is skewed toward shortness is suspect for growth stunting from such conditions as prevalent chronic infection (e.g., intestinal parasitism) or undernutrition.*	Growth charts for groups of children in the community	Children
Childhood injury control	5. By 19___ the incidence of childhood injuries, including home burns, poisoning, plumbism, and traumatic deaths, will be no greater than ___.	Injury incidence	Children
Childhood vaccine-preventable disease	6. By 19___ the incidence of ___†, or the absence of disease will be maintained.	a. Incidence b. Secondary spread	Children
Rhesus hemolytic disease	7. By 19___ rhesus hemolytic disease will be eliminated.	Incidence of rhesus hemolytic disease	Rh negative women
Birth defects, mental retardation, and genetic diseases	8. By 19___ drug-caused and environmentally caused birth defects, mental retardation, and genetic diseases will not exceed ___.	Incidence of drug-induced and environmentally induced birth defects	Women capable of bearing children (from the time of menstruation)
Process (actions and services)			
Women's health services	9. By 19___ the community will be served by an identifiable organized program of health care, including dental care, directed toward women and children, including necessary financial assistance for eligible individuals.	Existence of the program	All infants, children and youth, and women capable of bearing children (from time of menstruation)

*Based on model standards for community preventive health services, Washington, D.C., 1979, Centers for Disease Control, U.S. Department of Health and Human Services.

†Insert name of each officially designated vaccine preventable disease.

Continued.

MATERNAL AND CHILD HEALTH (MCH) OBJECTIVES AND ACTIONS FOR COMMUNITIES—cont'd

Focus	Objectives	Indicators	Population in need
Women's health services—cont'd	9a. By 19___ population subgroups whose morbidity and mortality statistics exceed those of the community by more than 20% will participate in comprehensive health service programs that address social and environmental as well as medical needs.	Extent of subgroup enrollment in such programs	Subgroups whose morbidity and mortality indicators exceed those of the community by more than 20%
	9b. By 19___ the community will have access (within 30 minutes for 70% of the population) to preconceptional, prenatal, intrapartum, and postpartum services.	a. Availability and accessibility of preconceptional, prenatal, intrapartum, and postpartum services b. Transport time to the nearest services site by the population in need of such services	All neonates and women capable of bearing children
	9c. By 19___ confidential pregnancy testing and counseling services will be available to all women in the community who wish to have such services.	Availability of services	All women of childbearing age
Genetic services	10. By 19___ the community will have access to a voluntary program of genetic services.	Availability of program	The community
Prenatal services	11. By 19___ at least 90% of pregnant women in the community will be receiving prenatal care during the first trimester of pregnancy, and 95% by the end of the second trimester.	Percent of women receiving prenatal care during the first and second trimesters	All pregnant women
Delivery environment	12. By 19___ 100% of deliveries will be planned to be performed by trained attendants in an environment chosen by the family as conducive to healthy birth outcome.	a. Percent of deliveries that were not planned to be attended or that were attended by unlicensed personnel b. Satisfaction of mother and family with the delivery environment c. Delivery outcome audits according to delivery sites	All births

Maternal death reporting	13. By 19___ 100% of all maternal deaths associated with pregnancy and childbirth will be reported to an official health authority within 1 month of occurrence.	Percent of deaths from pregnancy and childbirth reported within 1 month of occurrence	The community
Breast self-examination	14. By 19___ 80% of women will be provided instructional information about breast self-examination techniques.	Percent of women who have been provided breast self-examination information	Women over age 15
Postnatal home visits	15. By 19___ every postpartum mother and her infant, not receiving direct services from a primary care provider, will receive at least one postnatal home visit.	Percent of mothers and infants in need of visit who receive one	Mothers and infants not under the direct supervision of primary care providers
Child health services	16. By 19___ 90% of all children in the community will participate in a system that assures access to a full spectrum of health services, including dental services.	Percent of children in the community enrolled in comprehensive health care systems (e.g., private care, comprehensive center, etc.)	All children and youth
Process			
Immunization	17. By 19___ at least 90% of the 2-year-old population will have completed primary immunization for the officially designated vaccine-preventable diseases, and 90% of 2- to 21-year-olds will have received appropriate immunization boosters.	Percent of children completely immunized	All children by age 2
Screening	18. By 19___ 80% of the children in the community will be screened for disorders of vision and hearing by 3 years of age (gross screening should occur in the first year) and, as appropriate, diagnosed and treated. (See table on p. 131 for additional objectives on screening.)	a. Percent of children screened b. Percent of positive screens who are diagnosed and treated	All children by age 3
Poison control	19. By 19___ the community will have access to a poison control center.	Demonstrable access to such a center	The community (particularly children and youth)
Injury control	20. By 19___ the community will be protected by the enforcement of housing and building codes that have been developed to improve the injury-related morbidity and mortality patterns of the children and youth.	a. Existence of codes b. Extent of code enforcement	The community

Continued.

MATERNAL AND CHILD HEALTH (MCH) OBJECTIVES AND ACTIONS FOR COMMUNITIES—cont'd

Focus	Objectives	Indicators	Population in need
Prevention of child abuse and neglect	21. By 19___ parenting programs, commencing in the primary grades and continuing through the twelfth grade, will be available to all students attending public and private schools.	Percentage of schools that have parenting classes in grades 5-12	Students in grades 5-12
	21a. By 19___ the community will be served by a system that encourages the reporting and follow-up of 100% of children subjected to child abuse.	a. Presence of system b. Comparison of reporting system statistics with the expected statistics for the community	The community
	21b. By 19___ emergency family placements and respite care services will be available to provide care to 100% of the children in need.	a. Presence of services b. Time required for placement	Children and youth
	21c. By 19___ support services, such as parent anonymous groups or other innovative approaches, will be accessible and their outcomes evaluated.	Availability and use of programs	Families in need
Parental bonding-attachment	22. By 19___ a parental and infant bonding-attachment program will be available in 100% of hospitals providing delivery services in the community.	Percent of hospitals providing intrapartum care, including supportive services to mothers who choose breastfeeding, rooming-in for mothers who choose it, and early supportive contact between parents and newborn infants	All hospitals providing delivery services
Parenting skills	23. By 19___ programs that encourage foster parenting skills will be available for all parents or potential parents.	Availability and use of programs in schools, clinics, and other centers appropriate to both men and women	Parents and potential parents

SCHOOL HEALTH OBJECTIVES FOR COMMUNITIES*

GOAL: The school health program will be planned and implemented to ensure that each student and staff person is provided a healthful environment in which to work and study, together with needed preventive health services and health instruction.

Focus	Objectives	Indicators	Population in need
	Process (actions and services)		
Organization	1. By 19___ the official health agency or other appropriate governmental agency will ensure that necessary preventive health services for the school children are provided by the administration of the community schools, or, where services are not available, the appropriate governmental agency will provide them.	a. Statement of common goals and relative responsibility adopted by the school system and the official health agency or other appropriate governmental agency b. Availability of preventive health services (e.g., immunization services)	The community
	2. By 19___ the school district will designate a responsible official or functioning unit from within the school district or official health agency staff to be responsible for the planning, implementation, and evaluation of the district's school health program.	Designated official or unit	The school district
	3. By 19___ there will be a manual of policies governing the provision of health services, including health instruction, for each school in the community that has been approved by the responsible school administration and policy board.	Existence of manual	
Immunization	4. By 19___ the community's school system will establish, in accordance with appropriate state and local laws and medical–public health guidelines, requirements governing the minimum immunization status of its students against the officially designated vaccine-preventable diseases.	Existence of policy statement	

*Based on Model standards for community preventive health services, Washington, D.C., 1979, Centers for Disease Control, U.S. Department of Health and Human Services.

Continued.

SCHOOL HEALTH OBJECTIVES FOR COMMUNITIES—cont'd

Focus	Objectives	Indicators	Population in need
Immunization —cont'd	5. By 19___ and in each succeeding year, all school enterers will have complied with one of the following alternatives: a. 100% of primary and appropriate booster immunizations complete b. A remedial course to bring immunizations up to 100% has been initiated and certified by an appropriate provider c. Exemption for medical or religious reasons from immunization requirements	a. Percent of student body whose immunization has been recorded b. Percent of school enterers complying with criteria	All enterers to a school system
	6. By 19___ each school will have, and make use of, an area for isolation and observation of any ill child with a suspected communicable disease, pending exclusion or transfer to home or other facility.	a. Designated area b. Percent of schools with designated area	All schools
Health instruction	7. By 19___ the curriculum of the community's school system will include, as appropriate and at designated levels, material on the following: a. Growth and development of the human body b. Prevention of accidental injuries, and communicable, addictive, and environmentally caused diseases c. Chronic diseases and conditions d. First aid (e.g., cardiopulmonary resuscitation) e. The promotion of preventive health behavior through adequate nutrition, exercise, rest, and the establishment of a life-style conducive to good health and long life f. Sexual responsibility	a. Documentation that curriculum includes listed items b. Percent of classroom instruction time devoted to health c. A professionally trained health educator, at least at the district level	Each school system

	g. Appropriate use of the health care system (e.g., selection of health care provider, health care facility, and insurance)		
Screening	8. By 19___ 100% of children in the community will be screened, preferably before entry into school, to determine the existence of any conditions (including speech or perceptual handicaps) that may require special education services, and, as appropriate, be diagnosed and treated.	a. Percent of children screened b. Percent of positive screens who are diagnosed and treated	All preschool children in community
	9. By 19___ 100% of children who demonstrate school failure, truancy, underachievement, or discipline problems will receive a comprehensive health evaluation, including a psychosocial assessment.	Percent of children receiving such assessment	Children demonstrating school failure, underachievement, or discipline problems
	10. By 19___ all school children will be screened and referred for necessary diagnosis and treatment for deficient hearing and vision not less frequently than every 3 years during the elementary school years and on referral.	a. Existence of screening program b. Percent of children screened c. Percent of children referred for appropriate follow-up	All school children
School dental health	11. By 19___ all schools in the community's school system will have operational a comprehensive, prevention-oriented dental health program for 100% of school children. Elements of the program will include as appropriate to meet the particular needs of children of various ages the following: a. In fluoride-deficient areas, a fluoride mouthrinse or tablet regimen (NOTE: *Self-administered fluorides are not a substitute for either community or school fluoridation. Moreover, consideration should be given to a mouthrinse program even where community water supplies are fluoridated.*)	Existence of comprehensive, well-designed program	School children and parents

Continued

SCHOOL HEALTH OBJECTIVES FOR COMMUNITIES—cont'd

Focus	Objectives	Indicators	Population in need
School dental health—cont'd	b. Oral health assessments by a dental professional in combination with referrals for examination and treatment, and assistance in finding sources of dental care and financial support if needed c. Oral hygiene instruction and practice d. Dental health education for students and parents e. Dietary counseling for students and parents		
Cariogenic foods	12. By 19___ no highly cariogenic foods will be offered in any school food program or any vending machine in the community's schools.	Percent of highly cariogenic foods, such as those with excess sugar, available in the community's schools	School children and school personnel
Fluoridation	13. By 19___ all schools in the community's school system that are not served by a community water system and that enroll children who have fluoride-deficient drinking water at home will have fluoridated their water supplies and thereafter will regularly monitor and properly operate the fluoridation system to ensure that the optimum level of fluoride is maintained.	Existence of properly maintained fluoridation equipment	Children attending rural schools who have fluoride-deficient drinking water at home
Emergency services	14. By 19___ every school will have a procedure (including teacher orientation) known to all school personnel for the efficient handling of injuries and emergencies, including plans for the transfer of critically injured or ill children to an appropriate medical facility.	a. Existence of procedures b. Percent of teachers trained in emergency techniques	All schools
First aid	15. By 19___ there will be at least one person in each school designated to be responsible for first aid and necessary referral for sick or injured children.	Designated individual	School employees

Employee physicals	16. By 19___ all school employees will be required to submit evidence of their physical health, commensurate with their responsibilities, including freedom from active tuberculosis with employment.	Existence of policy concerning documentation of employee health	School employees
Health needs of the handicapped	17. By 19___ every school system will assure that the special health needs of the physically handicapped and special health needs of students with emotional, developmental or physical health problems, including pregnancy, are met.	Evidence of physical and programmatic adaptations and alternatives	Selected individuals in each school
Food service	18. By 19___ each school food service will comply with local and state codes for commercial food service and shall be regularly inspected by the health agency of jurisdiction.	a. Percent of schools in compliance b. Evidence of correction of deficiencies	All schools
Physical education and athletic safety	19. By 19___ the physical education and competitive athletic program of each school will include provision for the evaluation of each individual's appropriate level of participation, a plan for graduated conditioning, training in the prevention of injuries relevant to each type of activity, the provision of all appropriate safety equipment, and the handling of medical and dental emergencies, all in accordance with policies that have been reviewed and approved by the official health agency serving the community.	Percent of schools having evaluation policy	Students participating in school-sponsored athletics and physical education

FAMILY PLANNING OBJECTIVES AND MEASURES FOR COMMUNITIES*

GOAL: Pregnancy will occur by choice and under circumstances of lowest risk; the number of high-risk pregnancies will be reduced; unwanted fertility will be eliminated; and safe and efficacious fertility services will be available to persons desiring them.

Focus	Objectives	Indicators	Population in need
Family planning— general	**Outcomes (health status)**		
	1. By 19___ the number of unplanned pregnancies will represent less than ___ % of all pregnancies. NOTE: *The number of unplanned pregnancies can be estimated by survey or modeling techniques. One such model is described in "Actual Versus Desired Fertility," prepared by the Centers for Disease Control, 1978.*	a. Total births by age, race, and marital status of mother b. Unwanted births by age, race, and marital status of mother c. Children put up for adoption within 12 months of birth d. Elective abortions by age, race, and marital status of mother e. Women practicing contraception (childbearing age, exposed to pregnancy) (1) Within program (service statistics) (2) From all other sources (3) Prevalence of male and female sterilization	Women ages 12-44
	2. By 19___ high-risk pregnancies will be less than ___ % of all pregnancies.	Pregnancies in high-risk categories: a. Less than 18-year-old mother b. Greater than 35-year-old mother c. Less than 18 months between births d. Pregnancies out of wedlock e. Birth order greater than five f. Known genetic diseases g. Mother's health at risk (e.g., cardiac or renal problems) h. Fetal health at risk (e.g., maternal alcoholism or drug addiction, or employment in a hazardous occupation)	Women in categories a–h
	3. By 19___ the death-to-case rate from induced abortion will be less than ___ per 100,000 abortions.	a. Induced abortion–related deaths b. Percent of total abortions performed after twelfth week of pregnancy	Women obtaining induced abortions

Process (actions and services)

	Process (actions and services)		
Family planning information	4. By 19___ a mechanism will be in place in the community to inform all potential parents of the availability of community family planning resources.	a. Existence of mechanism b. Percent of adolescents exposed to information about existing family planning services c. Public service messages (tv, radio, newspapers, etc.) per year about family planning services d. Capacity in human service programs to refer clients to family planning services as appropriate	Men and women ages 12-44
	4a. By 19___ confidential pregnancy testing and counseling services will be available to all women in the community who wish to have such services.	Availability of services	Any women desiring services
	4b. By 19___ every facility with obstetrics capability (e.g., hospitals, ambulatory care centers, abortion clinics) will be providing information about family planning to all women terminating a pregnancy and, if possible, to their partners.	Percent of facilities with information programs	Women terminating pregnancies, and their partners
	4c. By 19___ the community will be served by an information program designed to a. Decrease the use of prescription high-dose oral contraceptives b. Decrease smoking among women who use oral contraceptives	Existence of program	The community
	5. By 19___ outreach capability will exist in the community to reach and make available services to all women who would enter the high-risk pregnancy group were they to become pregnant.	Agencies with identifiable outreach services (budget-personnel allocations)	Women in high-risk categories (a-h) and their partners

*Based on Model standards for community preventive health services, Washington, D.C., 1979, Public Health Service, U.S. Department of Health and Human Services.

SUMMARY

Maternal, infant, and child health are the foundation of community health promotion because they lay the base for health education, immunization, early diagnosis and treatment, and the development of health habits and "host resistance" upon which health in later years is built and sustained. In the spirit of disease prevention and health promotion, community maternal health is essential to successful infant health outcomes, which in turn provide the foundation for successful community health programs directed at children, youth, adults, and eventually the aged. Students or practitioners using this book are encouraged to review the status of their community by using the foregoing standards.

QUESTIONS AND EXERCISES

1. Why is death from puerperal sepsis virtually inexcusable at the present time?
2. Appraise this statement: The maternal health program is a phase of the general, overall community health program and not an independent program isolated from all other health measures.
3. Why is it desirable for a woman to have a premarital medical examination to determine her capacity for childbearing?
4. What is the reciprocal obligation of the expectant mother and society?
5. Why is the U.S. maternal mortality higher than New Zealand's even though obstetrics is just as far advanced in the United States as it is in New Zealand?
6. To what extent is legislation of benefit in maternal health promotion?
7. Appraise the economic factors in your community that are significant in maternal health.
8. Consider one of the leading causes of infant deaths and propose measures for reducing the number of infant deaths from this cause.
9. Where in the field of infant hygiene could time and funds for research be best invested?
10. Make an analysis of the causes of infant deaths in your county during the past 5 years and propose measures to improve the situation.
11. What are contributions of voluntary agencies to the infant health program in your community?
12. Propose a 5-year community program to educate parents in the advisability of taking apparently healthy children to their family physician, pediatrician, or child health clinic for a checkup at regular intervals.
13. What resources are available in your community for obtaining the correction of a defect in a child whose parents cannot afford the necessary services?
14. Evaluate this statement: The school assumes the role of the parent when it concerns itself with the pupil's health.
15. What official agencies are available in your community for helping a family with a child needing orthopedic services?
16. What nonofficial agencies are available in your community for helping a family with a child needing orthopedic services?
17. What are some of the special social and mental health problems associated with disability in childhood, and what is a community's responsibility in dealing with these by-products?
18. Take one or more of the objectives in the standards for community programs at the end of this chapter and determine an appropriate target date by using the indicators for your community.

BIBLIOGRAPHY

Albritton, R.B.: Cost-benefits of measles eradication, Policy Analysis 4(1):1, Winter, 1978.

American Academy of Pediatrics: The report of the Committee on Infectious Diseases, ed. 17, Evanston, Ill., 1974, The Academy.

Anderson, C.L., and Creswell, W.H.: School health practice, ed. 7, St. Louis, 1980, The C.V. Mosby Co.

Bruess, C.E., and Gay, J.E.: Implementing comprehensive school health, New York, 1978, Macmillan Publishing Co., Inc.

Chase, H.C.: Perinatal and infant mortality in the United States and six west European countries, Am. J. Public Health 57:1735, 1967.

Chinn, P.L.: Child health maintenance: concepts in family-centered care, ed. 2, St. Louis, 1979, The C.V. Mosby Co.

Cornacchia, H.J., and Staton, W.M.: Health in elementary schools, ed. 5, St. Louis, 1979, The C.V. Mosby Co.

Crawford, C.O.: Health and the family, New York, 1971, Macmillan Publishing Co., Inc.

Deutach, M., et al.: The disadvantaged child, New York, 1967, Basic Books, Inc., Publishers.

Ellis, R.W.B., and Mitchell, R.G.: Diseases in infancy and childhood, ed. 6, Baltimore, 1968, The Williams & Wilkins Co.

Fraser, G.R., and Friedman, A.I.: Causes of blindness in childhood, Baltimore, 1968, The Johns Hopkins Press.

Green, L.W., et al.: Guidelines for health education in maternal and child health, Int. J. Health Educ. Suppl. **21:**1, 1978.

Green, L.W., et al.: The school health curriculum project: its theory, practice, and measurement experience, Health Educ. Q. 7:14, 1980.

Iverson, D.C., editor: Promoting health through the schools: a challenge for the 80s, Health Educ. Q. 8:5, 1981.

Krugman, S., and Katz, S.L.: Infectious disease of children, ed. 7, St. Louis, 1981, The C.V. Mosby Co.

Levine M.I., and Seligman, J.H.: Your overweight child, New York, 1970, Hawthorn Books, Inc.

Mayshark, C., Shaw, D.D., and Best, W.H.: Administration of school health programs: its theory and practice, ed. 2, St. Louis, 1977, The C.V. Mosby Co.

University of Michigan School of Public Health: Comprehensive health care for children and families, Sixth Bi-Regional Conference, Ann Arbor, Mich., 1967.

U.S. Department of Health, Education, and Welfare, Public Health Service: Morbidity and Mortality Weekly Report 24(3):27, Jan. 18, 1975.

U.S. Department of Health, Education, and Welfare, Public Health Service: The Surgeon General's report on health promotion and disease prevention, background papers, Washington, D.C., 1979a, U.S. Government Printing Office.

U.S. Department of Health, Education, and Welfare, Public Health Service: The Surgeon General's report on health promotion and disease prevention, healthy people, Washington, D.C., 1979b, U.S. Government Printing Office.

U.S. Department of Health and Human Services: Promoting health, preventing disease: objectives for the nation, Washington, D.C., 1980, U.S. Government Printing Office.

U.S. Department of Health and Human Services: Better health for our children: a national strategy. The report of the Select Panel for the Promotion of Child Health, Washington, D.C., 1981, DHHS (PHS) Pub. No. 79-55071, 4 vols., U.S. Government Printing Office.

Whaley, L.F., and Wong, D.L.: Nursing care of infants and children, St. Louis, 1979, The C.V. Mosby Co.

World Heatlh Organization: Demographic yearbook, Geneva, 1979, The Organization.

Wynn, M., and Wynn, A.: The prevention of premature birth, London, 1977, Foundation for Education and Research in Childbearing.

6

ADOLESCENT AND ADULT HEALTH

Moderation in all things, but a binge of
something every day.

Anonymous

At the turn of the century, when the attention of the health professions was directed toward the prevention and control of communicable diseases, major emphasis was directed toward the child of school age. It soon became apparent that for proper control measures it would be necessary to go back to the preschool child. It then became obvious that the infant could not be neglected, and the child under the age of 1 year became the object of an intensive program of communicable disease prevention and control that soon expanded into an interest in all aspects of infant health. If everything possible was to be done for the infant, it would be necessary to consider prenatal factors, and this logically led to intensified efforts in maternal health.

With the advances in communicable disease control and the prevention of death in the early years of life, greater proportions of the population survived to adulthood and into old age. Now the chronic and degenerative diseases, usually most prevalent in adulthood, became the leading causes of death and disability. This shift in emphasis directed the attention of the health professions to the health of the adult population.

Adult health in the 1980s is a direct product

of the adolescent and child health of previous decades, from the historical perspective of primary prevention (see Chapters 1 and 5). From the epidemiological and ecological perspectives, adolescent and adult health are both products of the structure of communities and the distribution of community populations, and products of the cultural, social, organizational, economic, and technological forces that alter community environments (see Chapters 2 and 3). From the behavioral and educational perspectives, adolescent and adult health are products of all these things interacting with the attitudes, values, beliefs, and behavior of individuals (see Chapter 4). Fig. 6-1 summarizes these perspectives.

This chapter will work back from the current demographic and vital statistics on adults and adolescents to the alleged behavioral and environmental causes of social and health problems. From these social, epidemiological, and behavioral analyses (according to the model for community health diagnosis presented in Chapter 4) it should be possible to assess the prospects for health education and community health promotional programs that might alleviate some of these problems in the quality of life.

HISTORICAL AND DEVELOPMENTAL PERSPECTIVE (CHAPTERS 1 AND 5)

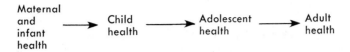

ECOLOGICAL AND EPIDEMIOLOGICAL PERSPECTIVE (CHAPTERS 2 AND 3)

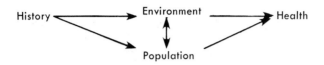

BEHAVIORAL AND EDUCATIONAL PERSPECTIVE (CHAPTER 4)

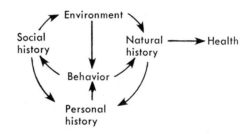

FIG. 6-1. The main features of the several perspectives from previous chapters are cumulative in their relevance to adolescent and adult health.

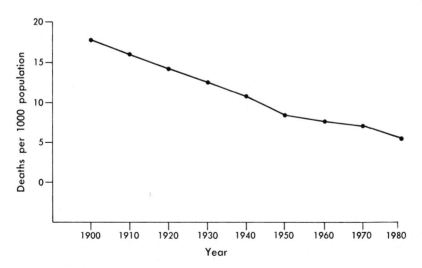

FIG. 6-2. Age-adjusted death rates, United States, 1900-1980.

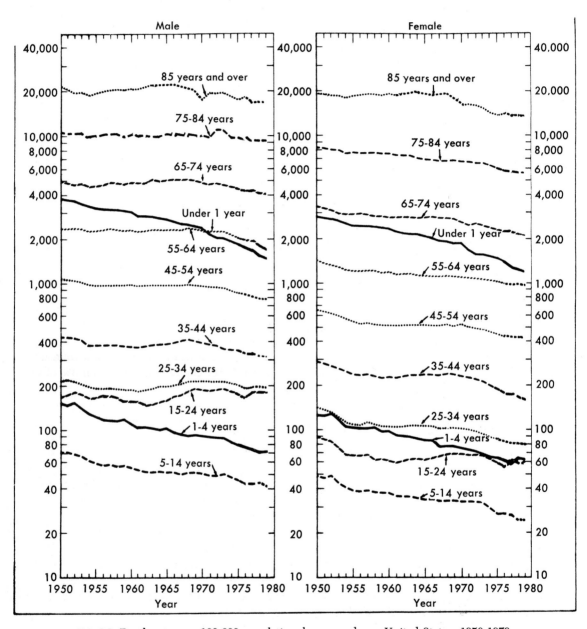

FIG. 6-3. Death rates per 100,000 population, by age and sex, United States, 1950-1979.

From U.S. Department of Health and Human Services.

DEMOGRAPHY OF HEALTH

The proportion of adolescents in most Western countries relative to the general population is on the decline, having reached a peak in the mid-1960s, as the postwar babies reached their teens. In 1976 the U.S. population estimates for the 10- to 19-year-old age group numbered some 42 million, or 19% of the population, but projections indicate that a steady decrease is expected to follow through the 1980s and beyond. The line between adolescent and young adult status is blurred by the lag between psychosocial and biological maturation. This makes it difficult to characterize the adolescent population by the usual developmental or chronological criteria.

People do not live longer than they did in 1900. At the turn of the century, some citizens attained the age of 100 years. Today, still less than 1% of the U.S. population reaches 100 years of age but over 10% is over 64 years of age, contrasted with 3.4% in 1880.

Fig. 6-2 shows the fall in age-adjusted death rates (such rates express most directly the probability of dying) from 1900 to 1980 in the United States. The rate of fall is decreasing, particularly in the adolescent and young adult age ranges, as shown in Fig. 6-3.

The recent increases in mortality among adolescents and young adults have been noted in other countries and have been attributed particularly to accidents, suicides, and homicides (approximately 70% of deaths of 12- to 17-year-olds in the United States). These increases will be shown in later sections to be caused in turn by another set of social, behavioral, and health problems, including alcohol and drug misuse, stress, and family disruption.

Even with the advance in postponing death and extending life expectation, the median age in the United States is only 29 years. It is expected to be 35.5 by 1999.

The ratio of females over males is increasing. The United States has 5 million more females than males. This excess is particularly noticeable in the older age groups so that among those over 64 there are only 722 males per 1,000 females. This discrepancy is the result of the higher death rates suffered by males in three of the leading causes of death—heart diseases, cancer, and accidents.

Certain economic, social, medical, educational, and community health problems are inherent in the changes in population, age distribution, and sex composition. Statistics on the causes of death and the incidence of various diseases of adults provide priorities that a guide to the adolescent and adult health programs should logically address.

PRINCIPAL CAUSES OF DEATH

According to the data in Fig. 6-4, the four leading causes of death in the United States now account for 72% of all deaths; over half of those are a result of cardiovascular disease. The 1979 list contrasts with causes of death prevailing in 1900, when influenza and pneumonia ranked first, tuberculosis second, heart disease third, and gastroenteritis fourth. The leading cause of death in 1900 is now relegated to sixth place, contributing less than 3% of total deaths, as opposed to 55% in 1900.

Significant as the decline in the general death rate for adults has been, of more immediate interest and value is an analysis of the principal causes of death at the present time. Such an analysis will be an aid in pointing out the particular health problems that exist in the adult age groups and the areas where special emphasis must be placed.

In all of the 11 leading causes of death (Fig. 6-4), measures of prevention now exist. It is estimated that at least 400,000 lives and $20 billion could be saved each year in the United States alone with proper application of these measures.

CARDIOVASCULAR DISEASE

Deaths in the United States in 1979 totaled 1,906,000, and 953,100 of them were from cardiovascular causes, a rate of 433 per 100,000 population. This rate peaked in 1963 and is

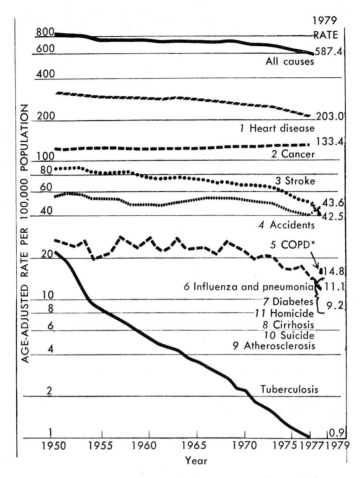

FIG. 6-4. Trends in the six leading causes of death in 1950 in the United States show major reductions in age-adjusted rates for heart disease, stroke, and the communicable diseases. Accidents have moved into third place, and a new set of chronic and violent causes of death have clustered in the top 11 causes of death with similar rates. The ranks *(1 to 11)* are based on numbers of deaths in 1979, which differ in rank from the age-adjusted rates shown by the trend lines.

From National Center for Health Statistics, U.S. Department of Health and Human Services.

now decreasing at more than 2% per year. Coronary (ischemic) heart disease is the greatest contributor, with two thirds of the cases, and stroke is responsible for one fifth. The common underlying pathological factor is atherosclerosis, a disorder of the blood vessels where the caliber of the vessel is narrowed and the elas-

ticity is decreased. This process is associated with aging, but the rapidity and the extent of involvement is extremely variable among different people. The resulting disease depends on which organ system is chiefly affected and how severely it is affected.

Heart disease continues to be the leading

cause of death in the United States, while cerebrovascular disease, or stroke, is the third leading cause of death (in number of deaths, fourth in age-adjusted death rates). For both these components of cardiovascular disease, the death rate has fallen dramatically since 1950. Between 1950 and 1970 the age-adjusted death rate for heart disease fell 18.0%, or an average of 1.0% every year. From 1970 to 1978 it declined another 18.0%, or approximately 2.5% each year. For stroke, the 1950 to 1970 decline was 25.0%, and the 1970 to 1978 decline, an additional 33.0%. These achievements can be attributed both to improvement in treatment of these conditions and to community health promotion activities that prevent and reduce their incidence.

Community action in reducing heart disease and deaths from stroke has a long history, during which the role of prevention has continually increased in emphasis compared with that of treatment. Major epidemiological studies conducted in the 1950s and 1960s have provided the evidence for defining the risk factors associated with heart disease and stroke and for developing intervention strategies that are associated with reduced morbidity. Smoking is one example. The 1964 U.S. Surgeon General's report on smoking and health was a bold step to address this major contributor to both heart disease and cancer. Efforts by communities to reduce smoking and the risks from smoking continue to expand and have produced positive results. Diet and obesity represent another area in which the U.S. government has continued to promote research and education. Management of high blood pressure is a third risk factor that warrants separate documentation in itself. With the identification of physical inactivity as a risk factor, communities began to promote the positive effects of physical fitness and activity. A recent national survey, for example, indicated that during 1979, 59% of adult Americans exercised regularly, and fewer adult males were smoking.

Coronary heart disease

Normal function of heart muscle is dependent on an adequate blood supply, which is provided by the coronary arteries. Narrowing of the caliber of these vessels is caused by deposits of cholesterol and fat beneath their inner lining. As the blood flow is consequently reduced, the patient may notice chest pain on exertion (angina pectoris). This condition may progress to fibrosis of the heart muscle, reduction of cardiac function, and ultimately, death. The narrowing of the coronary vessels may become so acute as to permit a blood clot (thrombus) to form, thus suddenly arresting the blood supply to a portion of the heart muscle. This is called a myocardial infarction, or heart attack, and results in the sudden death (within 2 hours) of the patient in almost one fourth of the cases. Two thirds of all heart attack victims survive their first attack, but of the fatalities 70% occur outside the hospital (that is, before the patient can reach the hospital).

Risk factors. Risk factors may be divided into modifiable (that is, those we can do something about) and nonmodifiable. Among the latter are age, sex, family history, and personality type.

1. Age. The incidence of heart attacks rises steeply from age 35 to 55 years and then falls as those susceptible to the disease are eliminated.

2. Sex. Males below 50 years of age are afflicted in a ratio of 4:1 compared to females. After 50 years of age the male excess is markedly reduced but still persists. This suggests some hormonal factor in the cause.

3. Family history. There is a strong familial tendency toward coronary heart disease, particularly on the male side. Families share many habits and customs of exercise, diet, and lifestyle; thus it is not clear whether this familial predisposition reflects a genetic or environmental cause.

4. Personality type. This is included as a nonmodifiable risk factor, for it has not been proved that it can be changed. People of a

striving, time-conscious pattern are labeled type A personality. They are involved in a chronic struggle against time or another person. There is no limit to the number of events these persons squeeze into a day. They have an intrinsic drive toward some goal that gives status and personality enhancement, and the achievement of this goal is opposed by time, persons, and things. Consequently, persons with type A personality often suffer frustration, are constantly in a hurry, and have free-floating hostility. Type A behavior is not characterized by worry but by overanxiety or hysteria. The converse of the type A personality is the type B personality, expressed by tranquility. Persons with type A personalities suffer higher rates of heart attack than those with type B.

Modifiable factors. Three factors—high serum cholesterol levels, high blood pressure, and cigarette smoking—have been identified as being positively correlated with increased rates of heart attack. Nations whose citizens have high serum cholesterol levels, chiefly the westernized countries, have heart attack rates much higher than countries such as Japan, whose people have low cholesterol levels. Cholesterol levels are closely related to the percentage of saturated animal fats in the diet. Alteration of the national diet is the most promising avenue to reduction of coronary mortality. High blood pressure is associated with increased risk of heart disease, and reduction of the pressure by diet and drug therapy reduces the risk. Cigarette smokers have an increased risk of heart disease; this is similarly reduced when they abandon the habit.

These three modifiable risk factors act in a synergistic fashion. Other variables, particu-

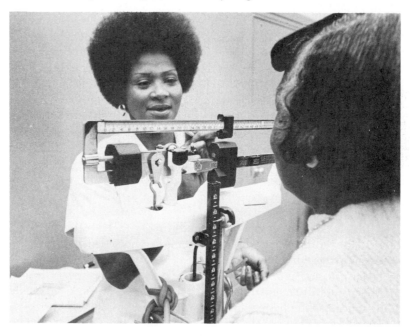

FIG. 6-5. Weight control and diet management are major strategies in adult health promotion, especially for patients with diabetes, hypertension, and heart disease. Public health nurses, nutritionists, physicians, and community health educators participate in these programs.

Courtesy Johns Hopkins Medical Institutions.

larly stress and sedentary habit, have been named as possible risk factors. Stress is difficult to measure either as a source or as a result of emotional tension. A period of severe stress or overfatigue is commonly identified as preceding a heart attack. Sedentary habit, or lack of exercise, is alleged to predispose to heart attacks. The evidence is inconclusive, except that in those who practice regular exercise the outcome of a heart attack is more favorable than in those who do not. The benefits of regular exercise are many and may include a reduced rate of heart attack, but this is not proved. Obesity is associated with increased frequency of heart attacks, particularly in the markedly obese. The difficulty is that such patients are frequently hypertensive, of sedentary habit, or diabetic, and it is difficult to identify which risk factor is operative.

In summary, coronary heart disease is multifactorial in origin. Atherosclerosis is usually present, together with elevated cholesterol, sometimes accompanied by other risk factors.

Hypertension

High blood pressure is widely prevalent in the United States, with 35 million Americans having systolic blood pressure readings of 165 or higher, or diastolic readings of 95 or higher. Another 25 million Americans have borderline hypertension. High blood pressure is the major factor contributing to strokes and is very significant in heart disease and renal disease. It has been estimated that hypertension costs the nation more than $8 billion per year in medical care costs, lost productivity, and lost wages. Furthermore, hypertension has been found to be highly correlated with reduced life expectancy: the higher the blood pressure, the shorter the life. Prevalence of high blood pressure among males and females increased between the 1960 to 1962 National Health Examination Survey and the 1971 to 1974 National Health and Nutrition Examination Survey—from 28.8% to 31.9% (age adjusted) of

the population between 35 and 74 years of age.

Federally funded studies in the United States in the late 1960s and early 1970s clearly demonstrated that high blood pressure could, however, be controlled and that reduced disease and death for middle-aged males would result. However, the national health examination surveys indicated that about 85% of individuals with high blood pressure were either unaware, untreated, or uncontrolled. In 1970 the Department of Health, Education, and Welfare (DHEW), through the National Heart, Lung, and Blood Institute, appointed a special panel to examine these problems and to recommend additional studies as needed. A large-scale study was recommended that would provide data on the effectiveness of antihypertensive therapy for both sexes, all races, and both young and middle-aged adults. The results of this large-scale study were reported in late 1979 and clearly indicate that the systematic, effective management of high blood pressure, especially when combined with effective patient education, can reduce the death rate for those with both severe and mild hypertension (Hypertension Detection and Follow-up Program Coordinating Group, 1979; Levine, et al., 1979; Morisky, et al., 1980).

In the early 1970s the National High Blood Pressure Education Program was initiated with participation by government agencies, private industry, voluntary health associations, and professional groups. This education program has been effective in decreasing the proportion of undetected cases of high blood pressure. Further, the proportion of those under treatment for whom blood pressure was controlled has also increased. The reductions in death from heart disease and stroke can at least partially be attributed to the success of the effort to control high blood pressure (Office of Disease Prevention and Health Promotion, 1981).

Following the initiation of the National High Blood Pressure Education Program in the United States, there was a considerable rise between 1973 and 1979 in the number of people having their blood pressures checked. But the number of people who stopped treatment in 1979—about one fifth of those who had high blood pressure—did not change significantly during the six-year period. Greater efforts are needed at the community level to provide follow-up and reinforcement for the continuing treatment of hypertension.

Almost three quarters of the total U.S. population surveyed in 1979 by the Public Health Service believed that high blood pressure was a "very serious disease." This represented a 16% increase over the 1973 figure, moving high blood pressure up in the public's perception of the most serious diseases to a ranking of fourth after cancer, stroke, and "heart conditions." Among blacks, understanding of its seriousness was 82% compared to the national average of 73%.

Americans' desire and ability to detect high blood pressure appear to be solidly entrenched, according to the 1979 survey conducted by the U.S. Public Health Service. Of those questioned in 1979, 83% reported having their blood pressure checked within the past 12 months, up from 77% in a similar survey in 1973. Among the black population in 1979, the number was 86%, up from 83%. In 1979 almost all persons (93%) recognized the existence of effective treatment for high blood pressure, and almost as many (84%) knew that medication effectively lowers blood pressure.

Although it is generally understood that hypertensive persons must stay on medication throughout their lives, in the 6 years between the 1973 and 1979 surveys, the number of hypertensive persons who stopped taking medication decreased only slightly, from 23% to 20%. In 1973 61% who stopped medication attributed their actions to a physician's instruction. By 1979 the percentage of those who gave this reason, while still high, had dropped to 41%.

Physicians maintain that side effects from medicine can be minimized, a concept borne out by the U.S. Public Health Service surveys. In 1973 and 1979 less than 10% of dropouts blamed side effects for their actions.

Even though there is strong medical evidence refuting the reliability of self-perceived symptoms for high blood pressure, a high percentage of hypertensive persons continued to believe that they can detect their own symptoms. Of those who stopped medication in 1979, 69% believed they knew their blood pressure was high. Among blacks who stopped medication, the percentage who thought they could detect symptoms was even higher at 83%. Among all the 1979 hypertensive persons who were questioned as to how they knew their blood pressure was high, 59% volunteered "dizziness," and more than half said "headaches."

The 1973 survey indicated that a high percentage of persons responded that they were able to sense their own blood pressure levels, but it was encouraging that in 1979 89% of the total population said it was likely that a person could have high blood pressure without obvious symptoms.

Physicians continued in 1979 to be the leading source of health information for the public (83%), followed by radio-television public service messages (63%), magazine articles (58%), television news (57%), and newspaper columns (53%). The 1979 survey also provided evidence that communication improved between professionals and patients on the subject of the meaning of blood pressure measurements and that a wider range of health professionals and community resources, besides physicians, is being used by patients to control their blood pressure.

The natural course of hypertension spans some 15 to 20 years, starting on the average around age 35 years and often ending in premature death around age 50 years. The duration of the disease is for the most part (75%) asymptomatic. When symptoms do occur they

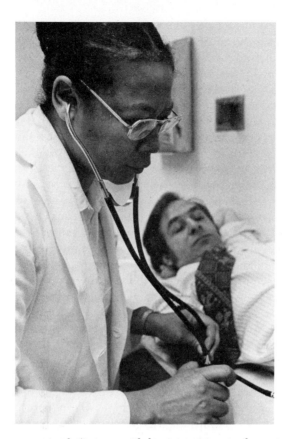

FIG. 6-6. Blood pressure control. Patients with hypertension must be assisted by community agencies to maintain a lifelong regimen of diet and medicine to prevent strokes and other cardiovascular complications.

Courtesy Johns Hopkins Medical Institutions.

are manifested by damage to the following organs—heart, brain, kidney, and fundus of the eye. Hypertension is the single most important risk factor for strokes, both hemorrhagic and thrombotic, and is a very important risk factor for heart disease. The cause of hypertension is unknown in 95% of cases. There is often a family history of hypertension, and relatives of hypertensive persons have been shown to be more likely to be hypertensive (especially children of two hypertensive parents). Obesity and salt consumption are correlated with hypertension, and both of these factors are modifiable.

The use of oral contraceptives may increase blood pressure also. Smoking and high blood cholesterol are not associated with development of hypertension, but the prognosis in hypertensive persons who smoke or have hypercholesterolemia is reduced. A great advance has been made in the treatment of hypertension with the introduction of effective drug therapy.

Hypertension lends itself well to community control, because community surveys can be performed to identify people who are hypertensive and do not know it. People can visit centers that have been set up in their community and have their blood pressure recorded, after which they can be referred for treatment if needed. (There are some 2,000 locally organized hypertension programs in the United States.) Once the cases are identified the problem then lies in patient education to effect compliance in taking the drugs to maintain normal levels of pressure. The benefits from the increasing number of hypertensive persons who have been brought under control because of efficient drug therapy has been demonstrated by reduced mortality and morbidity. This reduction is reflected in a decrease in the number of heart attacks in which hypertension was a factor and also, more importantly, in reduction of the number of cerebrovascular accidents, or strokes.

Stroke

The third ranking cause of adult mortality, following heart disease and cancer and preceding accidents, is stroke. Stroke is essentially the result of interference with the blood supply to the brain, which may be either gradual or abrupt. An artery of the brain may rupture, usually one with preexisting damage, the result of atherosclerosis. This is particularly likely if the patient has high blood pressure—the weakened vessel is inadequate to withstand the higher pressure. Such hemorrhagic strokes have a high fatality rate and are usually found among older people. A blood clot may form in the artery either from atheroma or from a clot formed elsewhere, such as in the heart itself, if there is a damaged valve there. The clot blocks the cerebral artery and deprives the brain tissue of oxygen. This type of stroke is termed *thromboembolic* and occurs in younger patients, possibly without such fatal results. Many people recover from the initial stroke, but they are often left with some residual disability. Despite devoted efforts of therapists and the perseverance of patients, complete recovery after stroke is uncommon. Particularly in

older people stroke is a major source of morbidity. The hope lies in prevention, chiefly by controlling hypertension.

CANCER

Found in all races and ages of humans and all other animal species, cancer is a group of diseases in which there is uncontrolled and disordered growth of abnormal cells. Cancer cells displace or destroy normal cells and, if not stopped, spread to other parts of the body. Thus cancer has two hallmarks—reproduction and invasion. Reproduction of cells is, of course, a normal biological function in growth and repair of tissues. Cancer cells, however, have a higher rate of cell growth than the normal tissues from which they are derived.

Cancer cells invade by three main mechanisms. The first is by direct spread or extension, growing into surrounding tissues and failing to respect the boundaries from which they are derived. Cancer cells may also invade lymph channels and be carried to distant parts of the body. The lymph channels meet at points where there are lymph nodes. There the cancer cells may enlarge and grow. The cancer cells may also be carried directly into the bloodstream, which enables them to reach distant parts of the body where they grow, attempting to reproduce the tissue of their origin. This new or secondary tumor is called a metastasis. The original tumor may be silent, that is, without symptoms such as pain or bleeding early in its life, and it may spread quickly. These factors make some cancers difficult to treat successfully and thus emphasize the necessity of early diagnosis, which is the objective of most community cancer control programs.

In 1979 there were about 410,000 deaths caused by cancer in the United States—20% of the total deaths. Both the number of cancer deaths and the proportion of total mortality in the United States accounted for by cancer have been increasing.

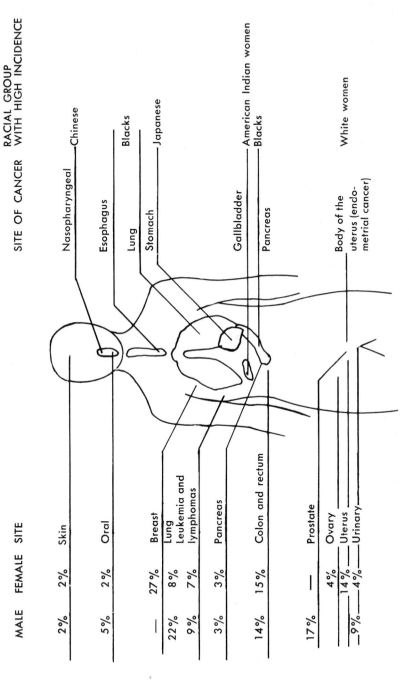

FIG. 6-7. Sex and racial propensities for cancer in different sites are revealed by the relative incidence in 1980 estimates. *Modified from American Cancer Society; and U.S. Office of Health Information, Health Promotion, and Physical Fitness and Sports Medicine.*

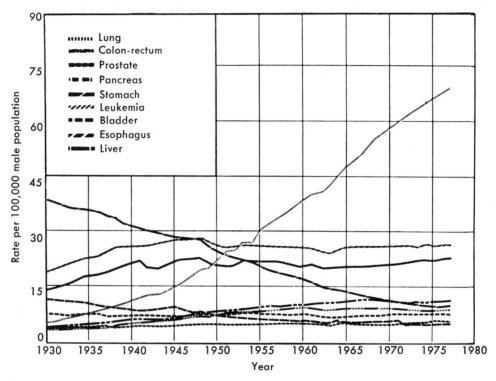

FIG. 6-8. Male cancer death rates by site, United States, 1930-1977. Rate for the male population is standardized for age in the 1970 U.S. population.

From National Vital Statistics Division and Bureau of the Census, United States; chart from the American Cancer Society, Inc., June, 1980.

Cancer is predominantly a disease of middle and old age; it is rare in children and young adults. Persons around age 70 account for a higher number of cases than any other age group. The risk of developing cancer increases with age. The male death rate exceeds that of the female. At the present time the chance of a person who is less than 20 years old developing cancer sometime during his or her lifetime is about one in four for males and slightly higher for females. The most common site in males, as seen in Fig. 6-7, is the lung, followed by the prostate gland. In females breast cancer is the most common, followed by colon cancer and rectal cancer, which is the third most common site in males. Surveys conducted in the United States since 1930 (Fig. 6-8) reveal that overall cancer has increased most rapidly in black males, whereas females of both races showed a decrease in overall cancer incidence. Cancer of the stomach has decreased in both sexes and both races, as has cancer of the cervix in females.

Lung cancer rates in most countries have increased dramatically in both sexes, with more recent increases in females bringing lung cancer almost even with breast cancer in the United States (Fig. 6-9). The increase up to 1965 in smoking among females produced an increasing rate of lung cancer among females. Females do seem to be quitting, though. From 1965 to 1976 the percentage of females in the United States who smoked remained almost stable at 32% to 33%. The proportion then

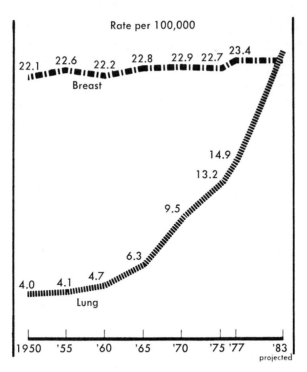

Rate per 100,000

22.1 22.6 22.2 22.8 22.9 22.7 23.4

Breast

14.9
13.2
9.5
6.3
4.0 4.1 4.7

Lung

1950 '55 '60 '65 '70 '75 '77 '83
projected

FIG. 6-9. The increases in female smoking up to 1965 in the United States will continue to yield increases in female lung cancer for several years, at least until it surpasses breast cancer.

From Office of the Assistant Secretary for Health, U.S. Department of Health and Human Services, 1980.

dropped to below 30.0%, and 1979 preliminary estimates indicate a level of 28.2%. One worry, however, is the fact that young females are picking up the habit at a stable rate. For the first time in history, for any age group, females ages 17 to 19 are smoking more than their male cohorts.

Much of the debt for increased smoking among females since World War II is yet to be paid. For males born this century, each successive age group has fewer cumulative years of smoking and lower smoking prevalence rates. Females born from 1921 to 1940, however, have much greater smoking rates. Barring a mass smoking stoppage, these generations of females will reach their older years with more years of smoking, more years of smoking non-

filter cigarettes, and higher totals of cigarettes smoked than females who preceded them. Coming years will show those effects in lung cancer and heart disease rates.

Risk factors for cancer include a familial tendency for the development of cancer, especially of breast, stomach, and large intestine. It is not known to what extent this is truly a genetic factor or whether it is caused by environmental factors such as diet, life-style, or occupation, which may remain similar from one generation to the next.

Repeated infections, particularly viral, are associated with cancer of the cervix. Radiation may also be a cause, stemming from industrial and medical uses of x-rays and radioactive devices. Older radiologists have been shown to have an excess mortality from leukemia. Uranium mine workers have been found to develop lung cancer at higher rates than does the general population. The atomic bomb survivers in Japan have experienced excessive mortality from leukemia.

The risk factor most clearly related to development of cancer is cigarette smoking. All the tissues in smokers that are exposed to the carcinogens in tobacco smoke have higher rates of cancer. These include the larynx, oral cavity, esophagus, lung, and urinary bladder. The impact of cigarette smoking is very large, both because of the prevalence of the habit (about 33% of adults in the United States are smokers) and because of the high relative risk of lung cancer that accompanies cigarette smoking.

Specific occupational hazards, such as asbestos, result in higher cancer rates. The contribution of air pollution is difficult to evaluate because of the long latent period for many cancers (20 to 40 years) between exposure and diagnosis of the cancer combined with the confounding effect of cigarette smoking.

Treatment and survival of cancer patients

Cancer may be treated by surgery, irradiation, and drugs. Surgery may range from simple local excision of the tumor to radical surgical exenteration of the tumor, the surrounding tissues, and the lymph nodes, so that the whole tumor area is excised. This may require diversion of the urinary or alimentary tract. Irradiation may proceed or follow surgery and may be applied by different emitters. Drug therapy may involve altering hormonal status if the tumor is hormonal dependent, and chemotherapy involves use of cytotoxic and antimetabolite drugs. The type of treatment used depends on many factors, such as the organ or origin of the tumor, the extent of invasion, the microscopic appearance, and the age and general health of the patient. Often a combination of two or more treatment methods are used, and a second or third course of treatment is frequently helpful. The dominant factor in the prognosis

for cancer patients is the stage at which treatment is first begun. The outlook is markedly improved if the cancer is treated when it is still localized, rather than spread to the neighboring lymph glands or distant organs of the body. Some examples of the superior 5-year survival rates for localized tumors compared with those that have spread are shown in Fig. 6-10, which demonstrates that if the number of cases diagnosed and treated in the localized form is increased, overall survival will increase.

Although cancer is probably the most feared diagnosis, it is one of the most curable of the chronic diseases today. For the more serious cancers, the overall survival rate is 41%, compared to 33% in 1955. Averaging in the relatively less dangerous skin cancers and early cervical cancer, the survival rate is increased to 58%.

Early detection of cancer

The most promising method of early detection is screening people who have no symptoms but who, by reason of their age, sex, occupation, or life-style, may be in a high-risk group. The validity of screening methods varies. Some have proved most effective, the outstanding example of which is the Papanicolaou (PAP) smear. Cervical cytology—the Pap smear—is both sensitive and specific in detecting precancerous changes in the cervix. The test is reliable, painless, inexpensive, and lacks morbidity; as a result it has achieved wide popularity among health providers and patients. The 5-year survival rate in the earliest, precancerous stage, of cervical cancer is 100%. Virtually all women can be saved if the diagnosis is made at this point, which can be done by the cervical smear technique. The community problem is that certain groups of women, including the old, the poorly educated, and those who are not assimilated into the community, do not seek out the screening test. Community efforts can be directed toward identifying these women and encouraging them to avail themselves of this preventive procedure.

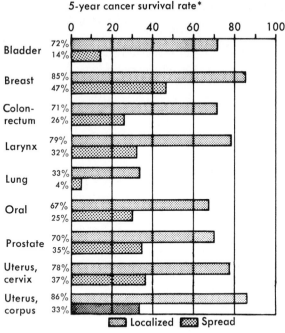

5-year cancer survival rate*

FIG. 6-10. The survival of cancer victims over the 5 years following diagnosis has improved with advances in treatment methods, but survival still depends primarily on early detection in well-organized community education and screening programs.

Modified from End Results Group, National Cancer Institute; and American Cancer Society, Cancer Facts and Figures, 1980.

In breast cancer two methods can be employed on a community basis. The most important is that of breast self-examination, which can be used by all women, examining their own breasts every month. The method is simple to learn and can be taught by demonstration, films, television programs, and printed material. Community health leaders can make everyone aware of this method. Soft tissue x-ray films or mammography holds great promise of identifying early tumors that are too small or inaccessible to palpate in women over 35. Mammography has reduced mortality from breast cancer in women over 50 years of age.

The gloomy outlook in lung cancer is slowly improving. Although we can identify persons of high risk, namely, men over 45 years of age who smoke more than one pack of cigarettes

daily, it is still difficult to detect lung cancer early. This is because x-ray film changes occur late, and lung cancer cells are difficult to produce and interpret microscopically. Not all tumors exfoliate cells that may be coughed up and recognized as cancer cells under the microscope. Periodic sputum cytology examinations in high-risk groups will become a community program if the present research trials prove the method feasible.

Colon and rectal cancers may be detected by the presence of blood in the stools. Sigmoidoscopy (direct vision of the lower bowel) and an x-ray examination of the lower bowel are indicated if blood is present. Tablets may be developed, which, when dropped into the toilet bowl, will give a characteristic color if blood is present in the stool. Such a mass screening

TABLE 6-1. Cancer-related checkup chart*

Test or procedure	Sex	Age	Frequency
Chest x-ray	Not recommended for any population		
Sputum cytology	Not recommended for any population		
Sigmoidoscopy (rectal examination)	M&F	Over 50	Every 3 yrs. (1)
Stool slide test	M&F	Over 50	Every yr.
Manual rectal examination†	M&F	Over 40	Every yr.
Pap test	F	20-65 (2)	Every 3 yrs. (3)
Pelvic examination	F	20-40	Every 3 yrs.
		Over 40	Every yr.
Endometrial (womb) tissue sample	F	At high-risk at menopause (4)	At menopause
Breast self-examination	F	Over 20	Every month
Breast physical examination	F	20-40	Every 3 yrs.
		Over 40	Every yr.
Mammography	F	35-40	1 baseline examination
		Under 50	Consult physician
		Over 50	Every yr.
Health counseling and cancer checkup (5)	M&F	Over 20	Every 3 yrs.
	M&F	Over 40	Every yr.

*From the American Cancer Society, Inc., 1980.
†Includes a single stool slide test.
(1) After two initial negative examinations a year apart.
(2) Pap test should also be done on women under 20 who are sexually active.
(3) After two initial Pap tests done a year apart are negative, high risk women should have more frequent Pap tests.
(4) History of infertility, obesity; failure of ovulation, abnormal uterine bleeding, or estrogen therapy.
(5) To include examination for cancers of the thyroid, testicles, prostate, ovaries, lymph nodes, oral region, and skin.

program offers the best hope of early detection of colon and rectal cancers at present.

The American Cancer Society, recognizing the costs and potential hazards of medical testing, issued in 1980 a protocol for fewer cancer-related checkups for symptomless people than it had recommended previously (Table 6-1). The American Cancer Society recommends screening for the asymptomatic population on a schedule graded by age and sex. High-risk groups by other criteria require more aggressive community outreach efforts to detect cancer in early stages.

Cancer research

Cancer research has the following three thrusts: (1) to discover the cause of the cancer so that preventive methods may be taken, (2) to pioneer new screening and education programs for early detection and the reduction of exposure to cigarettes and other risk factors, and (3) to improve results of treatment for persons with cancer. The public should not be persuaded to believe that if sufficient money is spent, the threat of cancer will be removed. The unfortunate fact is that, in cancers in which the cause has been discovered, the number of cases has actually increased. Lung cancer is the classic example, the cause being cigarette smoking, but prevention involves altering behavior, which is difficult to achieve. Many cancers may be prevented by modification of life-style to avoid known hazardous habits and customs and by the use of early detection methods already available. The community effort must be directed toward making people aware of this, rather than making them dependent on research results or cures at some future date.

DIABETES

One percent of the population of the United States, 2.2 million persons, have diabetes and are aware of this fact. An additional 3.3 million have diabetes and do not know it. Ninety-five percent of diabetic persons suffer the disease after the age of 40 years—maturity-onset diabetes. Diabetes should be viewed as a vascular disease as well as a metabolic disorder with altered carbohydrate metabolism. The morbidity of diabetes is caused by its vascular complications. Coronary heart disease rates are increased in diabetes. Specific preventable complications of diabetes include those for renal disease, and, if the retinal arteries are involved, diabetic retinopathy and blindness; amputations when blood supply to the limbs is decreased, usually in the foot and calf, with resulting gangrene; and perinatal morbidity and mortality due to diabetes in the mother.

Half of all diabetic persons may be treated by diet alone—one that is low in calories and fat. The remainder require insulin or oral hypoglycemic drugs. Community efforts are needed, for the prognosis in diabetes is related to the resources of the patients, their families, and the communities in which they live. Diabetics who are old, poor, or live alone do poorly. The duties of the community toward persons with diabetes are similar to those with hypertension. Screening programs to uncover the disease early, before it is symptomatic, are of prime importance. After the patients are identified, education is needed to assure adherence to diet and drug regimens.

ARTHRITIS

Arthritis and rheumatic diseases are the most common cause of lost work days annually in the United States, although the respiratory diseases account for the greatest number of episodes of sickness. It is difficult to determine the prevalence of arthritides because of the range of symptoms and the variability of diagnostic standards. If major mobility limitations are used, the prevalence of some arthritic symptoms is 3%. Rheumatoid arthritis is a systemic inflammatory disease with local joint manifestations, in which the small joints of the hands are often affected early. The disease pursues a chronic course marked by relapses and remissions. The sex ratio shows an excess of females, 2.5 to 1.0. Risk factors include lower socioeconomic status, infections, trauma, winter season, and social stress. The age of onset is young, between 20 and 45 years, commonly 30 to 40 years. In contrast, osteoarthritis affects older persons exclusively and occurs in larger, weight-bearing joints, hips, and knees. Trauma and obesity are antecedent factors. The community role includes employers providing work for those arthritic persons who are able to work, which is a surprisingly high proportion. Transport services from home to treatment facilities, home visits, and meals on wheels services are all vital to these patients.

As with each of the major chronic diseases (heart, cancer, diabetes, and lung diseases), the U.S. Congress has called for the establishment of regional comprehensive arthritis centers with two distinct purposes: (1) to develop and foster new methods for the prompt and effective application of available knowledge and (2) to develop new knowledge with which to combat arthritis. In response to this mandate the National Institute of Arthritis, Metabolism, and Digestive Diseases has developed, as some of the other National Institutes of Health, a program of multipurpose arthritis centers, each of which engages in research, education, and community demonstration projects.

The Multipurpose Arthritis Centers have a national distribution ranging from New Hampshire to Hawaii. Many of the projects underway in these centers could not have been started without the interaction of individuals brought together under the aegis of a Multipurpose Arthritis Center. Examples of major efforts of the centers include research into the genetic basis of arthritis; new advances in health services research, such as cost-effectiveness studies and analysis of disability; comprehensive education of allied health professionals; and research into the best methods of delivering arthritis health care and education to those least able to obtain it, such as the homebound individual and residents of the inner city.

PREVENTION OF CHRONIC DISEASE

The influence of medical treatment on established chronic disease is minimal in general. The thrust must be toward primary prevention (health promotion) and earlier diagnosis (secondary prevention). Patients, health professionals, and the community all have a role in this. Tuberculosis, hypertension, diabetes, syphilis, and gonorrhea can all be diagnosed early by simple tests and treated or controlled successfully. Screening tests, as shown in Table 6-1, are available for many diseases, such as cervical, breast, and colon cancers. The American Cancer Society has set a fine example in health education with the following seven danger signals:

1. Any sore that does not heal
2. A lump or thickening in the breast or elsewhere
3. Unusual bleeding or discharge
4. Any change in a wart or mole
5. Persistent hoarseness or cough
6. Persistent indigestion or difficulty in swallowing
7. Any change in normal bowel habits

Self-help groups. Patients suffering from certain diseases have been forming activist groups to aid others in a similar predicament. Parents of children with multiple handicaps and the spouses and children of patients have organized in various communities to identify community resources that may be available. Groups such as these remove fear and stigma of the disease and raise morale and achievement.

ADOLESCENT HEALTH

Adolescent behavior is often of greater concern to the community than adolescent health. Alcohol and substance misuse will be examined in Chapter 12 as "compulsive behaviors." The health-related behavior of greatest concern, although it does not show up in the mortality statistics, is the increase in sexual activity among adolescents, with its associated consequences of adolescent pregnancy and sexually transmissible diseases.

Teenage sex and pregnancy

About 1 million teenage women between the ages of 15 and 19 in the United States become pregnant each year; of these, 600,000 deliver, and of these, about 90% keep their babies. The 1979 national survey of metropolitan-area young women aged 15 to 19 years (Zelnik and Kantner, 1980) includes the following U.S. observations:

- Despite a greater percentage of teenagers who always use a method of contraception and despite a decline in those who never use birth control, the percentage of premaritally sexually active women who become pregnant has risen steadily, from 28.1% in 1971, to 30.0% in 1976, to 32.5% in 1979. The 1979 figure means that 16.2% of all women aged 15 to 19 become pregnant.
- Almost half (49.8%) of the teenage women surveyed in 1979 said they had had premarital sexual relations, up from 43.4% in 1976 and 30.4% in 1971. All the increase between 1976 and 1979 is attributable to white women, 47% of whom said in 1979 they had had premarital intercourse, up from 38% in 1976 and 26% in 1971. Of black women, 66% were sexually active in 1979 (66% in 1976 and 54% in 1971).
- The mean age at first intercourse remained stable between 1976 and 1979 and was, in 1979, 16.2 for all women (16.4 for whites and 15.5 for blacks).
- More than 26.6% of the sexually active

women never use contraception. About 62% of these become pregnant, thereby accounting for half of all premarital pregnancies among 15- to 19-year-olds.

- Although more teenagers today are using contraception, the proportions using a method are employing less effective methods than formerly, both at first use and in their later choice of method. Use of withdrawal among users has doubled as the initial choice of contraception, whereas initial use of the pill among users declined from 33% to 19%. Twenty-eight percent of teenage users in 1979 last used diaphragm, rhythm, or withdrawal, whereas last use of the pill and intrauterine contraceptive device (IUD) declined from 51% to 43% of users from 1976 to 1979.

- The proportion of premaritally pregnant women who marry during the pregnancy has fallen since 1976, from 23% to 16% while the proportion of unmarried pregnant women who choose to have abortions has risen since 1976, from 32% to 37%.

- An increase in premarital pregnancy combined with the changes in marriage and abortion has led to a slight rise in the illegitimacy rate among sexually active whites, but there is no change among blacks.

- Increases in use of contraception and abortion indicate that young women are increasingly trying to prevent unwanted pregnancies (and unplanned births). That they are somewhat less successful in preventing pregnancies than their counterparts in 1976 is in part a result of increased use of less effective methods of contraception.*

Although statistics for unplanned pregnancies of 18- to 19-year-olds appear to be improving, those for teens 17 and under continue to worsen, with teens aged 14 and under showing the most alarming increases. These very young mothers face the greatest risks of poor medical outcomes, discontinuation of education at too early an age, and high rates of repeat pregnancies. Pregnancy is the single most common cause of school dropouts among young girls and directly contributes to future diminished employment prospects and the probability of welfare dependence. Too often the pregnancy of a young teen leads to family tensions, early marriage and divorce, alienation from friends and relatives, loss of self-esteem, and may contribute to child abuse and both somatic and emotional disorders. Also, too little is known about the sexual behavior of adolescent males or why some adolescent couples use contraceptive techniques effectively and others do not.

Teenage smoking

A series of surveys in the United States shows significant drops in smoking among boys of all age categories, as well as among girls aged 12 through 16. Among girls aged 17 and 18, there has been a pronounced leveling off, with an increase of only 0.3% over the past 5 years. The overall decrease between 1974 and 1979 was 25% (Table 6-2).

---

*Adapted with permission from *Family Planning Perspectives*, Volume 12, Number 5, 1980.

TABLE 6-2. Percentage of smoking among adolescents in the United States

Age	Boys			Girls		
	1968	1974	1979	1968	1974	1979
12-14	2.9	4.2	3.2	0.6	4.9	4.3
15-16	17.0	18.1	13.5	9.6	20.2	11.8
17-18	30.2	31.0	19.3	18.6	25.9	26.2
12-18	14.7	15.8	10.7	8.4	15.3	12.7

Adolescent health education and services

As a complement to school health education and school health services, a major responsibility of community health education and ambulatory care services in the community is to recognize the special needs of adolescents beyond the classroom and the school. The developing sexuality and sexual activity of adolescents may not be acceptable behavior as judged by some members of society. Teenagers are confused by peer pressure, parental disapproval, their individual values, and their decision-making ability. This confusion may preclude their seeking help before they begin using alcohol or become sexually active, with pregnancy or automobile accidents already a possibility.

It is the responsibility of personnel of the ambulatory (walk-in) clinics and programs to be aware that teens who are seeking services will have different levels of information, education, and experience. Adolescents vary in their knowledge levels, attitudes, and behavior, so that no single program activity can meet all of their needs. Teens may or may not be living with their parents or attending school, and regardless of the family's income they may be unable to pay for medical services. Health services staff members must be prepared to deal with these variations in developmental levels, the social situations, the teenagers' degree of communication with the parents, the teenagers ability to plan, and their willingness to recognize the risks of alcohol, drugs, or sexual activity and to take preventive measures against pregnancy or driving.

The guidelines that follow were developed by the U.S. Department of Health and Human Services (1980) to assist community projects receiving federal support for adolescent health services.

- Adolescents often have vague and sometimes incorrect knowledge of drugs and sex. There is a need for open discussion of their ideas and beliefs about sex and reproduction; both sexes should be involved when possible. Teenagers need to be clearly informed in understandable terms of the possible results of sexual intercourse, alcohol or drug misuse, and of the health risks to both mother and child. Group discussions (rap sessions) may be an effective way for adolescents to gain the necessary information, but should not replace individual counseling. Adolescents should be told through media and outreach programs that they are welcome at the ambulatory care project, that their privacy is protected, their records are confidential, and education and counseling are free.
- Teenagers must be given sufficient knowledge at their level of understanding to make a responsible decision about engaging in sexual activity that may lead to pregnancy, to make an informed choice of a method of birth control, to be aware of possible side effects and contraindications of use of the various contraceptive methods, and to become thoroughly aware of the physical, emotional, and social consequences of sexual activity for both participants, their families, and their communities.
- Risk-taking with sex is often associated with other problems with which teenagers need help. Health care providers can assist by referring teenagers to employment agencies, alternative school programs, and drug or alcohol misuse agencies. Counseling services must be available to a teenager in urgent need of discussing problems. Delay in getting to "talk to somebody" can cause the person to change his or her mind about asking for help.
- A project should identify the resources of the community and other resources available under state and federal programs that are potential sources of assistance and cooperation. Projects can also use the materials and experience of national groups (e.g., March of Dimes, National Organiza-

tion for Women, Salvation Army) that are also dealing with the problem of teenage pregnancy. Local chapters of those organizations should be involved with the project's activity.

- Effective ways must be found to reach the teenage population. Techniques and means of contact need to be selected uniquely for the population, for example, teen-oriented radio stations, television, bulletin-board notices at teenage hangouts, school group activities, and youth groups. Some organizations have an interest in helping teens (e.g., Parent-Teacher-Student Association, the local school boards, churches, Big Brother and Big Sister organizations). Work with them can help to develop a broad base of support in the community. Work with the schools can promote educational programs to alert teenagers about health issues related to smoking, drugs, drinking, and adolescent sexual activity.

Develop community awareness. Projects should develop a plan for community education to increase awareness of adolescent pregnancy and its consequences. This can be done by

1. Publicizing the scope and implications to the community of teenage sexual or substance misuse activity (e.g., number of school dropouts due to pregnancy, number of teens with out-of-wedlock births, number of teen abortions, venereal disease rates, number of births to teenage girls, number of automobile accidents involving alcohol). On a broader scale, national data can be used.

2. Identifying community leaders and groups who can help to make contact with teens and remove barriers to their receiving services and continuing their education. These people could be school board members, social service workers, or youth workers. Parent groups can be highly effective in the review of materials and in initiating public action; parent groups may not have the same constraints as school administrators and teachers.

3. Developing programs for parents to educate them about the extent of teenage sexual or drinking activity, the knowledge and guidance teens may need, and where they can get information and help.

4. Providing a central source of information, resource material, and personnel. This could also mean helping libraries and bookstores acquire accurate and acceptable references, arranging displays for fairs and exhibitions, providing speakers for community groups, and notifying newspapers and radio and television stations of the availability of these resources.

Develop adolescent awareness. Teenagers today are faced with adapting to the mores of a rapidly changing society and, although lacking sufficient life experience in their developmental years, are forced to make decisions that can greatly affect their adult lives. It is the responsibility of health services staff members to be aware of the levels of information and education of the adolescents who come to them for services, so that the individual can be given appropriate knowledge of human reproduction, contraception, alcohol, drugs, or other information as appropriate. Sexually active teens need information about the specific family planning services available to them. Efforts must be made to reach teenagers, whether in the community or in family planning clinics. The following activities have been found to be effective.

1. Identify all access points for contact with adolescents (e.g., schools, homes, recreation centers, shopping malls, employment agencies, local hangouts, teen-youth programs, and radio and television).

2. Devise strategies to reach teens at their locations (e.g., put up posters at public places like sports arenas, educate adults working with teens about availability of counseling and referral, furnish spot announcements regarding family planning clinics for use by radio and television stations, send flyers to other health and social service agencies, and form discussion

panels for church groups or youth clubs).

3. Use audiovisual materials suitable to adolescents of different ages and different environments. Project developers should also be aware that many materials already are available in the United States from sources such as the National Clearinghouse for Family Planning Information, the National Health Information Clearinghouse, the Clearinghouse for Smoking and Health, and the National Clearinghouse for Alcohol Information. Materials developed locally should be age-appropriate and easily understood, with the information directed to assist teenage decision-making: whether to have sexual intercourse, how to choose a contraceptive, where and when to get tests for venereal disease or pregnancy. Teenagers can help with the preparation of some materials and can act as valuable "reviewers."

4. Make special effort to reach teens who are not in school. One approach is to identify hangouts such as bowling alleys, billiard parlors, hamburger stands, and beaches and swimming pools, and then establish rapport with the informal leaders.

5. Publicize the availability of services in terms that are meaningful to teenagers; teens may not know that family planning clinics, community health centers, or other ambulatory care projects are relevant to their needs. Teens need to know that family planning services are not only for adults or married couples.

Counseling. Counselors and educators should have thorough training in adolescent growth, development, and behavior patterns and be screened for their ability to relate to teenagers. The two major concerns of the counseling process are (1) to impart sufficient knowledge to help the individual make a responsible and intelligent choice about sexual intercourse and, if indicated, about a birth control method and (2) to instill the necessary motivation to enable the individual to follow through with the decision to use birth control.

Crisis counseling should be available to a teenager in urgent need of discussing his or her problems. Teens need more counseling than is usually provided for adults; many who come to the clinics are uncertain or worried about the risks they are taking. Teens should be encouraged to include their sex partners or friends in the counseling sessions. Males should be encouraged to come to the clinic for educational counseling services. If cooperation is lacking, educational materials should be sent to them by the teenage girl being counseled.

Complete and thorough discussions about sexual development, human sexuality, sexual reproduction, and the choices of contraceptive care must be given. Contraceptive methods discussed should include abstinence, natural family planning, barrier methods (diaphragms, condoms, and foam), as well as oral contraceptives and IUDs.

Services. An ambulatory care project should examine its service delivery system to evaluate its usefulness and attractiveness to adolescents. Many teenagers coming to the facility lack knowledge about many things: confidentiality of services, medical procedures, cost of services, and necessary follow-up of a positive pregnancy or venereal disease test. Teenagers are entitled to the full range of medical and other services offered by an ambulatory care project. To be encouraged to accept the project services, teenagers need special assurance that confidentiality will be honored. They are concerned with privacy, so services should permit anonymity, either with clinics made available through multipurpose health centers or with separate entrances or hours made for teen use. Appointments should be available on short notice; drop-ins should be seen, if the project has sufficient personnel. Teens should receive pregnancy testing or treatment for sexually transmitted infections as quickly as possible.

It must be made plain to teenagers that project services are free or low cost, and if there is a charge, they should be able to make deferred payments. The inability to pay for services, regardless of family income, is a serious deterrent to their seeking help. Many will pay for services if they can do so in installments and without being billed at home.

Pregnancy testing services are highly attractive to teenagers. Studies have shown that a pregnancy scare is often a prime motivation for a teenager to attend a family planning clinic. Providers wishing to attract teenagers should provide easily accessible pregnancy testing services and should not turn away or make a referral if the teenager requests only a pregnancy test and declines birth control assistance.

Staff members who work with teenagers should be sympathetic and sensitive to various teen-specific needs. They must avoid ambiguous language (e.g., they should not assume that sexual activity is understood by a teen to mean sexual intercourse). Teenagers need to know what will happen at the clinic and should be told what to expect during the physical examination.

Training. Family planning and health professionals who provide care to teenagers should have training that is specific to teenage needs. This training should cover adolescent growth and development, human sexuality, responsibilities of a sexual relationship, decision making on the use of contraceptives (for different relationships, ages, motivations, and development levels), health risks and problems specific to young females, responsibility of males, and alcohol and drug use and effects. Staff members may need special training in counseling or may need to supplement their skills by working with counselors who are alert and sensitive to the concerns of teenagers.

People outside the medical service disciplines who have contact and good rapport with adolescents should be enlisted to counsel and help disseminate information about family planning services. Some experienced providers suggest that the training of people who are other than medical professionals and who can communicate well with young people is an ex-cellent way to increase teen use of available services. Training for counseling should be thorough in all phases, with emphasis on the ability to communicate at the teenager's level of comprehension. It may be advantageous to have counseling given by a young person or one who appears young, for many adolescents will not express themselves nor listen to an individual who is not regarded as a contemporary. The training of volunteer peer counselors (other teens) is a technique that recognizes adolescent communication patterns. Teen counselors can be an important resource in the community.

Special efforts should also be made to develop on a community-wide basis education and discussion sessions for parents. Although much teen learning comes from peers, parents are keys to the development of values, attitudes, and the sense of responsibility of their children. Frequently parents are overlooked as important members of the team.

PROMOTION OF ADOLESCENT AND ADULT HEALTH

People must be educated and supported in developing and maintaining positive health-oriented behavior. Their health lies in their own hands, and diseases reflect life-styles.

In addition to the periodic health assessment or inventory, there are a number of contributions that individual citizens can make to their own health. The promotion of circulatory efficiency through physical activity adapted to one's capacity, regularity in living, relaxation, rest, proper nutrition, avoidance of extreme fatigue, avoidance of unnecessary exposure, avoidance of harmful substances, prevention of disease, immediate treatment of disease and disability that do occur, promotion of wholesome life interests, and attainment of emotional stability are all important in the promotion of a high level of health, the extension of the prime of life, and a greater life expectancy. Time, cost, and effort devoted to health promotion

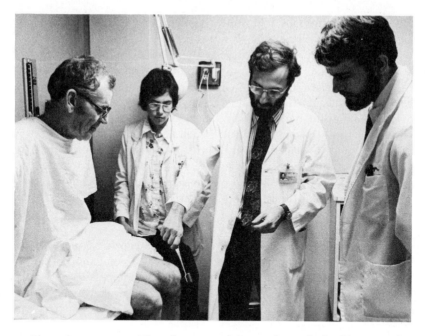

FIG. 6-11. Physical examination. The selective application of periodic health examinations can yield early detection of conditions for which later recognition could mean death or serious disability.

Courtesy Johns Hopkins Medical Institutions.

are well invested by communities and employers, as well as by individuals for themselves.

Basic to a community program of adolescent and adult health promotion is health education. This includes education of the person who is a patient, which is the responsibility of the attending physician and his or her staff; it includes family education, which is the joint responsibility of the physician and the public health department; and it includes community health education, for which the public health department and other nonmedical organizations have primary responsibility.

To be health-informed is not enough. Adults and adolescents must be health-educated in terms of having a fundamental understanding of health that they identify with themselves and apply to themselves. This means that citizens who value the health they now possess seek to understand how they can preserve and promote that health, and put into practice

those measures that will assure them of the highest level of health their native endowment will provide.

The model standards and objectives for community promotion and protection of adolescent and adult health are illustrated in the tables on pp. 163-168. The first table outlines the essential outcomes and services (process) expected in the control of chronic diseases in adults. The second table illustrates model standards and objectives for a communicable disease control program applicable to both adults and adolescents, but especially geared to adolescents. Other communicable and chronic disease control standards for communities will be illustrated in later chapters, and other behavioral problems in adolescence will be addressed in the chapters on community mental health (Chapter 8), community recreation and fitness (Chapter 9), and life-style and community health promotion (Chapter 12).

Text continued on p. 169.

CHRONIC DISEASE CONTROL OBJECTIVES FOR COMMUNITIES*

Focus	Objectives	Indicators	Population in need
Outcomes	1. By 19___ preventable deaths (or complications) associated with ___† will not exceed ___ per ___ population. NOTE: *Chronic conditions suggested for inclusion in outcome objectives are those that contribute significantly to the community's morbidity and mortality, and for which an effective preventive approach is available. Because of long latency periods and limited changes in incidence in the near term, outcomes for some chronic diseases, such as cancer, may need to be supplemented by measures more responsive to community programs. These could include complications, medical care utilization, and disability rates. However, communities should carefully consider the interrelationships of some of the suggested measures, for example, preventing premature death may increase the number of hospital days or the rate of disability from a given chronic disease. Similarly, reducing certain risk factors (e.g., smoking) will affect more than one outcome (e.g., the incidence of cancer, myocardial infarction, emphysema). Thus, while recognizing that reduction of morbidity and mortality is the appropriate goal for chronic disease control, communities may wish to stress risk factor reduction and process objectives.*	a. Hospital admissions rate associated with specific preventable complication b. Hospital days of stay associated with specific preventable complication c. Disability days–restricted days associated with specific preventable complication d. Incidence or prevalence with specific preventable complication e. Survival rates for populations with diagnosed conditions	The community or appropriate high-risk population

*Based on Model standards for community preventive health services, Washington, D.C., 1979, Public Health Service, U.S. Department of Health and Human Services.

†Insert specific chronic disease or condition, e.g.: Atherosclerotic and other cardiovascular disease (coronary artery disease, rheumatic heart disease, stroke, myocardial infarction); cancer, specific sites (lung, breast, bladder, gastrointestinal tract, cervix, oral cavity, etc.); chronic obstructive lung disease; diabetes and other metabolic disease; bone and joint disease (arthritis, spine); vision impairment (glaucoma, injury); hearing impairment (noise, chronic infection); neurological disorder; congenital anomalies; traumatic injury; cirrhosis; nutritional anemia.   *Continued.*

CHRONIC DISEASE CONTROL OBJECTIVES FOR COMMUNITIES—cont'd

Focus	Objectives	Indicators	Population in need
Surveillance-epidemiology	**Process**		
	2. By 19 — the community will be served by a surveillance-epidemiology system that can monitor those chronic diseases and conditions and the major risk factors associated with them that contribute significantly to morbidity and mortality and that are preventable.	Existence of system: a. Risk factor data specific for high-risk population segments. b. Chronic disease data (system should cover at least all elements for which outcome objectives have been developed)	The community or appropriate high-risk population
	2a. By 19 — the community surveillance and epidemiology system will permit measurement of the impact of community interventions. NOTE: *Certain chronic diseases may require large population bases to permit accurate monitoring of disease trends.*		
Preventive services	3. By 19 — the community will be served by preventive services designed to reduce the major chronic disease problems.	Existence of systems with linkage to program data sets	
	Illustrative activities—services (problem area affected)		
	3a. By 19 — : Promotion of smoking cessation (cancer, cardiovascular diseases, pulmonary disease).	Presence of —Physician education program —Public information program —Community policies regarding nonsmoking areas	
	3b. By 19 — : Promotion of prudent diet for high-risk groups (obesity, cardiovascular disease, diabetes, bone and joint disease).	Presence of —Nutrition education (family) —Physician education —Weight control services —Vending machine control	
	3c. By 19 — : Promotion of appropriate levels of exercise (cardiovascular disease, obesity, bone and joint diseases).	Presence of —Life-style education in schools —Physician education —Opportunities and facilities for public fitness programs	The community or appropriate high-risk population

			The community or appropriate high-risk population
	3d. By 19 ___ : Protection from hazardous occupational exposures (cancer, pulmonary disease, bone and joint disease, vision and hearing impairment, neurological disorders).	Existence of —Occupational health and industrial hygiene services	
	3e. By 19 ___ : Protection from environmental pollutants (cancer, pulmonary disease, hearing impairment).	Existence of —Environmental prevention programs, e.g., air quality, food protection, noise control, radiological health, water quality, solid waste	
Screening–early diagnostic services	4. By 19 ___ the community will be served by screening and early diagnostic services designed to interrupt the chronic disease process at the earliest possible stage.	a. Existence of 1. Physician education 2. Public information system to inform people of the availability of screening services and to promote their use 3. Preschool and school-based detection programs 4. Selected programs for high-risk adults, e.g., hypertension 5. Public assurance of referral, follow-up, and treatment services b. Number of individuals screened, positive, referred, diagnosed, and treated c. The timeliness of screening procedures (e.g., 90% of diagnosed cervical cancer should be no more advanced than Stage I).	
Access to services	5. By ___ the community will be served by a system that assures access to medical and other services for control of chronic conditions (e.g., hypertension, diabetes, arthritis).	a. Existence of system to assure access b. Existence of 1. Data on provider acceptance of referrals and new clients 2. Data on service availability and utilization	
	5a. By 19 ___ the community will be served by a system that assures access to rehabilitative services for those individuals with chronic conditions.	a. Existence of system to assure access b. Existence of 1. Vocational rehabilitation services 2. Education on availability of services 3. Data on service availability and utilization 4. Physical rehabilitation services	

OBJECTIVES AND ACTIONS FOR COMMUNITY CONTROL OF SEXUALLY TRANSMITTED DISEASES*

GOAL: The spread of sexually transmitted diseases and their sequelae will be prevented.

Focus	Objectives	Indicators	Population in need
	Outcomes		
	By 19 __ the incidence of __ † __ will not exceed __.	Incidence	The community
	Process		
Program management	1. By 19 __ each community will be served by a program for the control of sexually transmitted diseases, including a. Oversight, planning, and evaluation b. Consultation to physicians and others in clinics and the community c. Recognition of situations and cases requiring extraordinary attention	Availability of program	The community
Surveillance and reporting (syphilis)	2. By 19 __ the community will be served by a system for the routine reporting of all new cases of syphilis.	a. Existence of system b. Positive serologies that are reported c. Percent of positive serologies investigated d. Previously treated cases, not reported, named as contacts e. Percent of cases treated by private physicians and reported promptly (i.e., within time required by state statutes but not more than 3 days)	The community
	2a. By 19 __ all positive laboratory results will be reported and evaluated, and investigated where necessary, to ensure appropriate epidemiological treatment and follow-up.	Percent of reported positive laboratory results evaluated	
Gonorrhea	3. By 19 __ the community will be served by a system for estimating the incidence, prevalence, and demographic characteristics of its gonorrhea cases.	Presence of system that produces statistical reports of incidence and prevalence by demographic characteristics	The community

			The community
Other sexually transmitted diseases	4. By 19 ___ the community will be served by a system that assesses the extent of and potential need for a program to control sexually transmitted diseases other than syphilis and gonorrhea (e.g., genital herpes, nongonococcal urethritis and cervicitis, sexually transmitted hepatitis)	Existence of system	The community
Case follow-up	5. By 19 ___ the community will be served by qualified staff to interview and conduct contact investigations of every reported case of infectious and recently infectious syphilis and to determine reasons for the occurrence of congenital syphilis under 1 year of age.	Availability of qualified staff	
	5a. By 19 ___ all locatable infectious syphilis cases will be interviewed within 3 days of reporting, and 75% of contacts brought to examination within 2 weeks of the case report.	a. Percent of locatable cases interviewed within 3 days of reporting b. Percent of contacts brought to examination within 2 weeks of the case report c. Percent of congenital syphilis cases under 1 year that are investigated	The community
	6. By 19 ___ the community will be served by a procedure for bringing contacts of gonorrhea cases to diagnosis or treatment.	Presence of procedure (e.g., selective interviewing of cases, patient self-referral of contacts)	
Diagnosis and treatment (availability)	7. By 19 ___ there will be readily identifiable clinical resources conveniently available for the confidential diagnosis and treatment of the sexually transmitted diseases.	a. Inventory of appropriate community resources b. Telephone listings	The community
	7a. By 19 ___ at least one readily identifiable sexually transmitted disease information and referral system will be found within the community.	Presence of system	
	7b. By 19 ___ provision will be made for diagnosis and treatment services for all citizens, including minors, under which plan cost is not a deterrent to needed service.	Documentation of such plan and means of publicizing it to target populations	

*Based on Model standards for community preventive health services, Washington, D.C., 1979, Public Health Service, U.S. Department of Health and Human Services.

†Insert the name of the specific sexually transmitted disease, e.g.: syphilis, including congenital syphilis; gonorrhea, including opthalmia neonatorum; nongonococcal urethritis and cervicitis; genital herpes; sexually transmitted hepatitis; other diseases as appropriate. *Continued.*

OBJECTIVES AND ACTIONS FOR COMMUNITY CONTROL OF SEXUALLY TRANSMITTED DISEASES—cont'd

Focus	Objectives	Indicators	Population in need
Quality of care	8. By 19 __ all health care providers seeing suspected cases of sexually transmitted disease will have been provided the latest officially recommended practices for diagnosis and treatment.	a. Record of dissemination to all health care providers and clinics of recommended standards for diagnosis and treatment b. Percent of patients reported who have been treated according to recommended standards for diagnosis and treatment received adequate diagnosis and treatment	Health care providers
	8a. By 19 __ sexually transmitted disease treatment services will include surveillance for treatment failures.	a. Proportion of sexually transmitted disease treatment services that include surveillance (test-of-cure) for treatment failure b. Percent of treated patients receiving a test-of-cure c. Treatment failure rate	
Patient education	8b. By 19 __ persons suspected of having been exposed to a sexually transmitted disease will be counseled concerning its causes, dangers, and prevention.	a. Percent of public clinic attendees suspected of having been exposed to a sexually transmitted disease counseled concerning its causes, dangers, and prevention b. Clinic policies and staffing patterns	All sexually transmitted disease patients
Public information and education	9. By 19 __ education about sexually transmitted disease, including but not limited to causes, signs and symptoms, prevention, treatment, and personal hygiene should be incorporated into the educational curriculum for all junior and senior high school students and be a part of an organized community health education program directed toward high-risk groups (e.g., college students, homosexuals,).	a. Presence of a sexually transmitted disease component in education curricula b. Percent of schools providing sexually transmitted disease education c. Percent of students receiving sexually transmitted disease education d. Existence of a community education program, including involvement from community groups (e.g., youth-serving agencies, voluntary associations, industrial health units)	Students
Gonorrhea screening	10. By 19 __ the community will be served by a mechanism to assure the availability of gonorrhea screening for high-risk persons.	Existence of mechanism	High-risk persons

A community health education program, ideally, is organized under the direction of a competent health educator working from a community health center supervised by the community health department or other officially assigned agency. Programs of public health education are less effective with overt opposition from the medical profession. All program planning should include consultation with the medical society. The practicing physician has contributions to make to the health education phase of a community's health promotion program.

Health education must use a combination of methods and channels of communication—speaking, writing, demonstrations, radio, and television. It must recruit a variety of people who may have a contribution to make. It must enlist the services of concerned organizations—official health agencies, the medical profession, voluntary health agencies, service clubs, church groups, labor unions, parent organizations, neighborhood units, and other organized groups. A community health council composed of representatives from various community organizations can be a productive force in a community health education program. Such a council is an unofficial body reflecting community interests and needs. The council serves as a coordinating and catalytic agency in the community. Its function is to cooperate in the program, not to operate it.

The health education program must concentrate on specific health problems and at the same time must promote general health education. It must deal with the present but must project itself into a continuing program for future needs.

QUESTIONS AND EXERCISES

1. Why is the quest for health seemingly an endless journey?
2. How would the conquest of infection affect the incidence of the degenerative disease?
3. What is meant by a nondegenerative, organic disease?
4. Why is it important that effort be extended toward research in the treatment as well as in the prevention of the degenerative diseases?
5. What indications exist that adults are taking a more objective attitude toward diseases of the circulatory system?
6. Why is the death rate from vascular lesions affecting the central nervous system higher among females than among males, although males have a higher incidence of arteriosclerosis and hypertension?
7. Why does the United States not invest more money in research related to circulation in the human?
8. In the United States in 1900, nephritis ranked sixth as a cause of death with a specific rate of 88.6 per 100,000. Now more than 80 years later, the rate is about 4 per 100,000. To what do you attribute the decline in this specific death rate?
9. Propose a program for your community to decrease the incidence of cancer of the respiratory tract.
10. Why is it preferable to teach a respect for cancer rather than a fear of cancer?
11. Using only local funds and resources, design a community program to obtain early discovery of cancer through the regular medical examination of virtually all adults.
12. What additional services and faciliities are needed by your community for an adequate cancer control program?
13. Propose a program designed to discover all cases of diabetes mellitus in your community.
14. Survey the services and facilities available in your community for the diagnosis and treatment of arthritis.
15. What additional services and facilities are needed by your community for an adequate adolescent health program?
16. Apply any of the standards for community programs in chronic disease control or sexually transmitted diseases to your community, using the indicators to assess the current status of community efforts.

BIBLIOGRAPHY

Bachman, J., O'Malley, P., and Johnston, J.: Change and stability in the lives of young men: adolescence to adulthood, vol. 6, Ann Arbor, Mich., 1978, Institute for Social Research.

Bateson, G., Jackson, D., Haley, J., and Weakland, J.: Toward a theory of schizophrenia, Behav. Sci. **1:**251, 1956.

Becker, M., and Green, L.: A family approach to compliance with medical treatment: a selective review of the literature, Int. J. Health Educ. **18:**173, 1975.

Blane, H., and Chafetz, M.E., editors: Alcohol, youth and social policy, New York, 1979, Plenum Publishing Corp.

Blos, P.: The adolescent passage, New York, 1979, International Universities Press.

Coates, T.J., Petersen, A., and Perry, C.: Adolescent health: crossing the barriers, New York, 1981, Academic Press, Inc.

Cohen, S., editor: New directions in patient compliance, Lexington, Mass.,1979, Lexington Books.

Consumer self-care in health, National Center for Health Services Research Proceedings Series, U.S. Department of Health, Education, and Welfare, Public Health Service, DHEW Pub. No. (HRA)77-3181, Aug., 1977.

Cullen, J., Fox, B., and Isom, R., editors: Cancer: the behavioral dimensions, New York, 1976, Raven Press.

Elkind, D.: The child and society, New York, 1979, Oxford University Press.

Enelow, A.J., and Henderson, J.B.: Applying behavioral science to cardiovascular risk, New York, 1975, American Heart Association.

Evans, R.I.: Smoking in children and adolescents. Smoking and health: a report of the Surgeon General, U.S. Department of Health, Education,and Welfare, 1979.

Facts on the major killers and cripplers: diseases in the United States today, New York, National Health Education Committee, Inc.

Fass, M.F.: Thr role of health education in hypertension control, Fam. Commun. Health 4:73, 1981.

Goodstadt, M.S.: Alcohol and drug education: models and outcomes, Health Educ. Monogr. 6:263, 1978.

Haynes, R.B., Taylor, D.W., and Sackett, D.M., editors: Compliance in health care, Baltimore, 1979, The Johns Hopkins University Press.

Hypertension Detection and Follow-up Program Cooperative Group: Five-year findings of the Hypertension Detection and Follow-up Program, J.A.M.A. 242:2562, Dec. 7, 1979.

Institute of Medicine: Adolescent behavior and health: a conference summary, IOM Pub. No. 78-004, Washington, D.C., 1978, Institute of Medicine, National Academy of Sciences.

Jessor, R.: Health-related behavior and adolescent development: a psychological perspective. Paper presented at the U.S. Institute of Medicine conference on Adolescent Behavior and Health, Washington, D.C., 1978, National Academy of Sciences, IOM Pub. No. 78-004.

Kaplan, B., and Stamler, J., editiors: Preventive cardiology, Philadelphia, 1981, W.B. Saunders Co.

Kett, J.: Rites of passage, New York, 1977, Basic Books, Inc., Publishers.

Kolbe, L.: Comprehensive school health education: proposed policy guidelines. Report prepared for School Health Education Project, National Center for Health Education, San Bruno, Calif., 1979.

Konopka, G.: Young girls: a protrait of adolescence, Englewood Cliffs, N.J., 1976, Prentice-Hall, Inc.

Levi, L., editor: Society, stress and disease, vol. 2: childhood and adolescence, New York, 1975, Oxford University Press.

Levine, D.M., et al.: Health education for hypertensive patients, J.A.M.A. 241:1700, April 20, 1979.

Lincoln, R., Jaffe, F., and Ambrose, L.: 11 million teenagers, New York, 1976, The Alan Guttmacher Institute.

Maimon, L., et al.: Education for self-treatment by adult asthmatics, J.A.M.A. 241:1919, May 4, 1979.

Malmquist, C.: Handbook of adolescence, New York, 1978, Jason Aronson, Inc.

McKenney, J.M.: A model for the pharmacist's involvement in high blood pressure control, Fam. Commun. Health 4:53, 1981.

Morisky, D.E., et al.: The relative impact of health education for low- and high-risk patients with hypertension, Prev. Med. 9:550, July, 1980.

Muns, R.E.: Theories of adolescence, ed. 3, New York, 1975, Random House, Inc.

National Advisory Cancer Council: Progress against cancer 1970, U.S. Department of Health, Education, and Welfare, Public Health Service, National Institutes of Health, 1970.

National Center for Health Statistics: The association of health attitudes and perceptions of youths, 12-17 years of age with those of their parents, Vital and Health Statistics, Series 11, No. 161, March, 1977.

National Center for Health Statistics: Monthly vital statistic report, annual summary for the United States, 1979, U.S. Department of Health and Human Services, Public Health Services, DHHS Pub. No. (PHS)81-1120, 28(13): Nov. 13, 1980.

National Diabetes Advisory Board: The treatment and control of diabetes: a national plan to reduce mortality and morbidity, U.S. Department of Health and Human Services, Public Health Service, National Institutes of Health, NIH Pub. No. 81-2284, Nov., 1980.

National Heart, Lung, and Blood Institute, Division of Lung Diseases: Respiratory diseases: taskforce report on prevention, control, education, U.S. Department of Health, Education, and Welfare, Public Health Service, DHEW Pub. No. (NIH)77, 1284, March, 1977.

National Heart, Lung, and Blood Institute, Office of Prevention, Control and Education: Proceedings of the National Heart and Lung Institute Working Conference on Health Behavior, U.S. Department of Health, Education, and Welfare, Public Health Service, DHEW Pub. No. (NIH)77-868, 1977.

Office of Disease Prevention and Health Promotion: Prevention '80, Washington, D.C., 1981, DHHS Pub. No. 81-50157, U.S. Government Printing Office.

Office of Health Information, Health Promotion and Physical Fitness and Sports Medicine: Strategies for promoting health for specific populations, Washington, D.C., 1981, DHHS (PHS) Pub. No. 81-50169, U.S. Government Printing Office.

Parcel, G.S., Luttman, D., and Meyers, M.: Formative

evaluation of a sex education course for young adolescents, J. Sch. Health, 49:335, 1979.

Radius, S., Dielman, T., Becker, M., Rosenstock, I., and Horvath, W.: Adolescent perspectives on health and illness, Adolescence 15:375, 1980.

Schwartz, J.L., editor: Progress in smoking cessation: proceedings of the international conference of smoking cessation, New York, 1978, American Cancer Society.

Seidman, H., Silverberg, E., and Holleb, A.: Cancer statistics, 1976—a comparison of white and black population, New York, 1976, American Cancer Society, Professional Education Publications.

Shapiro, S., Strax, P., and Vener, L.: Periodic breast cancer screening: the first two years of screening, Arch. Environ. Health 15:547, 1967.

Squyres, W., editor: Patient education: an inquiry into the state of the art, New York, 1980, Springer Publishing Co., Inc.

Stamler, J., et al.: Epidemiology of hypertension, New York, 1967, Grune & Stratton, Inc.

Sugar, M., editor: Female adolescent development, New York, 1979, Brunner/Mazel, Inc.

Sutton, M.: Cancer explained: symptoms, signs and early diagnosis, New York, 1967, Hart Publishing Co., Inc.

Swisher, J.D.: Mental health—the core of preventive health education, J. Sch. Health 46:386, 1976.

U.S. Department of Health, Education, and Welfare: Self-reported health behavior and attitudes of youths 12-17 years, United States, vital and health statistics, Series 11, No. 147, DHEW Pub. No. (HRA) 75-1629, Washington, D.C., 1975, U.S. Government Printing Office.

U.S. Department of Health, Education, and Welfare: Adolescent health care: a guide for BCHS-supported programs and projects, DHEW 79-5234, Rockville, Md., 1979.

U.S. Department of Health, Education, and Welfare: Healthy people: the Surgeon General's report on health promotion and disease prevention, vol 2, background papers, Washington, D.C., 1979.

U. S. Department of Health and Human Services: Compendium of resource materials on adolescent health: interdisciplinary adolescent health training workshop series, 1977-1980, Rockville, MD., 1980.

Weinstein, M., and Stason, W.: Hypertension: a policy perspective Cambridge, Mass., 1976, Harvard University Press.

Weiss, S., editor: Behavioral medicine research, New York, 1981, Academic Press, Inc.

White, P.D., and Donovan, H.: Hearts: the long follow-up, Philadelphia, 1967, W.B. Saunders Co.

Windsor, R.A., Green, L.W., and Roseman, J.M.: Health promotion and maintenance for patients with chronic obstructive pulmonary disease, J. Chronic Dis. 33:5, 1980.

Zelnik, M., and Kantner, J.F.: Sexual activity, contraceptive use and pregnancy among metropolitan-area teenagers: 1971-1979, Fam. Plann. Perspect. 12:425, 1980.

7

COMMUNITY GERIATRICS

Our objective should be to die as
young as possible—as late as possible.

Anonymous

How far the gulf-stream of our youth may flow
Into the arctic regions of our lives—
For Age is Opportunity No Less
Than Youth Itself! Though In Another Dress,
And as the evening twilight fades away
The sky is filled with stars, invisible by day.

H.W. Longfellow from *Morituri Salutamus*

Gerontology and geriatrics both study the aging process, including biological, psychological, and social change. Gerontology concerns itself with the natural aging process and with pathological aging. Geriatrics deals with the care of the aged and concerns itself primarily with enabling old people to live productively and enjoyably. The research health scientist finds gerontology of special interest, whereas the applied field of community health deals more with geriatrics than with gerontology; hence this chapter will be concerned with health as an aspect of geriatrics. Health cannot be isolated from the total life of the citizen. Aspects of living that are indirectly related to health must be considered.

Aging could be thought of as a process that begins with conception. In practice, aging is regarded as that phase in life when bodily functioning begins to decline. Technically, then, it would be in order to describe everyone over the age of 30 as aging. The problem here is

with the particular health factors that are of special importance at a given age. Because the age of retirement is usually accepted as 65, it is customary to think of anyone beyond this age as being in the classification of "aged." Yet a person of chronological age 55 could be older physiologically than another individual of age 75. The arbitrary age of 65 is accepted in health circles as marking off a segment of the U.S. population that has health needs different from those of other segments. This is accepted even though it is acknowledged that many of the health problems that exist in the retired population could have been prevented or at least anticipated constructively with preretirement counseling. Furthermore, the average age of retirement is declining. For these reasons, we define the aged population at 60 and over for much of the discussion of community geriatrics.

Although health is a primary concern of the elderly, illness and old age are not synonymous. Data from national surveys indicate that the majority of the elderly in the United States see themselves as well, not sick. Over half of those over the age of 80 who are living in the community report that their health is good. In assessing their health status, the elderly compare themselves not with all people, but with their age cohorts, with those who are institutionalized and those who have died. There is a high correlation between the negative evaluation of health status and the degree to which an elderly person feels economically stressed, lonely, alienated, or useless.

In general, the elderly person who reports that he or she has good to excellent health is also more likely to report having a more positive psychological attitude, feeling more financially secure, having a high sense of the worth of things, feeling useful, and feeling personally secure and not being bothered by feelings of anger, tension, restlessness, or confusion.

THE AGING POPULATION

That the age distributions of Western populations are shifting toward the older group is general knowledge. The number of people in the United States over age 60 has increased in size from 4.9 million in 1900 to nearly seven times this number in 1977 (32.8 million), while the population under 60 years of age has increased at only one fourth this rate. Current Census Bureau projections indicate that the elderly will continue to grow at a faster pace than the rest of the population into the twenty-first century. The growth rate for the elderly population will slow somewhat around the turn of the century as the relatively smaller percentage of cohorts who were born during the Depression of the 1930s reach the age of 60. As persons born during the "baby boom" years reach the age of 60 early in the next century, most of the growth in the U.S. population will occur in the older age brackets. Between 1980 and

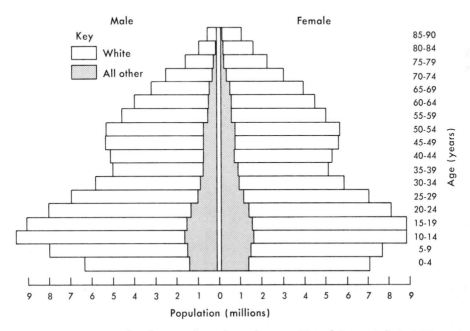

FIG. 7-1. Age-sex distribution of population by race, United States, July 1, 1980.

2035, the total population is projected to grow by about 40%, from 220 million to 304 million persons. The elderly population is projected to be more than double in size during this same period, from 33 to 71 million.

With these demographic changes, the average age of the U.S. population has risen from 23 years to over 29 years since 1900, and it is projected to climb to 38 years by the year 2035. At the beginning of this century, persons 60 years old and over represented 1 of every 16 persons. They now represent 1 of every 7 and, by the year 2035, will represent about one fourth of the total population. Among the population 25 years old and over, the elderly now represent one fourth of this age group and will represent over one third by the year 2035, when today's college students are in their seventies. Because of the rapidly dropping death rate and birthrate, the U.S. age pyramid, as shown in Fig. 7-1, is shrinking at the bottom and growing wider at the top.

The elderly merit an organized community program for the promotion of their health. Concern for the health of the older age segment of the population has been intensified by the rapid increase in the number of older people.

One third of the older population is very old, 75 years or above. This proportion will stay about the same for the foreseeable future if mortality remains constant. If it does, there will be about 12 million of the very old by the year 2000. If mortality continues to decline, however, the numbers of the very old may grow as high as 16 or 18 million.

A 65-year-old man can now expect, on the average, to live to 78; a women of 65, to 82. By the year 2000, life expectancies for 65-year-olds may increase by another 2 to 5 years. The gain in life expectancy during the twentieth century represents an outstanding achievement, but it brings with it substantial changes in the society as a whole and enormous challenges for communities. The increasing numbers of the "young-old"—persons in their late 50s, 60s, and early 70s, who are retired, relatively healthy and vigorous, and who seek meaningful ways to use their time, either in self-fulfillment or in community participation—challenge the community to use their talents both to enrich their own lives and to improve society at large.

A second set of community issues stems from the fact that there are even more striking increases in the numbers of the "old-old"—persons in their mid-70s, 80s, and 90s. An increasing minority of the old-old remain vigorous and active, but the majority need a range of supportive and restorative health and social services. The old-old of the 1980s represent a disproportionately disadvantaged group. The reasons are several, including the fact that this group includes many immigrants who were poorly educated and who have spent their working years at low-paying jobs. Many have been unable to accumulate savings or to build up sufficient equity in the Social Security system to sustain them adequately through their years of retirement.

Future populations of young-old and old-old persons will have different characteristics. They will have been better educated and will have received better medical care throughout their lives. Because their life experiences will have been markedly different from the present population of older people, their expectations of life, including their expectations of old age, will be different. As a result, programs suited to the young-old and old-old persons of today will need continuous revisions if they are to be suited to future populations.

FACTORS IN AGING

Aging is a natural process with a number of physiological changes, many of them merely a decline in the rate of functioning. A reduction in the metabolic rate of about 7% occurs every 10 years after the age of 30. There is a retardation of the rate of cell division, cell growth, and cell repair. Tissues, including their cells, tend to dry out. A fatty infiltration usually occurs with cellular atrophy, and a decrease in the speed of muscular response and a decline in muscular strength occur. With a reduction in the efficiency of circulation, endurance is adversely affected. Connective tissues suffer a decrease in elasticity, bones become more brittle as the amount of organic material becomes reduced, teeth lose their structural integrity, and functioning of the digestive system declines so that digestion proceeds at a much slower rate. Many people over age 60 produce no hydrochloric acid in their stomach. Some of the nutritional deficiency in the older individual can be attributed to poor digestion and inadequate absorption rather than a poor diet. There is a general decline in the functioning of the nervous system and special sense organs. Because of a delayed response to infection or any other disorder, illness tends to be extended in the older person.

The principal concern of health science, however, is with pathological aging, which means a hastening of the aging process by adverse factors affecting body functioning. Repeated insults to the body leave their toll. The prime of life, as we know it, could be extended and thus aging could be delayed if all factors that produce pathological aging could be prevented or dealt with summarily.

Low-grade infection, particularly of a chronic nature, takes a toll. Toxins from the environment also hasten the aging process. Extended critical illness from which an individual recovers nevertheless hastens aging. Deteriorating diseases such as hypertension, arthritis, and rheumatism tend to produce premature aging. Chronic tension, worry, and fatigue, associated with an inability to relax, can hasten the aging process. The stress syndrome masks a disturbance of biochemical functioning that can take a considerable toll in premature aging.

Inactivity can be a factor in producing pathological aging. The level of effectiveness that the circulatory system attains is dependent on regular activity to challenge the circulatory system and on the native endowment one may possess in the way of a circulatory system. Marked nutritional deficiency that results in emaciation over an extended period of time has a recognized adverse effect on the retention of the prime of life. Nutritional deficiency such as one observes in some of the underdeveloped nations of the world can have some effect on the aging process. Inadequacy of vitamins, proteins, and minerals in the diet can have an effect in producing premature aging. Cigarettes and excessive alcohol are the most clearly isolated agents contributing to more rapid degeneration today.

CHARACTERISTICS OF ELDERLY PEOPLE

It would be inaccurate to speak of a typical elderly person, although it would not be inaccurate to say that one could expect to find in many older people the following characteristics: (1) loss of status and an increased uncertainty about personal worth, (2) an insecurity associated with a feeling of inability to meet the demands of life, (3) apprehension about health, (4) difficulty in adjusting from a work routine to one of retirement, (5) an inability to find avenues of service that will provide personal gratification, (6) difficulty in meeting stresses created by social change, and (7) limited incentive for social participation.

Elderly people are eager to be useful in some capacity. Women make the transition into retirement more easily than men, partially because they have been preparing for the later years of life and usually have experienced a gradual transition into that phase. They have developed interests and associations that provide opportunity for useful service. Men, on the other hand, may find retirement an entirely new way of life and may find themselves floundering helplessly in an attempt to find some social grounds on which to tread. Life soon loses it objectivity for one who finds no purpose in day-to-day living. Preparation for retirement has become as important as preparation for employment.

STATUS OF THE ELDERLY IN THE COMMUNITY

Just as many of the health problems of the poor are related to problems of racism and class, and as some problems of women are related to sexism, so too are major problems of the aged related to "ageism." A community approach to the health of the elderly therefore must concern itself with public and professional attitudes toward aging and sterotypes about the aged. Institutional prejudice against age also exists to the extent that our community services and institutions discriminate against the aged in ways that threaten their access to preventive and health care resources. Community health programs attempt to adjust resources, communications, and organizational arrangements to meet the special needs of older people.

Each day the community sees its elderly people and may assume that they are living more enjoyably and effectively or more unhappily than they really are. Yet each community should make a critical appraisal of the status of its elderly citizens. Retirement provisions in America are still inadequate but are being improved rapidly. The Office of Research and Statistics, Social Security Administration, and Department of Health and Human Services, report that of citizens 65 years and older, 39% are retired (30% Social Security, 6% railroad retirement, 3% private pensions), 4% are living on veteran's benefits, 5% are on public assistance, 33% are living on the income of their employment, 15% are living on investment income, and 5% are supported by relatives. As the provisions of the Social Security program are broadened, a greater percentage of citizens over age 65 will receive old age and survivors insurance benefits, and a smaller percentage will be employed. Socioeconomic factors may even produce a retirement age of 60 for the general population. The earlier retirement age will pose additional problems unless better programs are promoted for preparing people for retirement.

Approximately half the men over age 65 are potential members of the labor force, and many of them prefer to work. Frequently it is not possible for them to continue in the type of work they were pursuing before retirement and it is necessary to learn a new type of work. Some find that their skills and trades have become obsolete, and for this reason have to find new types of employment. Many of these individuals have an adequate physical capacity as well as an adequate learning capacity to take up new jobs, but industries are reluctant to employ elderly workers because they tend to be slower and have a high accident rate and a higher rate of absenteeism. However, the older worker is generally meticulous in work, produces work of a high quality, and is extremely reliable. There is a need to lower work barriers for the elderly who are physically and mentally capable. Employment opportunities need to be increased for those elderly citizens capable of contributing to the community's economy. Part-time jobs have their merit, particularly when the elderly person supplements work with other community services and activities.

Personal adjustment is the key to satisfactory retirement. Workers must alter their lives when retirement is reached. Preparation for successful old age should begin at about age 40, with the development of a wide range of interests and channels of community service. Elderly persons must be supported to accept change, cultivate a range of interest, maintain a willingness to learn, and participate actively in community affairs.

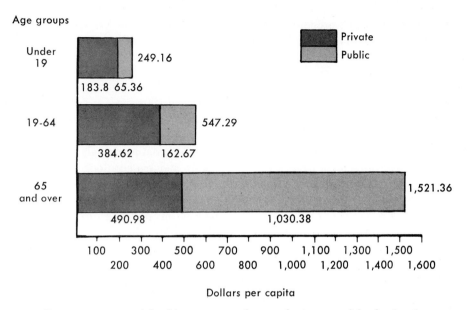

Age groups

FIG. 7-2. Per capita personal health care expenditures, by source of funds, for three age groups, fiscal year 1976, United States.

From U.S. Department of Health and Human Services, Health Care Finance Administration.

HEALTH PROBLEMS CREATED BY LONGEVITY

Fig. 7-2 reveals that many of the disorders in the later years, such as diseases of the heart, arteriosclerosis, and other degenerative diseases, require far more medical care than those of earlier years. The main problem becomes that of proper medical supervision for the afflicted individual, and government must bear a larger proportion of the bill for the aged. Primary prevention is still in order for certain infectious diseases, such as influenza and pneumonia, and for accidental deaths. Early detection and treatment (secondary prevention) of malignant neoplasms and hypertension could give these older citizens several additional years of life. Even individuals over age 60 who appear to be in excellent health should have a thorough medical examination once every 2 years. Certainly, those who obviously are not well should have periodic checkups more frequently.

Several disorders not commonly a cause of death nevertheless represent important problems for the aged. Arthritis and rheumatism, two of the principal causes of disability in the aged, can usually be treated to relieve patients of much of their pain and enable them to extend their activities. Disorders of vision are common among the aged. Some degree of correction is usually possible even though the individual's vision with glasses is not normal. When the loss of vision has progressed to a state where the individual is no longer able to read, records are available that enable the blind or near blind to enjoy hearing the literature or feature articles of the day that they would normally read. Loss of hearing in the later years of life is common. Hearing aids have been developed to the point where a much higher percentage of the hard of hearing are aided to hear adequately for customary needs. Deafness produces a feeling of loneliness. This increases the need to develop programs to provide whatever hearing can be obtained.

Mental health and mental disorders

Definitions of health and disease change not only with biomedical advances, but also with social and historical factors, for instance, with changes in social attitudes toward deviant behavior. These issues apply especially to attempts to distinguish mental health and mental disorder, as the next chapter will show. But for older people they pose growing social problems. It is estimated that some 15% of persons over 65 suffer from mental disorders, 5% from severe disorders. Alcoholism and drug misuse appear to be increasing among older persons. One striking fact is that, while this age group constitutes only 10% of the total population, it accounts for over 30% of all suicides. Criminal behavior, on the other hand, drops dramatically with age.

Physical health is a very important element in mental health, but so are social factors. Such social issues need continuing study, issues of how ethnicity, socioeconomic status, marital status, and rural-urban residence contribute to incidence and prevalence, to diagnosis, to cause, and to treatment of mental disorders. Workable models are needed for relating social and cultural factors to biological factors in ways that can lead to prevention as well as amelioration of disorders. For instance, industrialization and urbanization are often said to be producing greater social stresses and greater social isolation for older persons, and therefore more mental disorders. But this remains a moot point. The nature of social stress is not well understood, and studies indicate that social isolation is more often an outcome than a cause of mental illness in older people, as in younger adults.

Education and income are highly related to the type of mental illness and also to the type of treatment offered by mental health professionals. There is a relationship also between education and the extent to which people seek help, either professional or nonprofessional. In Western society at large, there has been a broadening range of problems for which people seek assistance and a rising level of expectation with regard to outcomes. At present, older people seem underrepresented in these patterns of social change. But as new cohorts of the old are increasingly well educated, their needs and expectations of the mental health system are likely to change.

The majority of functional psychiatric disturbances in old age (hypochondriacal states, paranoid reactions, and particularly the depressions) are responsive to appropriate treatment. Some 10% to 15% of organic brain syndromes are reversible (those due to coexisting physical illness or to drug intoxication, for instance). At the same time, older persons are dramatically underserved by community mental health centers, psychiatric outpatient clinics, and private psychiatric practitioners.

From the perspective of the mental health system as a whole, there have been striking changes in patterns of use of psychiatric facilities for different age groups. As mental health ideologies have changed, the mental health system has served a smaller proportion of older persons, with a great shift occurring after World War II from the use of mental hospitals to the use of nursing homes.

MEETING THE GERIATRICS PROBLEM

The health of the older age groups in the population has become recognized officially as a public health problem. The National Institute of Aging of the U.S. Public Health Service has been established in the United States to support research in gerontology and demonstrations in geriatrics. Plans and programs must originate with communities. Many state health departments have agencies for the promotion of the health of older citizens or administrative agencies to coordinate a statewide program for the promotion of the health and welfare of the aged.

The elderly, perhaps more than any other group in society, rely heavily on health and welfare resources. The lengthening period after retirement has exacerbated the problems of providing social and health services, maintaining income, and maximizing the ability of the elderly to function in society.

Present service systems are flawed. Communities are often unable to respond effectively and efficiently to the age-related needs of individuals and families. Service programs are often not flexible enough for the person in need; in fact, sometimes they are not available. Even when service programs are available, persons who need them may be unaware of them. State and federal resources are required to supplement the resources of most communities to meet the needs of their aged.

COMMUNITY ORGANIZATION AND THE AGED

The provisions of a community for the allocation of resources and social roles to the aged make a large difference in the quality of life and consequently in the health of the aged.

Social networks

The continued involvement of older persons in various social networks (such as family, friendship, work, leisure, religious, and other organizations) is considered a deterrent to feelings of isolation in later life. Dyadic or paired relationships (for example, a confidant) maintained over time seem to be of particular importance, but dyadic bonds have seldom been organized, except for the husband-wife relationship.

With advancing age there is a decline in number of roles, amount of interaction, and variety of social contacts. Less active persons, however, are likely to be older, in poorer health, and in more deprived circumstances, so it is not clear to what extent the decline is a cause or a consequence of the aging process. It is probably both, creating an isolation-aging cycle.

Communities cannot ignore the impact on the aged of declining involvement in various social networks. Activity and morale are influenced by the extent to which social networks encourage or discourage continued participation. Therefore a distinction must be made between voluntary and involuntary withdrawal. Furthermore, it is probably the quality of interaction, rather than the frequency, that is important.

Assessment of social networks in the community focuses on examining interpersonal connections between people, not on institutional structures, personalities, or life histories. In recent years the method has been used to seek an understanding of social conditions, problems, and behavior in all age groups.

Family networks

Among social networks, the family has been paramount. For instance, although social norms may stress nuclear family independence, older people remain linked to kinship networks both within and across generations. Most older people have close relatives within easy visiting distance, contacts are frequent, and it is children, particularly daughters, to whom older people turn for help.

The family has remained a strong and supportive institution for older people. Most older persons want to be as independent of their families as possible, but when they can no longer manage for themselves, they expect their children to come to their aid. Not only do such expectations exist, they are usually met. Patterns vary among social classes and ethnic groups, but most older persons see their children regularly, and a complex pattern of exchange of goods and services exists across generations, with ties of affection and ties of obligation remaining strong. Furthermore, elderly parents appear to have attitudes and values remarkably similar to those of their children and grandchildren.

A trend toward separate households for older persons has developed (*family* is not synonymous with *household*). Yet the latest national data show that the older the individual, and the sicker, the more likely the person is to be found living with a child. In 1970, of all persons aged 75 and over, 1 out of 5 women and 1 out of 10 men were living with a child— more than double the number who were living in institutions. The trend toward separate households will be affected by economic factors, housing policies, and the increasing number of families in which old-old persons have children who are themselves old. If more effective networks of supportive social and home health services are built, more intergenerational households in which both generations are old may emerge.

The structure of the family has changed in the past few decades, with larger proportions of older men and women married and living with their spouses, and with accompanying decreases in proportions of those widowed, divorced, and those who never married. At the same time, the absolute number of widows is increasing as the difference in longevity between the sexes grows greater. Whether these trends will continue in the next 25 years will depend on a host of social and economic factors, not least among them, changing attitudes toward divorce and remarriage and toward nontraditional forms of family life, such as communal living for people in their later years.

Friendship and membership ties

Friendship and membership ties complement kinship ties by relieving some of the burden of care from kin. The more characteristics neighbors have in common (such as socioeconomic status, marital status, and value orientations), the more integrated the friendship network. Gerontology has seldom elaborated on friendship patterns or sociability, or on the so-

cial contexts of work, leisure, and organizational participation. Voluntary membership in associations and participation in such organizations, including old-age clubs and senior centers, depend to a considerable extent on styles established earlier in life.

Church attendance drops off among the very old, but it is not clear how much this relates to such factors as health, residential location, or socioeconomic status. Nor is it clear how age-related factors relate to historical factors in affecting patterns of church attendance or patterns of private devotions. In what ways does church attendance among older people reflect broader social trends? To what extent do private devotions replace church attendance? Related questions concern the church as a social institution in the lives of older persons. To what extent and for what subgroup does the church perform a supportive social and psychological function?

In recent years more women have been assuming dual roles in the home and marketplace. Women have increased the time spent in paid work and have somewhat decreased the time spent in family roles, although not enough to compensate for the increase in paid work time. The allocation of men's time to work and family roles, on the other hand, has remained relatively constant. It appears that as the women's labor force participation increases, there is a net transfer of labor away from men and toward women. Many women are under considerable stress resulting from these dual roles, but their opportunities for social ties that will carry over into retirement have been multiplied.

Civic participation

Elderly people are less connected to the fabric of society because of their extrusion from their earlier roles, especially work and family, and thus are correspondingly more alienated from their community. Civic participation is a means of reestablishing this connection.

Within populations with similar educational, social class, and ethnic background, the political behavior, community organizational involvement, and volunteer activities are not noticeably different for older people than for younger people. Voting behavior remains remarkably consistent far into old age, older people do vote, and they tend to vote for the party for which they have always voted. There is no evidence of a voting bloc composed of the elderly. There has, however, been an enormous growth of lobby groups among the elderly. But their influence and representation are doubtful. Other than voting, participation in political activity is infrequent among older people.

The elderly who participate in community organizations appear to be a very select sample (who may represent their individual needs more than any constituency). The community organization often selects to represent in the community those elderly people who can be expected to go along with the organization's practices rather than those who might be critical.

Age-based organizations

An age-based organization is one that depends on, for its activities, the existence of older persons. The old are its members, its direct or indirect consumers, or its subjects of special concern. Such organizations exist in industrialized nations throughout the world. A few are active in U.S. politics, such as the National Council of Senior Citizens and the American Association of Retired Persons. Such organizations can play a role in shaping the issues of public policy debate; they gain access to legislators, administrative officials, and political party organizations, but few have yet displayed a capacity to organize a bloc of old-age votes consistently at the local or national level.

Aging as a concern of political systems

The aged first became a major concern of governments in the late nineteenth century.

The birth of the modern welfare state, with economic relief for older persons as a major feature, began in Germany in the 1880s, then spread to other industrialized countries, appearing relatively late in the United States with the enactment of the Social Security program in 1935.

Income-maintenance policies have undergone innumerable expansions in the intervening decades. The range of efforts for helping older persons has broadened. It now includes attempts to meet personal needs, such as shelter, medical care, and employment training, and group needs, such as better transportation and other community improvements. The evolution of governmental policies toward the aged can be traced to a number of factors, ranging from the efforts of individual reformers to various societal changes brought about by long-term economic and ideological trends. Organizations such as political parties, labor unions, economics elites, and professional and commercial organizations have found reason to advocate or oppose governmental action toward the aging.

Community programs

It is on the community level that functional programs must be formulated, because at higher levels the program will fail to touch individual elderly citizens and their families. Of necessity, the state or provincial program will be far removed from the individual who needs health services.

The problem of a community is basically threefold: (1) public education in the field of adult health, (2) integration of all services and forces in the community that have a service to offer elderly persons, and (3) the acquisition and provision of necessary services that the community does not now have available. A community health agency must be designated to determine the needs for health promotion and the approaches that should be used. The official community health center may not pro-

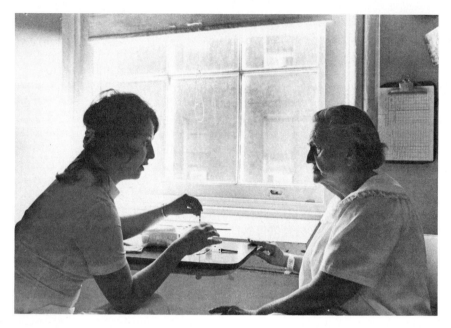

FIG. 7-3. Patient education for the elderly. Chronic conditions require long-term maintenance and self-care. To be highly effective, education must be individualized at some point in the process.

Courtesy Johns Hopkins Medical Institutions.

vide medical service, but may serve as an information, coordinating, and program promotion center.

Emphasis in the community program must be placed on public health education. The public needs to understand the nature of aging and the phenomena associated with advancing years. The public should understand what can be done to prevent some of the premature deterioration of aging and should have an understanding of measures for the prevention of diseases and disabilities of the advancing years. The public needs to be informed of the importance of self-care and medical supervision and the contribution that various individuals, agencies, and self-help groups have to make to the elderly citizens of the community. Perhaps most important, the public needs to adjust its unrealistic perceptions of the aged themselves.

A community program to promote the health

of elderly people must include attempts to provide the various services required for the treatment, hospitalization, and rehabilitation of those elderly people who have some disability. It must include provisions for activities that elderly people can enjoy through participation. For elderly people who are unable to pay for professional services the program should provide some means through which they may receive the professional services required.

Perhaps the greatest contribution such a program can make is to give the elderly a feeling that someone is concerned with their problems and that there is an agency in the community to which they can turn for guidance and assistance. Most elderly people in a community are self-sufficient or have members of their immediate family who can provide any advice or assistance that may be needed, but some have no such source of aid. These individuals would be greatly benefited by an effective community health program for the elderly.

Nutrition programs in the United States

In addition to promoting better health among older Americans through improved nutrition, health education, counseling, and the limited delivery of health services, nutrition programs help reduce the isolation of older persons by offering them an opportunity to participate in community activities and to combine food and friendship. The 1972 Amendments to the Older Americans Act of 1965 stated the situation for the United States in the following way:

Many older persons do not eat adequately because (1) they cannot afford to do so; (2) they lack the skills to select and prepare nourishing and well-balanced meals; (3) they have limited mobility, which may impair their capacity to shop and cook for themselves; (4) they have feelings of rejection and loneliness which obliterate the incentive necessary to prepare and eat a meal alone. These and other physiological, psychological, and social and economic changes that occur with aging result in a pattern of living which causes malnutrition and further physical and mental deterioration.

To meet this situation, there have been established throughout the United States nutrition program projects that provide at least one hot meal a day, at least 5 days a week, to Americans 60 and over and their spouses of any age. The meal must provide one third of the current recommended daily dietary allowances (RDAs) as promulgated by the Food and Nutrition Board, National Academy of Sciences–National Research Council. The U.S. Department of Agriculture provides a stipulated value of donated foods, or cash, or both, for each meal the nutrition program serves.

Community provision of meals in group settings is emphasized. Meal sites include schools, churches, community centers, senior citizen centers, public housing, and other public and nonprofit facilities where other supportive services may also be available. Outreach programs identify those older persons most in need. Escort and transportation services to bring participants to nutrition program project sites are also a part of the package the program provides.

Although the nutrition program by law is not a home-delivered meal activity, it does provide home-delivered meals to regular participants who from time to time are unable to attend the meal service site. In 1980 about 15% of all meals served were home delivered.

The program recognizes the need for a network of supportive services, including health services, information and referral, escort services, health and welfare counseling, and consumer education. The nutrition program projects act as centers of activity, attracting older persons to a place where, in addition to a nourishing meal, they have the opportunity to receive these services, as well as advice on such important matters as legal rights, housing, shopping assistance, income maintenance, and crime prevention. Older persons also have the opportunity for socialization and recreation and for volunteer service to others. Under the terms of the Older Americans Act, states are encouraged to make nutrition program projects part of the system of services coordinated through area agencies on aging.

An important part of the nutrition program is health and nutrition education, designed to direct attention to all health needs, including good nutrition. Such education makes older persons, project staff members, and volunteers aware of the relative values of food and their contribution to health and well-being, and can thereby influence selection, purchase, and preparation.

There are more than 1,100 nutrition program projects serving over 400,000 meals daily in approximately 9,000 sites. Meals served to persons representing minorities represent 22% of the total, and 67% of the meals are served to persons below the poverty threshold.

As a formula grant program, the National

Nutrition Program for Older Americans allocates to each state an amount that bears the same ratio to the total amount appropriated as its population aged 60 or over bears to the population of that age in all states. However, no state is allotted less than one half of 1% of the amount appropriated. Guam, American Samoa, the Virgin Islands, and the Trust Territory of the Pacific Islands are each allotted at least one fourth of 1% of the total appropriation.

In each state the nutrition program is administered by the state agency on aging, unless another agency is designated by the governor and approved by the U.S. Commissioner on Aging. The administering agency makes grants or contracts with public and nonprofit agencies, institutions, and organizations for actual provision and delivery of meals. Information concerning administration of the program is available from the state agencies on aging. State agencies administering the nutrition program must provide for advisory assistance that includes consumers of services rendered, members of minority groups, and persons knowledgeable in the provision of health, nutrition, and other supportive services.

Projects must serve primarily low-income persons 60 years of age and over and their spouses and other older Americans who are determined to be in greatest need. The state also must ensure that awards are made to initiate projects to serve minority, native American, and limited English-speaking individuals, at least in proportion to their numbers within the state. Meal sites are required to be located in urban areas that have heavy concentrations of target group older Americans and in rural areas that have high proportions of eligible older persons.

No one may be turned away from a meal for inability to pay, and there is no means test. All participants are given an opportunity to contribute to all or part of the cost of a meal. The nutrition program project councils, all of which contain participant majorities, establish either a contribution schedule based on resources or a single flat sum as a guide to the size of contributions. Each participant determines what he or she is able to contribute. Contributions are received in such a manner that the amount contributed is known only to the participant contributor.

HEALTH PRACTICES

Most elderly individuals follow a normal course of living, although perhaps in second gear rather than in high gear and with modification of some of the established health practices. The particular routine of living adopted by each of these individuals should be adjusted to his or her capacities, past mode of living, present needs, and life interests. Certain factors are common to virtually all.

Nutrition. While the quantity of food required by the person in the later years of life is not as great as in the earlier years, the qualitative needs are just as important. Diversity of proteins, a sufficiency of vitamins, and adequate minerals should be included in each day's diet. Food should be attractive because the sense of taste becomes dulled with age. In the later years of life the output of digestive enzymes is reduced and the rate of digestion is much slower. For this reason, many elderly people find that eating more frequently and eating less at each meal is a highly satisfactory practice. Self-medication of the digestive system and supplementary vitamins should be used only on the advice of a physician.

Activity. Unless a supervising physician advises otherwise, moderate activity is highly desirable for the normal elderly person. The general tone of body functioning that activity produces can be beneficial in producing a level of functioning near the maximum for the individual. Some degree of fatigue during the day is normal, but excessive fatigue can be harmful. Activity can be purposeful, such as tending a garden or performing other simple tasks, and can be productive. Not rigorous activity, but

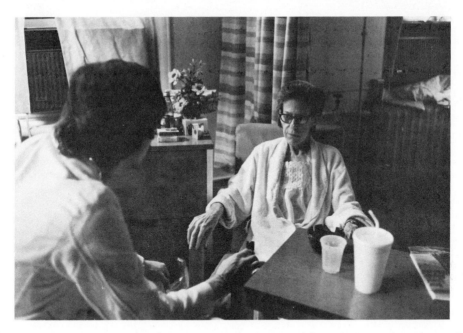

FIG. 7-4. Nutrition counseling. Before patients are discharged from the hospital, professional staff may lay the groundwork for follow-up home visits to assist patients.

Courtesy Johns Hopkins Medical Institutions.

moderately paced exertion, can be rewarding physically, emotionally, and socially.

Rest and sleep. Intervals of rest during the day should be coordinated with the tasks or activities requiring physical exertion. A mid-morning, noon, and midafternoon rest period will be adequate for some, but others may need more frequent rest periods. Some elderly individuals do very well without any particular rest periods. This is true of the somewhat restless individual who prefers to be occupied with some task.

Generally, as people get older they tend to sleep longer each day. The tendency is for the elderly person to go to bed earlier and to rise earlier than is the custom of the general adult population. Some seem to require less sleep than they did in earlier years. Each person in the old age group seems to adjust sleep to individual needs.

Safety. Physical injury and accidental death are high among people in the old-age groups. Slowed reaction time, poor vision, and the inability to adjust readily to changing situations make the old person more accident prone than younger individuals. Conditions in the home should be made as safe as possible. Living on one floor is an effective safety measure, because falls on stairs constitute a frequent cause of death for old people. Having well-lighted rooms and hallways, and even the use of continuous dim light through the night, can be effective safety measures. Old people have a high fatality rate in motor vehicle-pedestrian accidents. Many elderly people object to being squired or guided. Such objections may have to be overruled when special hazards exist and when the individual appears to have difficulty in adjusting to the tempo of traffic.

Bathing. Bodily cleanliness has an important psychological value for the elderly. A well-established living routine that includes bathing is

Text continued on p. 190.

Model standards for nursing homes and other community institutional services*

GOAL: Persons in institutional settings will have safe and healthful living conditions.

Focus	Objectives	Indicators	Population in need
	Outcome		
	1. By 19 ___ the number of premature deaths occurring in ___ will not exceed ___ † per year.	Mortality in excess of that expected	Institutionalized persons
	2. By 19 ___ the incidence of disease or infection attributable to the institutional environment will not exceed 1,000 person days per year for ___ †.	Morbidity	
	3. By 19 ___ the incidence of injuries attributable to the institutional environment will not exceed ___ per 1,000 person days per year for ___ †.	Injury rate	
	Process		
Health protection and promotion	1. By 19 ___ all institutions will conduct a health protection and promotion program as an integral part of their service for the resident population.	Percent of institutions with program	Institutionalized persons
	1a. By 19 ___ each institution will have established policies and procedures including provision for an intake health screening that will provide for the identification of health problems and needs for care and treatment.	a. Percent of institutions with such policies and procedures b. Percent of institutionalized persons screened	
	1b. By 19 ___ all institutionalized persons will be informed of their rights to and have access to medical, dental, and mental health care and treatment services.	a. Percent of institutionalized persons with access to such services b. Percent of institutionalized persons informed of rights to such services	

1c. By 19 — each institution will have established policies and procedures to provide residents with required pharmaceuticals, supervise the administration of medications as required, and control the use of pharmaceuticals in the institution.	Existence of policies and procedures
1d. By 19 — each institution will maintain an accurate, complete, up-to-date health record on each resident.	Percent of records meeting appropriate institutional review criteria
1e. By 19 — each institution will be served by a program of comprehensive environmental surveillance and maintenance.	Existence of service
1f. By 19 — each institution will be served by a communicable disease control program.	Existence of service
1g. By 19 — each institution will provide food that meets each individual's nutritional needs, including medically-indicated special dietary needs.	a. Existence of menu planning process b. Percent of medically indicated diets needed that are provided
1h. By 19 — each institution will provide, on a regular basis, exercise, activity, and recreational opportunities appropriate to the needs of the institutionalized persons.	a. Existence of recreational, exercise, and other activity opportunities b. Percent of eligible persons participating
1i. By 19 — each institution will designate specific management responsibilities, including responsibility at the executive level, to direct and implement the various elements of its health protection and promotion program.	Existence of policies and designated management assignments

*Based on Model standards for community preventive health services, Washington, D.C., 1979, Public Health Service, U.S. Department of Health and Human Services.

†Insert type of institution.

Model standards for home health services in the community*

GOAL: Residents of the community with illnesses or handicaps that restrict self-care but do not require acute care or continuous supervision will be able to continue living at home rather than in a health care institution for as long as desirable and feasible.

Focus	Objectives	Indicators	Population in need
Care of the sick and functionally disabled	**Outcome**		
	1. By 19___, ___ % of persons known to be in need of noninstitutional supportive services will receive the appropriate level of services.	Percent of persons in need of services who receive them	Chronically ill and functionally disabled
	2. By 19___ the percent of inappropriate placements in long-term care institutions will not exceed ___ .	Percent of inappropriate placements	
	Process		
	1. By 19___ the community will have access to the following home health services. (Recommend that an agency provide services a–e directly):	Availability of services	Chronically ill and functionally disabled
	a. Nursing		
	b. Home health aide		
	c. Physical, occupational, speech and hearing therapy		
	d. Social work		
	e. Dietary and nutrition services		
	f. Homemaker (or homemaker-home health aide)		
	g. Dental services		
	h. Chore services		
	i. Shopping services		
	j. Transportation		
	k. Respite care		
	1a. By 19___ the community will be served by a mechanism to assure the quality of the services delivered.	a. Assessment of home health services delivery system in the community (a possible model is the National League of Nursing criteria)	
		b. Licensure, where required by state law Scope of alternatives available	
	2. By 19___ alternatives to institutional placement will be available that make independent living in the home possible despite functional disability.		The community

Category	Objective	Indicators	Target population
	3. By 19 ___ the community will be served by a program to increase community and professional awareness of the range and sources of home health services and their appropriate use.	a. Existence of information and referral program in community b. Increases in number of referrals to home-health agencies c. Number of referrals to agency from noninstitutional sources: family, self, community agencies	Hospital patients
Cost control	4. By 19 ___ effective discharge planning will be provided for all hospital patients. (This planning should focus on returning the patient home with necessary nursing, therapeutic, and support services as early as possible.)	a. Existence of discharge planning component in hospital b. Percent of patients covered by discharge planning—less than 85% unsatisfactory c. Percent of screened patients appropriately referred to home health service systems from hospitals	The community
	5. By 19 ___ all levels of home health services will use personnel in an efficient, cost-effective manner.	a. Assessment of agency use of personnel in delivering home health services with regard to current state practices b. Assessment of licensing and credentialing mechanisms, practice acts for all types of home health personnel, and barriers to use and reimbursement, with recommended modifications where appropriate	
Disease control	6. By 19 ___ the official health agency or other appropriate governmental agency will have an established procedure for the investigation, follow-up, and prevention of communicable diseases that occur in the home health services environment.	Established procedures	Homebound individuals
Health education	7. By 19 ___ homebound individuals and those responsible for them will receive health education and health promotion counseling in the home, including counseling on physical and emotional problems.	Percent of homebound individuals receiving counseling	Homebound individuals

*Based on Model standards for community preventive health services, Washington, D.C., 1979, Public Health Service, U.S. Department of Health and Human Services.

a health asset for the elderly person. Because the old person's sensitivity to heat is reduced, it is sometimes desirable that a younger person test the temperature of the water in the tub or of the shower. Many old people have been severely scalded by bath water that they were not able to recognize as too hot until they had been badly burned.

Clothing. Clean clothing adapted to the season and needs perhaps represents a factor in mental health more than in physical health. Extremely important for the elderly is a feeling of pride, status, or worth. Dress can be used to advantage in creating the state of mind that a person is important. Personal appearance can do much to give the elderly the spark necessary for effective and enjoyable living.

Health practices of the elderly should be directed as much toward their mental and emotional needs as their physiological needs. Through health practices, it is possible to create in elderly persons the feeling that they are still very much a part of the community and that they have a significant, even important, role to play.

MEDICAL SERVICES

Most communities can provide the variety of medical skills necessary for the more complex problems of the aged by calling on the services of the various specialists available in the area. Interest in the health aspects of geriatrics has been rising steadily, but the question is still unanswered whether a new specialty is needed. Many physicians and other professionals are members of the American Geriatrics Society or the Gerontological Society. The membership of these two organizations has increased tenfold since 1950. Unfortunately, medical and nursing students have shown resistance to working with geriatric patients.

Special geriatrics clinics have been established in the United States. Their goal has been to offer coordinated medical and social services to the independent, working, elderly group to aid them in retaining their independence. Clinics in Wakefield, Rhode Island, and at the Peter Bent Brigham Hospital, Boston, have demonstrated the value of coordinated medical and social service. In addition to providing important diagnostic service to the elderly group, the geriatrics clinic is able to formulate and supervise a continuing program of health supervision for its clients. Other geriatrics clinics are being organized, particularly in the larger population centers. Out of these pioneering efforts to provide organized health supervision for elderly citizens may well evolve the type of community programs needed to deal with the growing problem of providing for the health needs of the aged. The special demonstration project of the Kips Bay-Yorkville Health District in New York illustrates the experimental efforts under way to gain an understanding of what might be done in providing for the health needs of the aged. Other examples are the Brooklyn Hebrew Home and Hospital for the Aged, and the Waxter Center for Senior Citizens in Baltimore.

These efforts and special projects are most laudable, but as yet most communities rely on the general hospital and medical services that are already available. Older people require proportionately more medical services than the general population.

NURSING HOMES AND HOME CARE

Nursing homes play an increasingly important role in the care of elderly persons. In 1973 the United States had 14,873 nursing homes and 6,961 personal care homes. These 21,834 homes had a total of 1,327,704 beds. Model standards for community health concerns with nursing homes are shown in the table on pp. 186 and 187.

Although it may be saddening to note that more than 1 million aged people in the United

States are in nursing homes, it is at the same time encouraging to note that over 19 million are not. Most of the geriatric concern has been with the 5% who are institutionalized. This has tended to bias popular and professional perceptions of what old age is like. We are guilty in the United States of "ageism" in our abandonment of many to nursing homes.

Public health departments have been lax in licensing nursing homes in the United States. While all 50 states have licensing laws, the requirements are below the minimum standards recommended by the Committee on Aging of the National Social Welfare Assembly. The National Association of Registered Nursing Homes has made laudable contributions to the improvement of standards, and the efforts of this organization should be supported and encouraged. The present situation still calls for legal action for providing desirable standards through licensing of nursing homes.

Nursing homes should be affiliated with general hospitals and should cooperate with general hospitals. In such an arrangement, physicians will have elderly patients moved from the general hospital to the less expensive nursing home, where they know the chronically ill can receive the necessary nursing care. Such an arrangement also means a greater likelihood that the majority of the patients in the nursing home will be under medical supervision.

Physicians, nurses, occupational therapists, and social workers agree that the aging who are ill should be cared for in their own homes as long as possible. Model standards for home health services in the community are shown in the table on pp. 188-189. Obviously, there are situations that make this impossible or undesirable, but when home conditions are acceptable, some chronically ill can be as well taken care of in the home as in the nursing home or the hospital. Visiting nursing services can be used to good advantage, especially when only part-time nursing service is necessary.

REHABILITATION

The ill or disabled elderly person needs more than custodial care. Chronic disease hospitals are not the answer, because they tend to create the conception of lifelong disability. When hospitalization is necessary for an aged person, the general hospital can usually provide all of the services necessary for the care and treatment of the patient, without creating the impression of cold-storage institutionalization. In the general hospital elderly patients should have a combination of medical care and rehabilitation to prepare them for their mode of living after they are discharged from the hospital. Both nursing and social service are necessary before patients are transferred home. Perhaps here the elderly person may need some supervision until a reasonable adjustment is made in terms of normal living routine. Even when the elderly person is in a domicile with other members of his family, social work services can be of value in aiding all concerned to understand what the needs of the elderly person are and how these needs are to be met.

COMMUNICATING WITH THE ELDERLY

Old people, like all members of society, must be able to read and grasp the meaning of a great deal of printed and optically projected material if they are to maintain a self-sufficient life-style. But it is not generally recognized that their lack of comprehension, when it occurs, may result from a sensory rather than intellectual failure.

One aspect of this sensory failure is the ways in which type style, type size, and layout of printed materials affect an older person's reading speed, ease of reading, and interest in written materials. Older persons both prefer and can read faster when shown roman rather than other styles of type. Roman type may be found in the New York Times and many school books. Increasing the type size beyond a certain point does not facilitate reading for older people.

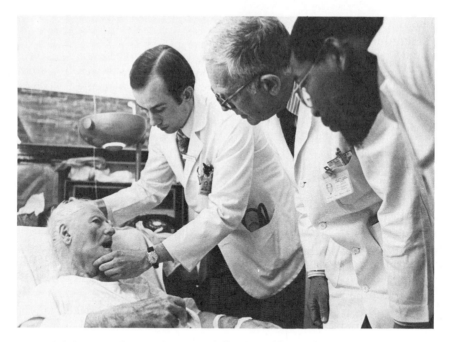

FIG. 7-5. Rehabilitation. The complications of illness in old age are compounded by economic loss and separation from family. Home-care programs sponsored by community agencies have proved their value in relieving some of these problems.

Courtesy Johns Hopkins Medical Institutions.

We know very little about specific benefits or costs of the communications media used to provide information about social services. Isolation from communication flows sometimes accompanies physical isolation. Communication by print—fliers, pamphlets, notices, newspapers, and the like—is the least effective substitute for face-to-face contact between older people and those responsible for interpreting laws, regulations, eligibility, and entitlements.

It is often incorrectly assumed that anything other than face-to-face communication is necessarily inferior. This assumption is incorrect because modern communications media, including the telephone, allow trade-offs between telecommunications and transportation, sharing of valuable human resources among underserved populations, and other benefits.

These media should be implemented as solutions ready and waiting to alleviate problems.

Over half the services provided to clients by public social service agencies are information exchanges of one sort or another and, hence, are directly amenable to enhancement by telecommunications. Some studies show that older adults watch television, on the average, 3 hours per day—slightly less than the average for the total population. On the other hand, some studies found that television viewing increases as an activity with age. Studies reported that a majority of 204 old people in the Age Center of New England saw television viewing as an important recreational activity; in fact, television viewing ranks first among all activities of the elderly, according to some surveys. It has been reported that old people prefer personal, nonfiction programs in which people like themselves play important roles, either as members of the studio audience or as contestants.

The older woman is far more likely than the older man to live alone. This isolation impairs communication, making both the diagnosis and the treatment of physical and mental illness more difficult in older women. Many women may be diagnosed as suffering from senile dementia when in fact they are lonely, isolated, and depressed. Loss of vision or hearing, which are common health problems of the aged, may increase communication problems and isolation from family and community and lead to misunderstandings and misdiagnoses.

Telephone reassurance provided by daily telephone contact with an older person who might otherwise have no outside contact for long periods of time can be an important service to the aged and their families. Persons receiving telephone reassurance may be called at a predetermined time each day. If the person does not answer, help is immediately sent to his or her home. Usually in the event of no answer, a neighbor, relative, or nearby police or fire station is asked to make a personal check. Such details are worked out when a person begins receiving this service. Telephone reassurance has been credited with saving many lives by the quick dispatching of medical help. An alert caller, in one case, noticed a slight slurring of speech in a client she talked with regularly. Although the client reported no difficulties, the caller reported the slurred speech to her supervisor who sent someone to check the situation personally. The client had suffered a heart spasm and was rushed to the hospital in time. Telephone reassurance generally costs little and can be provided by callers of any age from teenagers to older people themselves. It is sponsored by a variety of organizations and agencies in the United States ranging from women's clubs to police departments. For example, in Nassau

County, New York, residents of a home for the aged make calls to the elderly living alone. In Florida 102 older persons who cannot leave their homes are called daily by 42 senior center members. In Albuquerque, New Mexico, a hospital auxiliary and the Business and Professional Women's Club make daily calls. In Nebraska the State Federation of Women's Clubs sponsors telephone reassurance.

Radio and television have brought religious services into the home for elderly shut-ins, and this has been supplemented by the churches' providing additional, more personal, services to the shut-ins. These personalized services need not be of a strictly religious nature. Church people are in a strategic position to give the type of personal service that will help the older shut-in to attain and maintain the frame of mind and general well-being so essential to physical as well as mental health.

TRANSPORTATION

The physical environment links the elderly to the services, facilities, resources, and opportunities necessary for existence. Transportation is critical, whether for visiting and traveling, taking the individual to a health service or facility, or bringing a service provider to the individual. Transportation or the lack of it also influences the effectiveness of other services for the elderly. Basic priorities and accompanying funding for transportation will remain inadequate, forcing communities to choose between improvements for the elderly or for all travelers.

Mass transportation systems have become increasingly important with the general decline of the automobile as the primary mode of transportation. Further, automobile ownership declines with age. This decline is mostly a result of the lower incomes of the elderly, but it is also influenced by their decreasing physical and psychological ability to drive. Studies indicate a greater dependence on walking among the aged, but walking is limited by the inadequacy of pedestrian accommodations and security. Studies also indicate that public transportation is least adequate for those most in need of it—the physically frail, individuals with no friends or relatives to drive them, minority group members, and the poor.

Serious attention to the role of transportation in the lives of older persons is a comparatively recent development. The subject received minimum attention at the 1961 White House Conference on Aging. It emerged as a priority at the 1969 International Congress of Gerontology and the 1970 workshops sponsored jointly by the Administration on Aging and the U.S. Department of Transportation. The 1971 White House Conference on Aging ranked the question of transportation immediately after income, health, and housing. Another White House Conference on Aging was underway in 1981.

The U.S. Department of Transportation, the Administration on Aging, the General Services Administration, and many communities and civic organizations either now offer or are experimenting with various forms of assistance to help meet the transportation needs of America's older population.

U.S. federal support

The National Mass Transportation Act of 1974 included a number of provisions that aided older riders. The act required that any public transit system receiving capital assistance funds from the Urban Mass Transportation Administration of the U.S. Department of Transportation charge half fare or less for the elderly. Other programs administered by the Urban Mass Transportation Administration include research and development grants to test innovative approaches to transportation problems and funding for capital assistance and the acquisition of vehicles and other needed equipment.

The Federal Aid Highway Act of 1973 pro-

vided for a public transportation demonstration program designed to encourage the development, improvement, and use of public mass transportation in rural areas. Applicants for these demonstration funds must be either public agencies or public purpose (nonprofit) agencies or corporations, preferably with state or area-wide responsibilities. Although the program is designed for demonstrations for the general rural public, one criterion for project selection by the Federal Highway Administration is that the transportation system be adaptable to the needs of the elderly and handicapped. Organizations and agencies interested in demonstration projects can contact their state highway department, department of transportation, or agency on aging, all located in the state capitol, for information regarding the status of this program and possibilities for support.

There are several other avenues of assistance that can be used to provide transportation services for the elderly. Under Title III of the Older Americans Comprehensive Services Amendments, which authorizes support for state and community programs, the U.S. Administration on Aging awards grants to the designated state agencies on aging to assist state and local agencies in the development of comprehensive and coordinated services to the elderly. The designated state agency can identify potential sources of funding for transportation, provide advice on how best to plan for and implement a project, and coordinate efforts with other agencies and organizations that might be involved in planning and supporting transportation projects.

The state agency can also advocate for the use of existing transportation services on behalf of the elderly and help in efforts to secure revenue sharing funds to establish transportation projects for the elderly. Under certain limited circumstances, the state agency or possibly the Administration on Aging can provide direct project funding.

Community programs

Many states, provinces, and local areas operate diverse transportation projects ranging from the relatively inexpensive, informal use of volunteer drivers in small towns and rural areas to the use of sophisticated demand-responsive or regularly scheduled transit vehicles, often designed to meet the special needs of the elderly.

Free or reduced fares on public transportation vehicles are enabling the elderly in many parts of the United States and Europe to travel during midday, night, and weekend hours. All public transit operators in Pennsylvania, for example, participate in the state's free fare program, which is subsidized by the Pennsylvania Lottery. Many areas that permit older people to ride free during off-peak transit hours also offer reduced, but not free, fares during rush hours.

A project in St. Petersburg, Florida, called TOTE (Transportation of the Elderly) is providing service to the elderly and handicapped where little or none existed before. Eligible riders have access to specially equipped minibuses that offer door-to-door service, nominal fares, and transportation by advance reservation, weekly subscription, or telephone request, as well as charter service.

OATS (Older Adult Transportation Service) is a personal membership, door-to-door bus network operating in more than 80 of Missouri's 114 counties. Over 10,000 people are enrolled in the OATS system, which is a nonprofit corporation serving the elderly and medically handicapped. They pay a moderate annual membership fee plus a per-mile contribution for distance traveled. Although the system is rapidly growing into a statewide network, routes and schedules and certain policies are determined at the local level by county committees composed of volunteers. An additional 500 volunteers across the state regularly call or are called by OATS subscribers needing transportation. In fact, the expanding service could not exist without its heavy reliance on volunteers in a variety of roles.

LEISURE-TIME ACTIVITIES

The value of recreation and social participation is generally acknowledged, but for no group are these of greater health value than for the aged (see Chapter 9). With a great deal of newly found time on their hands, the elderly need activities that will occupy them profitably and enjoyably. Some have business interests, trade skills, voluntary association memberships, or a garden to occupy their attention and time, but many are in need of help in developing satisfying leisure-time activities. Most of the elderly seek and enjoy the companionship of others (Nystrom, 1974). A community can provide for individual instruction for recreation purposes, but provision for instruction and supervision on a group basis is usually more practical.

Small groups of elderly people can take up arts and crafts, music, dramatics, poetry, and creative writing. The mutual encouragement, the sociability, and the general elation that come from such participation can do more for many of these elderly people than can the physician or the hospital. On the other hand, participation in social activities and associations cannot be offered as a substitute for health care (Bull and Aucoin, 1975).

On a large group basis, concerts, lectures, dancing, parties, excursions, and outings can be highly important in the lives of the elderly and can contribute measurably to their outlook. Checkers, chess, cards, and shuffleboard are popular games that can be organized and promoted among the elderly. Zest for living is extremely important in the health of these persons. Social action groups such as the Grey Panthers provide a vehicle for productive participation, but in communities without such organizations the community should provide avenues for the development and promotion of a zest for living. This aids older people in their feeling of security, which is a primary need of every person, but it also brings returns to the community in the continuing participation of the aged in community life.

APPRAISAL

Community responsibility for the health of the aging population encompasses concern for the citizen's total living. Included in the program are medical services, hospital facilities, nursing home provisions, housing conditions, health education, health counseling, recreation programs, and provision of opportunities for individual and group participation in productive and enjoyable activities. The community health department alone cannot carry the whole program, but it can be the agency that integrates all community resources having a contribution for the elderly. As an established official agency, the health department can initiate action necessary for the promotion of the well-being of the aged.

QUESTIONS AND EXERCISES

1. What are some signs of "ageism" in your community?
2. Why must gerontology concern itself with social and psychological aging as well as with physiological aging?
3. In 1883 Chancellor Bismarck of Germany set 65 as the age of retirement. Appraise the current use of age 65 as the landmark for the classification of "aged."
4. List 20 persons of your acquaintance who are over 65 years of age. What percentage have good health, what percentage have fair health, what percentage are ill but up and around, and what percentage are disabled?
5. What percentage of this 20 have health impairments that could be corrected or at least reduced?
6. To what extent do changes in the economy affect the population age distribution of a county or a state?
7. What factors are essential if an individual is to be relatively "young" at age 75?
8. What is the general social status of the elderly people of your community and what is the significance of their social status in terms of their health?
9. To what extent is the community health program for the aged primarily a program of curing illness rather than health?
10. What does your state or provincial health department have in the way of an agency and a program for the promotion of the health of the aged?
11. What special activites in the interest of better health for the aged are carried on by your official community health department?
12. What are the voluntary health agencies of your community doing in behalf of the health of elderly citizens?
13. What are the contributions of other institutions such as churches of your community to the health and general well-being of the senior citizen?
14. How interested and how well informed is the general public in your community about matters relating to the health of elderly people?
15. What would be a good routine of daily living for a man or woman of age 70 without impairments?
16. Why are health practices recommended for elderly people usually directed more to their psychological needs than to their physiological needs?
17. State the reasons for and against establishing a special geriatrics clinic in your community.
18. To provide ideally for the health needs of its elderly citizens, what should your community provide in the way of medical and other services and in the way of hospital and other facilities?
19. In terms of community geriatrics in the United States, evaluate the role of the state certified nursing home, affiliated with a general hospital, and staffed with registered nurses.
20. What organized lesiure-time activites for the aged are now available in your community and what additional provisions should be made?

BIBLIOGRAPHY

Administration on Aging: Transportation for the elderly: the state of the art, DHEW Publication No. (OHD) 75-20081, Washington, D.C., 1975, U.S. Government Printing Office.
Alvarez, W.C.: Hazards leading to accidents, Geriatrics 28:76, 1973.
Anderson, H.C.: Newton's geriatric nursing, ed. 5, St. Louis, 1971, The C.V. Mosby Co.
Anderson, W.F.: Preventive aspects of geriatric medicine, J. Am. Geriatr. Soc. 22:385, 1974.
Atchley, R.C.: Retirement and leisure participation: continuity or crisis? Gerontologist 11:13, 1971.
Austin, M.J.: A network of help for England's elderly, Soc. Work 21:114, 1976.
Binstock, R.H.: Political consequences of aging, Philadelphia, 1974, American Academy of Political and Social Science.
Binstock, R.H., and Shanas, E., editors: Handbook of aging and the social sciences, New York, 1976, Van Nostrand Reinhold Co.
Birren, J.E., and Schaie, K.W., editors: Handbook of the

psychology of aging, New York, 1977, Van Nostrand Reinhold Co.

Brocklehurst, J.C., editor: Geriatric care in advanced societies, Baltimore, 1975, University Park Press.

Bull, C.N., and Aucoin, J.B.: Voluntary association participation and life satisfaction: a replication note, J. Gerontol. **30**:73, 1975.

Butler, R.N.: Why survive? Being old in America, New York, 1975, Harper & Row, Publishers.

Butler, R.N., and Lewis, M.I.: Aging and mental health: positive psychosocial approaches, ed. 2, St. Louis, 1977, The C.V. Mosby Co.

Byerts, T., editor: Housing and environment for the elderly, Washington, D.C., 1972, The Gerontological Society.

Cantor, M.H.: Life space and the social support system of the inner city elderly of New York, Gerontologist **15**:23, 1975.

Cowgill, D.O., and Holmes, L.D., editors: Aging and modernization, New York, 1972, Appleton-Century-Crofts.

Coyle, M.G.: Gynecological disorders of old age, Practitioner (London) **208**(1246):480, 1972.

Crisp, A.H., and Stonehill, E.: Sleep, nutrition and mood, New York, 1976, John Wiley & Sons, Inc.

Eisdorfer, C., editor: The psychology of adult development and aging, Washington, D.C., 1973, American Psychological Association.

Ellwood, T.W., and Oakes, T.W.: Failure by a group of elderly men to use a preventive health service, J. Am. Geriatr. Soc. **23**:74, 1975.

Havighurst, R.J.: The future aged: the use of time and money, Gerontologist **15**(1, Pt. 2):10, Feb., 1975.

Hyams, D.: The care of the aged, Westport, Conn., 1976, Technomic Publishing Co.

Kayser, J.S., and Minnigerode, F.A.: Increasing nursing students' interest in working with aged patients, Nurs. Res. **24**:23, 1975.

Kent, D.P., Kastenbaum, R., and Sherwood, S., editors: Research planning and action for the elderly: the power and potential of social science, New York, 1972, Behavioral Publications.

Klippel, R.E., and Sweeney, T.W.: The use of information sources by the aged consumer, Gerontologist **14**:163, 1974.

Kosberg, J.I.: Methods for community surveillance of geriatric institutions, Public Health Rep. **90**:144, 1975.

Kreps, J.M.: Lifetime allocation of work and income, Durham, N.C., 1971, Duke University Press.

Lawton, M.P.: Planning and managing housing for the elderly, New York, 1975, John Wiley & Sons, Inc.

Lewis, M.I., and Butler, R.N.: Why is women's lib ignoring old women? Aging Human Dev. **3**:223, 1972.

Lopata, H.Z.: Widowhood in an American city, Cambridge, Mass., 1973, Schenkman Publishing Co., Inc.

Marmor, T.R.: The politics of Medicare, Chicago, 1973, Aldine Publishing Co.

Mathieu, R.: Hospital and nursing home management, Philadelphia, 1971, W.B. Saunders Co.

National Center for Health Statistics: Current estimates from the Health Interview Survey No. 95, DHEW Publication No. (HRA) 75-1522, 1975.

National Institute on Aging: The older woman: continuities and discontinuities (report of the National Institute on Aging and National Institute on Mental Health Workshop), Bethesda, Md., 1979, Public Health Service Publication No. (NIH)79-1897.

National Institute on Aging: Special report on aging 1980, Bethesda, Md., 1980, Public Health Service, NIH Publication No. 80-2135.

National Institute of Child Health and Human Development: Research directions toward reduction of injury in the young and old, Bethesda, Md., 1973, DHEW Publication No. (NIH) 73-124.

Neugarten, B.L., editor: Middle age and aging: a reader in social psychology, Chicago, 1968, University of Chicago Press.

Neugarten, B.L.: Patterns of aging: past, present, and future, Soc. Service Rev. **47**:571, 1973.

Neugarten,, B.L., editor: Symposium: aging in the year 2000: a look at the future. Introduction. Gerontologist **15**(1, Pt. 2): (entire issue), 1975.

Neugarten, B.L., and Havighurst, R.J., editor: Social policy, social ethics, and the aging society (report prepared by Committee on Human Development, University of Chicago, for National Science Foundation), Washington, D.C., 1976, U.S. Government Printing Office.

Nystrom, E.P.: Activity patterns and leisure concepts among the elderly, Am. J. Occup. Ther. **28**:337, July, 1974.

Park, B.: An introduction to telemedicine: interactive television for delivery of health services, New York, 1974, Alternate Media Center, New York University.

Pastalan, L.A., and Carson, D.H., editors: The spatial behavior of older people, Ann Arbor, Mich., 1970, Institute of Gerontology, University of Michigan.

Peterson, D.A.: Life-span education and gerontology, Gerontologist **15**:436, 1975.

Pfeiffer, E., editor: Alternatives to institutional care for older Americans: practice and planning, Durham, N.C., 1972, Center for the Study of Aging and Human Development, Duke University Press.

Poon, L.W., editor: Aging in the 1980's: psychological issues, Washington, D.C., 1980, American Psychological Association.

Quirk, D.A., and Skinner, J.H.: IHCS: physical capacity, age and employment, Indust. Gerontologist **19**:49, 1973.

Reichel, W., editor: Clinical aspects of aging: a monograph of the American Geriatrics Society, Baltimore, 1977, The Williams & Wilkins Co.

Riley, M.W., Johnson, M., and Froner, A., editors: Aging and society, vol. 3, a sociology of age stratification, New York, 1972, Russell Sage Foundation.

Rosow, I.: Social integration of the aged, New York, 1967, The Free Press.

Schulz, J.H.: Providing adequate retirement income, Hanover, N.H., 1974, University Press of New England.

Shanas, E., Townsend, P., Wedderburn, D., et al.: Old people in three industrial societies, New York, 1968, Atherton Press.

Sigel, M.M., and Good, R.A., editors: Tolerance, autoimmunity and aging, Springfield, Ill., 1971, Charles C Thomas, Publisher.

Steinberg, F.U., editors: Cowdry's the care of the geriatric patient, ed. 5, St. Louis, 1976, The C.V. Mosby Co.

Sterne, R.S., Phillips, J.E., and Rabushka, A.: The urban elderly poor: racial and bureaucratic conflict, Lexington, Mass., 1974, Lexington Books.

Strauss, A.L.: Chronic illness and the quality of life, St. Louis, 1975, The C.V. Mosby Co.

Streib, G.C., and Schneider, C.J.: Retirement in American society: impact and process, Ithaca, N.Y., 1971, Cornell University Press.

Thurnher, M.: Goals, values, and life evaluations at preretirement stage, J. Gerontol. 29:85, 1974.

Tobin, S.S.: Social and health services for the future aged, Gerontologist 15:32, 1975.

Tobin, S.S., and Lieberman, M.A.: Last home for the aged, San Francisco, 1976, Jossey-Bass, Inc., Publishers.

Warren, H.H.: Self-perception of independence among urban elderly, Am. J. Occup. Ther. 28:329, 1974.

Zax, M., and Spector, G.A.: An introduction to community psychology, New York, 1974, John Wiley & Sons, Inc.

8

COMMUNITY MENTAL HEALTH

Sweet are the thoughts that savor of content;
The quiet mind is richer than a crown—
A mind content both crown and kingdom is.

Robert Greene

Mental disorder and mental health are no longer approached with trepidation and apprehension in most countries. More and more, society has learned to deal objectively with mental health and mental disorder. Many of the social movements of the 1980s, such as Women's Liberation, have as one of their main concerns mental health.

Knowledge in the field of mental health and mental disorder is advancing rapidly through the extension of research. Although more knowledge in this field is needed, if all of the knowledge now available were properly used, a highly effective community mental health program could be promoted. Such a program would concern itself with the mental health of the normal citizen, promotion of mental health, epidemiology of mental illness, mental disorder as a phase of social pathology, various types of mental disorder present in the population, medical and hospital resources available, and provisions for rehabilitation of those who have been mentally ill. The community aspects of alcohol and drug misuse will be considered in Chapter 12.

CONCEPT OF MENTAL HEALTH

For practical reasons, the term *mental health* is used to include emotional and social well-being as well as the mental state of the individual. Emotions are intense feelings with physiological as well as psychological components. A person is not just angry mentally. He or she also experiences certain physiological changes as an aspect of anger. Yet all of it must, in the final analysis, be appraised in terms of the mental state experienced by the individual. Social adjustment perhaps represents a phase of mental health rather than an independent entity. It must be acknowledged that some individuals of normal mental health live extremely limited social lives and perhaps have an adequate level of mental health. Nevertheless, to attain a high level of mental health in today's pattern of life, social relationships can be a major factor.

Mental health must be evaluated in terms of the individual's productive and enjoyable living. This, perhaps, is best expressed by a statement of Dr. Karl Menninger:

Let us define mental health as the adjustment of human beings to each other and to the world about them with a maximum of effectiveness and happiness. Not just efficiency, or just contentment—or the grace of playing the rules of the game cheerfully. It is all of these together. It is the ability to maintain an even temper, an alert intelligence, socially considerate behavior and a happy disposition. This I think is a healthy mind. [Menninger, 1953.]

No one lives perfectly efficiently, nor does any normal individual experience continuous happiness. The best that the normal individual can do is attain happiness occasionally, and then only for short periods. Nor would it be fair to label an occasional lapse of "socially considerate behavior" a mental disorder. Imperfect people in an imperfect world means that even the highest level of mental health is not perfect health. We deal here with a relative matter with varying degrees of mental health.

MENTAL HEALTH OF THE NORMAL POPULATION

By "normal" is meant that which is accepted as the usual and must be regarded as within a range. No two individuals are alike. Each is unique. Yet most of us, in terms of mental health, fit within the overall pattern or range accepted as the usual. This allows for the wide span of individual differences to be found among persons whose conduct is regarded as within accepted patterns. Within this range of normal mental health we find various degrees or levels. Some individuals function efficiently on a high level and derive unusual enjoyment in their living. They encounter frustration, disappointment, and failure, but with a minimum of friction. They freely and effectively use their abilities in harmony with life's demands and gain a maximum of personal satisfaction and enjoyment in their accomplishments.

Another group of individuals adjusts to frustration, disappointment, and failure quite readily and experiences but a moderate amount of disturbance in the friction they encounter in life. This is a very commendable quality of mental health and perhaps should be rated as good mental health. Doubtless, many of the individuals in this group could attain an excellent level of mental health with a better understanding and an organized effort.

A third group constitutes the majority of people in a normal population. These individuals are not mentally disordered, although they do experience occasional or even more frequent emotional upsets. Their distinguishing characteristic is that seldom do they seem to attain a dynamic level of adjustment in which they attain considerable accomplishment with an accompanying great amount of enjoyment. They tend to operate in second gear and live rather uninteresting, uninspired, and passive lives. They drag through life, getting a half-measure of what life really has to offer. These individuals possess a fair level of mental health. Many of them, through proper understanding and application, could elevate their mental health level to the good and even to the excellent status with community support.

To improve one's mental health, one must understand what motivates human conduct, the nature of emotional maturation, and the attributes of a well-adjusted personality. Persons need to understand why they do certain things, what gives rise to certain emotions, what they need to do to adjust to their emotional responses, and what personality qualities they need to fortify or develop. This is the area in which a community mental health program can provide its greatest service to the normal citizen. People of the community need a better understanding of mental health. This education can be provided through the various methods and devices available to community health personnel. Citizens need the benefit of mental health counseling by qualified mental hygienists. Some need guidance in special health problems they may encounter. Normal citizens in the community have a need for mental health services just as they have a need for services that promote physical health.

Disintegration of personality. No normal individual possesses all of the qualities of personality integration to a perfect or even near-perfect degree. Indeed, every normal person experiences emotional upsets and personality disturbances. Disease, pain, and fatigue are common causes of personality disintegration. Personal disaster such as the loss of an election, family disaster such as serious injury or death, and the mounting tensions of modern living may produce personality upsets even in the best integrated personality. The well-integrated personality tends to recover quickly from any disturbance. The poorly integrated individual not only is upset more easily but requires a longer time to recover even from a moderate disturbance. There are two good indications of the degree of personality integration. The first is the ability to meet challenging situations effectively, and the second is the ability to recover quickly from a stressful event.

MENTAL HEALTH PROGRAMS

A health matter becomes a public health problem when it is amenable to solution through public action. Many aspects of the mental health problem can be dealt with most effectively through public action. In the United States, state governments direct and finance most mental health programs. However, psychiatrists are not always cordial to the concept that mental hygiene is a public health responsibility.

Some U.S. psychiatrists feel that state hospital staffs should be responsible for all mental hygiene in the state. However, the psychiatric hospital is isolated from the community, and the hospital staff has neither the organization nor the experience to deal with integrated community action. Generally, psychiatric hospitalization is not a function of the state health department but is administered by a separate administrative agency such as a hospital commission. If public health departments were to administer hospitals for the mentally disordered, this function would soon dwarf other activities. Mental health promotion is a function of the state health department; severe mental disorders and care of the institutionalized mentally ill are the functions of psychiatrists and the hospitals for the mentally ill.

Many states, such as California, Minnesota, New Jersey, New York, and Vermont, have passed a Community Mental Health Services Act. Other states that have not enacted a specific mental health services act nevertheless have provided for the establishment of a statewide mental health program. A few states promote mental health as a component of existing programs, such as in the maternal and child health division of the state health department. However, an identifiable state mental hygiene agency within the state department of public health provides recognition of the importance of mental hygiene as a phase of public health service. Maryland gives prominence to the mental health program by naming the state public health agency the Department of Health and Mental Hygiene.

The division of mental hygiene, or some similarly designated agency, is charged with the primary responsibility for mental health promotion in many states. This division serves as the coordinating agency in the state for all statewide forces concerned with the promotion of the mental health of the general population. It cooperates with the various voluntary agencies and official agencies in the state that are engaged in some phase of mental health. It cooperates with the state department of education, the prisons, hospital commissions, and the hospitals. While its major concern is with the mental health of the normal individual, it does provide certain services directed toward assistance for the maladjusted—the mental health of the alcoholic, the narcotics addict, the delinquent, the criminal, the physically handicapped, the aged, and other segments in the population having special mental health problems. The division of mental hygiene may sponsor or support legislation on the subject of mental health, make statistical studies, provide library facilities, make mental health education materials available in other respects, provide consulting service to agencies or communities, set up workshops and seminars for professional personnel, sponsor special programs of mental health promotion, establish and promote mental health facilities, and otherwise serve as a general mental health resource for the people of the state.

Voluntary agencies such as mental health associations play an important role in providing leadership for those groups and individuals in the state who have an understanding of the general problem of mental health and a sincere interest in mental health promotion. Various professional organizations whose members deal professionally with services and problems having mental health aspects have been of particular value in pointing out the need for greater services in the mental health field and have provided leadership and support necessary for its attainment on a statewide basis. Frequently, it is a movement initiated by groups such as these that give rise to the establishment of an official mental health agency in the state devoted to the promotion of the mental health of the general public.

COMMUNITY MENTAL HEALTH PROMOTION

Most communities have provisions for institutionalizing the mentally ill, although facilities for early diagnosis and care are frequently in-adequate or totally absent. Very few communities have a well-organized, well-functioning program for the promotion of the mental health of the normal citizen. Large portions of the community's population have a vital interest in mental health promotion as it relates to their community, their neighborhood, their family, and themselves. Yet few want to see a mental health facility located in their neighborhood. Establishing a community mental health program means developing community support. Leadership can come from the local mental health association, from the community health council, and from other sources. Productive action usually requires long-range planning rather than a high-pressure "crash" program. Lay leadership is important, even though primary responsibility must rest with the official community public health agency. Interagency cooperation is necessary for the success of a program such as one in mental health, and full

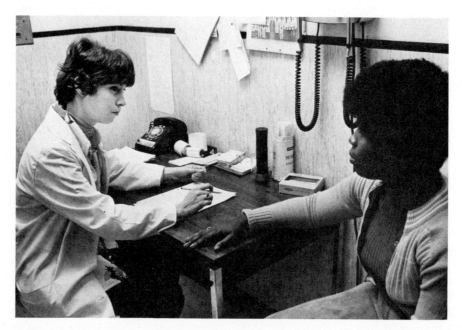

FIG. 8-1. Mental health promotion. Every clinical encounter offers opportunities for health workers to assist patients in coping with health problems and other sources of stress.

Courtesy Johns Hopkins Medical Institutions.

cooperation can be obtained only with public understanding, public interest, and public support.

Mental health needs

A survey of the specific mental health needs of a particular community would be essential to the determination of what the mental health program should be in that particular community. There are certain factors and certain mental health needs that are common to most communities, but within the community, specific factors that influence the mental health of individuals must be recognized and evaluated. Socioeconomic, neighborhood, and ethnic backgrounds, family relationships, child-rearing practices, community norms, and cultural values all represent factors determining the soil in which the mental health program is to be planted.

Adult mental health needs, as well as the special or difficult problems for which adults have a need for special assistance, are in the province of normal, everyday adjustment. Individual and family counseling services, marriage counseling, sessions for expectant parents, child study groups, parent discussions, guidance services for elderly citizens, promotion of cultural interests, recreation programs, and general health information services all represent desirable needs in a community. No one agency will necessarily provide all of the services to satisfy these needs, but by means of an integrated community mental health program, some agency or individual will provide for each of the various needs. While a major portion of a community health program is directed toward normal people in the normal walks of life, there will be mentally disturbed people in hospitals, patients under physicians' care, patients who have been released from psychiatric hospitals and are in the process of rehabilitation, and individuals who have come to the attention of community agencies and are under the direction of these agencies.

Child and youth mental health services will be provided largely through the schools. Most communities have other agencies that will provide for some of the mental health needs of children and youth. These needs may not appear to be extensive, but they are extremely important. They include psychological testing and diagnostic services; counseling services for children, consulting services for parents of the youngsters, mental health guidance services for youth, remedial programs in the school, an in-service mental health training program for teachers, mental health instruction as a phase of the basic hygiene program, and family life education. An effective coordinated community-school mental health program should devote its major attention to the mental health of the normal youngster but must also provide for the mental health needs of the delinquent, the emotionally disturbed, the mentally retarded, the academically handicapped, and the youngsters who are having adjustment difficulties.

Organization and administration

The effectiveness of any community mental health program will depend to a considerable extent on its planning, organization, and direction. A community may possess many resources for dealing with its manifold mental health needs, but unless some central agency exists that will crystallize the various services available, many needs that could be fulfilled will be neglected, many services will be inadequately provided, and there will be unnecessary duplication and even conflict in function. Setting up a central administrative agency does not mean that the various individuals, agencies, and services in the community will be hampered or otherwise obstructed in their functioning. Rather, it will mean a coordination of services available from the various agencies and individuals in the total program. This will help reduce duplication and fragmentation of services.

In a given community, a considerable number of people may have a contribution to make to the community's mental health program. Individuals with a smattering of knowledge or with a morbid curiosity about mental health may be willing volunteers or even persistent participants, but the public is entitled to protection from the charlatans and the incompetent in mental health as well as in other areas of health.

Community mental health center

The U.S. Community Mental Health Centers Act of 1963 authorized $150 million for fiscal years 1965, 1966, and 1967 for the construction of community mental health centers, which form the core of the U.S. national program. Allotments to states continued to rise to $235 million in 1980, based on population, financial need, and the need for community mental health centers. Funds were provided on a matching basis. The centers were expected to include the following:

Inpatient services

Outpatient services

Partial hospitalization, including day, night, and weekend care

Emergency services

Community services, including consultation with community agencies and professional personnel

Diagnostic, screening, and follow-up services.

Rehabilitation services, including vocational and educational programs

Precare and aftercare community services, including foster home placement, home visiting, and halfway houses

Alcohol and drug problem services

Training

Research and evaluation

Congress appropriated an additional $8 million for grants to aid in the preparation of statewide plans for comprehensive mental health programs (National Institute of Mental Health, 1970).

In 1980 President Jimmy Carter signed into law the Mental Health Systems Act, one of the very few health initiatives his administration was able to pry from Congress. The legislation gives states greater authority over mental health grants; it allows funding of programs other than the traditionally defined community mental health centers; it targets certain priority populations; and it puts more emphasis on prevention.

Citizen participation in community mental health

Democratic representative government is based on the idea that political, economic, and social processes must be responsive to the needs and aspirations of the people. The U.S. federal program of Community Mental Health Centers (CMHCs) was based on the premise that for a CMHC to be successful, it must be responsive to the viewpoints and problems of local communities. For this reason, the following mandate was included in the Community Mental Health Centers Amendments of 1975, U.S. Public Law 94-63:

The governing body of a community mental health center shall: (i) be composed, where practicable, of individuals who reside in the center's catchment area and who, as a group, represent the residents of that area taking into consideration their employment, age, sex, and place of residence, and other demographic characteristics of the area, and (ii) meet at least once a month, establish general policies for the center (including a schedule of hours during which services will be provided), approve the center's annual budget, and approve the selection of a director for the center.

Increasing citizen input into the process of making policy-level decisions for a mental health center is expected to improve the delivery of mental health services by making them more responsive, accountable, and flexible. But even though broadly based consensus and support would be beneficial to every health program of the community, many communities have been slow to respond to the particular needs of the people for whom these programs are carried out. Community action groups can work to promote innovative services or programs, change the goals and priorities of organizations as needed, and expand the rate and effectiveness of participation by citizens.

How can strong mental health boards develop pressure for action through governments, old and new organizations, lobbying, and advocacy? Steps in an idealized model of community action might answer this question for some boards. Face-to-face visits by board members with businessmen have been shown to be an effective activity for board members, but study of the community must be done before community development by mental health advocacy groups can be very successful.

Typical community awareness surveys address mental health needs and problems in the community, knowledge about community resources, and attitudes toward mental health issues. Data concerning the physical and environmental status of minority groups are important for citizen boards to consider, for these often correlate with mental illness and should influence the selection of priority target areas. The use of, and resistance and accommodation to, mental health services by minority groups in the community are important considerations in programming and delivering services. Alienation felt toward mental health agencies and services must be recognized among minority groups, if it exists; services should be designed to be attractive, responsive, and viable for all groups (National Institute of Mental Health, 1979).

Community health department mental health programs

Many U.S. county and city health departments have had a mental health division or section. Indeed, this has become a standard unit in the modern local health department. Frequently, this unit is organized as a clinic with a staff consisting of one or more psychiatrists, clinical psychologists, psychiatric social workers, health educators, and mental health nurse consultants. The staff provides consulting services for citizens who are normal, citizens who are mentally ill, and those who may be borderline cases. This service is extended to children as well as to adults. Marriage counseling and family counseling are frequently included in the services.

The staff provides diagnosis and recommends treatment. A limited amount of treatment may be provided, but the program is not designed for complete treatment. In some instances the mental health staff advises courts on matters relating to mental competence of people before the court. The staff may recommend rehospitalization and may assist in rehabilitation of a patient who has been released from a mental hospital.

The importance of a mental health unit in the community health department lies in its value as a resource for citizens who have a need for mental health consultation services. This gives citizens of the community a certain degree of security in the knowledge that competent mental health personnel are available when needed.

The value of the service provided by each agency in the community would appear to depend on the freedom each agency has to do its best work within the general community mental health program or organized mental health plan. The work of the general medical practitioner or the psychiatrist should be regarded as a part of the total community mental health program. Psychiatric clinics supervised by professional psychiatrists and staffed by other personnel will continue to be vital to the mental health needs of the community (Nash, 1975).

In addition to acting as the coordinating agency, the community public health department can point out mental health needs in the community that are not being met. It can assume the role of leader in obtaining the necessary services to fulfill the recognized needs. It can provide for the fullest use of voluntary services that are available in the community. It can serve as the liaison between segments of the public and the special mental health services these various segments of the public need. It can keep the community informed on matters of mental health, particularly in terms of services available, and how these services may be used.

Medical practitioners. Practicing physicians obviously have an important role in the mental health of the community. About 50% of general medical and surgical patients in the United States (33% in Ireland) are estimated to have some kind of emotional disorder. Further evidence that patients who come with physical ailments to their family physicians are in need of mental health guidance is reported by the U.S. National Association for Mental Health: of all patients who go to general hospitals for physical ailments annually, 6 million are suffering

from serious mental and emotional illnesses that are partly responsible for their physical complaints. Many individuals who would be classified as having normal mental health nevertheless have minor or moderate mental health problems and look to a physician as their consultant in dealing with these mental and emotional disturbances (Fig. 8-2). A citizen with a neurosis—under the supervision of a family physician, who understands the patient's total background—can usually adjust reasonably well to his or her situation and live a virtually normal life. In addition, the physician is frequently the first person consulted when a family suspects that one of its members is suffering from mental disturbance. General medical practitioners, although they do not profess to be specialists in psychiatry, nevertheless have an adequate background to be an important resource in the community mental health program if continuing education programs are made available.

Psychologists, health educators, and social

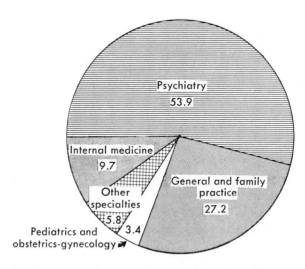

FIG. 8-2. Percent distribution of office visits for mental disorders, by most visited specialty, United States, 1975-1976.

From Advance Data from Vital and Health Statistics of the National Center for Health Statistics, U.S. Public Health Service, No. 38, Aug. 25, 1978.

workers usually have a background that gives them an understanding of the field of mental health, the mental health program, and their place and contribution in the field. Working in cooperation with psychiatrists, nurses, family physicians, and other professional people, psychologists, health educators, and social workers can make constructive contributions to community mental health through their understanding of various factors operating in the community and of the resources that can be drawn on to help the individual, the family, or the neighborhood (Wax, 1974).

Many small communities with limited professional mental health resources can draw on the facilities available in a large neighboring community. A reasonably well-organized mental health program, even in a small community, will have complete information on facilities available in nearby communities so that citizens in the smaller community can have the benefit of the highly trained pyschiatrist and other specialists who are most likely to be practicing in larger cities.

EDUCATION FOR MENTAL HEALTH

People today frequently find themselves incapable of making the necessary adjustments to the kaleidoscope of modern life without assistance. The base of the pyramid termed the community mental health program is community education in mental health. Such a program is directed primarily to the mental health needs of the normal individual and is positive in its approach. Its objectives are to promote wholesome attitudes toward mental health, to help people understand themselves as normal human beings, to show people how to manage and control stress, and to keep the community informed of the various mental health services and facilities that are available and how those services and facilities are best used.

A community mental health education program will function more effectively under the direction of an individual professionally pre-

pared in the field of community health education. An important function of the program director is that of enlisting and using the services of all qualified people or organizations in the community who can contribute to mental health education. This means organizing and administering a continuous program that provides for the mental health education needs of the various segments of the population. Resourcefulness and ingenuity are demanded, particularly when necessary resource people or organizations are not available.

As in other categorical programs, the function of health education in community mental health is to identify behaviors requiring development or change, to analyze the factors influencing these behaviors, and then to select or develop communications, community organization, and training methods to influence these factors. Examples of specific behaviors to which mental health education can be addressed are coping (Green, et al., 1978) and clinic dropouts (Barsky, Colpitts, and Green, 1979). It is estimated that approximately one third of the patients of community mental health centers drop out of treatment without staff approval or recommendation.

Community mental health education programs use discussion groups, pamphlets, radio, television, films, posters, newspapers, journals, institutes, and other materials and aids. Personal contacts between the health department and individual citizens in their homes are somewhat confined to public health nurses for purposes of conveying information or suggestions or advising the individual where certain information or services may be obtained. This service thus is not a consulting service, but rather an information service.

The development and use of clinical facilities in most U.S. communities for temporary hospitalization and care of mentally ill patients require public education even though the community relies on the state hospital facilities for its mentally ill who are in need of extended hospitalization. A developing trend is the establishment of long-term community care for the mentally ill. This could develop to a point where state hospitals will play a minor role or be abandoned. Most states have proprietary hospitals that specialize in the care of the mentally ill, but these facilities are used by a small and declining percentage of mentally ill patients. The necessary funds for the construction and maintenance of adequate community facilities depend on the understanding and the interest of the general public. The proper use of such facilities similarly requires public education.

MENTAL ILLNESS

It is essential that the public recognize that major mental illness is an important consideration in the mental hygiene program but that equally important is the mental health of normal individuals. Most people in a community are normal, although they have their mental upsets and emotional disturbances. Others in the community have mental and emotional deviations sufficiently severe to be disturbing but not constituting frank mental illness. Both the normal individual and the one with minor mental disturbances need consulting services of professional mental hygienists. The severely mentally ill are in need of special medical and hospital services, and this is the province of the psychiatrist or the medical practitioner. Psychiatry is that discipline or profession that concerns itself with the prevention, diagnosis, treatment, and cure of mental disorder.

The present psychosomatic approach indicates that the physical and psychological are interrelated and that mental disorders can have their genesis in a physiological disturbance. Mental illness, which was once regarded as primarily a problem of custodial care, is now regarded as a problem in medical care. This change has come about because of the development of specific medication in the treatment of mental disorder and the concept that a men-

tal hospital is a place where one can go for a short time for treatment. Cold-storage institutionalization has become obsolete, and today mental illness is regarded as truly remediable. Advances in the last decade indicate that a major breakthrough in the treatment and care of mental disorder has occurred and that the problem is yielding to the united efforts of the many disciplines attacking the problem. The general public is not yet aware that the success of chemotherapy in dealing with mental illness represents a landmark in the march of public health as important as the use of artificial immunization against infectious disease.

Epidemiology of mental illness

Epidemiology concerns itself with the occurrence of phenomena affecting human health and welfare. It is a discipline that deals with population-based rates, with the incidence and prevalence of a specific condition, with age distribution, and with changes in the occurrence of phenomena.

Admissions to mental facilities. In 1977 in the United States the total of 1,588,964 admissions to all inpatient mental hospitals was 25% more than the total number of admissions in 1971. In 1977 state and county mental hospitals had 414,703 admissions of mental and mentally retarded patients. Admissions to all physchiatric services in 1977 totaled 4 million, with 2.4

TABLE 8-1. Admission rates per 100,000 population to all inpatient and outpatient psychiatric services, by age, United States, 1971

Age (years)	Rate of admissions
Under 18	626.8
18-24	1936.0
25-44	1982.2
45-64	1315.7
65 and over	615.2
ALL AGES	1238.5

million in outpatient services. Males had higher admission rates to inpatient services, whereas females had higher outpatient utilization rates. The rates of admission by age groups are of interest (Table 8-1). In Ireland, one in five people surviving to 70 years and one in four surviving to 80 years will be admitted at least once to a psychiatric hospital.

Data on admission of patients by diagnosis give an indication of the principal causes of mental disorder afflicting the U.S. public (Table 8-2) and where people seek help for these conditions.

Whether mental disorder is on the increase in the United States is difficult to assess. More facilities are available, and people today are more inclined to use professional services and facilities. (Over 66% of all admissions to psychiatric hospitals in Ireland in 1976 were readmissions.) Chemotherapy has not reduced admissions significantly but does shorten the length of hospital stay and increases outpatient utilization.

Population in mental hospitals. From 1880 to 1955 there had been a steady increase in the average number of patients in state and county mental hospitals per 100,000 people in the United States. Since 1955 there has been a steady decline (Table 8-3). In 1955 the average daily census of the state and county mental hospitals for mental disease in the United States was 559,000—54% of patients in all hospitals. In 1956 for the first time in the history of the United States, there was a reduction in the number of resident patients in the state and county mental hospitals. On December 31, 1956, there were about 7,000 fewer patients in these hospitals than on December 31, 1955. This was the result of the successful use of chemotherapy in the treatment of mental disorder. The decline was particularly significant when one considers that between the years 1945 and 1955 there was an average increase of 10,000 patients per year in these mental hospitals. Each year since 1956 there has been a further decrease in the year-end census of patients in mental hospitals.

The incidence of the various mental disor-

TABLE 8-2. Admission rates per 100,000 population to all inpatient and outpatient psychiatric services, by diagnosis, United States, 1971

Diagnosis	Rate of admissions	
	Inpatient	Outpatient
Alcohol disorders	94.0	33.9
Depressive disorders	134.3	82.6
Brain syndromes	37.6	17.3
Schizophrenia	161.1	96.9
Drug misuse disorders	30.2	12.9
Other psychoses	9.8	9.1
Mental retardation	7.4	21.5
All other diagnoses	110.9	290.2
Undiagnosed	11.5	77.4
ALL DIAGNOSES	596.8	641.8

TABLE 8-3. Patients in state and county mental hospitals, United States, per 100,000, 1880-1977*

Year	Rate per 100,000
1880	32
1920	230
1940	364
1955†	390
1958‡	363
1960	343
1963	311
1965	287
1971	204
1977	201

*From National Institutes of Health: Utilization of mental health facilities, 1971, DHEW Publication No. (NIH) 74-657; and Health United States, 1980, DHHS Publication No. (PHS) 81-1232.
†Tranquilizers were introduced.
‡Antidepressant drugs were introduced.

TABLE 8-4. Mental disorders of patients in state and county mental hospitals, United States, 1972 estimate, by diagnosis and age

Mental disorders	Total	%
By diagnosis		
Schizophrenic reactions	110,469	40.4
Manic depressive reactions	8,240	3.0
Other psychotic disorders	7,612	2.7
Chronic brain syndrome	5,438	2.0
Senility diseases	27,674	10.0
Psychoneurotic reactions	7,944	3.0
Personality disorders	10,056	4.0
Alcoholism	17,538	6.3
Mental deficiency	23,440	8.6
All other diagnoses	54,458	20.0
By age (years)		
Under 25	34,376	12.6
25-34	29,792	10.9
35-44	34,209	12.5
45-54	42,947	15.7
55-64	60,027	22.0
Over 64	71,518	26.2
ALL PATIENTS	272,869	100

ders of patients in the state and county mental hospitals is portrayed in a report of the National Institute of Mental Health (Table 8-4). This report classified 272,869 patients in state and county mental hospitals in 1972. It represents the prevailing distribution of various types of mental disorders in the mental hospital population.

The epidemiology of mental illness extends beyond hospitalized patients. A considerable number of people being treated through outpatient clinics are mentally ill. The number of patients served through outpatient clinics will be increased substantially as new methods of treatment are developed.

Available records indicate that about 200,000 children in the United States are brought to mental health clinics each year. Obviously, not all of these youngsters are mentally ill. Many are poorly adjusted and can benefit from coun-

seling by the mental hygienist but would not be diagnosed as psychotic or even neurotic. The Department of Psychiatry, Columbia University, reports that 10% of public school children are in need of mental health guidance. This is not to be interpreted to mean that all of these children represent cases of mental disorder. Many people not classified as mentally ill nevertheless are in need of the services of mental health specialists.

Cost of mental illness

In 1945 the cost per patient in mental hospitals in the United States was $1.06 per day. In 1956 this figure had risen to $3.26 per day. In 1960 the cost had risen to $4.91, and in 1973 the cost per patient per day was $25.20. The financial burden of caring for the ill is considerable, but the price paid in other respects is even greater. Patients, their family, their neighborhood, their community, their employer, and the nation as a whole can be affected. Mental illness casts its shadow over all of us and makes prevention an attractive course for national policy (Harper and Balch, 1975).

Mental disorder and social pathology

Many factors contribute to the social pathology of a community, but most seem to relate to a failure in human adjustment. In some instances psychosis, in some cases a neurosis, and in other cases inadequate adjustment of an otherwise normal individual is fundamental to a particular social pathology. Mental disorder does not account for all crime, delinquency, alcoholism, drug misuse, narcotic addictions, divorce, child abuse, and suicide. Indeed, the greatest portion is caused by people who are regarded as normal. Yet these individuals, regarded as normal, are generally people with explosive tempers, exaggerated feelings of inadequacy, marked feelings of persecution, or people who are asocial or antisocial, highly suspicious, overly sensitive, impulsive, overly emotional, unstable, or unable to obtain self-gratification through the normal avenues of life.

A review of the extent of social pathology gives some indication of the magnitude of the problem in the United States.

- Approximately one out of every two marriages results in divorce.
- The United States has more than 2 million serious crimes each year.
- About 300,000 children between the ages of 11 and 17 appear in court in a year.
- Over 25,000 suicides are recorded each year.
- In one recent U.S. survey, 82% of those polled indicated that they "need less stress in their lives."
- In 1978 there were 5,100 deaths from suicide among people ages 15 to 24.
- In recent years suicide has ranked as the ninth leading cause of death for all age groups. It ranks as the second leading cause of death among youths 15 to 24. Increasingly, it is also an important cause of death among the aged.
- It is estimated that 200,000 to 4 million cases of child abuse occur each year and that 2,000 children die each year in circumstances suggesting abuse or neglect.
- Hundreds of thousands of cases of violent, but nonfatal, assault occur each year. These include instances of spouse abuse and rape.
- The death rate from homicide among black males ages 15 to 24 increased from 46.4 per 100,000 population in 1960 to 72.5 per 100,000 in 1978.
- Minority groups have a greater risk of death from homicide than whites. An estimated 60% to 80% of homicides occur as the result of personal disagreements and conflicts. Firearms were used in 63% of murders occurring in 1977, with handguns used in half of the cases.
- The emotional problems that adults in a California survey reported encountering in 1979 covered a range of subjects, including family problems—20%; spouse or partner—19%; work or school—18%; financial or business—16%; death of someone—15%; problems with self—13%; illness of self—13%; and illness of another—9%.

Factors in divorce. A successful marriage is partly a matter of personality adjustment. The individual who finds difficulty in adjusting to single life is ill-prepared to adjust to the complexities of married life. One needs but go over the complaints of wives and husbands in divorce actions to recognize the extent to which inadequate personal adjustment is the basic factor. A husband's complaints in divorce actions are revealing—wife's feelings are too easily hurt, wife criticizes me, wife is too nervous and emotional, lack of freedom in the home, wife is quick-tempered, wife nags, wife tries to improve me, wife complains too much, wife is not affectionate, wife is too argumentative, we cannot agree on choice of friends. Wives, on the other hand, offer these complaints—husband is nervous and impatient, husband criticizes me, husband is argumentative, husband is quick-tempered, husband doesn't talk things over, husband is selfish and inconsiderate, husband is touchy, husband doesn't show affection, husband is too demanding, our marriage is too confining, husband criticizes my choice of friends. These complaints, obtained from complaints filed in divorce proceedings, are an indication that personality, maturity, and adjustment are factors in marital stability.

Marriage counselors can provide a valuable service to a community for those individuals in marriage who are having difficulty in making an adequate marriage adjustment. More important is a community health service that assists people in problems of mental health before these people are married. Not all people in a community are in need of mental health counseling, and not all married couples need the services of a marriage counselor. A community

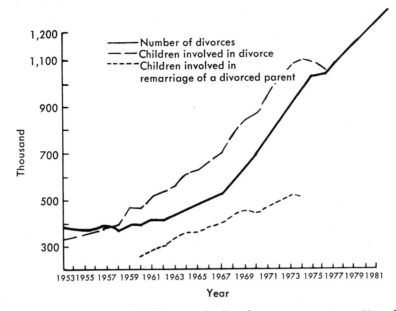

FIG. 8-3. Trends in divorces and children involved in divorce or remarriage, United States, 1953-1980.

From U.S. Department of Health and Human Services: Births, marriages, divorces, and deaths, Jan., 1981, DHHS Publication No. (PHS) 81-1120, Monthly Vital Statistics Report **30**(1):3, April 20, 1981.

health department that provides mental health counseling for normal people who do need such services will contribute not only to the general level of mental health but to the prevention of a great deal of social pathology in the form of broken families.

There were 1,170,000 divorces granted in the United States in 1979, for a rate of 5.3 per 1,000 population. The rate has increased steadily since 1958 when it was 2.1 divorces per 1,000 population. As shown in Fig. 8-3, the number of children involved in divorces has also increased since 1953 until recently when the delays in childbirth after marriage and the reduction in family size reduced the number of children affected by divorce.

Factors in suicide. Most information on the mental state of people who attempt to take their own lives is obtained from those people who failed in a suicide attempt. There is one successful suicide for every eight attempts, and

about 5% of those who fail are repeaters. The rate among men is more than three times that among women. Suicide is now the tenth leading cause of death in the United States. The suicide rate is low among certain groups. The rate is especially low among Mormons and Roman Catholics, and blacks rarely take their own lives. These data would indicate that the suicide rate can be influenced by conditioning in the individual's life. Studies indicate that perhaps 30% of those who take their own lives are actually mentally disordered. The remainder of suicides are largely the result of a decision that death is the best solution to a situation. For many of these there were coping possibilities that were not adequately explored. When life has lost its purpose or when the individual is badly frustrated, has lost self-esteem, or is depressed, an individual who lacks good personality integration may attempt to escape from reality by self-destruction.

Helping individuals over the immediate crisis, together with counseling that helps them to see the problem and its solution, will not only prevent a present attempt but will prevent further attempts at self-destruction. People who threaten suicide often carry out their threats. That persons threaten to take their own life is an indication of disturbance and of the need for assistance. Most suicides can be prevented if people recognize that the individuals are disturbed, take action to protect the individuals against themselves, and assist them in understanding and solving the situation. Persons who suffer marked depression are particularly in need of guidance during the period of depression. Highly sensitive persons may take their own life to hurt others. These individuals simply are too "thin-skinned" and sensitive for the rugged world in which they live. For these individuals, mental health counseling is long past due. If a community has adequate mental health counseling and a considerable number of citizens who recognize the various factors that indicate that a person is likely to attempt to take his or her own life, it can be predicted conservatively that suicide could be cut to one third of its present rate.

Mental illness among criminals. The first U.S. study made of the incidence of mental illness among criminals was conducted more than a quarter of a century ago by Dr. Bernard Glueck, who conducted the first penal psychiatric clinic at Sing Sing Prison. Dr. Glueck's examination of incoming prisoners revealed that 12% were frankly psychotic and that 19% were borderline cases. A subsequent study by the National Association for Mental Health in 11 state penitentiaries of 8,581 consecutive admissions revealed that 25.4% were psychotic and that 14.1% were borderline cases. An early recognition of mental illness might have prevented some of the crimes in which these individuals were involved. It is in this respect that informed citizens of a community could be of service in recognizing abnormal behavior that could be associated with violence.

Individuals who have a tendency toward violent outbursts of temper, who are overly suspicious, who have delusions of persecution, who are antisocial, or who are quarrelsome should be recognized as people who are more likely to be involved in actions of violence and destruction. Behind the wheels of automobiles a community will find people who are frankly psychotic as well as borderline cases. Antisocial individuals behind the wheel of a motor vehicle have little respect for the rights or welfare of others. They not only will inconvenience others, but their recklessness, impatience, carelessness, excitability, and lack of responsibility can be important factors in causing motor vehicle accidents. In terms of accident prevention, a motor vehicle driver's personality mold is more important than a mechanical ability to handle the car. This may force communities eventually to deny a motor vehicle operator's license to an individual because of a personality deficiency as well as because of driving deficiencies.

After a crime has been committed, courts properly refer a prisoner to a psychiatrist for determination of the prisoner's level of mental responsibility. This is a procedure with which most responsible citizens will agree. A corollary of this program is an effort to determine irresponsibility in individuals before they become involved in serious crimes. It is not possible to predict all people who may engage in crime, but repeaters have identified themselves as possible chronic criminals and have indicated the need to determine whether they are mentally ill. Others who show marked deviation in their behavior pattern should also be examined to determine the degree of mental and emotional responsibility they possess. Unfortunately, the legal machinery is frequently cumbersome, and threats to civil rights can be so great that people in the professional social field are hesitant to initiate any action to provide for the psychiatric examination and counseling of citizens who could be possible threats to the people of the community. It is possible to protect the rights of the individual whose conduct appears to deviate markedly from the normal and at the same time protect the welfare of the children and adults in the community (Kocher, 1976). This would truly be a program of prevention, both in terms of mental health and in terms of community protection.

PUBLIC RESPONSIBILITY IN MENTAL DISORDERS

The diagnosis of mental disorder is the province and the responsibility of qualified professionals. Unfortunately, the physician or psychologist frequently does not see the patient with a mental disorder until the condition is very far advanced or some crisis with serious consequences has occurred. There is a need in every community to provide the means by which people showing indications of mental disorder will be directed to professional sources for diagnosis, treatment, and care. This can be provided by having responsible people in the community informed on the early indications of mental disturbance or possible mental illness. The popular misconception that a mentally disordered person dresses oddly, has weird mannerisms, is likely to be maniacal, or talks foolishly must be displaced by a more realistic conception of the indications of mental disturbance. People in the parahealth fields, such as teachers and social workers, could be better trained to recognize some of the early indications of mental disorder. When this nucleus of professional workers coming in daily contact with the public is aided by other reliable citizens having an understanding of the early indications of mental disturbance, then a community possesses a valuable means by which individuals likely in need of diagnostic services and counsel are directed to services at an early stage when constructive and even preventive measures can be taken. In addition, such a group of informed citizens in a community can be the means by which tragedies such as child abuse and other forms of violence can be prevented (Jones, 1974).

Informed citizens can give responsible support to necessary programs for providing hospital clinics and other services necessary for the proper care and treatment of the mentally disordered. Well-informed people can lend the essential support to desirable legislation to promote an effective mental health program. They can also support the necessary official agencies, including courts, in their programs to deal with the mentally disturbed (Ruiz and Behrens, 1973).

MEDICAL RESOURCES

An appraisal of available medical resources in mental health must include clinics and professional personnel available to the general public, as well as psychiatrists, nurses, and other personnel available in psychiatric hospitals. An accurate accounting of all mental health services available to the general public is extremely difficult because of the number of human service workers who devote but a limited portion of their practice to the mentally disordered but who contribute a very important service. Most studies are limited to those clinics and practitioners primarily concerned with the mentally ill.

Community mental health centers are playing an increasingly important role in the treatment of mental illness. With the development of effective alkaloids for treating specific types of mental disorder, about one third of the patients now treated in clinics would have been hospital patients but are now able to remain at home. In addition, many patients hospitalized for chronic disorders can now be released to return to their communities under the supervision of a clinic or a physician. More than half of these clinics are located in the northeastern United States, which has about one fourth of the population. Qualified authorities maintain that there should be one psychiatric clinic for every 50,000 people, a standard that would require nearly doubling the full-time clinics in the United States.

With more successful treatment of the mentally ill and a declining population in psychiatric hospitals, the need for hospital staff becomes less, but the need for community workers becomes greater.

Employment of clinical psychologists for the care of the mentally ill is a more recent development, but the service that has been given by clinical psychologists indicates that there will be an expansion of this service in the future in schools, industry, and community agencies to forestall mental illness. With the expanding concept of community service in mental health, clinical psychologists should become increasingly important as the value of their services becomes better appreciated (Autor and Zide, 1974; Shochet, 1974).

REHABILITATION

Rehabilitation is the restoration to the fullest physical, mental, social, vocational, and economic usefulness of which an individual is capable. Total rehabilitation of persons who have recovered from mental illness may require only the services of their family physician or may require the well-integrated program of a rehabilitation team consisting of psychiatrist, psychologist, psychiatric social worker, nurse, occupational therapist, rehabilitation therapist, and family counselor.

The success of chemotherapy in the treatment of mental disorder is relieving the overcrowding in mental hospitals in the United States but is increasing the need for rehabilitation services. With specific measures for the treatment of mental disorder, a mental hospital has become a place where one can go for a short time for treatment. This revolution in the treatment of mental disease means that custodial care is being replaced by medical treatment. A patient who has been hospitalized for several years has a social adjustment to make

as well as a medical recovery. As the medication is effective in improving the patient's mental illness, the patient is permitted to visit a neighboring community under the guidance of a hospital attendant. After several escorted visits and observable improvement in adjustment to society, the patient is permitted to visit the community unescorted. When the patient's social adjustment and mental adjustment appear to be sufficiently advanced, the patient is permitted to return to his or her home and community, but only when adequate supervision is available. This means that both medical and social supervision must be provided.

A family physician may accept responsibility for the continuation of the treatment the patient has been receiving. Medical supervision may be arranged through a psychiatric clinic in the patient's community. Rehabilitation services also are needed to assist the recovered or recuperating individual to make the necessary social, economic, and other adjustments that normal living requires. Getting a job, finding social groups and interests, adjusting to the tempo of community living, and finding leisure-time activities may require the services of specially prepared people. Statewide clinic systems are emerging in the United States from the community mental health centers. State hospitals that presently have a rehabilitation service are establishing links with centers throughout the state where former patients in need of assistance may obtain rehabilitation services conveniently and promptly.

RESEARCH

It would be incorrect to say that research is the greatest need in the mental health field because hospital facilities, medical services, and other types of professional services are indispensable. Research has not received the attention in mental health that it has in most other areas of health. The 50 states in the United States, which properly provide millions of dollars for mental hospitals for the care of the

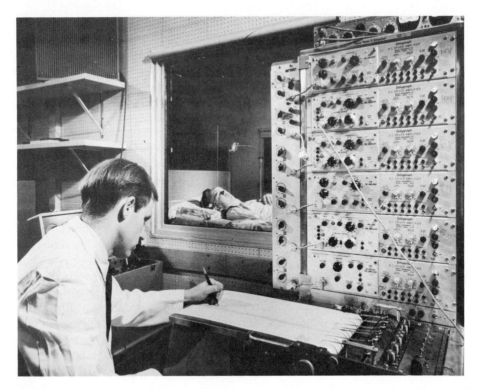

FIG. 8-4. Sleep studies. Today mental health research is far-reaching and uses sophisticated instruments. Using the electroencephalograph, it is possible to get recordings of brain wave changes during different phases of sleep, all of which can aid investigators in understanding the restorative functions of rest and stress reduction.

Courtesy National Institutes of Health.

mentally ill, appropriate for research only 1.5% of their total mental hospital budget. State mental health officials contend that from 4% to 7% of a state's annual budget for mental health should be allotted to research.

On a national scale the research program in the field of mental health is more encouraging, but the amount appropriated is still inadequate to do the job that is needed. Actual expenditures for research from the Alcohol, Drug Abuse, and Mental Health Administration (incorporating the National Institute of Mental Health) amounted to $141.2 million in 1980. The trend in appropriations for mental health research is shown in Fig. 8-5. An additional

$68 million is devoted to alcoholism and drug misuse. The mental health budget is diluted by pressures on the government to devote these resources to major social problems, including rape and other forms of violence as well as the problems of minorities and women. These are all important problems, but they are so complex as to diffuse scarce mental health resources for service as well as research.

As formidable as $141.2 million appears to be, it represents but a small fraction of the funds invested in research in other areas of health. The many recognized problems in mental illness that cry out for solution indicate that, as a nation, the United States ought to

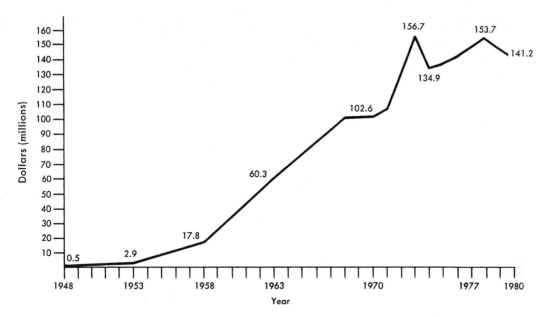

FIG. 8-5. Appropriations for mental health research, United States, 1948-1980.

From Forward Plan for Health, FY 1978-82, DHEW Publication No. (OS) 76-50046.

double or triple its efforts in mental health research.

The most fruitful area of research would be in the preventive aspect of mental illness. The use of alkaloids has enabled many individuals to remain at home who otherwise would have been sent to a psychiatric hospital for treatment. As important as preventive medication procedures are in dealing with mental illness, functional or psychological measures for the prevention of mental illness may be an equally productive field of research, but one in which little organized research has been completed.

Investigations into the cause, prevention, treatment, and cure of mental illness could be intensified if more resources were devoted to the pursuit. Research is also needed in the mental health of the normal individual. Advances in the health and medical fields in the United States in the past quarter-century have included only modest progress in the understanding of the mental health of the normal individual. Research in the motivation of human conduct, the genesis of emotional disturbance, the nature of mild deviations, procedures for improving and fortifying personality attributes, and the measures by which an individual of normal health may cope with stress are all in need of intensive study. Perhaps new methods of research need to be developed and more behavioral scientists prepared to do research in the mental health of the normal individual as well as in the problems of the mentally ill. Research on methods of mental health education will become more urgent as other research findings accumulate. Community leaders, particularly those in the health professions, must take the lead in emphasizing the need for intensive research in the field of mental health.

U.S. OBJECTIVES FOR 1990

Objectives for community mental health as developed by the U.S. Public Health Service are as follows. Other communities can adapt these to their mental health needs.

Improved health status

- By 1990 the death rate from homicide among black males ages 15 to 24 should be reduced to below 60 per 100,000. (In 1978 it was 72.5 per 100,000 for this group.)
- By 1990 injuries and deaths to children inflicted by abusing parents should be reduced by at least 25%. (Reliable baseline data are unavailable—estimates vary from 200,000 to 4 million cases of child abuse occurring in the United States each year.)
- By 1990 the rate of suicide among people ages 15 to 24 will be reduced 20% to 4,500 deaths, or 11 per 100,000. (In 1978 the rate was 12.4 per 100,000, or approximately 5,100 suicide deaths in this age group.)

Increased public-professional awareness

- By 1990 the proportion of the population that can accurately identify an appropriate community agency to assist in coping with a stressful situation should be greater than 50%. (Baseline data are unavailable.)
- By 1990 the proportion of adolescents who can accurately identify the existance of an accessible suicide prevention hot line should be greater than 60%. (Baseline data are unavailable.)
- By 1990 the proportion of the primary care physicians who take a careful history related to personal stress and psychological coping skills should be greater than 60%. (Baseline data are unavailable.)

Improved services-protection

- By 1990 to reduce the gap in mental health services, the number of persons reached by mutual support self-help groups should double from 1978 baseline figures. (In 1978 estimates ranged from 2.5 to 5 million, depending on how mutual support self-help groups were defined.)
- By 1990 stress identification and control should become integral components of the continuum of health services offered by the

majority of organized health programs. (Baseline data are unavailable.)
- By 1990, of the 500 largest U.S. firms, the proportion offering work-based stress reduction programs should be greater than 30%. (Baseline data are unavailable.)

Improved surveillance-evaluation systems

- By 1985 surveys should show what percentage of the U.S. population perceives stress as adversely affecting their health and what proportion of this percentage is trying to use appropriate stress control techniques.
- By 1990 surveys should show what percentage of the U.S. population understands the role of stress in health and has some knowledge about how to deal with it.
- By 1990 the existing knowledge base through scientific inquiry about stress effects and stress management should be greatly enlarged.
- By 1985 a methodology should have been developed to rate the major categories of occupation according to their environmental stress loads.
- By 1990 the reliability of data on the incidence and prevalence of child abuse and other forms of family violence should have been greatly increased.

QUESTIONS AND EXERCISES

1. With what phases of mental health should the community mental health program concern itself?
2. Why is social health properly regarded as a phase of mental health?
3. Describe some adult in your community who has excellent mental health and analyze the attributes he or she possesses.
4. Why is public health education fundamental to a community mental health program?
5. Give several examples of conduct by an adult that indicate emotional immaturity.
6. What can a community mental health program do to assist people in improving their social personalities?
7. Why do citizens with marked aggressions represent a special community mental health problem?

8. State the case for and against having the staffs of the state's mental hospitals in charge of the total state mental health program in the United States.
9. Why has a mental health program been slow in developing in your community?
10. Appraise the mental health program of the official mental hygiene agency of your own state.
11. What statewide voluntary mental health agencies function in your state and what are their programs?
12. Survey the mental health needs of your community.
13. Propose a program to meet the mental health needs of your community.
14. Based on the available data, make a prediction of the future epidemiology of mental illness in the United States.
15. Show how personality maladjustment can be the true cause of a divorce.
16. If you had good reason to believe that one member of a family of your close acquaintance was in need of psychiatric service, what measures would you take to bring this about?
17. If you had good reason to believe that one member of a family you did not know was in need of psychiatric service, what measures would you take to bring this about?
18. To what extent is it correct to say that every person has his mental measles and emotional chicken pox?
19. Evaluate this statement: "Research in the field of mental disorder will create the problem of preparing professional specialists in the field of rehabilitation."
20. What research is needed in the area of normal mental health?

BIBLIOGRAPHY

Autor, S.B., and Zide, E.D.: Master's level professional training in clinical psychology and community mental health, Profess. Psych. **5**:115, 1974.

Barsky, A.J., Colpitts, J., and Green, L.: Walk-in patients' decisions about follow-up care, J. Nerv. Ment. Dis. **167**:742, 1979.

Broskowski, A., and Baker, F.: Professional, organizational, and social barriers to primary prevention, Am. J. Orthopsychiatry **44**:707, 1974.

Butler, R.N., and Lewis, M.I.: Aging and mental health: positive psychosocial and biomedical approaches, ed. 3, St. Louis, 1981, The C.V. Mosby Co.

Clinebell, H.J., editor: Community mental health, Nashville, Tenn., 1970, Abingdon Press.

Dohrenwend, B.P.: Sociocultural and social-psychological factors in the genesis of mental disorders, J. Health Soc. Behav. **16**:365, 1975.

Faberow, N.L.: Bibliography on suicide and suicide prevention, Rockville, Md., 1972, National Institute of Mental Health, DHEW Publication No. (HSM) 72-9080.

Fairweather, G.W., et al: Community life for the mentally ill: an alternative to institutional care, Chicago, 1969, Aldine Publishing Co.

Green, L.W., et al.: Coping and self-care patterns of normal adults in response to mild symptoms of stress. Paper presented at American Psychiatric Association, Atlanta, May 10, 1978.

Grob, G.N.: State and the mentally ill, Chapel Hill, N.C., 1966, The University of North Carolina Press.

Grunebaum, H.: Practice of community mental health, Boston, 1970, Little, Brown and Co.

Halpern, W.I., and Kissel, S.: Human resources for troubled children, New York, 1976, John Wiley & Sons, Inc.

Harper, R., and Balch, P.: Some economic arguments in favor of primary prevention, Profess. Psych. **6**:17, 1975.

Jones, F.H.: A 4-year follow-up of vulnerable adolescents: the prediction of outcomes in early adulthood from measures of social competence, coping style, and overall level of psychopathology, J. Nerv. Ment. Dis. **159**:20, 1974.

Kaplan, L.: Eduction and mental health, rev. ed., New York, 1971, Harper & Row, Publishers.

Kline, J., and King, M.: Treatment dropouts from a community mental health center, Community Men. Health J. **9**:354, 1973.

Kocher, G.P., editor: Children's rights and the mental health professions, New York, 1976, John Wiley & Sons, Inc.

Lawrence, M.M.: Mental health team in the school, New York, 1971, Behavioral Publications, Inc.

Marmor, J.: Psychiatrists and their patients: a national study of private practice, Washington, 1975, American Psychiatric Association.

Menninger, K.A.: The human mind, ed. 3, New York, 1953, Alfred A. Knopf, Inc.

Murred, S.A.: Community psychology and social systems: a conceptual framework and intervention guide, New York, 1973, Behavioral Publications, Inc.

Nash, K.B.: Supervision and the emerging professional, Am. J. Orthopsychiatry **5**:93, 1975.

National Center for Health Statistics: Health resources statistics, 1974, DHEW Publication No. (HRA) 75-1509.

National Center for Health Statistics: Parent ratings of behavioral patterns of youths 12-17 years, United States, Vital and Health Statistics, Data from the National Health Survey, Series #11, No. 137, DHEW Publication No. HRA 74-1619, 1974.

National Institute of Mental Health: The comprehensive community mental health center, Rockville, Md., 1970, PHS Publication No. 2136.

National Institute of Mental Health, Alcohol, Drug Abuse, and Mental Health Administration: Serving mental health needs of the aged through volunteer services, Rockville, Md., 1974, DHEW Publication No. NIH 74-669.

National Institute of Mental Health: Citizen participation in community mental health centers, Rockville, Md., 1979, DHEW Publication No. (ADM) 79-737.

Panzetta, A.F.: Community mental health, myth and reality, Philadelphia, 1971, Lea & Febiger.

Resnick, H.L.P., and Hawthorne, V.C., editors: Suicide prevention in the 70's, Rockville, Md., 1973, National Institute of Mental Health, DHEW Publication No. (HSA) 72-9054.

Rosenzweig, S.: Compulsory hospitalization of the mentally ill, Am. J. Public Health **61:**121, 1971.

Ross, D.M.: Hyperactivity: research, theory and action, New York, 1976, John Wiley & Sons, Inc.

Ruiz, P., and Behrens, M.: Community control in mental health: how far can it go? Psychiatr. Q. **47:**317, 1973.

Shochet, B.R.: The role of the mental health counselor in the psychiatric liaison service of the general hospital, Int. J. Psychiatry Med. **5:**1, 1974.

Sutherland, J.D., editor: Towards community mental health, New York, 1971, Barnes & Noble Books.

Szaz, T.: The myth of mental illness, New York, 1961, Harper & Row, Publishers.

Task Force on Community Mental Health: Issues in community psychology and preventive mental health, New York, 1971, Behavioral Publications, Inc.

Wax, D.E.: A collaborative-interactive model for mental health consultation, Child Psychiatry Hum. Dev. **5:**78, 1974.

Welu, T.C.: Broadening the focus of suicide prevention activities utilizing the public health model, Am. J. Public Health **62:**1625, 1972.

Williams, C.L., Henderson, A.S., and Mills, J.M.: An epidemiological study of serious traffic offenders, Soc. Psych. **9:**99, 1974.

9

COMMUNITY RECREATION AND FITNESS

It is better to wear out than to rust out.

Bishop Richard Cumberland (1631-1718)

Recreation and exercise serve many purposes, including the contribution they make to health. The primary values of recreation and exercise include health promotion, prevention of certain disorders, and treatment of certain disabilities. Recreation and physical education personnel sometimes regard themselves as parahealth professionals.

Many individuals can provide for their own recreational needs. A large portion of the citizens in the community, however, are unable to fulfill an adequate portion of their needs without the benefit of an organized community recreational and fitness program.

THE PROBLEM

Fitness attitudes and practices have changed positively in the following ways:

1. More and more physicians prescribe exercise as a means of maintaining and enhancing health and as accepted therapy for many heart patients and the victims of other degenerative diseases.
2. Western society is in the midst of a genuine exercise boom—more bicycles than automobiles are being bought; sports fashion and athletic footwear have become major industries; and the number of

runners, skiers, and tennis players has tripled. Joggers, backpackers, and bicycling commuters, once sources of amusement or amazement, are commonplace in most communities (There are 17 million joggers, 20 million regular cyclists, 3.1 million raquetball and 14 million tennis players, and 26 million serious swimmers among America's 110 million adults.)
3. The number of young women participating in interscholastic and intercollegiate sports quadrupled between 1966 and 1976 in the United States.
4. Ninety percent of the Americans questioned in a national survey said that there should be physical education programs in elementary and secondary schools.

Despite these facts, pockets of public apathy, urban growth, and modern life-style continually threaten to neutralize physical fitness advances. Nearly half of adult Americans never engage in physical activity for exercise, according to a national survey. Older, poorer, and less-educated adults frequently have little understanding of the contributions that exercise can make to health, performance, or the quality of life. Millions of North Americans, and Europeans still are willing victims of schemes that promise fitness in a few minutes a day, without sweat or strain. One third of all American children and 62% of adults are overweight. The continuing financial crisis of schools and the trend away from required subjects have resulted in the loss of many physical education programs. A simultaneous trend toward "elective" physical education often results in students' taking courses that contribute little to fitness or development of progressive skills. Only one American child in three participates in the daily program of physical education recommended for fitness. Larger schools and larger cities often diminish opportunities for participation in sports and other active forms of recreation.

Recreation is an activity, pursued during leisure time, that is free and pleasurable and has its own immediate appeal. Therefore it is a behavior common to everyone regardless of employment status. Recreation has come to be viewed also as an emotional state or condition that flows from a feeling of well-being and self-satisfaction, and it is characterized by feelings of mastery, achievement, exhilaration, acceptance, success, personal worth, and pleasure. As such, it is not necessarily dependent on any physical or social activity.

A BRIEF HISTORY OF RECREATION IN THE UNITED STATES

A brief review of the history of recreation in the United States provides some insight into the nature of recreation and the roots of its problems. Recreation, as it is recognized today, is largely a reflection of three historical movements: the conservation movement, the urban parks movement, and the recreation movement. Although they all arose during the latter half of the nineteenth century, each has its own particular and separate history.

The conservation movement was based on a belief in the wise and balanced use of natural resources. The federal government played a leading role by helping to conserve large areas of open spaces and unique landscapes, beginning with the designation in 1864 of Yosemite valley as the first national park. The establishment of a national park and national forest system was perhaps the most notable accomplishment of the movement. The subsequent creation of the U.S. Forest Service in 1905 and the National Park Service in 1916 stimulated state and local park and conservation programs, as did increased federal conservation assistance during the New Deal administration of the 1930s.

The urban parks movement was nineteenth century American leaders' response to the effects of industrialization and immigration on the rapidly growing urban population. Landscape architects, typified by Frederick Law Olmsted, created a new legacy of public green spaces among the bricks and grime of America's maturing cities. Beginning with Olmsted's Central Park in New York City, the urban parks movement spread rapidly across the country. By the early 1900s most big cities had large urban parks, and municipal governments had become well-established parkland providers.

Unlike both the conservation and urban parks movements, initial support for the recreation movement came largely from private and philanthropic sources rather than from government, and was specifically aimed at producing social reforms. The movement originated in private settlement houses of major cities where play programs, notably the "sandgardens" of Boston in 1885 and Jane Addams' model playground at Hull House in 1892, successfully provided organized recreational opportunities for children of immigrant tenement dwellers. Largely because of the success of these programs, by 1907 local governments had begun assuming responsibility for providing similar neighborhood recreational programs. The recreation movement was again reinforced by the creation of the National Recreation Association in 1925 and by federal public works and social programs of the 1930s that placed emphasis on parks, recreation, and cultural opportunities.

The movement was also characterized in the 1920s and 1930s by the development of spectator sports and box-office attractions. These were decades that created glamorous films and professional athletics.

The nation's park and recreation efforts expanded rapidly after World War II in response to population growth, large incomes, and new housing developments. By the late 1950s, however, the existing parks and programs could not satisfy the increased demand. In response, Congress created the Outdoor Recreation Resources Review Commission in 1958, which stimulated a resurgence of federal interest in parks and recreation.

The 1960s brought expansive growth in the protection and development of natural resources and recreational services, as reflected in the creation of the Land and Water Conservation Fund and the National Wilderness, Wild and Scenic Rivers, and Trails Systems. Another development was the acquisition of new national park and recreation areas close to major urban areas and expanded state and local parkland acquisition.

During the 1970s, recreation expenditures increased at all levels of government. In some cases, however, these funds were unable to keep pace with price escalations that affect recreational land acquisition, capital development, energy supplies, and staffing or programming. The lack of a consistent national recreation policy continues to impede the provision of recreation, particularly for those programs of other government agencies that influence recreation. In addition, the late 1970s saw the adoption of several approaches designed to increase community support for urban recreation and fitness resources and programs.

The most pervasive influence on physical and recreational patterns in the United States has been television, which has substituted passive entertainment for creative recreation and sedentary recreation for physical activity. By the time a child reaches school age, he or she is watching an average of 23.5 hours of television per week, while adults are watching 44 hours in the same week, according to Arthur C. Nielson's ratings. A 17-year-old has logged at least 15,000 hours of television time, more than any other activity except sleep. This will include 350,000 commercial advertisements (70% of which on Saturday mornings are for junk foods).

A community is obliged to develop a recreational and fitness program providing for a wide diversity of participation. At present, the trend of the public is toward participation in physical activities, and the community finds it necessary to serve citizens who desire to occupy their leisure hours in more stimulating and outdoor pursuits. But recreation includes creative and esthetic interests as well as those of a predominantly physical nature. A community doubtless can exist without formal recreational and fitness programs, but the community enhances the quality of life and provides alternative to drugs and alcohol as leisure pursuits by having an organized recreational program that provides for many of the social, creative, esthetic, communicative, learning, and physical needs of its people.

RECREATION AS HEALTH PROMOTION

More effective and enjoyable living through recreation can contribute to mental, social, and physical health. By breaking from the dull, commonplace routine of existence, recreation contributes to a greater realization of the individual's potential for living. Recreation alone cannot produce a high level of health, but combined with other factors affecting health it can elevate health for normal individuals. For some individuals the mental health contribution of recreation is the greatest value. For other individuals the physical health values or the social values are most important. For the individual with a chronic disability or some disorder, recreation frequently proves to be of value in restoring health. The rehabilitation value of recreation is universally acknowledged (Cousins, 1979).

Mental health

The normal individual seeks self-gratification and self-esteem. Many individuals are able to find this in their regular vocations, but in this assembly-line age of automation, where individuals find themselves a cog in a big machine, they frequently derive little gratification from the product they help to turn out or the services they give. They will seek some other avenue through which gratification can be attained. Recreation is serving as the avenue through which many individuals obtain the emotional gratification that accompanies self-fulfillment.

The normal person seeks attention, approval, and praise. Achievement, mastery, skill, and superiority bring elation and produce satisfying emotions. Through recreation, an individual can achieve a high level of personal performance, can experience mastery, and can obtain attention, approval, and praise, all of which arouse emotions of pleasure and elation. Recreation can lift the individual into an experience in which the self is of importance. Self-esteem, so essential to a high level of mental health, can be attained through creative, esthetic, social, communicative, and learning activities as well as through physical activities.

Aggressions can be given an outlet in competitive games. Creative urges can be satisfied through programs in crafts, painting, dramatics, music, writing, and other arts. Relaxation may be achieved through passive activities such as reading, music appreciation, art appreciation, listening to addresses, and otherwise serving somewhat the role of the spectator rather than the active participant. On the curative side is the prescription of specific types of recreation for each patient as part of the therapeutic procedure in mental health counseling and psychiatric treatment. A recent study links physical fitness to high motivation, persistence, learning achievement, self-confidence, and social acceptance (President's Council on Physical Fitness and Sports, 1980).

Social health

Social health is an extension of mental health. To give meaning to life, normal individuals want friendship and companionship or association with others. The interaction with fellow human beings promotes a feeling of worth, a feeling of security from group acceptance, approval, and recognition. Social drives include the desire for new experiences, adventure, and identity with others.

Recreation provides opportunities for participation, companionship, recognition, and security. Recreation can contribute to the social health of people of all ages. It can elevate the feeling of personal worth in the person who already enjoys a high level of social health. It can elevate the level of social health for the individual whose social adjustment has been adequate but not satisfying. It can be a means by which the asocial individual can become comfortable in social situations. It can be a means for preventing or correcting antisocial tendencies. Boys and girls who already are delinquents are not so attracted to physical activity. Those who are not delinquents but vulnerable to delinquency can find both release and wholesome direction in recreational participation. Family recreation can be an aid in preventing delinquency. In the United States a Detroit study of over 2,000 court cases showed that 60% of the juveniles had little or no recreation within the family group, 32% experienced occasional family recreation, and only 8% participated regularly in family recreation.

Even highly individualistic recreation such as painting, instrumental music, crafts, and stamp collecting have social health values. To have an interest in common with others can provide vicarious social reinforcement to the "loner." A common recreational interest can bring a diversity of people together and promote a general understanding and appreciation of other human beings, which in turn will improve the individual's ability to adjust socially. Properly developed, recreation and fitness are means to fuller personal development, social as well as otherwise.

Physical health

A study of longevity in the United States has shown that regular exercise, in combination with six other health practices, can help increase life expectancy by as much as 11 years for men and 7 years for women. One of the physicians who wrote the study report declared that "the daily habits of people have a great deal more to do with what makes them sick and when they die than do all the influences of medicine" (Belloc and Breslow, 1972).

The study started with 7,000 subjects in 1965, and by 1973 there had been twice as many deaths among the men who exercised infrequently, if at all, as there were among those who exercised regularly (Belloc, 1973). The evidence is mounting that the physically fit live longer, perform better, and participate more fully in life than do those who are not fit. Regular, vigorous exercise adds to vibrant good health, and it enhances the capacity for enjoying life.

Whether the activity is one requiring vigorous, moderate, or light exertion, certain physical health benefits will accrue. Physical exertion inherent in many physical activities creates organic vigor and physiological well-being and increases physiological efficiency. Physical activity develops skill, dexterity, coordination, and stamina. A recreational program is not designed to develop circus strong men or professional athletes. Many recreational activities, however, will provide sufficient physical exertion to stimulate the body to a higher level of efficiency in its functioning if pursued with enough frequency and intensity. Efficiency in

functioning refers to that level which is desirable for normal needs and to take care of any emergencies or special demands that may be made of a person. For the person without circulatory or other serious defects, this generally means moderate exercise of 20 to 30 minutes duration at least four times per week. The actual amount of exercise that recreation should give an individual or group should be determined by general condition and the exercise the individual gets from daily vocational and other day-to-day living practices. An individual who adjusts activities to capacity and needs can gain certain established benefits, as shown in Table 9-1. Metabolism will be improved, circulation will function more efficiently, respiration will function more effectively, muscle tone and coordination will be improved, greater flexibility may be achieved, and general body efficiency will be improved. Usually, the greatest physical health benefits accrue from the improved circulation. The chronically tired person will find that a recreational activity that interests him or her will have a surprising effect in eliminating the chronic feeling of fatigue. What such an individual usually needs is stimulation rather than rest (Crisp and Stonehill, 1976).

Hospitals have been slow to recognize the value of recreation, but more than one fourth of the hospitals in the United States have organized recreational programs. Physical rehabilitation programs employ recreational activities. Actually, much of the occupational therapy in rehabilitation programs is basically a recreational program. The motivation that a particular activity can give to a rehabilitation patient is often the difference between inadequate and adequate recovery. The mental and physical stimulation that a recreational or fitness activity can give to a normal individual actually can be even greater for the individual who is recovering from extended illness or a disability.

Daily living no longer provides enough vig-

Table 9-1. Summary of how seven experts rated 14 sports and exercises. Ratings are on a scale of 0 to 3, thus a rating of 21 indicates maximum benefit (a score of 3 by all seven panelists). Ratings were made on the basis of regular (minimum of 4 times per week), vigorous (duration of 30 minutes to 1 hour per session) participation in each activity*

	Jogging	Bicycling	Swimming	Skating (ice or rolling)	Handball/squash	Skiing-Nordic	Skiing-Alpine	Basketball	Tennis	Calisthenics	Walking	Golf†	Softball	Bowling
Physical fitness														
Cardiorespiratory endurance (stamina)	21	19	21	18	19	19	16	19	16	10	13	8	6	5
Muscular endurance	20	18	20	17	18	19	18	17	16	13	14	8	8	5
Muscular strength	17	16	14	15	15	15	15	15	14	16	11	9	7	5
Flexibility	9	9	15	13	16	14	14	13	14	19	7	8	9	7
Balance	17	18	12	20	17	16	21	16	16	15	8	8	7	6
General well-being														
Weight control	21	20	15	17	19	17	15	19	16	12	13	6	7	5
Muscle definition	14	15	14	14	11	12	14	13	13	18	11	6	5	5
Digestion	13	12	13	11	13	12	9	10	12	11	11	7	8	7
Sleep	16	15	16	15	12	15	12	12	11	12	14	6	7	6
TOTAL	148	142	140	140	140	139	134	134	128	126	102	66†	64	51

*From Conrad, C.C.: How different sports rate in promoting physical fitness, Washington, D.C., 1978, President's Council on Physical Fitness and Sports, Public Health Service, U.S. Department of Health and Human Services.

†Ratings for golf are based on the fact that many Americans use a golf cart and/or caddy. If one walks the links, the physical fitness value moves up appreciably.

orous exercise to develop and maintain good muscle tone or cardiovascular and respiratory fitness. In homes and factories, and even on farms, machines have virtually eliminated the necessity for walking long distances or climbing stairs.

It is estimated that in 1850 human muscles supplied nearly one third of the energy used by workshops, factories, and farms. Today the comparable estimate is less than 1%. Television holds children in captive idleness for as much as 50 hours a week. Pervasive inactivity, together with poor living habits, has resulted in a serious national fitness problem in the United States. Obesity is epidemic. Children do poorly on tests of strength and endurance. Fifty-four percent of all deaths in the United States result from diseases of the heart and blood vessels—diseases that are associated with physical inactivity.

Although there are too few data to permit documentation of the exact effects of exercise and physical fitness in reducing risks of incurring illness, its absence (sedentary living) has been established as one of the factors that increases the probabilities of falling victim to cardiovascular disease. Regular physical activity is valued for providing a general sense of well-being, thereby reducing stress, which is also associated with heart disease. Also, people who exercise regularly are apt to smoke less and to be able to maintain their desired weight more easily. Friendships centered around their favored activity can constitute one element of the social support systems people appear to need for good health. For all these reasons, opportunities for a lifetime of regular physical activity is a general objective to be sought during the 1980s. This means that public recreation departments and interested private agencies sponsoring physical activity programs should include the development of physical fitness and sports skills for all age groups and that health professionals should encourage their patients to engage in appropriate exercise.

NATURE OF RECREATION

Recreation is a diversion for the enjoyment an activity gives an individual. What may be a job to one individual can be recreation for another. Recreation usually is a leisure-time activity in which the rewards are personal rather than monetary. At least the monetary reward is a minor factor or even immaterial. Recreation can be an esthetic experience, an academic experience, a sporting experience, or any other diversion from the routine of daily life.

Recreation provides relaxation needed by people who are fatigued mentally and physically. Relaxation may take many forms. For some, social gatherings are relaxing. Others require strenuous activity. Still others prefer crafts or music or some other sedentary activity. Recreation provides experiences in the enjoyment of beauty, opportunities for serving others, and sharing interests, skills, and fellowship with others. Many adults derive considerable gratification from the service they can give in helping others in the community enjoy recreation. Recreation provides opportunity for creative activities. The job of creation is one of the richest experiences humans can have. Recreation can be mentally challenging. Discussion groups, forums, play writing, nature study, chess, and other similar activities can afford wholesome mental stimulation. Many individuals find very little opportunity for group participation in their normal vocational pursuits but find in recreation the opportunity to satisfy their need for group participation. Recreation can promote fellowship of a sincere type and can provide adventure. The planning as well as the participation in recreational pursuits can be invigorating.

SCOPE OF RECREATION

With the changing concept of recreation, it was inevitable that the scope of recreation would expand. From the limited philosophy of recreation as a diversion in sports and allied activities, recreation can now be found to extend into intellectual activities, communicative interests, creative and esthetic activities, and social activities. In attempting to indicate the various activities in each of these categories, it is recognized that a specific activity may well be considered as being in all of these categories. For purposes of delineation and convenience, a particular classification will include those activities whose primary function is in that particular category even though they may serve other purposes.

Physical activities

Recreational activities whose primary purpose is to provide physical exertion, weight control, and exercise include both team and individual events.

The number of calories per minute that might be expended by an individual pursuing physical activities is dependent on many variables, such as physical build, age, skill at the activity, and adverse circumstances, for example, a strong wind while running, waves while swimming, or an awkward partner while dancing. Table 9-2 is a comparative guide to the relative benefits to expect—in terms of weight loss and cardiovascular conditioning—based on Morehouse and Miller (1976).

Intellectual activities

Many recreational activities that are primarily intellectual or learning in nature have other values, although their primary attraction is in the intellectual stimulation or the opportunity for learning that they provide. These include amateur radio, astronomy, classes, coin collecting, chess, collecting of scientific materials, debates, discussion groups, educational games, educational television, exhibits, fairs, first aid, forums, interest groups, language study, mu-

TABLE 9-2. Calories and oxygen per kilogram body weight expended per minute in various activities*

Activity	Calories	Oxygen use (ml)	Activity	Calories	Oxygen use (ml)
Walking, 2.0 mph	2.8	9	Chopping wood	9.0	22
Bicycle riding, 5.5 mph	3.2	13	Skiing (cross-country), 3.0 mph	9.0	24
Walking, 3.5 mph	4.8	14	Swimming/sidestroke, 1.0 mph	9.2	45
Dancing/fox-trot, slow	5.2	17	Figure skating	9.5	41
Table tennis	5.8	22	Racketball or handball	10.2	42
Swimming/breaststroke, 1.0 mph	6.8	29	Running (jogging), 5.7 mph	12.0	35
Bicycle riding, rapid	6.9	31	Running, 7.0 mph	14.5	38
Dancing/rhumba or disco	7.0	20	Running, 11.4 mph	21.7	60
Swimming/crawl, 1.0 mph	7.0	38	Swimming/crawl, 2.2 mph	26.7	65
Tennis	7.1	40	Swimming/breaststroke, 2.2 mph	30.8	67
Skating, 9.0 mph	7.8	41	Swimming/backstroke, all-out competitive running, skiing, rowing, 2.2 mph	33.3	69
Horseback riding/trot	8.0	20			
Swimming/backstroke, 1.0 mph	8.3	40			
Gardening/digging	8.6	20			

*Data assembled and estimated from Morehouse, L.E., and Miller, A.T.: Physiology of exercise, ed. 7, St. Louis, 1976, The C.V. Mosby Co.

seums, ornithology, reading, scouting, stamp collecting, and tours.

Creative and esthetic activities

All creative and esthetic activities will have some aspects of a learning experience and will depend on intellectual application. There are certain activities, such as the following, that particularly satisfy the creative urge of people and provide special opportunities for exercise or esthetic experiences: aerobic and ballet dancing, clay modeling, dramatics, drawing and painting, group singing, instrumental music, jewelry making, leathercraft, metalcraft, music appreciation, needlework, photography, pottery, puppetry, sculpturing, weaving, and woodworking. One could also justifiably include some activities of the 4-H Club program and Cooperative Extension Service.

Social activities

Although virtually all recreation includes some social aspects, some activities, such as the following, are planned primarily for their social value: backgammon, card games, carnivals, church nights, circuses, concerts, C.B. radio, disco dancing, festivals, folk dancing, hobby clubs, and holiday parties.

The array of recreational activities suggests that a person who could not find one particular recreational interest indeed would be destitute. With the variety of recreational outlets now available, it is not surprising to find many people with several recreational interests who are able to get physical, intellectual, creative, esthetic, and social benefits.

VALUES IN RECREATION

Many people associate fitness with good physical performance, not with good health, improved appearance, or better performance on the job and in the classroom. This is especially true among the poor, the elderly, and the less educated.

For some people, vocation and other interests and activities seem to be adequate to provide them with the necessary motivation and gratification in living (Warr, 1976). Whether these individuals would live more effectively and enjoyably if they would engage in some form of recreation would be difficult to determine. Many of these individuals live so effectively and enjoyably already that it would be difficult to bring about very much improvement. Perhaps community services that some of these individuals give, in effect, serve as recreation, particularly as related to their life's vocation. For some individuals in the community, recreation merely serves to fill time. If this is a value in recreation, it is of a negative type, because if means only spending time. In the context of health promotion, recreation is a positive force in that it is a profitable investment of time. It provides values for the individual, the family, the group, and the community.

The main benefits people see in their leisure activities are partly a function of how physical the activity is. In a 1979 national survey of adults in Ireland, respondents were asked what they felt to be the main benefits of their leisure activities, as seen in Table 9-3. The most commonly articulated goal of leisure activities related to seeking rest, relaxation, and peace of mind, an aspect that tended to be emphasized to a greater extent by married rather than single people and particularly by those in the age range of 25 to 44 years.

In addition to dealing with the concept of "leisure" in the broadest sense, the Irish survey posed a number of questions relating specifically to the taking of exercise and the levels of interest and involvement in sporting activities of one sort or another. Four out of ten Irish adults claimed to take voluntary exercise outside the framework of organized sporting activities. Young adults in Ireland are much more likely to take physical exercise than those in the older age groups. There also is a distinct socioeconomic bias showing that 6 out of 10 white-collar workers take voluntary exercise, while only 4 out of 10 laborers and a quarter of

TABLE 9-3. Perceived main benefits of own leisure activities by adult public of the Republic of Ireland, 1979*

Perceived benefit	Total (%)	Voluntary exercise	
		Taken (%)	Not taken (%)
To rest/relax/peace of mind	44	41	46
Pleasure/sense of achievement	33	37	30
Contrast to regular work	14	14	13
Keeping active/physical fitness	10	19	4
Companionship/meeting people	9	9	9
To be out in the fresh air	5	7	3
To cultivate the mind	4	5	3
To pass the time	2	2	1
Don't have much leisure time	2	1	2
To reduce weight	1	2	-
Other answers	1	1	2
Don't know/no reply	7	4	9

*From Health Education Bureau Newsletter, Republic of Ireland, Dublin, Autumn, 1980.

TABLE 9-4. Leisure activities of the past week, by sex, in a national survey of the Irish Republic adult population, 1979*

	Men (%)	Women (%)
Watch television at home	88	89
Read or listen to music at home	73	86
Go for a drink in a pub or hotel	55	28
Knit/sew/household maintenance/do-it-yourself	26	54
Go out training/running/ any other exercise	27	17
Go dancing	19	17
Attend lectures/classes/ special interest groups	13	18
Go to the cinema/theatre	12	14
Indoor games/chess/ bridge, etc.	14	10

*From Health Education Bureau Newsletter, Republic of Ireland, Autumn, 1980.)

those from farming backgrounds take voluntary exercise. However, laborers, blue-collar workers, and farmers who are gainfully employed are much more likely to be involved in physical exercise as part of their work pattern than are the white-collar workers.

Respondents in the Irish survey were asked how they had spent their time, apart from their work or routine responsibilities, over the 7 days prior to the interview (Table 9-4). It was revealed that television viewing and listening to music are dominant nonwork activities, and only 27% of the men and 17% of the women had taken some form of voluntary exercise.

A large majority of Irish people are convinced that their leisure activities tend to have a beneficial effect on their physical well-being. About 1 in every 25 Irish adults admits that leisure activities might contribute negatively to physical well-being. Older men and women tend to be less assured or enthusiastic as to the likely beneficial effects of their leisure activities. Again, white-collar workers are more likely to be convinced of the beneficial effects of leisure activities than are laborers, blue-col-

TABLE 9-5. Perceived physical and psychological benefits of the athletic activity in which respondents claiming some regular physical activity engaged most, by level of activity, U.S. adult population, 1978*

Q: Now I want to ask you about some of the possible benefits that (ACTIVITY) has provided for you personally. For each item I read, please tell me whether for you personally it has been a major benefit of (ACTIVITY), a minor benefit, or no benefit at all.

	Total active (890)	High active (220)	Low active (354)	Gap between high/low active (—)
Physical benefits perceived	%	%	%	%
Am healthier in general	65†	74	53	+21
Have increased stamina	52	60	44	+16
Am physically fit	52	73	37	+36
Have become stronger	44	57	34	+23
Have improved coordination	43	53	42	+11
Lost weight	24	29	20	+9
Require less sleep	16	24	11	+13
Drink less than before	8	9	5	+4
Psychological benefits perceived				
Feel better in general	80	83	77	+6
Psychological effects in general	57	61	53	+8
Am less tense than before	53	62	47	+15
Sleep better	52	54	46	+8
Am more relaxed than before	50	58	42	+16
Feel less tired than before	45	55	36	+19
Will let me live longer	43	50	34	+16
Look better	42	48	37	+11
Concentration has improved	36	44	34	+10
Have become more disciplined in general	33	46	27	+19
Have a better self-image than before	33	38	28	+10
Have gained confidence	33	39	28	+11
Have improved outlook on life	32	35	27	+8
Am better able to cope with life's pressures	29	34	25	+9
Productivity has improved	28	39	23	+16
Am more assertive than before	27	31	24	+7
Think more creatively	25	28	21	+7
Smoke less than before	11	13	8	+5
Able to enjoy a better sex life	18	28	13	+15

*From The Perrier Study: Fitness in America, conducted by Louis Harris and Associates, Inc., New York, 1979, Perrier, Great Waters of France, Inc.

†Percents shown are those claiming each item was a "major benefit" of their physical activity.

lar workers, or those from farming backgrounds.

Individual benefits

For the individual, recreation provides adventure, physical activity, a feeling of belonging, skill, release of tension, relaxation, participation, challenges, accomplishment, mastery, success, creativity, stimulation, diversion from boring routines, elation, and a fullness of living. Doubtless, all of these can be acquired or experienced in pursuits other than recreation, but living in a highly organized and mechanized world, it becomes increasingly necessary for people to satisfy many personal needs through activities outside of work and normal living pursuits.

The particular benefits perceived by individuals in relation to their most common physical or athletic pursuits are more intensely felt by those whose level of activity is greater than a minimal or cursory involvement. Table 9-5 shows the personal responses of 890 adults who engaged in some physical activity, among 1,510 Americans surveyed in 1978. This table also contrasts the top 220 active people with the bottom 354 in terms of level of activity, showing a greater perceived benefit in each of 8 physical benefits and in each of 19 psychological benefits.

Family benefits

In an age in which there is a growing tendency to disperse the family rather than consolidate family living, recreation could serve to integrate family action (or unmarried coupling) through joint interests. Social changes tend to make the promotion of family recreation an increasingly difficult task. Mothers complete childbearing at an early age and thus experience an early release from maternal duties. Still young enough to accept career employment, family consolidation is reduced. Well-established neighborhoods have given way to a tendency for friendships based on special interests. Groups are not often organized on a neighborhood basis. With the increasing complexity of social services and social structure, the resulting overorganization tends to disrupt the family. Family-centered fun is heavily inclined toward commercialized amusements. Children and parents tend not to participate in common events. The child has his or her interests and recreational needs met in day-care centers, athletic groups, music, art, scouting, and similar activities.

Many activities exist in which both the children and the parents have potential interest and can participate. Some degree of promotion may be necessary ("The family that plays together stays together"), but frequently an interest exists that merely needs to be activated. In other instances, interest can be developed among all members of the family so that participation by all is realized. Camping seems to be a most popular family recreation, but other activities are as appealing and rewarding. Music, painting, photography, crafts, picnics, hiking, motor trips, boating, swimming, fishing, folk dancing, skating, skiing, bowling, tennis, golf, gardening, church activities, and special family nights suggest the variety of activities that lend themselves to total family participation and consolidation.

Benefits inherent in family (or couple) recreation are apparent. To participate as a group, to enjoy common experiences, to share the gratifications of accomplishment, and to pioneer together in new ventures will promote the physical, mental, emotional, and social well-being of the individual and the members of the family. The sense of belonging that recreation cements is highly important in family integration. With each member being an individual in his or her own right and free to pursue interests within the group, joint recreational participation is a highly valuable experience in adjusting to the needs, opinions, well-being, and respect of the other members.

The family dynamics of fitness activities are

TABLE 9-6. Attitudes toward children's involvement in fitness of activities among Americans who have children, by physical activity level of parent responding, 1978*

Q: How important is it to you that your son(s)/daughter(s) (READ FIRST ITEM ON LIST)—very important, somewhat important, or not important at all?

(No. of respondents:)	Respondents with sons				Respondents with daughters			
	Total (433)	Nonactive (150)	Active (283)		Total (408)	Nonactive (148)	Active (260)	
	%	%	%		%	%	%	
Grow up with a deep concern about staying in top physical shape	93†	97	91		93	92	94	
Be active in sports and athletics	89	83	92		82	74	87	
Play competitive sports	68	66	69		51	48	53	
Work to become a sports star	24	25	23		22	25	20	

*From The Perrier Study: Fitness in America, conducted by Louis Harris and Associates, Inc., New York, 1979, Perrier, Great Waters of France, Inc.
†Percentages are of those mentioning "very" or "somewhat" important.

reflected in the ways in which parents seek fitness and sports for their children. Whether or not they are active themselves, many parents today are eager that their children be both concerned and involved with physical fitness. Also, the increasing involvement of women in sports has influenced parental attitudes. With the exception of certain competitive sports or contact sports, parents are almost as eager for their daughters to be involved in athletics as they are for their sons, as seen in Table 9-6.

Most of the parents in the American Perrier survey felt it was either very or somewhat important that their sons or daughters "grow up with a deep concern about staying in top physical shape." Actual involvement in sports was given an almost equally high priority. Eighty-nine percent of parents with sons and 82% of those with daughters felt it was important that their sons and daughters be active in sports and athletics. In both instances, the active parents placed more emphasis on involvement than did the nonactive parents. The survey also showed that competitive sports are much less important to parents—particularly in relation to daughters—than that their children simply be active in sports. Still , the majority wanted to see their sons (68%) or daughters (51%) involved in some type of competitive sports activity. The parents were least enthusiastic about their children working "to become a sports star."

Swimming, tennis, and running, are preferred sports for sons and daughters alike. Parents generally prefer their sons to be involved in traditionally male sports, such as baseball (53%), swimming (48%), basketball (46%), football (30%), bicycling (27%), running (24%), tennis (24%), and track and field (20%). For their daughters, parents prefer involvement in swimming (60%), tennis (35%), bicycling (34%), gymnastics (32%), dance (28%), ice skating (23%), softball (19%), bowling (19%), volleyball (18%), walking (17%), running (17%), and basketball (17%).

The activities least preferred by parents for sons are boxing (33%), football (25%), wrestling (23%), mountain climbing (22%), hockey and karate (14% each), judo (12%), and weight lifting (10%). The strongest parental reactions against daughters' involvement are in relation to wrestling (48%), football (39%), boxing (38%), weight lifting (34%), mountain climbing (22%), hockey (19%), and judo and karate (17% each).

Group benefits

Social grouping in Western societies has undergone considerable change. In some areas there has been a regrouping, but some of the primary groups of past decades still continue. For all groups, recreation can have special significance so long as the human species is gregarious. Recreation provides one avenue through which this gregariousness can express itself. Association with others of the same status, of the same special needs, and the same interests can be made possible through recreation. In many instances recreational activities present the best means for providing opportunities for group participation and association. Engaging in common recreational pursuits rewards members of the group with a richer experience in group participation, in group adjustment, and in an understanding of people of like interests and pursuits.

The child group, the adult group, and the aging group have different recreational interests and different recreational needs. Age grouping, however, is not always the pattern on which group recreation is based. The physically handicapped with a great deal of time on their hands have special group recreational needs. People with impaired vision or hearing are not like everyone else in their need for special group recreational opportunities. The mentally retarded can benefit from opportunities for group recreation.

Formal groups find recreation an ideal vehicle for the promotion of group solidarity, morale, motivation, and attainment. Informal groups, where more individuality remains, find recreational activities that will permit individual development within group participation. Organized groups, characterized by individual sharing, and unorganized groups, characterized by a lack of cohesiveness, have equal need for recreational activities. For one, recreation provides opportunities for cooperative service to members of its group. For the other, recreation provides a community of interest that tends to hold the group together.

Whether recreation serves as a primary activity of a group or serves an ancillary role by providing a unity of interest and participation, recreation raises the general value and significance of the group to its members. In this respect, recreation is a means to an end rather than an end in itself. It is a means to achieve a greater significance of the group.

Community benefits

Whether leisure time is put to good use may be the best single index of the community's cultural level. Strictly speaking, community achievement is only a composite of individual achievement. The happiness, physical health, character development, and morale of a community are but an expression of these qualities on a composite basis in its citizens. Through its social processes, a community can do much to establish the general standard or pattern of community living. People respond in terms of what is expected of them. In this highly industrial age, a community that provides opportunities for recreational activity is laying the foundation for a wholesome community atmosphere. A community that provides alternatives to the tavern or the gambling hall will find its efforts reflected in greater interest in community affairs and social life. Time, effort, and funds put into community recreation and fitness are an investment in community stability, integration, and higher social values.

Economic benefits

In the United States the amount of personal income available for, and spent on, recreation has continued to increase and is rising faster than consumer spending as a whole, despite inflation. A total of $218 billion was spent on leisure activities in the United States in 1980. Recreation vehicles, such as trailers, boats, mobile homes, and snowmobiles, are the only form of leisure that appears to have declined since the mid-1970s, probably because of fuel prices. One household in ten owns some kind of boat. Total expenditures on recreational vehicles totaled $5.6 billion in 1976, but only $1.9 billion in 1980. Each year over $3 billion are spent on fishing and hunting. While travel and vehicular recreation has declined because of energy shortages, price increases, and incipient recession, the impact of recreation will continue to be felt in economic growth. The trends in participant activities are shown in Table 9-7.

The stimulus of recreation affects all levels of the economy. In the United States jobs in the service sector of recreation in particular have

TABLE 9-7. Trends in participant activities in the United States between 1973 and 1979*

Activity	No. (in millions) participating	
	1973	1979
Swimming	107.2	105.4
Bicycling	65.6	69.8
Camping	54.4	60.3
Fishing	61.2	59.3
Bowling	38.2	43.3
Boating	32.6	37.9
Jogging, running	†	35.7
Tennis	20.2	32.3
Pool, billiards	32.9	31.9
Softball	26.4	28.5

*From A.C. Nielsen Company, Sports Participation Studies conducted in 1973 and 1979.

†The question about jogging or running and racquetball was not even asked in 1973, reflecting the substantial increase in recognition as well as participation in these two most rapidly growing and valuable forms of physical activity. Roller skating and soccer appear to be additional newcomers to the list of the 1980s among the 30 most popular participant activities.

been growing at a faster rate than jobs in all industries, including other service industries. Another significant impact of recreation on the U.S. economy is the generation of federal, state, and local revenues through sales, income, property, amusement, and gasoline taxes. For example, depending on its proximity to private property, parkland can have a positive or negative impact on property values. Generally, however, recreation improvement enhances the monetary value of nearby properties.

Employers and businesses also gain important economic advantages from investments in recreation and exercise facilities for their employees. The assumed benefits include reduced absenteeism, fewer serious health problems, improved worker productivity, reduced insurance premiums or benefits paid, and improved morale of workers, resulting in better recruitment and less turnover and consequent expenses in training.

The provision and maintenance of recreation services is a sizeable component of local, state, and federal government budgets. Local government spending for recreation has consistently held at around 2% of county and municipal budgets.

PROGRAMS

In affluent, urbanized communities, planned programs must provide the physical activity that everyday life no longer supplies. Regular exercise and participation in sports must become part of a way of life for young and old alike. Homes, schools, employers, and voluntary agencies must join in providing leadership and facilities.

In the United States the national physical fitness program sponsored by the U.S. Office of Health Information, Health Promotion, and Physical Fitness and Sports Medicine, and by the President's Council on Physical Fitness and Sports has the following mission:

1. A population committed to physical fit-

ness and possessed of the knowledge and skills to achieve it.
2. Acceptance by parents, schools, recreational agencies, and sports organizations of their special responsibilities for fitness.
3. Recognition by communities and employers that fitness facilities and programs should be a part of the residential and work environments.
4. Maximum use of all resources—human and material, public and private—for physical fitness.

More specific U.S. objectives for accomplishment by 1990 are listed at the end of this chapter. The task of the federal government in fitness programs is to educate, advise, and encourage. The responsibility for action rests usually with parents, school administrators, teachers, coaches, recreation supervisors, civic and business leaders, and others at the community level. Some states have a Governor's Council on Physical Fitness.

Classification on a basis of who controls or promotes the activity or on the basis of who participates will tend to overlap. An activity regarded as a phase of a public recreational program may be classed as commercial recreation, and in another instance, may properly be classed as private recreation. In most North American and European countries, public recreation appears to be growing faster than commercial or private recreation, but all types of programs are undergoing some growth.

Commercial entertainment

Making a precise demarcation between recreation and entertainment is difficult, even impossible, but a general distinction can be made. Recreation involves actual participation, while entertainment has a connotation of the individual's being a spectator or enjoying the activity vicariously. In recent years it has become fashionable in some circles to condemn entertainment of all kinds. The term *spectatoritis* has been tagged to the growth of television and attendance at athletic and other spectacles. If leisure time were devoted entirely to being entertained, there would be justification for criticism and concern. Most people are participants in a vast variety of activities, and a reasonable balance between active participation in some activities and being a spectator at other activities can have a great deal of merit. The empathy, the exhilaration, and the enjoyment that come from watching the most highly skilled perform can have educational as well as other value. Commercial entertainment is big business. Unfortunately, for some, commercial entertainment is a complete substitution for recreation. Rather than condemn commercial recreation as damaging to a country's moral fiber, the constructive approach to the situation is to prepare people for, and provide the means for, recreational skill and interest. Commercial entertainment includes music, television, radio, professional sports, high school and collegiate athletics, theatricals, concerts, movies (cinema), horse racing, fairs, circuses, and a number of other activities in which people derive enjoyment merely from being spectators. In 1980, in the United States, approximately 350 million admissions to sports events were recorded, compared to 210 million in 1966. Most popular were thoroughbred horse racing (49.6 million), automobile racing (47.7 million), and major league baseball (43.6 million).

Commercial and semipublic recreation

Private investments have provided recreational facilities in response to recreational needs of citizens. The primary purpose in the promotion of the enterprise has been to obtain a business profit. Nevertheless, many of these enterprises provide admirable services for the community. Some of these commercial recreation enterprises actually may be semipublic in nature, but the vast majority of them are available to the general public. Semipublic recreation usually is made available through organizations that reserve their facilities for their own

members, but on occasion make their facilities available to others. Athletic clubs, golf clubs, tennis clubs, and social clubs may be in this category. Billiards, bowling, roller skating, ice skating, skiing, miniature golf, golf, swimming, canoeing, and horseback riding are illustrations of commercial and semipublic recreational activities that can serve as one component of a community's recreation program. In the overall evaluation of any community's recreation program, facilities available for public recreation on a commercial basis must be given full consideration.

Private recreational and fitness programs

In providing recreational opportunities in a community, sports groups and social organizations that limit their facilities and services exclusively to their own members should not be underestimated. From the standpoint of community recreation, these members are privileged to enjoy the kind of recreational opportunities one might hope everyone could enjoy. Even when organized primarily for recreational purposes, most of these private organizations serve more than one function. Private clubs for golf, swimming, boating, riding, hunting, skeet shooting, tennis, skiing, skating, bowling, billiards, and dancing often include creative, social, and esthetic activities.

Public recreation

Providing recreation has become an accepted public service. Providing opportunities for recreation does not mean that all recreation must be planned or in any sense formal. It would be tragic if a nation should reach a stage where the public depended solely on official agencies for all recreational and fitness activities. Indeed, it is a justifiable apprehension that, particularly among youngsters, there is too little opportunity for self-created recreational activity.

Recreational services in urban areas are primarily the responsibility of the local government. Localities generally have the authority to zone and acquire land and to provide public services, including recreation. Traditionally, they have done so in the United States, and studies show that local governments want to retain these roles. However, it is becoming more and more difficult for local governments to perform these functions alone. Political fragmentation often makes solutions to the problem of providing open space on a regional scale very difficult; it requires a cooperative approach that individual jurisdictions are sometimes reluctant to undertake. The increasing disparity in wealth of communities—poor core cities surrounded by wealthier suburbs—results in inequitable recreational services. Thus local solutions are sometimes impossible and often inadequate. The assistance of higher levels of government is often necessary.

Some states and provinces now are actively providing, or assisting local government to provide, urban recreational opportunities. Most states concentrate their park and recreation efforts on acquiring open space of regional or statewide significance. The potential is great for states and provincial governments to play a major role in urban recreation. In the United States, states could identify priority urban recreational needs, work with local governments to develop comprehensive strategies to alleviate identified deficiencies, and assign Land and Water Conservation Fund priority to urban recreational projects. States can also encourage localities in metropolitan regions to work together to develop regionwide open space strategies. States can also provide technical assistance to local groups.

A great deal can be done locally to improve recreational lands and services without any assistance from state, provincial, and federal governments. The following local and state courses of action are classified by objectives, based on suggestions made by local officials and other local people to the U.S. Department of the Interior (1978). They include actions by both public and private (for-profit and nonprofit) providers. In many cases these suggestions are currently being successfully carried out in localities, states, and provinces in the United States, Canada, Europe, Australia, and New Zealand.

Conserve open space for its recreational value. Local governments and private organizations must work together

- To develop procedures for multijurisdictional, public-private conservation of open space, through mechanisms such as fee acquisition, purchase of easement, management strategies, or establishment of regional resource conservation and recreation authorities with independent taxing and management roles.
- To transfer derelict land, tax-delinquent land, surplus highway rights-of-way, and other land not presently in productive use to park agencies through land exchange, purchase, or long-term, no-fee leases.
- To make maximum use of lands associated with public water supply reservoirs to meet urban recreational needs.
- To adopt regulations for new residential, business, or industrial development and redevelopment that require either the dedication of parklands, provision of recreational facilities, or payment of money to a public recreation fund.

In addition, state or provincial governments could

- Require local jurisdictions to prepare plans to implement regionwide open space strategies as a prerequisite to receiving state and federal funding assistance. Funding assistance for such plans could come from state or federal grants.
- Pass legislation authorizing local governments to require mandatory dedication of parkland or payments to a recreation fund by developers.

Provide financial support for parks and recreation. The National Urban Recreation Study carried out by the U.S. Department of the Interior (1978) revealed that good management, well-trained staff, and adequate financial support are suffering from cutbacks in local support. Satisfaction with recreational opportunities in the urban areas studied was more dependent on the existance of good programs and imaginative leadership than on large acreages or elaborate facilities.

Accessible facilities, diverse programs, year-round operation, and good maintenance are critical determinants of citizen satisfaction with community recreation. These elements all require substantial numbers of competent staff and a steady source of funds to sustain them. Hiring freezes and staff cutbacks have occurred in a majority of park and recreation departments over the last 5 years in the United States, resulting in reduced program opportunities and facility maintenance, while demands for recreational facilities and programs have increased.

Ways in which communities and state or provincial governments could address these problems are the following:

- Evaluate user fee policies and identify ways to increase recreation revenues through user fees and concession royalties.
- Earmark a portion of local tax revenues for parks and recreation.
- Hire grants experts to ensure that the local government is taking advantage of all appropriate nonlocal sources of assistance.
- Adopt legislation giving local governments full authority to set tax rates and issue bonds.
- Adopt legislation authorizing localities to deposit revenues earned from specific park and recreational activities (i.e., concessioners, golf, etc.) in accumulated capital outlay funds that can be used only for similar park and recreational activities.
- Increase state and local tax incentives for donations of land, easements, and money.
- Make state payments to local jurisdictions as a replacement for local tax losses to preserve park and recreation use of otherwise commercially developable land.
- Create local public trusts and foundations to receive donations that will assist in land preservation or provide programs and services.
- Provide funds for land acquisition and development by a combination of public and private providers.

Provide close-to-home recreational opportunities. Most people, especially in urban areas, want recreational opportunities within walking distance of home. By far the most frequent reason given in most surveys asking people why they are not getting enough exercise is "lack of time" or "too busy." For children and older adults the problem is one of transportation.

Many urban neighborhoods lack a variety of year-round programs and facilities that are responsive and available to all residents. About three fourths of the neighborhoods sampled in field studies reported dissatisfaction with neighborhood opportunities (U.S. Department of the Interior, 1978).

Recreation in urban areas includes a wide array of programs provided by many organizations in a variety of locations. Urban recreational opportunities encompass participant and spectator sports, environmental education, arts and cultural programs, "just relaxing" in the parks, and many others. These opportunities are provided by local governments, schools, private voluntary groups, and commercial organizations. They are found in parks; community and senior citizen centers; service centers of nonprofit, voluntary agencies; and in other public and private facilities. Indoor recreational facilities and community centers play a critical role in providing recreational services. General purpose community centers serve as neighborhood meeting places, are usable throughout the year, and often have supervised recreational programs not always available at outdoor sites.

Actions that can be taken by local governments and community groups to assure greater accessibility of recreational resources are

- To establish priorities that recognize the location of potential users when considering new recreation land acquisition.
- To use streets closed to traffic, rooftops, parking lots, utility rights-of-way, water supply reservoirs, and so on, to provide nearby recreation in heavily developed and densely populated areas.
- To use mobile recreation units where appropriate.
- To coordinate park planning and public transit planning to ensure that new parks and fitness facilities are accessible by public transit.
- To improve public transit service to parks and fitness facilities during weekends and evenings, which are times of peak recreation use.
- To plan for maximum pedestrian and bicycle access to new parks as an alternative to automobile access.
- To ensure that transit-dependent people have real input to the transportation planning process.
- To develop a comprehensive inventory and plan for all parks and physical improvements as a first step toward removing or modifying architectural barriers for the physically handicapped.
- To provide specialized staff and equipment for the handicapped, senior citizens, and young children to help them make better use of park facilities and programs.

Public recreation will be expanded very little in the years immediately ahead, with the exception of snow- and water-based facilities. Particular attention must be given to recreation for adolescents and for the elderly in the community.

Leadership

In the United States the President's Council on Physical Fitness and Sports (PCPFS), an outgrowth of the President's Council on Youth Fitness, was established in 1956. The first council grew out of concern about the poor performance of American boys and girls on standardized physical fitness tests. Subsequently, it was recognized that the fitness problem permeates all age groups. In 1963 the council was directed to begin promoting adult fitness. Today the PCPFS addresses its efforts to all ages, including the elderly, and its activities are part of national preventive health efforts under the direction of the U.S. Office of Health Information, Health Promotion, and Physical Fitness and Sports Medicine (OHIHP).

Fitness Canada, the federal lead agency for Canadian programs in physical fitness, has an annual budget three times greater than that of the PCPFS and OHIHP. Extensive mass media campaigns, materials, and grants in support of local programs, and federal support for national organizations developing specialized programs in physical fitness have been the ways in which Fitness Canada has provided leadership.

The Health Education Bureau of the Ireland Ministry of Health and Social Welfare sponsors an annual Health Race for over 100 bicyclists to tour over 900 miles of the country. The bicyclists arrive in each of eight district towns during Health Week that have a variety of health and fitness events sponsored by the local Junior Chamber of Commerce. Local activities include cycle rallies, community jogging, lectures, and films on aspects of health, sporting events, and lifesaving demonstrations.

Cycling events are equally popular in other European countries, some of which are following Ireland's example of sponsoring an annual Health Race to give high visibility and media attention to health promotion and fitness, in much the same way that marathons and health fairs have been used for community health promotion in the United States. The only concern with the government sponsorship of a cycling event for this purpose is that it conveys the impression that the government is recommending bicycling as a preferred form of exercise.

The facts, however, are that bicycling is the most hazardous of all vehicular activities in number of injuries, and it is not the most efficient of the alternatives such as swimming and running in achieving cardiovascular and respiratory fitness. A manual prepared by the OHIHP (1980) on organizing community events for health promotion outlines steps in the planning and conduct of events such as health fairs and marathons.

The greatest weakness in community recreational and fitness programs is in leadership. Of the more than 17,000 communities in the United States, fewer than one third have full-time recreational leaders. It must be pointed out that while full-time recreational leadership is essential to an effective recreation program, the employment of a full-time recreational leader does not in itself guarantee effective or even adequate leadership. Many recreational positions are political plums or are handed to a professional athlete to supplement the pay he receives for playing football, cricket, hockey, baseball, or basketball for the city team. Some recreational leaders have drifted into the field through close association with recreation on a voluntary basis. To like children or to be interested in recreation does not in itself indicate that a person has the necessary qualifications for good recreational leadership. Recreation has become a professional field, and more than 150 institutions of higher learning in the United States are granting degrees. At least 143 institutions are granting bachelor degrees, 80 are granting masters degrees, and 29 are granting doctorates or directorates in the field of recreation. An additional 70 junior colleges are offering courses.

The professional preparation of the recreational leader is built on a broad foundation in the liberal arts and sciences. On this foundation the college recreation major includes studies in American culture, government, city planning, public relations, community health, social group work, counseling, speaking, social recreation, hospital recreation, club work, sports programs, recreational dramatics, recreational music, photography, graphic and plastic arts, first aid, organization and administration of recreation, and field experience.

Areas and facilities

Physical fitness and recreation are national, state, provincial, county, community, neighborhood, group, family, and individual matters. Recreation is promoted at all governmental, economic, and social levels. On a national or a state level, in general, lands in the United States have been made available to provide recreational facilities for the general public.

On the local level in the United States, however, communities have been rather short-sighted. Frequently, recreational areas have had to give way to roads, housing developments, or other needs. Recreation needs more land, not less than it already has. Many communities, through zoning, require that any extended housing development set aside areas for recreation. All community planning should encompass recreational needs, long range as well as immediate. It is necessary that communities look forward to the possible recreational needs of the next quarter or even half century in anticipation of population increases. Community parks, playgrounds, swimming pools, beaches, golf courses, tennis courts, and other recreational facilities have become a recognized responsibility in community services and planning. More extended use of school facilities is both necessary and sensible. The school athletic fields, playgrounds, gymnasiums, and pools are part of the community's recreational facilities, and their use should be incorporated into the community recreational and fitness programs.

In the growing cities in the United States the greatest need is for development of new parkland and facilities; in the older cities lack of funds for programs and maintenance has restricted recreational opportunities and has resulted in the loss of large investments in park facilities as these facilities deteriorate and become unusable.

Rehabilitation of existing facilities is a great necessity in large, older cities and their suburbs. Neglect of short-term investments in maintenance has produced the necessity for large expenditures to accomplish essential renovation and redevelopment. Soaring energy prices make rehabilitation and modernization a high local priority, but current rehabilitation efforts are hampered by the fiscal distress of older core and satellite cities.

Recreational deficiences in the large, economically hard-pressed cities are unlikely to be corrected through local efforts or through existing federal programs, insofar as parks and recreational agencies in these cities are having difficulty competing for public dollars. These cities are often receiving less money to provide recreational services than they did 5 years ago with the severe budget cuts in the U.S. Department of the Interior.

COMMUNITY RESOURCES AND EDUCATION

Many people are not aware of the many recreational opportunities and activities that exist in their community. Those who are aware of their community's recreational program generally do not recognize the many untapped recreational and fitness resources that could be used in their community. There are groups and organizations making no contribution to the community recreational program who could contribute measurably to both the extensiveness and effectiveness of the community's recreational program. While a comprehensive recreational program does call for the expenditure of funds, many aspects of community recreation require little or no expenditure of money. Organizations having facilities and members who are willing to contribute their services can add appreciably to the community's recreational activities. It is not just a matter of accepting those who are willing to volunteer, but of recruiting all the individuals who may have

a contribution to make toward the program. By enlisting the cooperation and active participation of all the people in all the organizations and agencies in the community that might make some contribution, it is possible to have an extensive community-wide recreational program without huge expenditures on the part of any individual or group.

Some ways in which community action can expand the use of existing recreational and physical fitness resources are among the following:

- Use school buildings that have been closed because of declining enrollments for recreation and fitness.
- Consider the potential for joint recreation use in the planning stages for all new or expanded school and park facilities.
- Develop reciprocal, no-fee policies that encourage both park use by school groups and school use by park groups.
- Assist in providing services required to open school facilities to the public for recreational purposes after school hours; this will overcome present constraints on joint use, such as prohibitive custodial and maintenance costs.
- Encourage joint use for recreation, wherever possible, on lands and facilities committed to other private and public purposes, including federal properties, utility rights-of-way, and the property of institutions and private corporations.
- Encourage use of local park and recreational facilities for a wider range of human delivery services (i.e., health information, consumer protection, and nutrition).

In addition, states or provinces and national agencies could support the local use of facilities in the following ways:

- Provide financial and technical assistance programs to encourage the development of full service community centers, including strategies to use both public and private resources to provide human services, including recreation.

- Examine laws and funding programs to see how they can be used to encourage multiple use at the local level.
- Give priority, whenever possible, to meeting close-to-home recreational needs in state- or province-administered or state- or province-assisted planning, acquisition, and development projects.
- Certain groups demonstrate disproportionately low rates of participation in appropriate physical activity, including girls and women, older people, physically and mentally handicapped people of all ages, inner city and rural residents, people of low socioeconomic status, and residents of institutions. Target new programs on these groups.
- Education and information measures could include using television and radio public service announcements to provide information on appropriate physical activity and its benefits; providing information in school and college-based programs and information in health care delivery systems, including incorporation of queries about exercise habits into the routine clinical history; encouraging health care providers, especially in community health centers and other organized settings, to prescribe appropriate exercise in weight loss regimens as a complementary treatment modality in the management of several chronic diseases, and to give patients 65 years and older and the handicapped more detailed information on appropriate physical activity together with warnings about starting up exercise too fast; adopting an exercise component by community service agencies (such as the American Red Cross or the American Heart Association); assuring that all programs and materials related to diet and weight loss have an active exercise component; and tailoring education programs to the needs and characteristics of specific populations.
- Service measures could include providing physical fitness and exercise programs to school children and ensuring that those programs emphasize activities for all children rather than just competitive sports for relatively few; providing physical fitness and exercise programs in colleges; providing worksite-based fitness programs that are linked to other health enhancement components (e.g., smoking cessation, nutrition improvement) and that have an active outreach effort; and incorporating exercise and fitness protocols as regular clinical tools of health providers.
- Technological measures could include increasing the availability of existing facilities and promoting the development of new facilities by public, private, and corporate entities (e.g., fitness trails, bike paths, parks, pools); and upgrading existing facilities, especially in inner-city neighborhoods, and involving the population to be served at all levels of planning.
- Legislative and regulatory measures could include city council support for bicycle and walking paths for use in trips to work and school; developing and operating local, state, provincial, and national park facilities that can be used for physical fitness activities in urban areas; increasing the number of school-mandated physical education programs that focus on health-related physical fitness; establishing local councils on health promotion and physical fitness; and allowing expenditure of funds for fitness-related activities under nationally funded programs guided by national regulations.
- Economic measures could include tax incentives for the private sector to offer physical fitness programs for employees; encouraging employers to permit employees to exercise on company time or giving employees flexible time for use of facilities; and offering health and life insurance policies with reduced premiums for those who participate in regular, vigorous physical activity.

Relative strength of the measures

Programs most likely to be successful in recruiting new participants to appropriate physical activity include those that offer services and facilities to individuals and economic incentives to groups and individuals. On the other hand, programs that can more easily be implemented include those related to the provision of public information and education and improving the linkages with other health promotion efforts. The effectiveness of all measures is handicapped by the limitation in knowledge with respect to the relation between exercise and physical and emotional health; the optimum types of exercises for various groups of people with special needs; and the appropriate way to measure levels of physical fitness for various age groups.

Legal agencies

Tax-supported organizations are regarded as legal agencies in the United States. The state conservation department providing park, camping, hunting, and fishing facilities is an example of a legal agency on the state level that serves as a valuable resource in recreation. On the county and city level, county- or city-park boards, schools, and public libraries are resource agencies. A city recreation commission, formally organized by the city council with a staff of full-time professional recreational personnel, should be the hub about which the entire community recreational program rotates. The commission's program can be financed with at least 2% of the city's annual budget. While various recreational activities do produce some revenue, such income is merely an incidental factor in maintaining the program. Cities today accept recreation as a necessary and proper community service and must appropriate funds for its promotion.

Social groups

People with common interests and needs tend either formally or informally to form groups to promote their common interests.

This is notably true of recreational interests. These groups usually are limited in their numbers and usually serve only their own members but contribute appreciably to recreation in a community. Dance groups, jogging groups, bridge groups, groups of young married couples, and similar organizations are to be found in most communities. Each group in its own way meets certain recreational needs for its own members. Some social groups undertake to promote recreational activities that will be available to others than members of the group. Out of one social group, many groups may develop to enhance the overall recreational and fitness programs of the community.

Religious groups

Recreational activities sponsored by religious groups usually are conducted on a high level, not in competition with legal agencies, but as a supplement to the program of the legal agencies. The Young Men's Christian Association, the Young Women's Christian Association, Boys' Clubs of America, B'nai B'rith Hillel Foundations, Jewish Community Centers, Diocesan Youth Councils, Boys' League, National Catholic Youth Council, Christian Endeavor, Epworth League, and Methodist Youth Fellowship are examples of religious groups that promote outstanding recreational and fitness programs in the United States. Health and fitness are integral to most religious and philosophical systems.

Business and industry

Apart from their commercial interests in manufacturing, marketing, and servicing recreational and health-related products and facilities, employers have many reasons for contributing to the recreation and fitness of their employees, both at the worksite and in the community. Although existing programs are too new and too few to provide much statistical data, accumulating evidence from research shows that workers taking part in regular physical activity programs miss fewer workdays when they do get sick, are less vulnerable to accidents, have a higher overall work output, and suffer fewer emotional disorders and physical disabilities.

The most extensive research on employee fitness programs has been carried out in the Soviet Union, where the tangible economic benefits of regular exercise have been repeatedly documented. Russian experts found that working people who exercise regularly produce more, visit physicians less, and seem to be more immune to industrial accidents.

The benefits of a good fitness program take more subtle but no less significant forms. National Aeronautic and Space Administration employees who participated in a fitness study in Houston, Texas, reported a general sense of well-being that improved their attitudes about their work and enriched their leisure time. Even more significant, the results of medical tests bore out the perceived benefits of the program. Those who reported improved stamina, for example, showed marked improvement in cardiovascular performance. Similar results were reported for the employee fitness programs of the New York State Education and Civil Service Department, where risk factors were reduced, health problems eased, and employee absenteeism cut down.

The first true fitness program in a U.S. firm began in 1894 at the National Cash Register Company in Dayton, Ohio, when the president authorized morning and afternoon exercise breaks for employees, then proceeded to install a gymnasium and built a 325-acre park for National Cash Register people and their families. Since then, company-sponsored recreational facilities have become commonplace.

Today more than 400 companies in the United States provide fitness programs for their employees. Some companies subsidize community facilities such as parks or the programs of the YMCA rather than developing separate facilities at their own sites.

Some companies hesitate to launch fitness programs because they fear they will be liable for injuries to employees. Studies and on-the-site experience, however, show that this risk is minimal; where health-fitness programs are properly designed and supervised, the risk of accident is negligible. Anything a company does for its employees—whether a company outing or softball league—involves some liability. A fitness program should be recognized as an integral part of the job, under which the employee is fully protected by Workmen's Compensation or private insurance.

The experiences of Canada and the United States employee health promotion and fitness programs have been documented and summarized in guidelines available from Fitness Canada as well as the U.S. Public Health Service. A brief summary of the main features of successful programs in work settings should illustrate the characteristics common to effective health promotion and fitness programs in other community settings.

High-level support. Employee fitness programs, like other institutional or membership programs, will not succeed without the support and encouragement of the administration of the company and the labor organization to which employees belong. The fitness program must be perceived as a necessity, not a luxury, and there must be a substantial personal and financial commitment to its success, not merely passive tolerance of its existence.

Strong leadership. A competent person who is knowledgeable and committed to the program must be in charge, although a health-fitness director may work full time or part time. Volunteers from within the company should be recruited and trained, but most successful programs have professional leadership with solid training in the principles of exercise as well as in group and individual motivation and education.

Accessibility. Exercise facilities must be convenient to the workplace, or they will not be used. This includes changing and showering areas as well as the exercise facility itself.

Availability. Failing to offer fitness programs

at times when most employees can take advantage of them is a sign of hollow commitment. Ideally, the fitness facility should be available throughout the day with a concentration of group programs in the middle of the day. As more and more companies offer flextime schedules, and as more employers provide release time for fitness activities, it is feasible to offer a wide range of programs throughout the day.

Screening and assessment. All employees should have access to health assessment whether or not they intend to participate in a company fitness program. Screening and assessment should be voluntary and totally confidential. High-risk individuals can be identified through screening, but it is imperative that employees feel confident that their jobs will not be in jeopardy. Low-cost screening that includes blood pressure measurements and blood chemistry analysis, strength and body fat testing, and endurance testing should be available. Programs can also be augmented by more sophisticated medical techniques, such as exercise stress tests.

Recordkeeping. Good records should be kept of individual activity and progress so that improvements can be noted and reinforced. Carefully organized and readily available records help maintain a high level of performance and attendance.

Group exercise. The companionship of a group lends a social aspect to a fitness program that provides mutual support and motivation. Many people do prefer to exercise alone, so programs should not be limited to group activities. A balanced program will include activities such as jogging, swimming, calisthenics, and stationary cycling for those who wish to work out individually.

Challenging physical program. Participants need to be aware that cardiovascular improvement requires a sustained elevation of the heart rate, that muscles need to be stressed, and that joints must work through their full range of motion. Fitness programs should be vigorous and sustained. An atmosphere with games and lazy warm-ups is enjoyable, perhaps, but neither the company nor its employees will gain the same benefits.

Motivation and incentives. Merely offering space and time for a fitness program is not enough. The company should put its employee communications and incentive programs into its fitness activities. The job of the health promotion or fitness director includes designing a program of motivation and incentives. Cash prizes and silver trophies are neither necessary nor appropriate, but a variety of small tokens that recognize achievement are welcome. Companies have successfully used a variety of motivational techniques, including bonus payments, vouchers or premium reductions, program certificates, participation pins, and organized competitions.

Organization. Maintenance of facilities is essential to the success of a fitness program. The showers must work, towels must be available, the gym should be open on schedule, and the exercise leader should be on hand. In other words, the fitness program and its facilities should be as well organized as the plant or office in which the participants work.

Visibility and promotion. A company that agrees to undertake an employee fitness program needs continually to promote the program. The health or fitness director should use bulletin boards, newsletters, house organs, and verbal and written messages from management and labor leadership to keep the program visible and stimulate employee interest.

Continuity and extension. Fitness programs should not be static or committed to one set way of doing things nor end at the company gate. Employees should be encouraged to keep active during their leisure hours, to participate in community recreational activities, and to maintain the healthful habits of moderation in diet, smoking, and drinking. Perhaps the most important ripple effect of a good company fitness program is seen in such satellite activities as stress reduction, alcohol, drug and smoking cessation programs, nutrition counseling, and weight control programs. Many companies find that fitness programs are particularly successful when they include the spouses of employees. Such activities as Saturday morning workshops, nutrition and exercise lectures, and combined fitness sessions lend themselves to such participation.

Enjoyable program. If the fitness routine itself does not offer variety, companionship, stimulation, and pleasure, participation will drop and the program will fail. This does not mean that the program should slacken its demands for vigorous activity. But fun, as well as physical benefit, should be of paramount concern to the program's professional leader.

Youth-serving agencies

Over 250 organizations in the United States are working with children and youth under 25 years of age. The areas in which these organizations serve are so diverse that it would be difficult to imagine any recreational needs that are not provided. To name a few of these organizations would indicate the extensiveness of the list; 4-H groups, Future Farmers of America, Future Homemakers of America, Boy Scouts, Girl Scouts, Camp Fire Girls, Boys State, Girls State, youth centers, settlement houses, Big Brothers of America, and American Junior Red Cross is but a partial list. Scores of boys' and girls' groups, hosteling, and other groups indicate the many agencies created to serve the youth of America. The important thing is that each community organize, support, and promote the particular youth-serving agencies necessary to provide the leisure-time activities essential for the best development of the children and youth of the community.

Service groups

Nationally known community service groups have continuing fitness and recreational programs, either competing or cooperating with another agency or sponsoring the program themselves. Equally important is that these service groups can be called on to support any worthwhile recreational program in the community. This is a resource that is ever present. Rotary clubs, Lions Clubs, Kiwanis, Exchange Clubs, Soroptimists, women's groups, Grange, Parent-Teacher Associations, and other service organizations provide a diversity of services in their communities in the United States, not the least of these being the promotion of recreational and fitness programs.

Neighborhoods

Recreational activities grow out of group interests. An actual or potential neighborhood interest can serve as a catalyst in initiating and extending recreational activities. Many of these enterprises are self-starting, but others need leadership to crystallize the interest that exists and to implement the contribution of the group. Interest in having a playground developed in the neighborhood can be a starting point from which an extensive neighborhood recreational program can be developed. When a playground already exists in the neighborhood, interest may be present or can be generated in expanding both the facilities and the activities that are carried on at the playground.

Special interest groups

In a typical community, one is likely to find a number of groups having special recreational interests, such as gardening, music, dramatics, chess, stamp collecting, and photography. Through these groups, others can be encouraged to develop new interests or to enjoy an interest they already have. There is something contagious about an intense interest in some fascinating or challenging hobby or avocation. As people become exposed to all possible recreational outlets, there is a greater likelihood that they will find those particular activities that will appeal to their particular abilities and temperament.

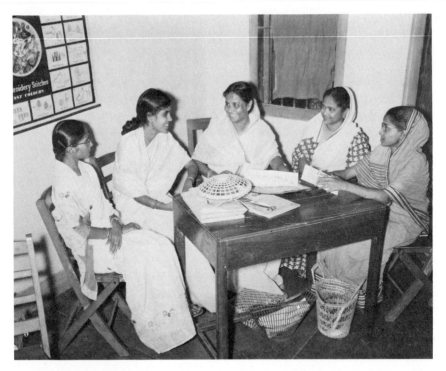

FIG. 9-1. Special interest groups are universal. In this sewing group in Dacca, Bangladesh, women discuss health and family planning concerns as well as embroidery stitches.

Courtesy Public Health Education Research Project, University of California, Berkeley.

Other community resources

Labor unions, industrial firms, retail business houses, the Chamber of Commerce, and fraternal organizations promote and support various recreational enterprises. All of these establishments find that providing recreation is one of the finest services they can contribute to their constituents. In any community it is possible to discover public-spirited organizations that will respond to reasonable requests for support of any worthwhile community enterprise. These are the organizations that, with very little fanfare, play an extremely important role in the year-in and year-out promotion of the well-being of the community. These organizations may take an active role and actually administer a recreational or fitness program of their own, or their participation may be limited to financial or other support. Resources

for the promotion of recreation are rarely more than partially tapped in most communities. To use all possible resources, three things are usually necessary. The first is a worthwhile program; the second is qualified leadership; and the third is an informed community.

Actions that communities can take to strengthen planning, leadership, and public education include the following:

- Employ professionals to do recreational services planning, as well as fitness program and facility planning, on a continuing basis.
- Improve coordination between planning and implementation efforts to ensure realistic plans and responsive action to meet identified needs.
- Coordinate recreational planning with other human service planning; coordinate

park and facility planning with overall land use planning, physical fitness, and health planning.

- Develop cooperative programs between resource agencies and local education advisors so that park and recreational resources become an instrument for environmental teaching as an extension of the community health education program.
- Adopt policies and provide in-service training programs that result in sound environmental management.
- Use local parks as year-round, close-to-home, urban environmental laboratories for all age groups to study natural systems. Use other facilities such as wastewater treatment centers, streets, and utilities to study the interaction between humans and their environment.
- Broaden the scope of interpretive programming to address local environmental issues; sponsor public forums on land use planning, energy conservation, and environmental management programs to involve the public in the decision-making process.
- Encourage residents to assume responsibility for making neighborhood parks safe by giving them a role in park supervision and maintenance.
- Publish information on comparative local recreation preferences and needs throughout the state or province.
- Conduct citizen participation and preference surveys to determine recreation deficiencies.
- Authorize and encourage the use of school bond monies for the development of environmental and health urban areas.
- Recruit inner-city personnel through an office of volunteerism to lead interpretive environment education in the urban environment. Sponsor training programs for urban volunteers by using resources of local professional interpreters.

Physical fitness through recreation will increase in importance with the increase in lei-sure time and the extension of life expectation. Many factors enter into the extension of community fitness and recreational programs. Understanding by the public, qualified professional leadership, and adequate facilities must advance more rapidly than during the past decade if the recreational program is to serve the needs of expanding populations.

U.S. OBJECTIVES FOR 1990

The *Objectives for the Nation* developed by the U.S. Office of Disease Prevention and Health Promotion can serve as a useful guide to other nations and to communities in establishing realistic goals for the decade of the 1980s. Objectives for physical fitness and exercise are as follows.

Reduced risk factors

- By 1990 the proportion of children and adolescents ages 10 to 17 participating regularly in appropriate physical activities, particularly cardiorespiratory fitness programs, should be greater than 90%. (Baseline data are unavailable.)
- By 1990 the proportion of children and adolescents ages 10 to 17 participating in daily school physical education programs should be greater than 60%. (In 1974 to 1975 the share was 33% in the United States.)
- By 1990 the proportion of adults ages 18 to 65 participating regularly in vigorous physical exercise should be greater than 60%. (In 1978 the proportion who regularly exercised was 35% in the United States.)
- By 1990 50% of adults 65 years and older should be engaging in appropriate physical activity, for example, regular walking. (In 1975 about 36% of older Americans took regular walks.)

Increased public-professional awareness

- By 1990 the proportion of adults who can accurately identify the variety and duration of exercise that most effectively promotes

cardiovascular fitness should be greater than 70%. (Baseline data are unavailable.)
- By 1990 the proportion of primary care physicians who include a careful exercise history as part of their initial examination of new patients should be greater than 50%. (Baseline data are unavailable.)

Improved services-protection

- By 1990 the proportion of children and adolescents ages 10 to 17 participating in systematic and scientifically determined physical fitness assessment programs should be greater than 70%. (Baseline data are unavailable.)
- By 1990 the proportion of companies and institutions with more than 500 employees that offer employer-sponsored fitness programs should be greater than 25%. (In 1979 about 2.5%, or 400, of the companies in the United States had formally organized fitness programs.)

Improved surveillance-evaluation systems

- By 1990 data should be available with which to evaluate the short-and long-term health effects of participation in programs of appropriate physical activity.
- By 1990 data should be available to evaluate the effects of participation in programs of physical fitness on job performance and health care costs.
- By 1990 data should be available for regular monitoring of national trends and patterns of participation in physical activity; including participation in public recreation programs in community facilities.

QUESTIONS AND EXERCISES
1. Appraise the statement, "How a people uses its leisure time is an index of its vitality and an indication of its future."
2. To what extent is recreation a vehicle for health promotion?
3. To what extent is recreation a vehicle for the treatment of disabilities?
4. Why is recreation and fitness growing as a community enterprise in the United States?
5. What recreational and fitness activities are available in your community?
6. Indicate how recreation can promote social health.
7. Why does the public place so much emphasis on recreation of a physical nature?
8. By the use of examples, indicate how an activity that is not recreational for one person may be of recreational value for another person.
9. Identify some person who does not appear to need a recreational outlet, and analyze the factors that account for the absence of recreational needs.
10. Compare the recreational needs of two individuals who have widely different vocations.
11. Why is an intellectual activity recreational to one person but an unenjoyable task for another person?
12. Propose some measures to extend family recreation in your community.
13. How can group interests in your community be used to expand the community's recreational program?
14. What alternatives to the tavern and gambling hall does your community offer its citizens?
15. What role does commercial entertainment play in your community?
16. To what extent does commercial recreation contribute to the total recreational program of your community?
17. What recreational activities are provided publicly in your community?
18. What areas and facilities are available in your community?
19. What additional areas and facilities should be provided?
20. What is your contribution to your community's recreational program?

BIBLIOGRAPHY

Anderson, F.E.: Art for all the children: a creative sourcebook for the impaired child, Springfield, Ill., 1978, Charles C Thomas, Publisher.
Azarnoff, P., and Flegal, S.: A pediatric play program: developing a therapeutic play program for children in medical settings, Springfield, Ill., 1980, Charles C Thomas, Publisher.
Barrett, S.L.: Parties with a purpose: a handbook for activity directors, Springfield, Ill., 1980, Charles C Thomas, Publisher.
Belloc, N.B.: Relationships of health practices and mortality, Prev. Med. 2:67, 1973.
Belloc, N.B., and Breslow, L.: Relationships of physical health status and health practices, Prev. Med. 1:409, 1972.
Burton, E.C.: Physical activities for the developing child, Springfield, Ill., 1980, Charles C Thomas, Publisher.

Collins, D.R., and Hodges, P.B.: A comprehensive guide to sports skills tests and measurement, Springfield, Ill., 1978, Charles C Thomas, Publisher.

Conrad, C.C.: How different sports rate in promoting physical fitness, Washington, D.C., 1978, President's Council on Physical Fitness and Sports, Public Health Service, U.S. Department of Health and Human Services.

Cousins, N.: Anatomy of an illness as perceived by the patient: reflections on healing and regeneration, New York, 1979, W.W. Norton & Co., Inc.

Crisp, A.H., and Stonehill, E.: Sleep, nutrition and mood, New York, 1976, John Wiley & Sons, Inc.

Cunningham, D.A., and Hill, J.S.: Effect of training on cardiovascular response to exercise in women, J. Appl. Physiol. 39(6):891, Dec., 1975.

D'Onofrio, C.N., and Wang, V.L.: Cooperative extension and rural health education, Health Educ. Monogr. 3(1):4, 1975.

Dulles, F.R.: History of recreation: America learns to play, ed. 2, New York, 1970, Appleton-Century-Crofts.

Effect of exercise alone on obesity, (editorial), Br. Med. J. 7:1976.

Erben, R., and Mantek, M.: Health, leisure and holidays, Int. J. Health Educ. 16:1, 1973.

Farina, A.M.: Developmental games and rhythms for children, Springfield, Ill., 1980, Charles C Thomas, Publisher.

Fletcher, G.F., and Cantwell, J.D.: Exercise and coronary heart disease: role in prevention, diagnosis, treatment, ed. 2, Springfield, Ill., 1979, Charles C Thomas, Publisher.

Friedberg, P., and Berkeley, E.P.: Play and interplay: manifests for new design in urban recreation, New York, 1970, Macmillan Publishing Co., Inc.

Froelicher, V.F.: Does exercise conditioning delay progression of myocardial ischemia in coronary atherosclerotic heart disease? Cardiovasc. Clin. 8(1):11, 1977.

Gould, E., and Gould, L.: Arts and crafts for physically and mentally disabled: the how, what and why of it, Springfield, Ill., 1978, Charles C Thomas, Publisher.

Graney, M.J.: Media use as a substitute activity in old age, J. Gerontol. 29:322, May, 1974.

Gray, D., and Pelegrino, D.A.: Readings in recreation and parks, Dubuque, Iowa, 1972, William C. Brown Co., Publishers.

Hjelte, G., and Shivers, J.S.: Public administration of recreational services, Philadelphia, 1972, Lea & Febiger.

Hodson, J.L., and Buskirk, E.R.: Physical fitness and age with emphasis on cardiovascular function in the elderly, J. Am. Geriatr. Soc. 25:385, 1977.

Humphrey, J.H.: Child development through physical education, Springfield, Ill., 1980, Charles C Thomas, Publisher.

Humphrey, J.H., and Humphrey, J.N.: Sports skills for boys and girls, Springfield, Ill., 1980, Charles C Thomas, Publisher.

Ismail, A.H., and Montgomery, D.L.: The effect of a four-month physical fitness program on a young and an old group matched for physical fitness, Eur. J. Appl. Physiol. 40(2):137, Jan. 10, 1979.

Iso-Ahola, S.E., editor: Social psychological perspectives on leisure and recreation, Springfield, Ill., 1980, Charles C Thomas, Publisher.

Kraus, R.G.: Recreation today, program planning and leadership, New York, 1972, Appleton-Century-Crofts.

Lucas, C.: Recreational activity development for the aging in homes, hospitals, and nursing homes, Springfield, Ill., 1978, Charles C Thomas, Publisher.

Martin, D.E., and Gynn, R.W.H.: The marathon footrace: performers and performances, Springfield, Ill., 1979, Charles C Thomas, Publisher.

Michel, D.E.: Music therapy: an introduction to therapy and special education through music, Springfield, Ill., 1979, Charles C Thomas, Publisher.

Morehouse, L.E., and Miller, A.T.: Physiology of exercise, ed. 7, St. Louis, 1976, The C.V. Mosby Co.

Morris, J.N., Chave, S.P., Adam, C., et al: Vigorous exercise in leisure-time and the incidence of coronary heart-disease, Lancet 1:333, Feb. 17, 1973.

Nystrom, E.P.: Activity patterns and leisure concepts among the elderly, Am. J. Occup. Ther. 28:337, 1974.

Olszowy, D.R.: Horticulture for the disabled and disadvantaged, Springfield, Ill., 1978, Charles C Thomas, Publisher.

Pacific Mutual Life Insurance Company: Health maintenance, New York, 1978, Louis Harris and Associates, Inc.

Paffenbarger, R.S., and Hale, W.E.: Work activity and coronary heart mortality, N. Engl. J. Med. 292(11):545, March 13, 1975.

The Perrier Study: Fitness in America, conducted by Louis Harris and Associates, Inc., New York, August 1979, Perrier, Great Waters of France, Inc.

Polednak, A.P.: The longevity of athletes, Springfield, Ill., 1979, Charles C Thomas, Publisher.

President's Council on Physical Fitness and Sports: Proceedings of the National Conference on physical fitness and sports for all, Washington, D.C., 1980, Public Health Service, U.S. Department of Health and Human Services.

Radocy, R.E., and Boyle, J.D.: Psychological foundations of musical behavior, Springfield, Ill., 1979, Charles C Thomas, Publisher.

Saltin, B., Blomquist, G., Mitchell, J.H., et al.: Response to exercise after bed rest and after training, Circulation 38(suppl. 17):1, Nov., 1968.

Shea, E.J.: Ethical decision in physical education and

sport, Springfield, Ill., 1978, Charles C Thomas, Publisher.

Sherrill, C.: Creative arts for the severely handicapped, ed. 2, Springfield, Ill., 1979, Charles C Thomas, Publisher.

Sidney, K.H., Shepherd, R.J., and Harrison, J.E.: Endurance training and body composition of the elderly, Am. J. Clin. Nutr. **30**(3):326, March, 1977.

Straub, W.F., and Felock, T.: Attitudes toward physical activity of delinquent and nondelinquent junior high school age girls, Res. Q. Am. Assoc. Health Phys. Educ. **45**:21, March, 1974.

Thomas, G.S., Lee, P.R., Franks, P., and Paffenbarger, R.S., Jr.: Exercise and health: the evidence and implications, Cambridge, Mass., 1981, Oelgeschlager, Gunn & Hain, Publishers, Inc.

U.S. Department of the Interior: National urban recreation study: summary report, Washington, D.C., 1978, Heritage Conservation and Recreation Service, National Park Service.

U.S. Department of the Interior: The third nationwide outdoor recreation plan: the executive report, Washington, D.C., 1979, Heritage Conservation and Recreation Service, National Park Service.

U.S. Office of Health Information, Health Promotion, and Physical Fitness and Sports Medicine: Toward a healthy community: organizing health events, Washington, D.C., 1980, Office of the Assistant Secretary for Health, U.S. Department of Health and Human Services.

U.S. Office of Health Information, Health Promotion, and Physical Fitness and Sports Medicine: Taking action for fitness: a guide to selected information resources, Washington, D.C., 1981, National Health Information Clearinghouse, DHHS (PHS) Pub. No. 81-50164.

Verducci, F.M.: Measurement concepts in physical education: an introduction, St. Louis, 1980, The C.V. Mosby Co.

Warr, P.E.: Personal goals and work design, New York, 1976, John Wiley & Sons, Inc.

Weininger, O.: Play and education: the basic tool for early childhood learning, Springfield, Ill., 1979, Charles C Thomas, Publisher.

10

COMMUNICABLE DISEASE CONTROL

The prevention of preventable disease is the first purpose of a wisely governed state.

Erastus Brooks (1881)

Civilization has not conquered the infectious diseases, but through increased understanding of the nature and epidemiology of infection Western society has succeeded in controlling them. It would be entirely realistic to predict that eventually society will control so effectively the organisms that cause disease that infectious diseases will be a minor health problem. Even today infectious diseases as a cause of death are far less important than the degenerative diseases. Public health's knowledge of and ability to control infectious diseases are far greater than the knowledge and means of controlling personal behavior. Indeed, the remaining gains in communicable disease control will depend largely on behavior and therefore on health education.

NATURE OF COMMUNICABLE DISEASE

Disease is a harmful departure from normal. A communicable disease is one that can be transmitted from one human being to another or from lower animals to humans. Communicable diseases are produced by organisms that not only are parasitic but are pathogenic, or disease-producing. Most pathogens of humans are microorganisms, although some, notably the worms, are multicellular forms and can be seen with the unaided eye. Infectious disease represents a reaction of the host to the invader. The interaction may destroy the pathogen as well as produce abnormalities in the host, even to the point of causing the death of the host.

Infection and disease

Infection is the successful invasion of the body by pathogens under such conditions as will permit them to multiply and harm the host. The mere presence of organisms or toxins in the human body does not constitute disease. A person may be harboring millions of pneumococci in his or her lungs without having disease. He or she may have billions of streptococcus organisms on the skin without having disease. Only when the pathogens cause harm to the body can the condition be classed as a disease.

*Dis*infection consists of killing or removing organisms capable of causing infection. Disinfection mechanisms destroy pathogens by dehydration or desiccation, hydrolysis or hydration, coagulation of cell proteins, oxidation, and destruction of enzymes. For practical purposes, disinfectants possess the following desirable properties:

1. They do not damage human tissue.

2. They produce a minimum of pain.
3. They have a high germicidal effect and are quick-acting.
4. They are not affected by alkalies or acids.
5. They are low in cost.

Disinfection by the use of chemicals is the usual method. Here, the time element, concentration of the chemical, and temperature are important. The particular sensitivity of the tissue affected must always be considered in the use of a particular chemical antiseptic. Diluted alcohol is an example of a disinfectant in everyday use. Physical disinfection includes the use of such agents as ultraviolet radiation, sound waves, and electron treatment. While all of these procedures have certain limitations, experimentation in their possibilities may lead to benefits far beyond what is now realized in their use.

Bacteriostasis is an arrest in the multiplication of pathogens and in their metabolism. Thus toxin production by the invading organism is reduced or ceases completely. Sulfonamides arrest bacterial action by depriving the organism of the material that it must have to carry on normal metabolic processes. This bacteriostasis enables a human's phagocytes to destroy the pathogen.

Antibiosis, such as produced by penicillin, expresses a direct antagonism to specific organisms. The antibiotics have had spectacular effects in combating certain pathogens, but they have not proved to be the panacea many in the medical sciences at first contended. Despite their magnificent contribution to the battle against infection, the antibiotics have limitations. Bacteria develop resistant strains in response to antibiotics. This mutation, or adaptability by the bacteria limits the use of antibiotics. Resistant strains of bacteria are found particularly in hospital-acquired (nosocomial) infections, whereas an infection with the same organism acquired outside the hospital may be sensitive to the same antibiotics and respond well. Indiscriminate use of antibiotics, without proper indication, increases the proportion of resistant organisms. Newly developed antibiotics should be used only against organisms that have been shown to be sensitive to them and resistant to earlier antibiotics.

Contamination and decontamination

Contamination is the presence of pathogens of humans or nonpathogenic organisms, such as *Escherichia coli* of the alimentary canal in humans, on inanimate objects. Thus articles of clothing, a door handle, a spoon, a glass, milk, or water may be contaminated. Since certain organisms, such as *E. coli,* live in the intestines of humans, the presence of these organisms indicates presence of human discharges. Contact with a possibly contaminated object— and thus with pathogens from the alimentary tract of humans—is a present danger. The *E. coli* count is used as a standard in sanitary science and as such is a valuable index in terms of possible danger to humans, even though the *E. coli* bacterium itself is not a pathogen.

Decontamination means the killing or removing of pathogens and *E. coli* in or on inanimate objects. More drastic measures can be used here than are used in disinfection. Boiling, the use of steam, pasteurization, high levels of dry heat, long exposure to the sun, and highly concentrated chemicals are used.

TABLE 10-1. Reported cases of selected communicable diseases, United States, 1900 and 1980*

Disease	1900	1980
Diphtheria	147,991	5
Malaria	184,165	1,933
Smallpox	102,128	0
Typhoid fever	35,994	501

*From National Center for Health Statistics (1900 data); and Centers for Disease Control, Morbidity and Mortality Weekly Report **29**(52):710, Jan. 9, 1981.

INCIDENCE OF COMMUNICABLE DISEASES

Dramatic progress has been made in the control of infectious diseases. A comparison of reported cases of selected communicable diseases in the United States in 1900 and 1980 will indicate the extent of the gain (Table 10-1). In appraising the general decline in the number of reported cases of these selected diseases, an added weight must be given to the increase in population from 1900 to 1980; the population in 1980 was 180% greater than it was in 1900.

To dispel any idea that communicable diseases no longer are a problem in Western countries, one needs but study a table of reported cases of communicable diseases in 1976 and 1980 (Table 10-2). These figures would in-

dicate that the United States has not reached the point where its citizens can be complacent about communicable disease. Communicable disease still exists in epidemic, pandemic, and endemic forms.

Epidemic (Greek— *epi* upon, *demos* people) refers to a considerable number of cases of a particular disease in a rather limited locality such as a city. What constitutes the number of cases that would classify an outbreak as an epidemic is highly flexible, depending on the particular disease and the size of the community. In a city of 12,000 people, 10 cases of measles would not be an epidemic, but in a community of 200, that number of cases of measles might be regarded as in epidemic form. Ten cases of paralytic poliomyelitis in a city of 12,000 would be regarded as an epidemic.

TABLE 10-2. Recent progress in reported cases of specified notifiable diseases, United States, 1976 and 1980*

Disease	1976	1980
Botulism	29	70
Brucellosis	282	176
Chickenpox	182,250	186,913
Diphtheria	146	5
Encephalitis, infectious	1,616	1,134
Gonorrhea (excluding military personnel)	996,468	1,012,835
Hepatitis, infectious	41,263	59,402
Malaria	451	1,933
Measles (rubeola)	39,585	13,430
Meningococcal infections	1,534	2,716
Mumps	20,964	8,531
Pertussis (whooping cough)	925	1,651
Poliomyelitis	9	9
Psittacosis	71	106
Rubella (German measles)	12,090	3,837
Syphilis (excluding military personnel)	23,499	27,516
Tetanus	68	74
Trichinosis	89	126
Tuberculosis	32,549	27,983
Tularemia	146	226
Typhoid fever	384	501
Typhus fever, tick-borne (Rocky Mountain spotted fever)	892	1,136

*From Centers for Disease Control, Morbidity and Mortality Weekly Report **25**(52):650, Jan. 7, 1977; and **29**(52):710, Jan. 9, 1981.

TABLE 10-3. Deaths from infectious diseases, United States, 1970 and 1979*

Cause of death	No.	
	1970	1979
Bacillary dysentery (shigellosis) and amebiasis	89	30
Enteritis and other intestinal infections	2,567	350
Hepatitis, infectious (viral)	1,014	650
Influenza	3,707	590
Measles (rubeola)	89	0
Meningococcal infections	550	390
Pertussis (whooping cough)	12	20
Poliomyelitis	7	20
Septicemia	3,535	8,350
Streptococcal sore throat and scarlet fever	29	30
Syphilis	461	180
Tuberculosis	5,217	1,980
All other infections and parasitic diseases	3,079	3,320

*From Monthly vital statistics of the United States, Provisional Statistics, Annual Summary for the United States, 1979, 28(13):140, Nov. 13, 1980.

Pandemic (Greek— *pan* all) indicates a considerable number of cases of a disease in a wide geographical area such as a state, a section of a nation, the entire nation, a continent, or the world. Thus the outbreak of influenza in 1918 to 1919 was classed as a pandemic. Despite the advance in communicable disease control, no country is completely safe from pandemics.

Endemic (Greek— *en* in) refers to a decidedly limited number of cases in a markedly localized geographical area. The term is sometimes limited to diseases peculiar to a particular area.

Infectious diseases in the United States still account for a high death toll (Table 10-3). The table shows the progress and setbacks against infectious and parasitic diseases, which accounted for less than 1% of the total deaths in 1979.

CLASSIFICATION OF INFECTIOUS DISEASES

Many bases exist for the classification of infectious diseases. Each classification has its merits, and none is without some deficiency or other. From the standpoint of practical community disease control and community health promotion, the best classification would likely be one that incorporates at least a suggestion of how the disease is transmitted. The classification presented here perhaps does not do this in the strictest sense, yet it does serve the practical needs of those who are concerned with control of infectious diseases in the community (Table 10-4). Public understanding of these modes of transmission would go far toward controlling them.

It will be noted that in Table 10-4 some diseases are listed in more than one classification. Thus tuberculosis properly can be classed both as a respiratory disease and an open lesion disease. Smallpox also can be classified both as a respiratory and an open lesion disease. In both of these infectious conditions, the avenue of spread can be from the respiratory tract or from the lesions that these infections produce.

Respiratory diseases

It is not surprising that diseases of the respiratory tract rank far ahead of the other classes of diseases that plague people. In some re-

TABLE 10-4. Classification of infectious diseases

Respiratory diseases	Alvine discharge diseases	Vector-borne diseases	Open lesion diseases
Cerebrospinal meningitis	Amebic dysentery	African sleeping sickness	Anthrax
Chickenpox	Bacillary dysentery (shigellosis)	Encephalitis	Erysipelas
Coryza	Cholera	Malaria	Gonorrhea
Diphtheria	Hookworm	Plague	Scarlet fever
Influenza	Paratyphoid	Psittacosis	Smallpox
Measles (rubeola)	Poliomyelitis	Rabies	Syphilis
Pertussis (whooping cough)	Salmonellosis	Relapsing fever	Tuberculosis
Pneumonia	Schistosomiasis	Rocky Mountain spotted fever	Tularemia
Poliomyelitis	Typhoid fever	Schistosomiasis	
Rubella (German measles)	Viral hepatitis	Tularemia	
Scarlet fever		Typhus fever	
Smallpox		Yellow fever	
Streptococcal sore throat			
Tuberculosis			

spects, the respiratory tract is as exposed as the skin but without the defenses of the skin. Diseases of the respiratory tract are particularly prevalent in the temperate zone but exist universally. Usually acute, they pose a constant threat to the population. Only in recent years has society been reasonably effective in controlling them.

Infectious diseases of the respiratory tract follow a characteristic cycle of periods—incubation, prodrome, fastigium, defervescence, convalescence, and defection. An understanding of the typical course or cycle of a respiratory disease is helpful in controlling disease. Such knowledge points out what factors are operating at a given stage and where and what control measures should be taken.

Incubation starts with the invasion of the causative agent. Organisms multiply in the host during the incubation period, but no symptoms occur in the host. An infectious respiratory disease is normally not communicable during this period, although evidence indicates that chickenpox and measles may be transmitted to other hosts during the last 2 or 3 days of the incubation period. Length of the incubation period varies from disease to disease and from one person to another with the same disease. Generally, the more severe diseases have a short incubation period and the less severe diseases have a longer incubation period, although exceptions to this general tendency do exist.

The prodrome period begins with the first symptoms in the host and usually lasts about 1 day. Symptoms of this period are similar for all of these respiratory infections and resemble those of the common cold. It is difficult to make a definite diagnosis at this stage because of the similarity of symptoms for all of these diseases. From a community health standpoint, there exists a great danger of disease transmission during this highly communicable stage. With the assumption that they "just have a cold," patients continue their normal routine of

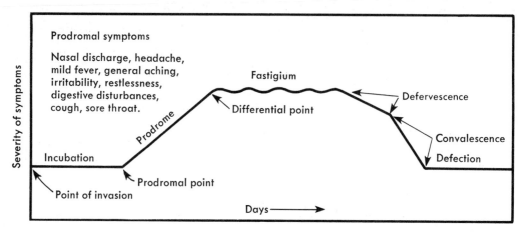

FIG. 10-1. Course of an infectious respiratory disease. The graph portrays the course of all respiratory diseases. Control of spread is most difficult during the prodrome and convalescence periods when the infected person may be up and around.

Adapted from Anderson, C.L., and Creswell, W.H., Jr.: School health practice, ed. 7, St. Louis, 1980, The C.V. Mosby Co.

life and unknowingly expose a considerable number of people. Effective public education is necessary to alert people to the danger of disease transmission during the prodrome period.

Fastigium is the period during which the disease is at its height. Differential symptoms and signs appear, making accurate diagnosis possible. Although a highly communicable stage, the fastigium does not represent a serious disease control problem. Because patients are at home or in a hospital, they expose only those who serve their immediate needs.

Defervescence indicates that the disease is declining in the severity of symptoms, although a relapse may occur.

Convalescence represents a recovery period. New problems in preventing disease spread arise because patients feel well enough to be up and about and expose those they come in contact with.

Defection represents the period during which the organisms are being cast off. It may run concurrently with the period of convalescence. Termination of defection is the signpost for the termination of isolation.

Alvine discharge diseases

Control of infections of the alimentary canal is essentially a problem in sanitation. Dysentery, typhoid fever, and other *Salmonella* infections are the principal alvine discharge diseases of consequence in North American and European Countries. *Salmonella* infections other than typhoid fever are rarely fatal, but the incidence is much higher than is generally recognized. Many cases of digestive disturbances, "intestinal flu," and "summer complaint" technically should be classed as *Salmonella* infections. Environmental control measures for alvine discharge diseases will be covered in Chapters 13, 14, and 16.

Vector-borne diseases

"Vector-borne diseases" is a better designation than "insect-borne diseases" because not all diseases in this classification are transmitted by insects. All of these diseases are normally transmitted to humans by means of an intermediate host, including rodents, bats, dogs, cows, snails, birds, fleas, and ticks. These diseases pose a far greater problem in the tropics than in Western countries where only a few exist and then only in endemic form. Intensive campaigns in these affected geographical regions have brought such vector-borne diseases as malaria, rabies, and Rocky Mountain spotted fever under control. Community control measures for vector-borne diseases will be discussed in Chapter 17.

Open lesion diseases

Syphilis and gonorrhea are the open lesion type of disease of primary importance in community health. Infection transfer in this class of disease normally entails direct contact with the open lesion or site of infection. In addition, only certain tissues, such as the mucous tissues, are specific for the organisms causing these diseases.

Tuberculosis and smallpox, as well as some other diseases producing skin eruptions, technically may be classed as open lesion diseases. The causative agents of these diseases leave their reservoir via the lesion of the infection.

ERADICATION OF SMALLPOX

Smallpox has been called the most devastating and feared pestilence in human history, a disease that has raged through densely populated areas, infecting and killing up to 50% of those who were not already survivors of the previous smallpox epidemic. From the fifteenth through the eighteenth centuries, as the New World was explored and as improved transportation and the need for commerce ended the isolation of many remote areas, smallpox epidemics followed, decimating populations. Early Asian writings indicate that the disease was prevalent in the more densely populated parts of Asia long before that time and probably reached Europe around the sixth century. Estimates vary as to the early death rate, but references to 20% to 50% fatalities among those who contracted smallpox appear in documents about various epidemics in the seventeenth and eighteenth centuries. By the middle 1700s smallpox was a problem in the United States, was believed to account for 10%

of all deaths, and was the leading cause of infant death. Even George Washington bore the scars of smallpox. The transmission of the disease from the sick to the well had been observed, and quarantine was the major weapon to prevent its spread. That immunity could be acquired from surviving a previous infection was also known, and the practice of acquiring immunity by deliberately being inoculated with a light case of smallpox by a physician predates Edward Jenner's discovery, which was published in 1798, by more than 75 years. This technique, called variolation, represented an early folk medicine practice that was widely used in England after being popularized by Lady Mary Wortley Montague and independently came into practice in America before the Revolution. Jenner's convincing documentation of the fact that smallpox immunity could be obtained through inoculation with much milder cowpox and his prediction that this practice would result in "the annihilation of smallpox" began a quest that, 182 years later, has succeeded.

Despite the growing widescale use of smallpox vaccination in the 1800s and early 1900s, the disease remained endemic throughout the world, and those who were not immune ran a high risk of being stricken sometime during their lifetimes. Following World War II, however, the concept of worldwide eradication gained new supporters as smallpox was successfully eliminated from North America, Europe, and a number of other countries that were willing and able to vaccinate the reservoirs of nonimmune individuals in population centers and to prohibit travelers from crossing their borders without evidence of smallpox vaccination. In 1959 the World Health Assembly passed a resolution directed at smallpox eradication, and the World Health Organization (WHO), UNICEF, and other organizations offered help to those countries willing to undertake mass vaccinations. It was not until 1966 that the commitment to worldwide eradication of smallpox was backed up with budget and bilateral agreements sufficient to make the goal of eradication by 1976 feasible. In 1967 there were still 33 countries where the disease was considered to be endemic, and cases attributed to travel through these areas had been reported in 11 other nations. By 1970 only 21 countries reported cases, and 16 did so in 1971.

The worldwide campaign to eliminate smallpox employed a multifaceted approach. Techniques of mass vaccination programs were improved, and costs decreased, with the development of the jet injector gun and the bifurcated needle. Production and quality control of vaccines were also greatly improved. Epidemiological techniques and the enlistment of hundreds of thousands of public health workers who detected cases, tracked down contacts, and vaccinated entire populations in areas where cases occurred contributed greatly to the success of this effort. A highly developed surveillance and containment technique was used, whereby these workers moved rapidly into any area in whch a case was detected, sealing off the spread to other areas, isolating and treating the patient, and finding and vaccinating contacts.

By 1974 the fight to eradicate smallpox was down to the "infected village" unit of measurement, with Afghanistan's last case reported in 1972, Pakistan's in 1974, Nepal's in April 1975, India's in May 1975, and the last in Asia was in Bangladesh in October 1975. Ethiopia's last reported case occurred in 1976, and the last cases in Kenya and Somalia were reported in 1977. A laboratory accident in England in 1978 produced the last verified case of smallpox. The Global Commission for the Certification of Smallpox Eradication required that a 2-year period pass without any cases before the disease could be considered to have been eliminated. That period ended in 1980, and the smallpox virus is considered to be extinct.

The expenditures for smallpox eradiction from 1967 to 1979 by the international community are estimated at nearly a third of a bil-lion dollars, a small amount in comparison to the annual costs the disease inflicted only 50 years earlier. The United States has been a major contributor to the effort, providing nearly a fourth of the WHO and bilateral aid budget, as well as the services of epidemiological consultants from the Public Health Service's Centers for Disease Control who provided technical assistance to individual countries and assisted the WHO Global Smallpox Eradication Program.

SEXUALLY TRANSMITTED DISEASES

Although the two major venereal diseases, syphilis and gonorrhea, are spread in essentially the same way, they present very different clinical and epidemiological patterns. In addition to ensuring effective diagnostic and treatment services, control programs incorporate the similarities as well as the differences in these two diseases. The methodology for syphilis control has been developed over a long period of time and has been demonstrated to be effective in reducing the incidence of disease when rigorously applied. However, gonorrhea control methodology is still in the developmental stages and is further complicated by the following factors: (1) the short incubation period of gonorrhea, (2) its asymptomatic nature in the majority of females and some males. (3) the frequency with which patients become reinfected because of a lack of immunity, and (4) the developing resistance of the causative organism to available antibiotics.

The major thrust of gonorrhea control programs is screening by bacteriological culture of all females for asymptomatic gonococcal infection, followed by prompt treatment if they are infected.

The syphilis control program involves reporting cases, their treatment, and follow-up and interviewing patients for contact information. Named partners are traced, tested, and treated to interrupt the transmission of disease within the community. The basic technique in syphilis control is contact investigation.

An element common to the control of both diseases is programs for venereal disease information and education. These program efforts are designed to create an awareness of the venereal disease problem and control methods and to inform the general public of the tragic consequences of these diseases. The focus is on increasing self-referrals for diagnosis and treatment and on expanding screening, contact tracing, and diagnostic and treatment programs within the community.

Syphilis and gonorrhea represent examples of the difficulty of prevention and control of sexually transmitted disease, even when the cause is known. The organisms are sensitive to drugs, yet behavioral factors are involved, with the resulting epidemic for gonorrhea shown in Fig. 10-2. Between 1965 and 1975, the number of reported cases of gonorrhea in the United States tripled. Since 1975, however, reported cases have leveled off with only a 1% increase since 1975. The recent improvement is attributed to federal assistance to establish state and local gonorrhea-prevention programs.

Genital herpes infections are very common, with an incidence of $^1/_2$ to 1 million new cases annually, with several million recurrences each year. No effective treatment is currently available for this painful condition; periodic recurrences are the rule. Herpes-complicated pregnancies often result in abortion, stillbirth, or severe neonatal infection; neonatal herpes results in death or permanent disability in two thirds of the cases.

Hepatitis B is caused by a virus with many different modes of transmission, including sexual transmission. Homosexual males are at very high risk; nearly 60% attending sexually transmitted disease clinics show evidence of past or present hepatitis B infection. This same popu-

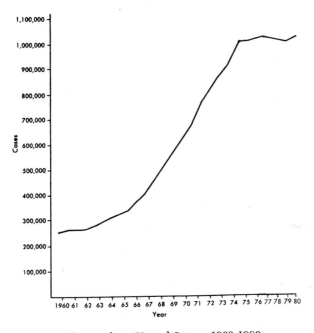

FIG. 10-2. Number of cases of gonorrhea, United States, 1960-1980.

From Centers for Disease Control, Public Health Service: Morbidity and Mortality Weekly Report **26***(1):6, Jan. 14, 1977;* **28***(45):603, Nov. 16, 1979; and* **29***(52):710, Jan. 9, 1981.*

lation is also at high risk of several other sexually transmitted diseases, including amebiasis and giardiasis. These and other sexually transmitted diseases have placed great strain on the resources of local health departments in the United States during the 1970s and will continue to do so in the 1980s.

Total costs for sexually transmitted diseases in the United States vastly exceed $1 billion annually. Costs for the most common reported sexually transmitted disease, gonorrhea, were estimated to total over $770 million in 1978.

Prevention-promotion measures

Education and information measures. The most fundamental component of a community program to control sexually transmitted diseases is education and training that includes clinical experience in schools for health professionals; education and information about sexually transmitted diseases for school children before and during the time they are at highest risk; preservice and continuing professional education for both health providers and health educators to deal with sexually transmitted diseases in a confidential, nonjudgmental fashion; and improved public understanding of sexually transmitted disease risks and confidentiality of treatment through effective and continuous campaigns using mass media. The measures may be mass directed or targeted to special groups such as women, children, adolescents, minorities, groups with special language needs, and other risk groups; and they may include the counseling of patients being treated for sexually transmitted diseases regarding complications and measures to avoid future infection and the use of peers, who are often adjuncts to educate and counsel adolescents about sexually transmitted diseases.

Service measures. The second level of community strategy is the provision of diagnostic and treatment services for patients with sexually transmitted diseases and their complica-

tions. Also included in secondary prevention and control are detection and referral methods, such as counseling infected patients and tracing and treating their contacts: screening for selected sexually transmitted diseases; and encouraging joint availability of services among related programs such as sexually transmitted diseases, family planning, and maternal and child health.

Technological measures. Properly used condoms are the best known measure for persons engaging in sexual activity to avoid acquiring or transmitting many of the sexually transmitted diseases. A vaccine for hepatitis B is being tested for efficacy; vaccines for gonorrhea and genital herpes are at an earlier stage of development.

Legislative and regulatory measures. Community agencies need to determine the magnitude of the sexually transmitted disease problem and establish objectives for inclusion in their annual implementation plans. Health planning and development agencies need to make certain that the health plan addresses gaps in education and service delivery regarding sexually transmitted diseases.

Other regulatory activities to support community control might include the examination of health professionals' knowledge of sexually transmitted diseases and competency in dealing with sexually transmitted diseases by specialty boards, certifying agencies, and other regulatory boards; the repeal of statutes and ordinances that inhibit the advertising, display, sale, or distribution of condoms; and regulations mandating information about sexually transmitted diseases as part of school health education programs.

Economic measures. The two most needed economic supports for sexually transmitted disease services would be prevention-related activities that are exempted from coinsurance or deductible provisions of health insurance and prepaid health plans with financial incentives for sexually transmitted disease promotion-prevention activities, including management of contacts who are not members of the plan.

Relative strength of the measures.

- Readily available quality clinical services without stigma form a necessary substrate for other clinic-related prevention activities.
- Early diagnosis and treatment of sexually transmitted diseases among patients attending clinics, contacts, and those identified in screening programs is highly effective in preventing transmission of the diseases and in limiting their disabling complications.
- Persons who properly and consistently use condoms experience lower rates of sexually transmitted diseases.
- As vaccines are developed and introduced, they can be effectively administered in the health care system.
- Mass and targeted education and information measures appear to be the only way to modify hardened public opinion and to reduce sexually transmitted disease ignorance and apathy.
- Education and training of health professionals and health educators is a necessary first step toward effective sexually transmitted disease service measures.

THE MICROBIOLOGY OF CAUSATIVE AGENTS

Not all parasites of the human body are pathogenic to humans, but all pathogens of humans are parasites of humans. Some of the parasites in humans—for example, *E. coli*—produce no antagonistic action. However, these inhabitants of the large intestine do not live in symbiotic relationship with humans because they do not return some benefit for the benefits they receive. Some pathogens may produce so slight a disturbance in humans that the host is not aware of the disturbance. Even in a carrier condition a pathogen may produce some disturbance in the host.

A pathogen is a poor parasite because it arouses the host. It is analogous to a burglar arousing the household that he is preying on. The response of the host is usually a defense reaction, basically of a chemical or immunological nature.

Infecting organisms

The vast majority of organisms pathogenic to humans belong to the plant kingdom, specifically of the phylum Thallophyta. Bacteria constitute the greatest number of pathogenic organisms, as shown in Table 10-5. Rickettsiae are small bacteria, and viruses are ultramicroscopic forms. Certain true fungi, including the molds, are also pathogenic to humans, although they may produce infestations as well as infections in that they live on the body as well as in the body. In the animal kingdom certain protozoa and a few metazoa are pathogens of humans. There are many classifications of pathogens, such as the taxonomy in Table 10-5, depending on which criterion or particular criteria are given more weight. For the purposes of the various people working in community health, a classification that can be readily applied to existing conditions, such as Table 10-6, would be most logical. Of necessity, such a classification must overlook certain microbiological or taxonomic criteria in the interest of functional needs.

Specificity of infecting organisms. A typhoid bacillus is derived only from a preexisting typhoid bacillus. The virility but not the species may change from generation to generation of a particular type of organism. The severity of the reaction the organism produces in human hosts may rise or subside with subsequent generations of the organism, but the action will always be similar in its basic nature. In addition to specific action, many organisms are harmful

TABLE 10-5. Microbiological classification of the major pathogens of humans

Plants		Animals	
Organisms	Diseases	Organisms	Diseases

Bacterium
(split fungi)
Bacillus
(rod-shaped)
	Diphtheria
	Bacillary dysentery
	Pertussis (whooping cough)
	Tuberculosis
	Typhoid
		Protozoan (one cell)
		  Ameba
		  Plasmodium
		
		Spirochete (spiral)
			Dysentery
			Malaria
			
			Syphilis

Coccus
(spherical)
	Furunculosis (boils)
	Gonorrhea
	Scarlet fever
	Streptococcal sore throat
		Metazoan
		  Roundworm (e.g., ascaris)
		  Tapeworm
		  Trichinella
			Trichinosis

Spirillum (spiral-shaped)	Cholera Rat-bite fever	Schistosome	Schistosomiasis
Rickettsia (small bacteria)	Rocky Mountain spotted fever Typhus fever		
Virus (ultramicroscopic)	Chickenpox Coryza Influenza Measles (rubeola) Mumps Poliomyelitis Rabies Smallpox		
True fungus Mold Yeast	Mycosis Tinea (ringworm) Blastomycosis Dermatophytosis		

only to specific types of human tissue. This basic tendency of all pathogens to be specific accounts both for the manner in which the organism functions and the reaction it produces in the host. In some respects the diphtheria bacillus may resemble the typhoid bacillus and in some respects the diphtheria bacillus may produce a somewhat similar reaction in the host, but the two different organisms have definite identities. This specificity of infecting organisms is a universal phenomenon.

Mode of action. Most pathogens injure human tissue by the toxins they produce. In their normal metabolic processes these pathogens produce substances that happen to be injurious to certain human tissues. Some organisms—for example, diphtheria bacillus—produce toxins that diffuse through the permeable membrane of the bacterium and for this reason are called exotoxins. Other pathogens—for example, typhoid bacillus—produce a toxin that does not diffuse through the impermeable membrane

TABLE 10-6. Means of pathogen transmission

Indirect contact			Direct contact
Airborne	**Water- and food-borne**	**Vector-borne**	
Anthrax†	Botulism†	Glanders†§	Anthrax†
Cerebrospinal meningitis*‖	Brucellosis†	Jaundice, infective*	Brucellosis†
Chickenpox*	Cholera*	Malaria*	Gonorrhea*
Encephaolmyelitis, equine†	Diphtheria*	Plague*	Rabies†
Influenza*	Dysentery, bacillary*	Relapsing fever*	Smallpox*
Measles*	Hoof-and-mouth disease‡§	Rocky Mountain spotted	Syphilis*
Mumps*	Poliomyelitis*‖	fever*§	Tetanus*
Pneumonia†	Schistosomiasis	Tularemia*	Tuberculosis†
Psittacosis†	Streptococcus*	Typhus fever*§	Tularemia*
Tuberculosis†	Tuberculosis†	Yellow fever*§	
Typhus fever*‡	Tularemia*		
	Typhoid fever*		

*Infects humans only.
†Infects humans and animals useful to humans.
‡Infects animals or birds only.
§Artificially transmissible by air in laboratory.
‖Means of transmission unknown.

that encloses the organism and for this reason are called endotoxins. When an organism of this type dies, its enclosing membrane undergoes changes that make it permeable to the toxins.

A small proportion of pathogens invade the tissues directly. Some of the protozoa such as the malaria plasmodium and the spirochete of syphilis, as well as some viruses and rickettsiae, invade human cells and bring about cellular change and, possibly, destruction.

Reservoirs of infection

Pathogens are relatively fragile organisms that survive only in a highly selective medium. A reported case of a new host for a particular type of organism means that the organism had been harbored in a medium favorable to the organism's survival, multiplication, and functioning. The medium in which organisms are thus harbored must possess moisture, relatively high temperature, nutrients, and an absence of light. It is rather easy to classify the reservoirs of organisms that affect people—those living hosts that provide an excellent medium and thus harbor these pathogens.

Human reservoirs. The human body is the greatest reservoir of organisms pathogenic to other human beings. This is the genesis of the time-tested question when a new case of disease is discovered—"Where is the other case?" Thus the human reservoir is the source of the greatest danger of infection. *Frank cases*, or persons obviously ill with a disease, may be of great danger to an individual but not to a community. Although the individual who nurses the ill person may be greatly exposed to the disease, the community can be effectively protected by preventing transfer of infection from the known reservoir to other possible hosts, once the reservoir has been located. *Subclinical infections*, variously referred to as missed, abortive, or ambulatory cases, constitute a great community danger because the affected individuals may continue their normal daily routine. An ambulatory patient with diphtheria, scarlet fever, dysentery, or smallpox could unknowingly expose and infect a considerable number of associates before the source of the new cases of the disease is located. *Carriers* are individuals who harbor and disseminate a pathogenic organism without themselves experiencing recognizable symptoms. The longer the duration of the carrier status, the greater the danger to the community. Chronic or per-

manent carriers carry a long-time threat; however, once they are identified, control measures can be instituted that will minimize and almost remove the danger of communicating the disease to others. A convalescent carrier or transient carrier can be a serious danger to those in the immediate environment. Although the period of communicability may be relatively short, a sufficient number of people can

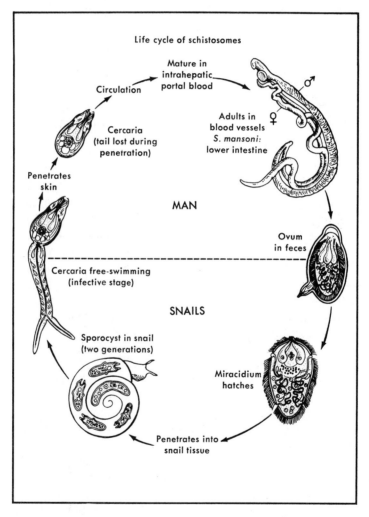

FIG. 10-3. Life cycle of schistosomes: a complex cycle involving alternate human and snail hosts.

From National Institutes of Health, Research Resources Reporter, Feb., 1981.

be infected by one such carrier to set off a chain reaction that may fan out and encompass a considerable number of new hosts.

Lower animals. Only a few species of lower animals harbor organisms pathogenic to human beings, and these are principally domestic animals. Rodents also serve as reservoirs of organisms that produce disease in humans. Society has the necessary means to protect the human species against diseases such as anthrax from sheep and cattle; glanders and tetanus from horses; hoof-and-mouth disease from cattle; brucellosis from cattle, swine, and goats; tuberculosis from cattle; trichinosis from swine; psittacosis from parrots and parakeets; rabies from rodents, canines, and bats; and Rocky Mountain spotted fever and tularemia from rodents.

Schistosomiasis, an organ-damaging and sometimes fatal disease whose victims number 200 million worldwide, is caused by a tropic-loving parasitic worm whose life cycle takes it from snail to water to human, during which time it grows to be up to 1 inch long, lays vast numbers of eggs, and has sexual unions that can last 30 years or more. The eggs of the threadlike parasite are hatched in humans, passed through stools, and often end up in fresh water where they develop into larvae. This preadult form searches out and infects a snail (the disease is sometimes called snail fever), only to be released again into water where it must burrow into a host within 24 hours, or die. (The cycle is shown in Fig. 10-3.) Damage to human hosts is caused by the great number of eggs produced by the adult worm. The eggs eventually lodge in the liver and result in a nonalcoholic and reversible form of cirrhosis of the liver. The tissue becomes inflamed and enlarged, triggering engorgement of the spleen and damage to other abdominal organs. Effects also include infection of the bladder and kidney and a slow sapping of energy. Thriving where water supplies are not adequatey treated by modern purification methods and where life styles do not always follow optimum habits of hygiene, schistosomiasis is one of the scourges of the Third World. The devastating effects of the disease have been felt throughout the Middle East, Africa, Latin America, the Caribbean, and Asia. Health education campaigns to control this disease have had to struggle against time-honored cultural and agricultural practices that cannot be easily challenged, especially in the face of economic hardships.

In the technical sense, the plant kingdom actually does not function as a reservoir of infection for humans. In considering hookworm and tetanus, however, there is some justification for the contention that soil may serve as a reservoir for the pathogens of humans.

Escape of organisms from reservoir

The fact that a particular pathogen is harbored in a particular host is important from the standpoint of disease spread, but the organism must escape from the reservoir if other potential hosts are to be endangered. For some diseases, the mere fact that a person harbors the causative agent in itself represents no danger or a danger only under most unusual circumstances. A person with trichinosis is not endangering the health of others unless for some reason they should become cannibalistic. The causative agent of trichinosis, being in the skeletal muscle of the human, has no avenue of escape. Likewise, a person who is an active case or carrier of malaria does not pose a danger to those about him under ordinary circumstances. The causative agent of malaria normally does not escape from the reservoir that harbors it. The organism can escape and endanger others only via the female *Anopheles* mosquito, a blood transfusion, or perhaps the common use of a hypodermic needle among drug addicts.

It is a common observation that most of the pathogens of humans escape from the human body. The avenue of escape depends on the site of infection. The respiratory tract represents the most common and most dangerous avenue of escape. While an individual harbors an infection of the respiratory tract, it is realistic to assume that the escape of the organism is a continuous process. The organism escapes by use of such vehicles as droplets from coughs and sneezes, eating utensils, or the human hands. Escape via the intestinal tract would be through discharges of the colon and via the urinary tract through the urine. Open lesions provide an easy means of escape. With tubercle bacilli this is true whether it is a lesion of lung tissue or of the surface of the body. Likewise, the open lesion of syphilis, gonorrhea, and common furunculosis (boils) provide ready means of escape for the pathogens that produce the lesion. Mechanical escape of organisms from the human body is possible by insects that bite or suck, but here the organism must be aided by a specific vector or intermediate host.

Preventing the organism from escaping from the reservoir obviously provides one means of communicable disease control. Efforts must be based on microbiological knowledge of the nature of the organism and epidemiological knowledge of the specific avenue through which it must escape, and transfer or spread to a new host.

THE EPIDEMIOLOGY OF INFECTION

Once the organism has escaped from the reservoir it still must be transferred to a new host if a new case of the disease is to occur, or if the organism is to survive and spread. The normal pathogens of humans do not walk or run or swim or fly. They must be transported by some vehicle. This transfer can be effected from person to person either directly or indirectly.

Direct transmission. Organisms can be transmitted directly from one person to another without an intermediate object. This requires intimate association usually, but not necessarily physical contact. Thus coughing and sneezing can be a direct means of transmitting organisms from one person to another without physical contact being involved. This accounts for the

high incidence of respiratory diseases in crowded living areas.

Indirect transmission. When an intermediate object is involved in the transmission of disease from the reservoir to a new host, the mechanism is classed as indirect transmission. Such a transfer involves no particular close relationship between the reservoir and the new host. There are, however, two basic requirements for indirect transmission. The first of these is that the organisms involved must be virile enough to survive a long time outside of a living body. Thus highly resistant organisms such as those causing typhoid, tetanus, and anthrax are most likely to be transmitted by indirect means. On the other hand, highly fragile organisms such as those causing meningitis, syphilis, and gonorrhea are less likely to be transmitted by an intermediate object except under most unusual and highly favorable survival circumstances. A second requirement for indirect transfer of infection is the existence of a favorable vehicle of transmission. It may be a specific living form of life, such as a mosquito, or a highly favorable substance for growth of the pathogen, such as milk. In a high proportion of diseases that can be transmitted by indirect means, for its survival the specific organism requires a specific medium or decidedly limited media and these media must be existing under certain circumstances and must be providing certain conditions.

Vehicles of transfer

The expression "vehicles of pathogen transfer," refers to the objects that make the transfer from the reservoir to a new host. They might also be referred to as routes of infection insofar as they represent certain pathways by which the organisms are transferred. Vehicles of transfer may be animate or inanimate.

Vectors. Animate vehicles are spoken of as vectors. These are intermediate hosts of the organism and represent the connecting link between one case of a disease and a susceptible new host. Transfer by vectors can be either biological or mechanical. In a biological transfer the organism spends part of its life cycle in the body of the intermediate host. Biological vectors are specific for specific diseases. Malaria is transmitted only by the female *Anopheles* mosquito, yellow fever by the *Aedes aegypti* mosquito, typhus fever by the louse, plague by the flea, and Rocky Mountain spotted fever by the tick. When a vector makes possible the mechanical transfer of organisms, such specific action does not prevail. In this instance the vector comes in contact with infectious agents that mechanically become attached to the vector's body, legs, or other parts and thus are transmitted.

In unusual cases a vector that normally produces a biological transfer may also effect a mechanical transfer. Normally, the *Anopheles* mosquito harbors the plasmodium of malaria for about 14 days while the pathogen goes through a life cycle. The resulting young forms are then introduced into a host. This is true of biological transfer. However, the *Anopheles* mosquito can get some blood from feeding on a human being with malaria, leave this reservoir, and immediately attach to a new host, where the organisms from the original reservoir can be mechanically introduced. This would be a mechanical transfer.

From the standpoint of knowledge of how to block the transfer of infection via vectors, society is well equipped. Theoretically, it would be possible to eliminate all disease transfer via vectors, but it is not possible to apply this knowledge because of the practical problem of extensiveness involved. Epidemiolgy knows how these vectors operate and how they can be destroyed, but, with the almost limitless number of vectors, public health has to concentrate on the destruction and other control of vectors in specific geographic areas or high-risk populations where the incidence of vector-borne diseases is pronounced.

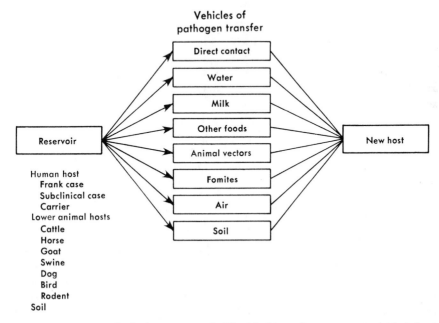

FIG. 10-4. Routes over which diseases travel. The blocking of routes over which infectious diseases travel prevents pathogens from reaching potential susceptible new hosts.

Inanimate vehicles of disease transfer pose a special problem as society becomes more complex and people congregate in ever greater numbers in restricted areas. If an inanimate object is to serve as a vehicle of pathogen transfer it must have certain characteristics; otherwise, the organism will not survive the interval between the time it comes into contact with the object and the time it is transmitted to the new host. If the organism is to survive and remain sufficiently virile to set up a new infection, the time interval during which the organism is carried by the medium must be relatively short. The medium must be moist, bland, warm (near 100° F, or 38° C), and exist in relative darkness. Water, milk, other foods, air, fomites, and soil are the recognized inanimate vehicles of disease transfer.

Water. Water serves as a medium for the transfer of organisms from the human alimentary tract. Typhoid, paratyphoid, cholera, and bacillary dysentery are transmitted via water. Organisms normally do not multiply in water, yet an organism such as the typhoid bacillus can live for 2 or 3 weeks in relatively cool water. Public health has developed the necessary measures to protect communities against disease transmission via water. Filtration and chlorination of community water supplies have been effective in controlling water-borne diseases.

Milk. Milk is an excellent medium for several organisms pathogenic to people. Contamination of milk can come from three sources. The first is infection within the udder from a disease with which the cow suffers, such as brucellosis and bovine tuberculosis. The second is infection within the udder by organisms accidentally introduced into the udder by a human being. Septic sore throat and scarlet fever are typical of this type of contamination. The third is direct contamination of the milk by a human being after it has left the cow. Thus a milk handler harboring diphtheria, typhoid, or dysentery bacilli may introduce the organism into the milk in the course of milk processing. Through herd testing, dairy sanitation, and pasteurization, public health has been able to prevent the spread of infectious disease via the vehicle of milk.

Other foods. Other foods can be a means of transmitting pathogens but are not offenders as often as the lay public believes. For solid foods to serve as a vehicle of disease transfer, they must be moist, nonacid, not cooked, and handled a great deal. If a clerk in a bake shop, through handling, should leave typhoid bacilli on baked goods, the likelihood is rather remote that these few organisms would survive over the considerable length of time that would intervene before the pastry is eaten. This does not suggest that a typhoid carrier should be working in a public bake shop, but it does indicate that disease transfer by this means is not as frequent as is commonly thought. There are three common sources of contamination by food. The first of these is food handlers conveying organisms to the food by coughing or by their hands. The second is contamination during growth, such as shellfish developing in a body of water contaminated with typhoid bacilli. The third is from infected animals, such as the transmission of trichinosis and tapeworm. Here, however, proper cooking would destroy pathogens. This is the key to protection against transfer via the common foods. Boiling or heating to the boiling point will destroy the usual pathogens that may be transferred via food.

Air. Air as a vehicle of disease transfer is not ideal. The dryness, low temperature, and light of the air are highly unfavorable to pathogenic organisms. Droplets from sneezing and coughing may give pathogens a moist vehicle that will help them survive long enough to set up an infection if they are inhaled into the respiratory passage of a new host. Measles and chickenpox appear to be more readily transmitted by this means than any of the other known respiratory diseases. A cubic foot of air may contain a considerable number of pathogens, but they would be so attenuated before being inhaled into the respiratory tract of a person that the likelihood that they would set up an infection in the new host is somewhat limited.

Fomites. Fomites are inanimate objects—other than water, milk, food, and air—that might be vehicles of disease transfer. The term embraces such things as clothing, bed linen, books, toys, handrailings, and similar objects. Fomites are no longer regarded seriously as vehicles of disease transfer because they do not provide a good medium for pathogens. It is possible however, that a patient, by handling an object, may leave a considerable number of organisms on the fomite and, if another person immediately handles the same object and gets his hands up to his mouth, the fomite may serve as a vehicle of spread. Increasing use of disposable items in the health care field minimizes this route.

Soil. Soil may harbor the organisms that cause hookworm, tetanus, anthrax, and botulism. Each of these presents a particular type of control procedure, but by the use of immunization, boiling, wearing of clothing, and other procedures, humans have various effective means for preventing soil from being an actual vehicle of disease transfer.

In any situation where an intermediate object is the vehicle for the transmission of disease from a reservoir to a new host, it should be possible to block that route and thus prevent disease spread. In practice, however, human beings do not use the knowledge available to them, primarily because of a lack of understanding or because of carelessness or indifference. Through proper education of the public and the exercise of community control, it is possible to reduce the transfer of disease via animate and inanimate objects. In practice, public health officials find that the control of the social contact route is a much more difficult task than the control of disease spread by vectors or inanimate objects.

Entry of organisms into new host

Arrival and entry are not synonymous. When the organism arrives at the place of the new host, it still has to find its proper port of entry and must overcome certain body barriers. Pathogens producing respiratory diseaes must arrive at the mouth or nasal entry to the respiratory tract. Likewise, the organism causing an infection of the alimentary canal must find its way to the mouth. Even when such an organism finds its way into the alimentary canal, acid in the stomach may destroy the organism. Direct infection of mucous membranes such as occurs in gonococcus infection requires that the organism come in contact with mucous membranes. Although the hookworm can go through the unbroken skin and mosquitoes can penetrate the skin sufficiently to introduce pathogenic organisms, nevertheless percutaneous infections generally require a cut or an abrasion of the skin if the organism is to enter the body and create an infection.

Defenses of the host

After leaving the reservoir, being transferred to the new host, and by chance reaching the right port of entry, the pathogen still encounters a series of defenses the new host possesses. Indeed, virile organisms in a large number must enter the new host if all of the defenses of the new host are to be overcome and infection produced.

Resistance. The nature of resistance is expressed as the ability of the host to ward off pathogens. General resistance against infection is nonspecific in that the various human resistance factors serve as barriers or are antagonistic to all pathogens of humans. The skin serves as a mechanical barrier, and its natural acid state provides a further defense against pathogens that usually require a neutral or alkaline medium. The secretion of mucous tissue serves as a defense against most, and in a sense, all pathogens. The ciliated epithelium tissues of certain passages such as the respiratory tract provide an added defense, as the cilia tend to propel organisms to the the exterior of the passageway. Acidity of such structures as the stomach, bladder, urethra, and vagina provides additional resistance to infection. Leukocytes with their phagocytic action destroy foreign organisms and perhaps represent the strongest human defense against infection. Lymph nodes filter out infectious organisms and are capable of destroying them. A highly important defense, not generally recognized as such, is the ability of the body to produce an elevated temperature or fever. The optimum temperature for most pathogens is about 100° F (38° C), which is the approximate normal temperature of the human body. In elevating the temperature by only 2 degrees, the body is able to inactivate the pathogens so that they are unable to multiply and carry on normal metabolism involving toxin production. During this stasis, the phagocytes of the body are able to engulf and destroy the pathogens.

It is apparent that from time to time small numbers of pathogens enter the human body without setting up infections. The human body's general resistance is normally able to provide the necessary defenses to prevent infection.

Immunity and susceptibility. The concept of immunity and susceptibility distinguishes the status of the host regarding defense against specific diseases. The host with no specific resistance is termed *susceptible* and may be converted to immunity status by a variety of mechanisms. Complete resistance is termed *immunity* and is specific for a particular disease. Immunity is dependent on the presence of specific substances in the body that are most easily identified in the bloodstream but are present in all tissues. These chemical substances are called antibodies and may be in the form of antitoxin, which neutralizes a particular toxin, agglutinin, which causes organisms to clump together, or precipitins, which produce a disintegration of pathogenic organisms.

Active immunity exists when an individual's own body produces the necessary antibodies. This occurs either through the actual attack of the disease or by artifical introduction of the necessary antigenic substance into the body by vaccination or immunization. An antigen is a substance (for example, toxin) that, when introduced into the body, causes the formation of antibodies.

Passive immunity is "borrowed" immunity and exists when antibodies produced in some other individual or animal are introduced into a person. The duration of passive immunity is relatively short because the protective substances tend to disappear, not to be replaced by the individual's own body action. Passive immunity is employed when a susceptible person has been exposed to a disease and there is insufficient time to produce active immunity. The injection of convalescent serum into a susceptible child exposed to measles would give the child temporary immunity or at least measles with very mild symptoms. The infantile immunity that a child experiences during the first 6 months of life is an example of natural passive immunity in that antibodies from the mother's bloodstream diffuse through the membranes of the placenta into the bloodstream of the fetus. The immunity exists only while the mother's antibodies survive in the child. No stimulation of the child's tissues to form antibodies occurs.

Natural immunity expresses the concept that a species has a genetic immunity to a particular disease to which some other species is susceptible. Mammals are immune to many of the microorganisms that cause infection in birds. Domestic animals are susceptible to some diseases, such as distemper, to which humans are immune. Likewise, domestic animals are immune to diphtheria, smallpox, typhoid fever, and other infectious diseases to which humans are heir. These are examples of natural immunity in species. Fortunately, the human species possesses an immunity to a vast number of microorganisms that conceivably could be disease-producing except for the human body's distinctive biochemistry. Communities are able to to add to this general protection or defense by offering artificial immunity to those diseases to which specific populations could be susceptible.

Acquired immunity comes either from having an attack of a disease or from artificially inducing a body reaction to produce the necessary protective antibodies. In humans second attacks are common in such diseases as influenza, pneumonia, gonorrhea, streptococcal sore throat, and the common cold but are relatively rare in such diseases as chickenpox, diphtheria, measles, poliomyelitis, scarlet fever, smallpox, typhoid fever, and yellow fever. Artificial active immunity is available for diphtheria, tetanus, pertussis, smallpox, poliomyelitis, typhoid fever, cholera, Rocky Mountain spotted fever, measles, German measles, mumps, and influenza. Various immunization schedules are in use (see Chapter 5).

Because no cases of smallpox have been reported since 1979, smallpox vaccination has been discontinued in many countries. There is a greater threat to human life in possible complication from vaccination than in not being immunized. The spread of an epidemic through a population is determined by the immune-susceptible ratio. When the supply of susceptibles is exhausted, the epidemic ceases. In the case of smallpox, the pathogen itself was isolated from susceptible populations until the agent-host chain was broken with the isolation of the last case in Somalia.

Agent-host-environment

The outcome of disease in the individual is determined by the interaction of agent, host, and environment. The agent may be of high virulence or present in high dosage. The host defenses may be compromised by age or concomitant disease, or the immune system may be affected by drugs given for chronic disease.

Agent

Host ⟷ Environment

The environment may be hostile in respect to climate, such as air pollution. In intervention, action may be applied at any of the three points. Resistance of the host may be enhanced by nutrition or by vaccination, for example. The agent may be directly attacked by chemicals or antibiotics, and the environment may be altered by sanitation.

This model may also be used to consider other conditions in addition to infectious diseases, such as automobile accidents, where the agent is the automobile, the host is the driver, and the highway is the environment.

EPIDEMIOLOGICAL PRINCIPLES OF DISEASE CONTROL

Epidemiology is the study of the distribution and determinants of disease in the population. The unit of study is not the individual, as in microbiology and clinical medicine, but the community. Epidemiology compares and contrasts, studying both sick and well groups. Variables such as age, sex, race, and occupation are analyzed in an attempt to determine which are found frequently in the sick yet are found rarely in the well. The validity of the conclusions reached is subject to statistical tests. Epidemiological methods may be used to study chronic as well as infectious diseases. Disease in the community is first categorized by time, place, and person. By studying the time of onset in an epidemic, a shared event, such as a meal, may be identified. It can then be determined if this particular meal was attended by many of the sick persons but by few of a comparison group of well people. Food histories may then be assembled and a suspect vehicle identified. The place of the epidemic may help to identify the offending vehicle, such as the density of cases in an area sharing a common water supply, or cases predominantly on the route of a mobile food vendor. The personal characteristics of those afflicted in an epidemic may point to its cause, for example, they might share a common exposure to toxic inhalants in an industrial plant or to asbestos fibers in construction work.

Legal authority

Communicable diseases are controlled through the exercise of police power, which is the authority or power of the people, represented by government, to do whatever is necessary for the protection and general well-being of the public. Basically, sovereignty or ultimate authority rests with the people, who vest it in the state or province to exercise for them. The state or province may in turn delegate police power to counties or parishes to exercise within their geographical boundaries. Municipalities may be granted a charter that gives broad authority, including police power, to do whatever is necessary for the well-being of the people within the political limits of the borough, villages, town, or city. It is clear that the authorities have the power to take the necessary measures to control communicable diseases within their limits. Likewise, counties have the authority to exercise control measures outside corporate municipalities. Municipalities and counties usually assign some authority to schools to carry out some control measures, such as isolation of infected or infested children.

The state or province reserves its power to take necessary action on an area basis for the protection of the public against the spread of communicable diseases. In practice, the state or province enters into communicable disease control practice in a broad advisory capacity to the community governmental units and by direct action when communicable diseases spread beyond a single county and become a threat to a considerable portion of the population. It is apparent that the state or province does not usually step in and take action unless local authorities are unable to cope with the situation or unless the state or province is requested by local authorities to assist in the problem of disease control.

In the exercise of police power, the one governing principle recognized by the courts is that whatever action is taken must be reasonable. Thus it may be reasonable for health authorities to isolate an individual in his home for a period of 5 days when he suffers from a diagnosed case of a certain communicable disease, but a court may rule that it would not be reasonable to require that patient to be removed to a hospital and isolated there for 2 weeks. Actually, the science of epidemiology has advanced to a point where the action taken is usually reasonable because it is based on sound principles of statistical probability, microbiology, and medical science. Further, citizens today are saved from a great deal of inconvenience suffered by their grandparents because modern public health science has displaced much of the guesswork applied in disease control less than half a century ago.

In exercising police power, health authorities cannot ignore the personal and religious rights of the individual, but courts have been reluctant to censure public health official action exercised reasonably in the interest of the general population. Courts have ruled that while official health boards cannot require a person to be immunized in opposition to relgious beliefs, action of health officials in imposing quarantine on some nonimmunized people when an epidemic threatens the community is just and reasonable. In the present era, however, control measures are so highly effective that if a relatively small percent of the population is not immunized against a disease, the fact that 85% of the people are immune virtually limits the spread of the particular disease by means of immunity level. From the standpoint of public health administration, communicable disease control is a much less difficult task than it was half a century ago. The present scientific approach to epidemiology encompasses certain well-established, effective measures of action.

Segregation of reservoir

An effective program of communicable disease control must direct itself to preventing the spread of disease and increasing the resistance of the new potential host. Logically, preventing the spread of disease is the most desirable and the most profitable in results in terms of the extended effort. Theoretically, perfect prevention of spread would mean perfect control of communicable diseases. It is possible to establish certain barriers around a reservoir of infection and thus block the spread of the disease.

Isolation. The oldest communicable disease control measure is the segregation of an infected person or lower animal until danger of conveying infection has passed. Isolation can be a highly effective control measure, but in practice isolation will occasionally fail resulting from variability in the duration of the communicable state and from human failures in observing regulations.

When bacteriological methods are used to determine the interval of isolation, the termination of the communicable state can be made with precision. Laboratory examination of the secretions of a patient with tuberculosis will establish the presence or absence of the tubercle bacillus and thus determine the continuance or termination of isolation. Likewise, examination of secretions from the nose and throat in a patient with diphtheria will provide an accurate bacteriological determination of whether isolation should be terminated. If two smears from the nose, taken 24 hours apart, and two smears from the throat, taken 24 hours apart, are all found to be negative, isolation can be terminated with assurance that the patient is in a noncommunicable state.

Laboratory examination of respiratory secretions will also indicate whether viable streptococci are present and will thus serve as a marker for the continuance or termination of isolation. Laboratory examinations of the excretions of patients with typhoid fever and dysentery likewise can give a reliable indication of whether isolation should be continued or ter-

minated. Typhoid, however, poses a special problem because a typhoid carrier tends to discharge the bacilli intermittently. In some cases, positive fecal specimens may be a month apart. The use of laboratory methods to terminate isolation requires that a good laboratory and a qualified technician be available and that the tests be practical.

An arbitrary period of time for isolation is far more common than the use of laboratory methods for determining the period of isolation. The arbitrary time designated by law or by board of health regulations is usually based on practical experience through observation. To designate too short a period of isolation would mean exposing others and would thus, defeat the true purpose of isolation. The longer the period of isolation, the greater the safety, but the greater the injustice because many patients reach a noncommunicable state long before the maximum isolation period is reached. No definite rule applies; for this reason, great variation is found from state to state or province to province and even from community to community. To set an inflexible isolation period would make no provision for individual variation. For this reason, the usual practice is to set a minimum time that experience has demonstrated will be ample in perhaps 80% to 90% of the cases, and then leave to the discretion of the attending physician the need for extending the isolation in individual cases. An arbitrary period of isolation can be quite satisfactory for diseases such as measles and chickenpox where no convalescent carriers occur, but unsatisfactory for a disease such as scarlet fever where convalescent carriers are always a possibility.

Isolation has certain limitations. Hidden cases—those never reported by parents—are not technically under isolation. Missed, subclinical, or ambulatory cases—those so mild that no medical services are obtained—are not subjected to isolation measures. Carriers of a disease do not usually have overt symptoms and thus are not identified as potential hazards. In addition, during the early or prodrome stage of a respiratory disease, individuals may not be ill enough to remain home; yet they are in a highly communicable state and capable of communicating the disease to others. In all of these cases isolation will not be applied.

Quarantine. The detention of susceptible individuals who have been exposed to a communicable disease is called quarantine. These individuals are often spoken of as "contacts." Nonsusceptible people are not included as contacts. Quarantine is infrequently used in disease control at present because the individual is rarely in a communicable state during the incubation period of a disease. As a consequence, not until first symptoms appear does the individual represent a danger, and, at this point, isolation can be imposed. Measles and chickenpox are exceptions in that they may be communicable during the last 2 or 3 days of the incubation period. However, even in the case of these two diseases, quarantine is of questionable control value.

When quarantine is imposed, the period of time is based on laboratory findings, the maximum incubation period, or both. Thus if several laboratory specimens are negative, the person is released from quarantine, or if the usual incubation period for the disease in question is 7 days, then after the seventh day following exposure to the disease the subject is released from quarantine if no disease symptoms are exhibited.

Reducing communicability. Treatment of a patient limits the reservoir and therefore represents an important procedure in communicable disease control. Medical treatment of patients can be highly effective in reducing communicability of certain diseases. Through the use of chemotherapy and antibiotics, syphilis can be rendered noncommunicable.

Reservoir eradication

Logically, the most permanent and thus the most desirable measure of communicable disease control would be the complete elimination of the reservoir. This is possible when the lower animals serve as reservoirs of organisms pathogenic to humans. Bovine tuberculosis has been eliminated in the United States by an orderly widespread program of testing cattle and then slaughtering those that are reactors. A similar program now under way seeks to eliminate all lower animals harboring *Brucella* organisms and thereby prevent undulant fever in humans.

Paradoxically, the principle of reservoir eradication can be applied to the human: not the entire individual but the particular organ harboring infectious organisms is eliminated. This procedure is directed to the carriers of disease. The major obstacle in the promotion of this program lies in the unwillingness of carriers to submit to the necessary surgery. A high percentage of typhoid carriers are rendered a noncarrier by the removal of the gallbladder. Health officials and the family physician can explain to the carrier that there is a strong likelihood that, by having the gallbladder removed, the carrier may no longer have to be bound by restrictions imposed by health regulations. However, no absolute guarantee can be made that the surgery will eliminate the source of typhoid bacilli in the carrier.

Sanitation

Environmental control measures are directed toward the vehicles of disease transfer and are effective in limiting the spread of such diseases of the intestinal tract as hepatitis, typhoid, paratyphoid, dysentery, salmonellosis, staphylococcus infection, and cholera. In the control of these diseases, the application of the principles of sanitation of water supplies, milk, and other foods and to sewage disposal has played an important role in the reduction of the incidence of alvine discharge diseases since the beginning of the century. Sanitation has been effective also as a measure in controlling vector-borne diseases such as malaria and yellow fever. By destroying the breeding places of the vectors and by the use of effective insecticides, programs in sanitation can effectively control the spread of insect-borne diseases.

Sanitation is ineffective and of little value in the control of such respiratory diseases as measles, chickenpox, scarlet fever, streptococcus sore throat, diphtheria, smallpox, and pertussis. Decontamination measures may possibly be of some value in preventing spread of the respiratory diseases, although their actual effectiveness has never been scientifically determined. Concurrent decontamination and terminal decontamination are still practiced on the assumption that contaminated fomites may, under certain circumstances, be a mode of respiratory disease transmission.

Increasing resistance of new host

Even though organisms of sufficient number and virility to establish infection should invade a new host, measures still may be taken to pro-

tect the host and prevent further spread of the disease. Passive immunization can give transient emergency protection. Before this procedure is employed, it must be ascertained that the person actually was exposed and is susceptible to the disease. Because passive immunization lasts but a few weeks, it provides only a stopgap for a particular situation when no other measures are feasible. Passive immunization has one marked disadvantage in that the serum usually used may sensitize the individual so as to set up the future danger of an anaphylaxis— extreme reaction to a second exposure to the foreign serum. For this reason, passive immunization is not regarded as a good community project to be used on a widespread basis. In practice, it is used only for selected cases.

Modification of the severity of a disease should be regarded as a control measure. Dis-

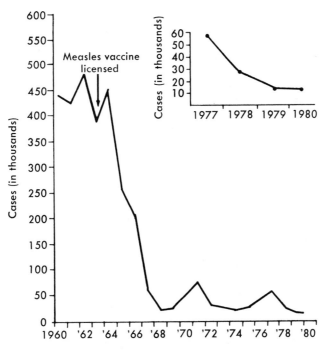

FIG. 10-5. Reported cases of measles, United States, 1960-1980.

From Centers for Disease Control, Public Health Service: Morbidity and Mortality Weekly Report **29***(49):660, Dec. 12, 1980; and* **29***(52):690, Jan. 9, 1981.*

eases such as diphtheria and scarlet fever can be modified by treatment, and by this procedure communicability can be reduced.

From the practical standpoint, the obvious approach is to immunize all prospective new hosts. This means artificial immunization of all children against such diseases as diphtheria, pertussis, and poliomyelitis.

Immunization of children and adults has provided the most dramatic examples of epidemiological control of infectious diseases, as in the example of smallpox eradication, which combined immunization with isolation and quarantine. More exclusive use of immunization has accounted for the spectacular drops in poliomyelitis and measles in the past 20 years, as illustrated for measles in the United States in Fig. 10-5. Measles is now a candidate for possible eradication, at least in some countries.

No communicable disease control program will be perfect. The application of present knowlege, methods, and techniques can yield a near-perfect result. Any communicable disease control program requires constant effort and analysis. What has proved to be effective will be continued. What can be improved will be changed. The decline in the incidence and death rates of the various infectious diseases is mute evidence that society has devised successful, although not perfect, means for preventing disease spread. Effective though present measures may be, there is still room for improvement, although public health workers do not expect to see the millenium when no infectious disease plagues society.

DISEASE CONTROL RESOURCES AND MEASURES

Many individuals and agencies serve in one capacity or another in the control of communicable diseases. Legal authority for the control of communicable diseases rests with the official health agencies, yet the medical profession, the hospitals, clinics, voluntary health agencies, and the schools all play important roles in disease control. In practice, official health agencies welcome the cooperation and assistance of individuals and agencies competent to assist in the general problem of disease control. Health education of the public is fundamental to effective communicable disease control measures, and official health agencies recognize that the supplementary health education contributed by other agencies is highly valuable in the general control program. Indeed, health education of the public represents the primary approach of the official health agencies in controlling diseases. In the philiosophy of modern community health, a department of health that must rely continually on its legal authority for an effective program would be regarded as an outdated and ineffective agency.

Personal hygiene and health habits

Individual behavior continues to be a factor in infectious diseases, particularly among those spread by person-to-person contact. Evidence for the continuing importance of proper hygienic measures is illustrated by outbreaks of illness associated with improper food handling both in private homes and institutions. Correct use of condoms is an effective measure in the prevention of sexually transmitted diseases. Similarly, simple handwashing techniques will prevent the transmission of many bacterial illnesses in both the hospital and the home.

Certain practices such as smoking, alcohol consumption, poor nutrition, drug misuse, and stress place people at increased risk for acquisition of infectious diseases and subsequent morbidity and mortality. Alcoholics are known to be at higher risk for several infectious diseases, including pneumonia (e.g., *Klebsiella pneumoniae*). Smokers are at risk, in particular, for pulmonary diseases such as bronchitis and pneumonia. Drug addicts are at risk both for hepatitis B and for endocarditis (most commonly caused by staphylococcal infection). Poor nutrition, particularly in children, puts them at risk for gastroenteritis and respiratory illnesses, secondary to infectious pathogens. Finally, studies indicate that stress will put people at risk for many kinds of illness, including infectious diseases.

Community health education and health promotion programs directed at these health practices and life-styles will contribute to the control of infectious diseases, even though this may not be the primary objective of such programs. Community health education interventions designed to support behavior conducive to infectious disease control could occur at any of the following five steps when people (1) become more susceptible (life-style behavior), (2) become exposed (hygienic behavior), (3) become infected (protective or prophylactic behavior), (4) become symptomatic (seeking medical care), or (5) suffer complications or relapses (adherence to prescribed medical regimens). These first three steps are primary prevention steps, and the last two are secondary prevention steps.

The need for immunization against typhoid fever and Rocky Mountain spotted fever should be determined by the prevalence in a specific area or of special danger to particular individuals such as nurses, public health workers, or foresters.

Community education

Fundamental to the effectiveness of any measures designed to control communicable disease is an effective continuous program of community health education. Government authority is necessary but not sufficient for a high level of effective disease control.

Public awareness. A community health education program that is keeping its citizens informed about the nature, spread, and control of communicable diseases will have ready a highly potent means to check the spread of any infectious disease that may break out. Knowledge not only helps in the prevention of disease but also in the proper control when disease does occur. In addition, a well-informed public will not be stampeded by scare rumors or fantastic reports such as fatal reactions to immunization. Further, a good community health education program will assist in obtaining funds for the promotion of immunization and other control measures. Community health education means combining various resources available. The printed word, the spoken word, visual aids, and demonstrations can be employed. The need is not an appeal to the emotions but an appeal to reason through understanding and an appreciation of the obligation to one's community, neighbors, family, and oneself.

Official health agencies in the United States

Legal responsibility and authority for the control of communicable diseases rests with the tax-supported agencies on the national, state, and community level.

Public Health Service. The Public Health Service of the U.S. Department of Health and Human Services has responsibility for the prevention of disease coming from outside the country. This encompasses international quarantine of harbors and air fields. In addition, the Public Health Service has responsibility and authority for the prevention of spread of disease between states. In this capacity the Public Health Service has jurisdiction over travel of infected persons as well as the shipment of infected animals and contaminated articles such as meat. In addition, the Public Health Service has supervision over the shipment of biologics via interstate carriers. The Public Health Service also grants assistance to states in dealing with severe epidemics of special disease problems. This is more a professional service courtesy than a legal obligation. Similar federal or central agencies serve these national functions in other countries.

State health departments. Communicable disease control measures within states are through their divisions of communicable diseases, laboratory services, and sanitation. State sanitary codes set up provisions for isolation and quarantine, vaccination, reporting of communicable diseases, examination of school children, exclusions from school, hospitalization standards, treatment of syphilis, protection of water supplies, disposal of human wastes, and protection of foods for sale. The state health department laboratory serves the medical profession and other qualified individuals in the diagnosis of disease and in the termination of isolation when laboratory tests are of value. In addition, routine laboratory services such as water and milk analysis are valuable in disease control. The state health department gives assistance to local health agencies when severe epidemics occur or when special disease problems exist. Under most circumstances the state health department has authority to step into a local situation only on invitation from the local health authorities.

Local health agencies. District, county, and city governments touch the individual citizen and, because of their close relationship with the people, represent the most important and most effective resources for disease control. Community health agencies may set up their own communicable disease regulations or codes to exercise within their own boundaries. These regulations may not be in conflict with the state regulations nor establish lower standards than those of the state regulations, but the local standards may be higher than those of the state. Essential to an effective program of local control, the health department must have an informed public and must work cooperatively with the medical profession, the schools, and all other agencies and individuals having a role in the control of communicable diseases.

Physicians' reporting of communicable disease cases is made as easy and effective as possible. As a practical measure, physicians use the telephone in reporting diseases, particularly the more serious diseases. Official isolation of a patient is done through the attending physician, who also is contacted concerning the release of the patient from isolation. A health department representative informs the family of official isolation requirements and usually places responsibility on the family for the observance of these requirements.

The most difficult disease control problems arise when no physician has been called. However, health department staff members, through their contacts in the community, will usually have information channeled to them about families having illness. Public health nurses particularly will get such information and will visit the reported family. In addition to the information they may give the family on the care of the illness, they will also likely refer the matter to one of the medical physicians on the health staff, who will make the necessary diagnosis for official control purposes.

Communicable disease control measures on the local level must be carried out every day of the year. Educating the community in the prevention and control of disease is a never-ending task. It goes on when there is not a single known case of infectious disease in the community as well as when an epidemic exists. It requires the promotion of immunization, particularly of infants and preschool children. It calls for constant attention to the community water supply, sewage disposal, food handling, and vector control. It involves special programs at different times of the year when seasonable communicable diseases are most prevalent. Communicable disease control is but one phase of the total official community health program, but it commands the best efforts of the local health department.

Schools

Within their own premises, schools have the legal authority and the responsibility to take reasonable measures for the prevention and control of communicable diseases. In cooperation with the local health department, the medical profession, and the parents, the school can contribute to the control of communicable disease by the promotion of immunization, the early recognition of signs of infectious disease, and the effective control of exclusions from school and readmissions to school. This requires school personnel who are versed in the fundamentals of communicable disease control and who have an appreciation of the schools' obligation to the students, the family, and the community in controlling infectious disease.

In general, immunization as a requirement for admission to school is regarded as a local measure and is left to the discretion of local school boards. Courts have upheld the right of a local board of education to require immunization as a condition for school admission when exceptions are made on religious grounds. As a general practice, the local board of education requires immunization against diphtheria, pertussis, tetanus, measles, rubella, and poliomyelitis as a requisite for school entrance.

Through inspections, reviews, and observations of children, teachers are able to detect early indications of possible communicable disease. Early detection of disease will result in early isolation of the pupil with greater protection to other youngsters in the school. The child with indications of communicable disease should be segregated immediately. An emergency rest room should be available where the child can lie comfortably on a cot. Parents are usually informed by telephone that their youngster is not feeling well, and it is suggested to them that the youngster be brought home. Informing the parents and enlisting their confidence and cooperation in the exclusion of the child is a desirable courtesy. However, the school has a responsibility to exclude any youngster who appears to have a communicable disease. This principle is clearly stated in the case of Stone v. Probst, in which the court said: "Pupils who are suffering or appear to be suffering from a communicable disease may menace the well-being of all pupils and therefore should be denied the privilege of school attendance."* After the child has been taken home by a member of the school staff or other designated person, responsibility for futher isolation of the youngster legally rests

*Supreme Court of the State of Minnesota, 165 Minn., 1925, 361,206 NW 642; appeal from the District Court, Hennepin County.

with the local health department. Consequently, the school keeps the local health department informed on all matters relating to the illness of children who have been excluded from school. A high degree of cooperation betweeen school and health department is necessary if the interests of the community are to be served best by both agencies.

In the event of an epidemic, the school works cooperatively with the community health department and is governed by the regulations and recommendations of the health department staff. In practice both health and school officials are reluctant to close the schools during an epidemic. Usually, with the schools in session, it is easier to control the spread of disease through morning and noon inspections of the children and constant observation throughout the day. Likewise, the opening of school in the fall is not delayed because of an epidemic. Experience has demonstrated that opening the schools and applying control measures that include the school are as effective as any other means for limiting the spread of disease. Occasionally, for efficiency reasons, a school may be closed when such a high percentage of youngsters is absent that the schoolwork will have to be repeated for the benefit of those who were absent. As an illustration, more than 70% of the students in a high school were absent because of influenza on a Wednesday. After consultation with the health department, school officials closed the school until the following Monday. This, however, was an education or economic measure rather than a communicable disease control measure.

Voluntary health agencies

In the United States all non-tax-supported voluntary health agencies that receive their financial support from private sources have neither a legal responsibility nor, strictly speaking, an official status except as they may be incorporated under the laws of a state or otherwise recognized. Yet the voluntary health agencies serve an important role in communicable disease control. Normally, a voluntary health agency is organized to deal with one specific health problem or a disease. From its founding, the National Tuberculosis and Respiratory Disease Association, now the American Lung Association, devoted itself to public health education by keeping the public informed and urging the public to take certain measures. As a supplement to this basic public health education program, the American Lung Association has sponsored testing programs and research. On the local level, the state associations in many instances have branched out into the broader field of health education, encompassing fields other than tuberculosis. Through the years, the efforts of this voluntary agency have contributed measurably to the battle against tuberculosis, even though it has never undertaken to contribute financially or otherwise to the treatment of patients. Its mission is now devoted to a broader range of lung diseases, having reduced the incidence of tuberculosis by about 5% per year.

The National Foundation, almost from its outset, has given direct financial assistance to families having a member afflicted with poliomyelitis. The National Foundation has also promoted research and an extensive public health education program. Its March of Dimes revenues are now devoted to a broad range of birth defects, again because its original mission in communicable diseases has been largely accomplished. Several other national and local voluntary health agencies in the United States also contribute to community communicable disease control programs. In the main, their contribution has been that of educating the public and supporting the official and other health agencies engaged in matters of health that include disease control.

Medical resources

Health professions. The keystone in the entire communicable disease control program is the practicing professionals who diagnose and

supervise the disease case. In the treatment and supervision of the patient and in instructions to the patient's family, physicians and nurses represent the first line of defense against the spread of communicable disease. Further, through advocacy of immunization and by immunizing as a routine part of medical service to the family, the practicing health professional daily makes an invaluable contribution to communicable disease control in the community.

Clinics and hospitals. A special arm in the community communicable disease control program is represented by the clinical and hospital services that exist in the community. Clinics, whether of the broad service type or of a specialized nature, serve as an immunizing and diagnostic service for special tests or other highly specialized techniques. The availability of such a medical center lends confidence and assurance to the public and community health service alike that the highest level of medical skill is available when a crisis or other unusual situation arises. Special immunization clinics may be set up when an epidemic threatens. An outbreak of typhoid fever may justify setting up immunization clinics. This is particularly true during disasters such as floods.

Hospitals may not be an indispensable agency in communicable disease control, because most patients with a communicable disease remain at home. However, circumstances may arise that make it not only highly desirable but imperative that a patient be hospitalized.

Prevention-promotion measures for immunizable diseases

Education and information measures. Community health education should include the following: provide useful immunization information to all mothers and new parents through hospitals, physicians, and others; aim educational programs at members of the health care professions; include discussion of immunization and preventive measures in school health curricula; enlist day-care centers, senior citizen centers, and churches to provide immunization information to parents and to older people; use the mass media for immunization activities; and continue the use of volunteers.

Service measures. Community health centers and other medical care settings can contribute to the control of immunizable diseases by adopting standardized official immunization records; developing and using "tickler" and recall systems to ensure that children return for immunizations on schedule; making immunizations available without financial barriers in all health care settings as a part of comprehensive health services; and continuing the use of indigenous volunteers.

Legislative and regulatory measures. Further organizational supports should include the following: enforcing existing school immunization requirements and extending them to include children at all grade levels in both public and private schools, as well as in organized preschool settings; including coverage of immunization as a health insurance benefit not subject to deductible provisions; requiring carriers under any national health insurance plan to reimburse for immunization services; requiring immunization as a condition of employment (e.g., in health care institutions); and including rubella immunization as a service routinely offered in family planning clinics, primary care clinics, and hospitals.

Economic measures. Related economic supports for vaccine-related behavior include reimbursing for immunizations under public and private health insurance plans; providing vaccines free to all health care providers as long as they do not charge for it; and providing economic incentives to health care providers and vaccine recipients.

Relative strength of the measures. The uniform and forceful implementation of school immunization requirements is one of the most effective means of improving immunization levels currently available. Enforcement of such requirements to the point of exclusion from school has resulted in the highest achievable immunization levels of school children and the lowest reported levels of diseases such as measles. One problem with this measure is that it does not assure that all preschool children are adequately immunized before the time of entry to school. Other potential regulatory measures, such as immunization requirements for employment in hospitals, address specific problems in selected population groups and are less effective.

Continuing education and motivation of the general public and health providers about the need to continue routine immunization and the accompanying need to accept the minimal risk of severe complications associated with some vaccines are essential to maintain and extend prevention of these diseases. Experience developed from the recent Childhood Immunization Initiative in the United States has demonstrated the importance of mass media and volunteer promotion of routine immunization to parents and children.

• • •

That society has made progress in the battle against infectious diseases is apparent. To be lulled into the complacent frame of mind that the battle has been won would be foolhardy and even tragic. The battle against infectious diseases goes on, day in and out. Research must find answers to many problems and questions as yet unsolved. In the meantime, communities employ the knowledge, methods, and techniques now available and thus hold the incidence of infectious diseases to a practical minimum.

U.S. OBJECTIVES FOR 1990

The practical minimum to which the incidence of communicable diseases can be brought is best expressed in the form of quantifiable goals or objectives for some specified date in the future. The goals in *Promoting*

Health, Preventing Disease: Objectives for the Nation (1980), recently developed by the Public Health Service, can be interpolated to represent achievable 10 year averages for communities in nontropical countries of the Western world. The objectives for the decade in relation to infectious disease control, immunization, and sexually transmitted diseases are listed under five levels of outcome. The logic is a hierarchy of objectives beginning with ultimate health status improvements and working back through (1) improved health behaviors or reduced risk factors required to achieve health status; (2) improved public and professional awareness, knowledge, beliefs, or attitudes required to predispose appropriate health behavior; (3) improved services, incentives, or protection required to enable or reinforce appropriate behavior or risk factor control; and (4) improved surveillance and evaluation systems required to track the progress of programs or detect outbreaks of new problems.

Improved health status

- By 1990 the annual incidence of hepatitis B should be reduced to 20 per 100,000 population. (In 1978 it was estimated to be 45 per 100,000 population.)
- By 1990 the annual incidence of reported tuberculosis should be reduced to 18,700. (In 1980 it was 27,000 or 8 per 100,000.)
- By 1990 the annual incidence of reported pneumococcal pneumonia should be reduced to 115 per 100,000 population. (In 1978 it was estimated at 182 per 100,000 population.)
- By 1990 the annual incidence of bacterial meningitis should be reduced to 6 per 100,000 population. (In 1978 it was estimated at 8.2 per 100,000 population.)
- By 1990 the (risk factor–specific) incidence of nosocomial infections in acute care hospitals should be reduced by 20% to 4% all admissions and by a similar percentage in long-term care and residential

care facilities. (In 1979 5% of all patients suffered nosocomial infections.)
- By 1990 reported measles incidence should be reduced to less than 500 cases per year—all imported or within two generations of importation. (In 1980 there were 13,430 measles cases reported.)
- By 1990 reported mumps incidence should be reduced to less than 1,000 cases per year. (In 1980 there were 8,531 mumps cases reported.)
- By 1990 reported rubella incidence should be reduced to less than 1,000 cases per year. (In 1980 there were 3,837 rubella cases reported.)
- By 1990 reported congenital rubella syndrome incidence should be reduced to less than 10 cases per year. (In 1979 there were 48 new cases of congenital rubella syndrome born.)
- By 1990 reported diphtheria incidence should be reduced to less than 50 cases per year. (In 1979 there were 65 diphtheria cases reported, but this objective was already achieved by 1980 when there were only 5 reported cases of diphtheria.)
- By 1990 reported pertussis incidence should be reduced to less than 1,000 cases per year. (In 1980 there were 1,651 pertussis cases reported.)
- By 1990 reported tetanus incidence should be reduced to less than 50 cases per year. (In 1980 there were 74 tetanus cases reported.)
- By 1990 reported poliomyelitis incidence should be less than 10 cases per year. (In 1980 there were only 9 poliomyelitis cases reported.)
- By 1990 reported gonorrhea incidence should be reduced to less than 700,000 cases per year. (In 1980 there were 1,012,835 cases reported.)
- By 1990 reported incidence of gonococcal pelvic inflammatory disease should be reduced to 75,000 cases per year. (In 1978

estimated cases per year were 150,000.)

- By 1990 reported incidence of primary and secondary syphilis should be reduced to 17,500 cases per year, with a reduction in congenital syphilis to 60 cases per year. (In 1979 the reported incidence of primary syphilis was 22,000 cases per year, while reported congenital syphilis was 105 cases per year.)
- By 1990 the incidence of serious neonatal and maternal infection (e.g., disseminated herpes encephalitis, chlamydial pneumonia) due to sexually transmitted agents, especially herpes and chlamydia, should be reduced to 350 cases of disseminated neonatal herpes and 15,000 cases of neonatal chlamydial pneumonia. (In 1979 about 700 cases of disseminated neonatal herpes and 30,000 cases of chlamydial pneumonia were esimated to have occurred.)
- By 1990 the incidence of nongonococcal urethritis and chlamydial infections should be reduced to 1,875,000. (In 1979 2,500,000 cases were estimated to have occurred.)

Reduced risk factors

- By 1990 the proportion of sexually active men and women who are protected by properly used condoms should increase to 25% of those at high risk of acquiring a sexually transmitted disease. (In 1979 the estimated share was less than 10%.)

Increased public-professional awareness

- By 1990 each junior and senior high school student should be receiving accurate, timely education about sexually transmitted diseases. (Currently, 70% of school systems provide some information about sexually transmitted diseases but the quality and timing of the communication varies greatly.)
- By 1985 all health care providers seeing suspected cases of sexually transmitted diseases should be capable of genital herpes diagnosis by culture, therapy (if available), and patient education; hepatitis B diagnosis among homosexual men, prevention through a vaccine (when proved efficacious), and patient education; and nongonococcal urethritis diagnosis, therapy, and patient education. (Baseline data are unavailable.)
- By 1990 prior to leaving the hospital, all mothers of newborns should receive instruction on immunization schedules for their babies. (Baseline data are unavailable.)

Improved services-protection

- By 1990 95% of licensed patient care facilities should be applying the recommended practices for controlling nosocomial infections. (Baseline data are unavailable.)
- By 1990 surveillance and control systems should be capable of responding to and containing (1) newly recognized diseases and unexpected epidemics of public health significance and (2) infections introduced from foreign countries.
- By 1990 at least 60% of people in populations designated as high-risk targets should be immunized within 5 years of licensure of new vaccines. Potential candidates include otitis media (*Streptococcus pneumoniae* and *Hemophilus influenzae*); selected respiratory and enteric viruses; meningitis (group B *Neisseria meningitidis*, *S. pneumoniae*, and *H. influenzae*).
- By 1990 at least 90% of all children by age 2 should have completed their basic immunization series—measles, mumps, rubella, polio, diphtheria, pertussis, and tetanus. (In 1978 completion varied from 50% to 90%.)
- By 1990 at least 95% of children attending licensed day-care centers and kindergarten through twelfth grades should be fully immunized. (In 1979 the immunization level was about 90% for first school entrants and lower overall.)

- By 1990 at least 60% of high-risk populations should be receiving annual immunization against influenza. (In 1979 about 20% of high-risk populations were immunized.)
- By 1990 at least 60% of high-risk populations should have received vaccination against pneumococcal pneumonia. (Baseline data are unavailable.)
- By 1990 at least 50% of people in populations designated as targets should be immunized within 5 years of first licensure of new vaccines. (It currently ranges up to 9 years.)
- By 1985 the nation should have a system in place to mount mass immunization programs in the face of possible epidemics of influenza or other epidemic diseases for which vaccines may exist.
- By 1990 no comprehensive health insurance policies should exclude immunizations. (Baseline data are unavailable.)
- By 1990 one half of major industries and governmental agencies will be providing sexually transmitted disease services (education and appropriate testing) within their health promotion–disease prevention programs. (Baseline data are unavailable.)

Improved surveillance-evaluation systems

- By 1990 data-reporting systems in all states should be able to monitor trends of common infectious agents not now subject to traditional public health surveillance (respiratory illnesses, gastrointestinal illnesses, otitis media) and to measure the impact of these agents on health care cost and productivity at the local and state levels and by extension at the national level.
- By 1990 the extent of epidemics of respiratory and enteric viral illnesses should be predicted within 2 weeks after they appear through community-wide sentinel surveillance systems.
- By 1990 all state health departments should be linked by a computer system to federal health agencies for routine collection, analysis and dissemination of surveillance data, rapid communication of messages, and epidemic aid investigations.
- By 1990 laboratories throughout the country should be linked for monitoring infectious agents and antibiotic resistance patterns and for disseminating information.
- By 1990 at least 95% of all children through age 18 should have up-to-date official immunization records in a uniform format that uses uniform definitions of completion at immunization. (Baseline data are unavailable.)
- By 1990 surveillance systems should be sufficiently improved so that at least 90% of those hospitalized and 50% of those not hospitalized with vaccine preventable diseases of childhood are reported, and that uniform case definitions are used nationwide. (Baseline data are unavailable.)
- By 1985 data in statistical aggregates should be available and sufficient to determine the occurrence of nongonococcal urethritis, genital herpes, and other sexually transmitted diseases in each local area and to recommend approaches for preventing sexually transmitted diseases and their complications.

COMMUNITY OBJECTIVES

To translate the U.S. goals for 1990 to community health program plans, the following exercise is recommended for application by the student or local health planner in a specific community. The appropriate year between now and 1990 can be inserted and target levels of disease prevention or program accomplishment specified. Implementation plans should follow from these specific objectives.

Immunization

- By 19__ the incidence of (insert name of each officially designated vaccine-preventable disease) will not exceed _____, or the absence of disease will be maintained.

- By 19___ and in each succeeding year, at least 90% of the 2-year-old population will have completed primary immunization for the officially designated vaccine-preventable diseases.
- By 19___ and for each succeeding year, all school enterers will have complied with one of the following alternatives: (1) 100% of primary and appropriate booster immunizations complete, (2) remedial course to bring immunizations up to 100% has been initiated and certified by an appropriate provider, (3) Exemption for medical or religious reasons from immunization requirements.
- By 19___ the community will be served by a system to monitor the immunization status of at least the following subgroups: 2-year-olds, school enterers, or older children (e.g., secondary school attendees).
- By 19___ the community will be served by a system that ensures that individuals in need of vaccine for particular vaccine-preventable diseases (e.g., tetanus, influenza, rabies) receive them.
- By 19___ the community will be served by a system to detect rubella antibody deficiency in women and to encourage their immunity before conception.
- By 19___ the community will be served by a public awareness program concerning the need for primary and booster immunizations.

Sexually transmitted diseases

- By 19___ the incidence of _____*_____ will not exceed _____ .
- By 19___ each community will be served

by a program for the control of sexually transmitted diseases that includes oversight, planning, and evaluation; consultation to physicians and others in clinics and the community; and recognition of situations and cases requiring extraordinary attention.

- By 19___ the community will be served by a system for the routine reporting of all new cases of syphilis.
- By 19___ the community will be served by a system for estimating the incidence, prevalence, and demographic characteristics of its gonorrhea cases.
- By 19___ the community will be served by a system that assesses the extent of and potential need for a program to control sexually transmitted diseases other than syphilis and gonorrhea (e.g., genital herpes, nongonococcal urethritis and cervicitis, sexually transmitted hepatitis).
- By 19___ the community will be served by qualified staff members to interview and conduct contact investigations of every reported case of infectious and recently infectious syphilis and to determine reasons for the occurrence of congenital syphilis under 1 year of age.
- By 19___ all locatable people with infectious syphilis will be interviewed within 3 days of reporting, and 75% of contacts will be brought to examination within 2 weeks of the case report.
- By 19___ the community will be served by a procedure for bringing contacts of gonorrhea cases to diagnosis or treatment.
- By 19___ there will be readily identifiable clinical resources conveniently available for the confidential diagnosis and treatment of the sexually transmitted diseases.
- By 19___ at least one readily identifiable sexually transmitted disease information and referral system will be found within the community.
- By 19___ provision will be made for diagnosis and treatment services for all citi-

---

*Insert the name of the specific sexually transmitted disease, for example, syphilis, including congenital syphilis; gonorrhea, including ophthalmia neonatorum; nongonococcal urethritis and cervicitis; genital herpes; sexually transmitted hepatitis; or other diseases as appropriate.

zens, including minors, under which plan cost is not a deterrent to needed service.

- By 19___ all health care providers seeing suspected cases of sexually transmitted disease will have been provided the latest officially recommended practices for diagnosis and treatment.
- By 19___ sexually transmitted disease treatment services will include surveillance for treatment failures.
- By 19___ persons suspected of having been exposed to a sexually transmitted disease will be counseled concerning its causes, dangers, and prevention.
- By 19___ education about sexually transmitted disease, including but not limited to causes, signs and symptoms, prevention, treatment, and personal hygiene, should be incorporated into the educational curriculum for all junior and senior high school students and be a part of an organized community health education program directed toward high-risk groups (e.g., college students, homosexuals).
- By 19___ the community will be served by a mechanism to assure the availability of gonorrhea screening for high-risk persons.

Tuberculosis

- By 19___ the new tuberculosis case rate will not exceed _____ .
- By 19___ at least 95% of new positive sputum tuberculosis cases reported will be negative within 6 months.
- By 19___ each community will be served by an agency responsible for overall tuberculosis prevention and control activities, including maintenance of surveillance system and case registry to ensure reporting of positive bacteriology from laboratories and prompt reporting of cases from private physicians and medical care facilities; development of effective monitoring systems to evaluate the quality and effectiveness of tuberculosis activities; consultation with

physicians and others in the community; collection and analysis of surveillance assessment data; and coordination of overall tuberculosis control activities in the community, including recommendations on the allocation of resources.

- By 19___ outpatient tuberculosis care services will be accessible to the community, and acute and long-term care facilities will be identified, accessible, and available.
- By 19___ at least 90% of all patients for whom two or more drugs are recommended will complete their prescribed therapy.
- By 19___ at least 90% of infected close contacts and other high-risk tuberculin-positive individuals will be placed on preventive therapy and will complete the recommended course of therapy.
- By 19___ for close contacts of infectious cases, at least ___ % of those under 15 years of age will be placed on preventive therapy, regardless of tuberculin status, and will complete the recommended course of therapy.

QUESTIONS AND EXERCISES

1. What distinction can be made between infectious disease and communicable disease?
2. Evaluate this statement: "If effective methods of immunization were developed for all of the communicable disease, humankind would eliminate the communicable diseases with which it is now plagued."
3. Recall three recent outbreaks of communicable disease you observed or otherwise were acquainted with. Do you class these outbreaks as endemic, epidemic, or pandemic?
4. What communicable respiratory diseases are most likely to appear in epidemic form in your community?
5. What disease do you predict will cause the next world-wide pandemic?
6. To what extent is there justificatication for saying that an epidemic is evidence of an inadequate public health education program?
7. Is pasteurization of the community milk supply less necessary today than it was 30 years ago?
8. Enumerate the various services your health depart-

ment provides in its communicable disease control program. Use the community objectives from the preceding pages as a checklist.

9. What are the various organizations or agencies in your community contributing to communicable disease control?

10. What steps should an ordinary citizen take when he or she has evidence that a case of communicable disease may exist in a household where no physician has been called and no precautions are being taken to prevent possible spread of the disease?

11. What is being done and what further should be done in your community to prevent the spread of communicable diseases via foods other than milk or water?

12. From the standpoint of public health education, how would you change this prevailing attitude: "It's just a cold"?

13. Why should passive immunization be rejected as a community-wide procedure?

14. An individual diagnosed, with laboratory confirmation, as having syphilis refused free treatment and was isolated in the county jail. Evaluate the action taken by the county health department.

15. What disadvantages in respect to communicable disease control does a democracy have that a dictatorship does not have?

16. Why does undulant fever exist in the United States, when slaughtering all brucella-infected cattle, swine, and goats would prevent the disease in humans?

17. Is there any evidence that new infectious diseases are appearing?

18. Design an experiment or study to show whether non-fatal infections shorten life expectancy.

19. Make a general comparison of the incidence of communicable disease cases and deaths in the United States in 1980 and predicted in 2000.

20. Estimate the date by which selected community objectives not already accomplished in your community might be expected to be accomplished. Consult with appropriate officials and health professionals to justify your estimate.

BIBLIOGRAPHY

American Public Health Association: Control of communicable diseases in man, ed. 13, New York, 1981, The Association.

Burton, L.E., and Smith, H.H.: Public health and community medicine for the allied medical professions, ed. 3, Baltimore, The Williams & Wilkens Co.

Centers for Disease Control, Public Health Service: Model standards for community preventive health services, a report to the U.S. Congress from the Secretary of Health, Education, and Welfare, Atlanta, 1979.

Centers for Disease Control, Public Health Service: Morbidity and Mortality Weekly Report 30(1): entire issue, 1981.

Green, L.W., Wilson, R.W., and Bauer, K.G.: Objectives for the nation in disease prevention and health promotion and requirements to measure our progress. Proceedings of the 18th National Meeting of the Public Health Conference on Records and Statistics: New challenges for vital and health records, Washington, D.C., 1980, National Center for Health Statistics, DHHS Pub. No. (PHS) 81-1214.

Krugman, S., and Katz, S.L.: Infectious diseases of children, ed. 7, St. Louis, 1981, The C.V. Mosby Co.

Lilienfeld, A.M.: Foundations of epidemiology, ed. 2, New York, 1980, Oxford University Press, Inc.

National Center Health Statistics: Facts at your fingertips: a guide to sources of statistical information on major health topics, vol. 4, Hyattsville, Md., 1980, Public Health Service.

National Center for Health Statistics: Monthly Vital Statistics Report 30(1): entire issue, 1981.

Sartwell, P.E.: Preventive medicine and public health, ed. 2, New York, 1980, Appleton-Century-Crofts.

Top, F.H., and Wehrle, P.F., editors: Communicable and infectious diseases, ed. 8, St. Louis, 1976, The C.V. Mosby Co.

U.S. Bureau of the Census: Directory of federal statistics for local areas: a guide to sources, Washington, D.C., 1981, U.S. Government Printing Office.

U.S. Bureau of Health Planning and Resource Development: Data aquisition and analysis handbook for health planners, 2 vols., Springfield, Va., 1977, National Technical Information Service.

U.S. Department of Health and Human Services, Public Health Service: Promoting health, preventing disease: objectives for the nation, Washington, D.C., 1980.

Weise, F.: Health statistics: a guide to information sources, Health Affairs Information Guide Series, vol. 4, Detroit, 1980, Gale Research Co.

World Health Organization: World health statistics annual, vol. 2: Infectious diseases: cases, deaths, vaccinations, Geneva, 1980, The Organization.

World Health Organization: World health statistics report, vol. 2: Current data, Geneva, 1980, The Organization.

11

COMMUNITY SAFETY AND INJURY CONTROL

As a despoiler of expected years of life, a producer of human misery, a waster of national financial and other economic resources, and a degrader of the quality of human existence, accidents probably rank first among all health problems of American people.

Norvin Kiefer, M.D.
Equitable Life Insurance Company, New York

Many agencies in a community concern themselves with safety, often with a special interest in one aspect such as home, occupational, recreational, motor vehicle, school, or fire safety. These agencies make their most effective contribution to community safety when there is a well-organized, well-integrated community safety program. This is a role and a service the official community health department can provide.

EPIDEMIOLOGY OF INJURIES

Any attempt to quantify the morbidity and mortality associated with injuries is fraught with difficulties. A standardized definition of *injuries* does not exist, nor is there a unified reporting scheme that would allow the consistent analysis of these events. These shortcomings and others make the magnitude of the problem unknown. The establishment of long-range objectives in some communities may have to be deferred until baseline data can be collected and the appropriate injury control methods can be identified.

The preferred term today is *injury control*

rather than *accident prevention* because an accident is an unintentional occurrence that may or may not produce a human injury. Many accidents occur that have no human involvement at all. Community health is concerned with preventing deleterious effects on human populations, in this case, injuries. Some injuries are inflicted intentionally rather than accidentally. Homicide, rape, assault, battery, child abuse, and suicide all inflict injury. Human *injury* is the health problem rather than *accident prevention*, which is not always a health problem. Nor is it always necessary to *prevent* accidents to prevent human injury. Some of the most effective community safety programs are ones that limit the impact of accidents, as in the use of seat belts, rather than preventing the accidents. Three specific types of accidental injuries—falls, burns, and drownings—have been demonstrated to be preventable occurrences. Six special settings or environments (highway, home, farm, occupational, school, and recreational environments) are useful sites in which to concentrate preventive efforts.

Accidental injuries and deaths in the home,

recreational, and farm environments, and those associated with motor vehicles, represent a public health problem of cardinal significance for which no strong national preventive focus exists in many countries. As with disease control problems, morbidity and mortality from injuries are amenable to reduction through an epidemiological and educational approach. A community program employing this type of approach to the prevention and control of accidental injuries in the residential and recreational environments, on farms and in other worksites, on the highway, and in schools will focus on those groups at high risk, most particularly children, adolescents, young adults, the elderly, and those exposed to environments that increase their risk of injury.

Components of a community safety and injury control program should include a surveillance system, epidemiological investigations, standards setting, public education, environmental reforms, and professional training. The primary national role should be one of providing leadership, direction, technical and financial assistance, and information to support injury prevention actions undertaken by state (or provincial) and local health agencies. State or provincial health agencies can serve as the organizational apex to coordinate the flow of resources and expertise. The local community role is one of innovation and implementation of injury prevention techniques.

Community health priorities might appropriately include the following types of injuries: motor vehicle, falls, drownings, burns, and poisonings. Injuries disproportionately affect certain age groups, particularly children, adolescents, young adults, and the elderly. Males suffer a much higher total accidental death rate than do females. The poor suffer a higher proportion of injuries than other income groups.

Accidents are the third leading cause of death in the United States; however, among people aged 1 to 38 years, they are the leading cause of death. Thirty percent of Americans

will be injured each year. Of 95,690 accidental deaths and 9,900,000 disabling injuries in the United States in 1978, the ranking was the following:

	Deaths	Disabling injuries
Motor vehicle	51,500	2,000,000
Home	23,800	3,600,000
Work	4,590	2,300,000
Public recreation	15,800	2,000,000

The ranking for frequency of all accidents was home, work, motor vehicle, and recreation.

Motor vehicle injuries

In the United States there were approximately 18.1 million accidents and 51,900 deaths from motor vehicle accidents in 1979. Motor vehicle mileage was up 4%. The death rate per 100,000,000 vehicle miles was 3.4, a 3% increase from 1976. After more than a decade of steady decline, the traffic fatality rate

TABLE 11-1. Traffic fatality rates in the United States increased in 1977 after a decade of decline*

Year	Deaths	Death rates per 100 million vehicle miles of travel
1965	49,163	5.54
1966	53,041	5.70
1967	52,924	5.50
1968	54,862	5.40
1969	55,791	5.21
1970	54,633	4.88
1971	54,381	4.57
1972	56,278	4.43
1973	55,511	4.24
1974	46,402	3.59
1975	45,853	3.45
1976	46,700	3.31
1977	49,500	3.38
1978	51,500	3.39
1979	51,900	3.40

*From National Safety Council, 1980.

TABLE 11-2. Despite occasional reductions in the annual number and cost of traffic accidents in the United States, the trend continues upward*

Year	Accidents (millions)	Costs (billions of dollars)
1965	13.2	8.9
1966	13.6	10.0
1967	13.7	10.7
1968	14.6	11.3
1969	15.5	12.2
1970	16.0	13.6
1971	16.4	15.8
1972	17.0	19.4
1973	16.6	20.2
1974	15.6	19.3
1975	16.5	21.2
1976	16.8	24.7
1977	17.6	30.5
1978	18.3	34.3
1979	18.1	35.8

*From National Safety council, 1980.

TABLE 11-3. Age distribution of deaths with motor vehicles, United States, 1978*

Age	No. of deaths
0- 4	1,600
5-14	3,200
15-24	19,000
25-44	14,500
45-64	7,700
65-74	3,200
74+	2,700

*From Centers for Disease Control, U.S. Department of Health and Human Services, 1978.

has increased in recent years, as seen in Table 11-1. Disabling injuries in 1978 numbered about 2,000,000. Costs, including wage loss, medical expense, administrative and claim settlement costs of insurance, and property damage amounted to $34.3 billion (Table 11-2).

Over one third of the deaths, were from accidents in urban areas (cities and towns with more than 5,000 population); about two thirds were from accidents in rural areas and towns under 5,000 population. There were approximately 8,800 pedestrian deaths, a 1% increase from 1977, and 43,100 nonpedestrian deaths, an increase of 6% from the 1977 figure. Age distribution of deaths with motor vehicles in 1978 in the United States is shown in Table 11-3.

Age, sex, and alcohol are significant variables in accidents. While psychological factors may also play a role, they are very difficult to separate from cultural and social components of behavior.

Age and sex. Male motor vehicle occupants in the 15- to 24-year age group have an exceptionally high death-to-injury ratio. Age difference in resistance to injury and in the ability to survive a given injury influence the age distribution of injuries and death. As a result, decreased ability to survive crashes is a major factor that causes older persons to be overrepresented among fatally injured drivers. It is important to separate the effect of age on the initiation of an event from the effect of age in the outcome of the event.

Half of all deaths of white males aged 20 to 24 years are caused by injuries. Over one third of all deaths in this age group are caused by automobile accidents alone. The influence of age is demonstrated by comparing the distribution in the 50- to 54-year age group, where only 2.4% of deaths are the result of automobile accidents.

Alcohol. The most important human factor known to be causally related to all types of accidents and a factor in over half of all fatal injuries is alcohol. It is a factor that increases the severity of the outcome and makes it harder for a passenger to escape from a burning or submerging car. It makes emergency treatment difficult and obscures the diagnosis.

Size of vehicle. Statistics in the United States indicate that drivers under age 25 run an 87% greater risk of being injured in a subcompact-

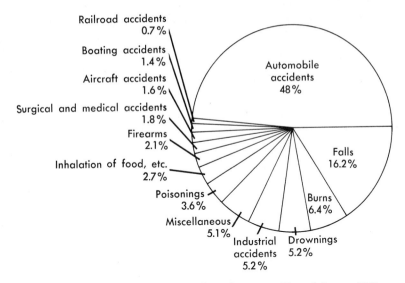

FIG. 11-1. Distribution of fatal accidents by cause, United States, 1971.
Data from Vital Statistics of the United States, vol. 2, 1973.

size car than in a full-size one. Nearly two thirds of the drivers under age 25 already drive small cars in the compact and subcompact classes. About 44% of older drivers do also. All age groups in the United States are expected to suffer increased motor vehicle fatalities with increased use of foreign import cars and as car manufacturers trim weight to meet progressively tougher federal gas mileage requirements and consumer preferences. The nation may well pay for these fuel economics with thousands of additional deaths and injuries, unless people drive less often and shorter distances. Particularly dangerous is the combination of small cars and inexperienced young drivers. Small, lightweight cars do not provide nearly as much crash protection as heavier vehicles. Heavy trucks contributed to 22% of fatal accidents in 1977, behind passenger cars with over 67% involvement in fatal crashes that year. Many of these fatalities were the result of large trucks colliding with passenger vehicles of all sizes.

Under current legislation in the United States, automatic safety equipment will not be required in small cars until 1984. Projecting at today's rates, a continued increase in injury and death rates can be expected until then.

The trend for motorcycle safety is most dramatic with the repeal of helmet laws in many of the states that had previously passed them. The incidence of head injuries is 81% for helmetless cyclists. The case fatality rate among injured cyclists is up 310% over 1978.

Burn injuries

More than 1 million Americans are burned each year, over 60,000 severely enough to be admitted to a hospital. Of those admitted to a hospital, about 15% are likely candidates for intensive burn care. The annual cost of providing intensive burn treatment is about $11,000 per patient. Projection of those figures to the total United States would place annual patient costs of specialized burn treatment at about $100 million.

About two thirds of burn injuries resulting in hospitalization occur in the home, with about one fifth occurring in the workplace. For both injuries and deaths, the first decade of life is a period of high risk. Other high-risk periods are the early working years and the years after 50. Older people experience scalding from bath water because their skin is less sensitive to the heat.

Each year about 5,000 deaths in the United States result from burns and fires—predominantly house fires—and an additional 1,300 Americans die from other kinds of burns such as scalds and electrical burns. Scalds cause about 40% of hospital admissions for burns.

Burn injuries occur about twice as frequently in males, and the rate of occurrence in the black population is about three times that of whites. A simple environmental intervention shown to be effective in reducing scalding in the home is to lower the temperature on hot water heaters. This can be accomplished both through regulation of manufacturers and through community health education.

When the statistics from the United States are compared with those from other industrialized countries, the fire incidents, casualties, and income loss per capita for Americans rank among the highest in the world. (U.S. Department of Commerce, National Fire Prevention and Control Administration, 1978). In addition to the 6,300 burn deaths, about 310,000 persons are injured by burns each year. Dollar losses from fires are estimated at $4.2 billion in direct property loss and $9.4 billion in other costs each year. In terms of years of life lost, burns rank second only to traffic accidents among all accidental causes of death. It is estimated that the years of life lost from burns in the United States each year approach 225,000.

An examination of the main fire killer—residential fires—shows that 56% of the fatal fires and a substantial number of burn injuries are cigarette-related, frequently from people falling asleep while smoking in bed. Painful recovery, disability, and disfigurement are among the tragic consequences.

Fall injuries

In 1978 falls killed 13,690 Americans and injured about 11 million. The mortality from falls has been declining in recent years.

In a study of 28,596 emergency room visits to one hospital, 1,740 (6%) of the visits were the result of injuries resulting from falls. Of these, 1,740 individuals (42%) had at least 1 preexisting health problem (e.g., obesity, cardiovascular disease, arthritis) known to predispose people to falls. Nearly half of children's emergency room visits related to injuries are caused by falls, mostly in the home (Centers for Disease Control, 1978b).

Over half of fatal falls occur in the home; 57% of fatal falls are by people over 75 years of age. Older people who survive falls are more likely to be injured with fractures than are younger people. Alcohol impairment is implicated in many falls.

Violent deaths

Homicide. Next to motor vehicle accidents, injuries from firearms cause the greatest number of violent deaths from traumatic injury in the U.S. population. In 1978 there were 31,000 deaths from gunshot wounds, or about 14 per 100,000 population. By contrast, in England and Wales in 1976 there were fewer than 300 deaths from gunshot wounds, or about 0.6 per 100,000 population.

Striking failures of prevention to date are in reducing the rates of homicides and suicides in the population. Murder is more common among the poor and minority groups. Among the age group 15 to 19 years of age, homicide rates for white males and white females have increased the most (Fig. 11-2). For the male population of races other than white, the age-adjusted rate for homicide peaked in 1972 (83.1 per 100,000); and for those in this population 15 to 19 years of age, the homicide rate peaked in 1971 (60.2 per 100,000). Alcohol, again, is often implicated.

Fig. 11-2 also shows wide differences in rates

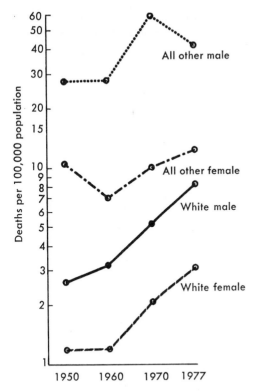

FIG. 11-2. Homicide rates for persons 15 to 19 years of age, according to race and sex, United States, selected years 1950-1977.

From National Center for Health Statistics: Computed by Division of Analysis from data compiled by Division of Vital Statistics, U.S. Department of Health and Human Services, 1980.

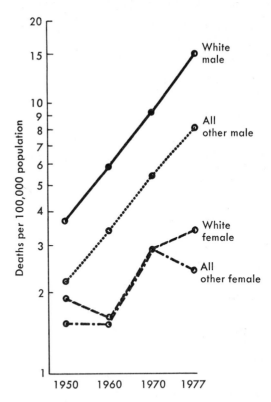

FIG. 11-3. Suicide rates for persons 15 to 19 years of age, according to race and sex, United States, selected years 1950-1977.

From National Center for Health Statistics: Computed by Division of Analysis from data compiled by Division of Vital Statistics, U.S. Department of Health and Human Services, 1980.

according to race and sex. In 1977 young black males were five times more likely to become victims of homicide than young white males, and young black females were more than four times as likely to become victims as were young white females.

From 1960 through 1974, handgun sales quadrupled to more than 6 million a year; during the same period the homicide rate increased from 4.7 per 100,000 to 10.2 for the overall population and from 5.9 to 14.2 for people 15 to 24 years of age.

Suicide. Young white males are at much higher risk of suicide than other males of the same age (Fig. 11-3). As with homicides, young females are at consistently lower risk of suicide. The increase in the rate of suicide is much greater among young males than among young females. Firearm use has been increasing at a much faster rate than other means of suicide. Over half of the 31,000 deaths in 1978 from gunshot wounds in the United States were suicidal.

INTERVENTION TO REDUCE INJURY

Intervention may be directed at the agent, host, or environment. Most effort is directed at the host, for the urge to reform and alter other people's behavior is strong. Investigation frequently reveals the cause of accidents to be human error. Unfortunately, this approach to injury control is the least rewarding of the three available. Consideration of automobile-related injuries illustrates this point. Three classes of people—young males, alcoholic persons, and elderly people—are most likely to be involved in automobile accidents, and these three groups are particularly resistant to education programs. For the amount of effort expended, the results of education programs for the general population are disappointing. Seat belts are used by less than half of the people who have them, despite their recognized efficacy in reducing injury.

Much more rewarding is intervention at the agent level modifying it so that the potential harm is lessened and the product made safer. This has been done to a limited extent in the automobile. Medication containers have been designed so that children cannot open them and poison themselves. Children's pajamas are made of flameproof fabric. Safety is now built into the design of many products. The doctrine of manufacturers' liability for harm resulting from faulty design or operation has done much to accelerate this trend. Legal accountability for products used by the public has forced companies to incorporate safety features. Ralph Nader is recognized for his early crusading efforts on behalf of consumer safety in the United States.

The most effective site of intervention is the environment. The environment should be modified so that it is safe and is designed so that accidents will rarely happen, and that when they do, little harm will result.

Highway environment

The most obvious and familiar example of environment is the highway. By using a wide median strip featuring a sturdy guardrail, fatal accidents can be immediately and permanently reduced. Safe access and exit ramps, clear signs, lighted junctions, and rest areas contribute to safe driving (Table 11-4). Other safety features well known to highway engineers and now available, such as frequently struck highway structures being covered with compressible materials such as a collection of oil drums filled with sawdust, also reduce injuries. This principle can be applied to pedestrian areas, which may be made safe by nonslip surfaces, grading, and lighting. The environment in industrial areas may be modified to increase safety by reduction of air and noise pollution and the use of guardrails. The environmental changes necessary for safety frequently involve enforcement of existing regulations (for example, the 55 mph speed limit in the United States) or enactment of new legislation. Such radical changes need to be preceded by information campaigns to educate the public as to the benefit of the change proposed. Once a measure has been successfully enacted, the people may not appreciate the benefit to the public health that ensues, and such laws are

TABLE 11-4. Classifying highway crashes and countermeasures*

	Human	Vehicle and equipment	Modification of environment
Precrash	Alcoholism control programs	Improved braking ability for heavy trucks	One-way street
Crash	Safety belt usage	Bumpers that reduce crash forces	Removal of unyielding structures from the roadside
Postcrash	Emergency medical care	Extrication	Emergency systems

*Adapted from Haddon, W.: A logical framework for categorizing highway safety pheonomena and activity, J. Trauma **12**(3):193, 1972.

sometimes rescinded. The laws for safety restraints in cars and motorcycle helmets have been reversed in many states in the United States.

Safety belts are effective in preventing injury and death, but only about 30% of automobile occupants in the United States use them. A study by the Highway Safety Research Center of the University of North Carolina demonstrated that lap-belted drivers had 43% fewer serious and fatal injuries than their unbelted counterparts in frontal impact crashes when all crash types and speeds were combined. Australia has reduced crash injuries substantially with the enforcement of mandatory seat belt use.

Passive restraint systems (air bags) have dramatically demonstrated the ability to cushion and decelerate people, including children, during crashes. As a result, the U.S. Congress has mandated passive restraint systems to be placed on all new automobiles sold in the United States by 1983, but an extension of this deadline is sought by the Reagan administration.

Motorcycle helmets have been known for over 30 years to reduce head injuries and death, but in 1977 the repeal of laws in 22 states that required helmet use produced an increase in motorcycle rider fatalities of one third in those states.

Tractor fatalities have been reduced in those areas where large farms regulated by the Occupational Safety and Health Administration (OSHA) are required to have rollover protective structures on tractors. But most farms do not fall under OSHA's jurisdiction. Tractors have been associated with 40% of the work-and nonwork-related injuries on Wisconsin farms. More than one half of these deaths result when tractors overturn and crush the operator.

Home environment

Each year about 24,000 people in the United States lose their lives as the result of an accident in the home, and about 3.6 million more

suffer disabling injuries. The health implications are starkly apparent.

At home the most dangerous area for accidents is the bedroom, because it is most often the site of falls, chiefly among older people. The second most dangerous area is the kitchen.

Community home safety programs. The combination of residential burns, falls, poisoning, cuts, drowning, and violence means that more people are injured in the home than in motor vehicle accidents, yet few communities have an organized continuing program of home safety promotion. In addition to the prevention of injuries, home safety programs could make inroads on the deaths that occur as a result of accidents in the home.

Some communities have an established fire prevention program that is laudable even though limited to one phase of home safety. In the United States, Cincinnati, Ohio, has a "Target System" of fire inspections supported by a Tactical Inspection and Educational Unit. Inspections are made of structures by assigned members of each fire company. Frequency of inspections is determined by the "Target" or category of the structure, and the five categories are determined by the inspectors based on the nature of the occupancy and the past inspection record. In the poorest category, inspections are made as frequently as every 2 weeks. When persuasion does not result in getting hazards corrected, court action may be taken against noncompliance with fire department orders.

In some communities the fire department encourages citizens to request fire inspection by the department staff. This is often associated with Fire Prevention Week. These programs are not to be discouraged, but obviously such piecemeal home safety programs are not adequate. A community-wide home safety program spanning all aspects of home accident prevention is the urgent need.

Because education is a basic ingredient of home safety promotion, the health education

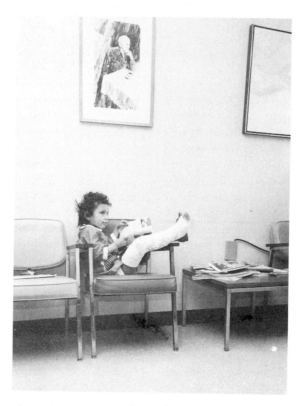

FIG. 11-4. Childhood accidents. Home safety, school, and community injury control programs tend to be too broadly oriented to rare or minor problems. More focus on the specific age and occupational groups experiencing specific types of injuries in specific environments is needed.

Courtesy Johns Hopkins Medical Institutions.

division of the community health department can provide the leadership and responsibility for a community program to prevent injuries in the home. With the health department spearheading the program, safety activities and contributions of organizations (for example, the fire department) and individuals can be correlated with the efforts of the health department. A community-wide home safety council can serve as a sounding board and an entree to the public and their homes.

Most home injuries are caused by some combination of improper practices and unsafe conditions. Safety promotion in homes must be directed toward the correction of practices and conditions. An extensive and intensive program

of education of the public must precede any action directed to correction of physical circumstances. This means the use of all possible media of communication and the promotion of special measures for alerting the public to the need for safety in the home.

Once the interest of the public has been aroused, the next step will be home safety surveys by householders themselves. Participation by the individual citizen is the key to effective home injury prevention. A *home safety survey* form should be delivered to all households and to other structures in the community. Such a survey should be a simple form based on conditions and practices of importance in safety, especially applicable to older homes.

Basement and laundry

1. Are all flues, stovepipes, and chimneys clean and tight?
2. Are combustible surfaces near stoves, furnaces, and vents insulated?
3. Is kindling wood stored at a safe distance from the furnace?
4. Are furnace fires started without the use of gasoline, kerosene, or other explosive materials?
5. Are ashes always placed in metal containers?
6. Are old newspapers and other inflammable materials removed promptly from the basement?
7. If the laundry floor tends to be damp, is a rubber mat provided?
8. Are cords that are exposed to water coated with rubber?
9. Are soap powder and other detergents kept off the floor to prevent slipping?
10. When not in use, are electrical appliances disconnected from the wall socket?
11. Are the basement and laundry room adequately lighted?
12. Are all gas connections checked twice a year to detect leaks or defects?
13. Are noninflammable cleaning fluids used and only out of doors?
14. Is a regular place provided for tools?
15. Is a smoke detector installed in the basement or laundry?

Kitchen

1. Is the floor clean and free from hazards such as upturned linoleum edges?
2. Are matches in metal containers and out of children's reach?
3. Is a short, sturdy stepladder used for reaching high places?
4. Are electrical appliances disconnected from the wall when not in use?
5. Is the electric iron rested on a proper stand when not in use?
6. Are the handles of pots and pans on the range turned out of the reach of children?
7. Are receptacles with water emptied immediately after using?
8. Are all gas connections checked twice a year to detect leaks or defects?
9. Is care taken to prevent gas flames from being extinguished by liquids boiling over or by drafts?
10. Are knives and other sharp instruments kept out of the reach of children?
11. In using a knife, do you always cut away from the body?

Living room and dining room

1. Are small rugs anchored so that they do not slip on polished floors?
2. Are the edges of rugs prevented from curling?
3. Is there a storage place for toys, and are they kept there when not in use?
4. Is nonskid wax used on floors?
5. Are chairs and other furniture in good repair?
6. Are scissors kept out of reach of small children?
7. Are pins and razor blades wrapped and disposed of properly?
8. Are extension cords placed where they will not be tripped over?
9. Are open wall sockets plugged?
10. Are all electric fixtures of an approved type and in good condition?
11. Is a sturdy stepladder used in reaching high places?
12. Are cigarette stubs extinguished and placed in convenient noninflammable containers?
13. Is a screen placed in front of a fireplace?

Stairs

1. Are stairs well lighted and unobstructed?
2. Do light switches operate from top and bottom of the stairs?
3. Is carpeting fastened securely to the floor and in good repair?
4. Is there a strong handrail on at least one side of the stair?
5. Are there secure gates at the bottom and top of stairs to protect young children?

6. Are all members of the household careful not to carry heavy loads on stairs?
7. Do the aged live entirely on the first floor and avoid the use of stairs?
8. Is the bottom step on the basement stairs painted a luminous white?

Bathroom

1. Is a rubber mat placed in the tub and a handhold installed on the wall?
2. Are electric fixtures made of porcelain, plastic, or other insulating material?
3. Are portable appliances and cabinets moved to an out-of-the-way place when not in use?
4. Are medicines and poisonous substances placed in a locked cabinet or other place inaccessible to children?
5. Are all poisons kept in clearly marked containers?
6. Is the label of every bottle containing poison double checked under clear light before the poison is used?
7. Are little children never left alone in the bathroom?

Bedroom

1. Is the passageway from the bed to the door unobstructed?
2. Are dresser drawers and closet doors always closed when not in use?
3. Are window screens securely installed?
4. Are electric heaters disconnected at the wall before the occupant goes to sleep or leaves the room?
5. Is there a convenient light switch for emergency night use?
6. Is it a practice never to smoke in bed?
7. Are safeguards provided to prevent children from falling out of cribs or beds?
8. Are smoke detectors installed in or near bedrooms?

Garage, yard, and porch

1. Are garage doors open while the car motor is running?
2. Is there a safe place to store garden equipment?

3. Is rubbish burned in a metal container on windless days and are children kept away?
4. Is the ladder of sound construction and properly anchored when used?
5. Are snow and slush promptly removed from porch and walks?
6. Is ice covered with sand, ashes, or other gritty materials?
7. Do the porch steps have a strong handrail?
8. Are the porch steps and walks unobstructed?

A survey is a means to an end, not an end in itself. A follow-up to correct unsafe conditions and practices is the logical corollary to the survey. Through the various media of communication, continuous emphasis must be placed on the importance of corrections if this approach is to yield tangible results.

Objective data may be obtained on injuries and how they occur in the home by providing all households with a form for reporting the time, place, factors involved, and the nature of the injury. These collective data can be highly meaningful in pinpointing where emphasis should be placed in the home safety program.

Fires. Residential fires kill about 8,000 Americans and injure 32,000 more annually. Nearly 8 out of 10 U.S. fire deaths happen at home, and more than half of them are in one- and two-family homes, according to the National Fire Protection Association—all the more reason to make fire safety a household concern.

More than half of the 800,000 home fires in the United States occur between midnight and 6 A.M.. Cigarettes, cigars, and pipes are still the major culprits, most often igniting in living rooms and bedrooms. They may smolder for several hours, but it takes only 2 to 4 minutes after ignition for combustible materials to go up in roaring flames that release poisonous gases. Unfortunately, all this can happen undetected by a sleeping family.

Without a doubt, smoke detectors can often

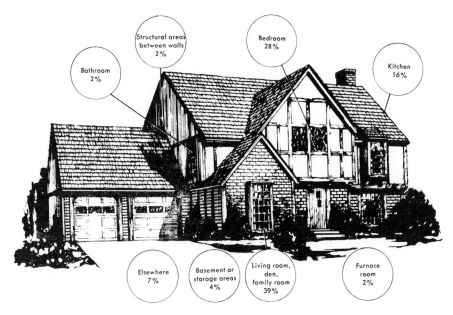

FIG. 11-5. Most fatal residential fires start in the rooms where people spend most of their time.

From National Fire Protection Association statistics, National Safety News, Aug., 1980.

mean the difference between life and death. Recent technology has produced a ready assortment of low-cost alarms. Smoke detectors are particularly effective in detecting fires in their early stages. Smoke detectors, as their name implies, are designed to detect the presence of smoke particles in the atmosphere. In the early stages of fires, smoke often develops before there is any appreciable increase in temperature, and smoke inhalation is a major cause of fire deaths.

The distribution of fire locations among houses that have burned shows that the majority of fires start in the three rooms where people spend most of their time—living room, bedroom, and kitchen—in that order of frequency (Fig. 11-5).

Poisoning. An estimated 400,000 children under the age of 5 are accidentally poisoned each year in the United States. One fourth of these children will be retreated for poisoning. Considerable progress in reducing the frequency of child poisoning has been achieved with special childproof lids on medicine bottles and household chemicals.

Farm environment

Safety on the farm is a complexity of occupational, home, motor vehicle, and recreational safety. From the standpoint of occupation, about one fifth of all industrial accident deaths occur in farming in the United States. The number of accidental deaths in farming, which is higher than in any other industry, is partially explained by the number of persons engaged in farming. On a basis of deaths per 100,000 workers, farming ranks third, exceeded only by mining and construction.

Agricultural work covers a wide variety of jobs depending on the farm products, farm size, its location, and availability of help. The work is seasonal and often demands long hours, physical strength, and quick execution. Farm workers usually perform multiple job functions, frequently without adequate safety instruction. Many times children, young adults, and uneducated laborers perform urgent work on family farms using a wide variety of heavy equipment, dangerous machinery, and intricate production methods. Farm families and workers are often exposed to the elements and may become vulnerable to sun, heat, and cold. Rural living and farm work also expose these persons to dangerous animals, toxic plants and insects, pesticides, and hazardous and volatile chemical compounds.

In the United States, state departments of agriculture and federal extension services carry on programs for promoting farm safety. Farm organizations such as the Farmers Union and the Grange also have continuing and special farm safety programs. These programs of action are usually supported by a variety of statewide safety education programs that include farm safety education. The state department of education usually promotes statewide safety education in the schools of the state, and farm safety is included in the program, particularly in the farm areas.

In the United States in 1976, 1,900 accidental work deaths occurred on farms. Of these, 1,500 (78%) involved farm residents and 400 (22%) involved nonresident workers on farms. Since 1973 there has been a 30% reduction of deaths among nonresidents, a probable benefit of the OSHA regulations. Unfortunately, there has been no reduction in work deaths among farm residents. Of the approximately 8 million individuals at risk in agricultural settings, only about 1 million are covered by OSHA regulations, which address only those farms that employ 10 or more persons.

Farm accidents. Farm life places the agricultural family in a variety of situations with unique problems in safety. Machinery poses a special hazard. U.S. Department of Agriculture studies provide interesting data on farm accidents (Table 11-5). These data can be compared with data for nonfarm people presented

TABLE 11-5. Fatalities on farm and comparable nonfarm fatalities, United States*

Cause	Farm (%)	Nonfarm (%)
Machinery	34.1	5.6
Drowning	15.0	22.3
Firearms	12.0	3.8
Falls	9.1	35.6
Blows	5.7	4.7
Animals	4.9	0.1
Electric current	3.4	3.4
Lightning	2.5	0.4
Poisoning	1.7	1.1
Suffocation	1.4	1.0
Other	5.0	17.0
TOTAL	100.0	100.0

*Data for farm accidents are from the U.S. Department of Agriculture; nonfarm data are estimates by the National Safety Council.

by the National Safety Council to indicate how fatal accidents on farms differ from fatal accidents not on farms. This epidemiological method identifies where the greatest emphasis should be placed in safety promotion on the farm. The U.S. Bureau of Agricultural Economics presents further information on the location of accidents causing injury to farm residents. It is thus apparent that accidents pose a special problem for the farm population, calling for more effective action than thus far has been expended.

Home	16%
Barn	22%
Elsewhere on farm	34%
Road or street	11%
Elsewhere or unknown	17%

Prevention of farm accidents. Preventing farm accidents includes the prevention of home accidents as well as the prevention of accidents elsewhere on the farm. A program of prevention must be vested in the farm families through self-direction as an outgrowth of an intensive and extensive program of farm safety education. Correlated with safety education should be a *farm safety survey* that farm families themselves can use profitably.

Farmyard

1. Do farmyard driveways provide a clear vision for automobile drivers and pedestrians who may use them?
2. Are automobiles driven slowly in the farmyard?
3. Is the parking place provided for automobiles one that will promote safety in backing out or in driving away?
4. Are unused lumber and materials piled or properly put away?
5. Are bins, racks, gates, and fences in good repair?
6. Are postholes and other holes properly covered or barricaded?
7. Are highly inflammable materials, sharp objects, and rubbish disposed of properly?

Buildings

1. Are all buildings in good repair?
2. Are stairs and ladders in good contition and free from obstruction?
3. Are all loose boards nailed down?
4. Are slippery floors covered with sand, straw, or other materials to prevent slipping?
5. Do only qualified people climb the silo, windmill, barn, or other high places?
6. Are hayloft and other openings properly covered or barricaded?
7. Is smoking in the hay barn prohibited?
8. Are smoke detectors installed?

Equipment, machinery, tools, and supplies

1. Are dangerous tools locked up away from the grasp of children?
2. Are insecticides and other poisons properly locked up?
3. Is gasoline stored separately in a proper tank?
4. Is a definite place assigned for all tools and equipment?
5. Are handles on tools secure?
6. Are children not allowed on farm machinery while the motor is running or while the team is hitched to it?
7. Is the motor shut off when the operator is not in the seat?
8. Are all machines and motors stopped before repairs are attempted?
9. Are all pulleys, hoisting equipment, and parts required to hold heavy loads inspected carefully before being used?
10. Is machinery properly stored and kept in good repair?

Animals

1. Do only qualified people handle livestock?
2. Are dangerous animals properly penned?
3. Is a lead staff always used in handling bulls?
4. Are animals always approached by speaking to them to avoid frightening them?
5. Are children properly instructed in necessary safety measures to avoid being injured by animals?

Combined with the home safety survey, this farm safety survey can be used as the basis for an evaluation of hazards and safety in farm life. All farm families should be encouraged through health education to take the time necessary for safety surveys and to follow up the survey by correcting the hazardous conditions and practices revealed by safety surveys.

A local committee of key leaders in agriculture leads and coordinates efforts in farm safety. In some communities a farm safety committee under the community safety council coordinates the efforts of organizations and individuals in farm health promotion. More than 20 organizations participate in farm safety on the local level in the United States. Agriculture Extension Service, Grange, Farmers Union, Farm Bureau, Future Farmers of America, 4-H clubs, and Future Homemakers are but a few of these. Meetings, campaigns, contests, demonstrations, and studies are the channels through which these organizations operate in safety promotion.

In the United States most states have full- or part-time farm safety specialists. With a professional safety expert working with a farm safety council, statewide programs serve to bolster local efforts as well as to promote special safety programs.

Occupational environment

Industrial safety refers to injury control in a branch of trade or production on a wide geographical stage, such as in the steel industry or automobile industry. Occupational safety refers to injury control within the confines of a single operational unit. It is an intramural program, such as the safety program in a chemical plant. Industrial safety is of value because of the pooling of experience and know-how among the various units within an industry. Yet it is on the local operational level where accidents must be prevented and where a safety program will yield the greatest results in injury control.

Of the major safety programs, occupational safety appears to have made the greatest progress in injury control in the United States. Although the enactment of Workmen's Compensation laws beginning in 1912 made safety economically profitable, management and labor have more than a business interest in safety promotion. Management and labor are interested in protecting the lives and health of employees. The effectiveness of safety programs is attested to by the drop in the injury frequency rate for companies reporting to the National Safety Council. The lost-time disabling injuries per 1 million person hours of work dropped from 31.87 in 1926 to 5.90 in 1970. This is a remarkable accomplishment, but more recent data show some setbacks.

Congress passed the 1970 Occupational Safety and Health Act (OSHA), which makes mandatory the reporting of occupational injuries and illnesses by employers. A new system of uniform reporting and recording has resulted in more complete reporting. During 1976 to 1977, the number of work-related injuries increased from 5 million to 5.3 million, and the number of workdays lost increased from 32.5 million to 35.2 million. Generally speaking, industries with the highest accident frequency rates (disabling injuries per 100,000 work hours) also have the highest severity rates (days lost per 1 million work hours). By their very nature, certain industries such as mining, marine transportation, quarrying, and construction tend to be hazardous. Other industries have a minor degree of hazard. Data for a total industry are of value in a local operation, but each plant or place of employment must deal with the hazards it has in its own operation.

In any consideration of occupational accidents, it must be pointed out that workers suffer more accidental deaths and injuries off the job than they do on the job. Further, the probability of an injury incurred at work being fatal is only half that for injuries incurred away from work.

Prevention of occupational injuries. Organization, a planned program, expert direction, and the enlistment of all personnel are the ingredients of an effective injury control program in occupations. Usually the program consists of the following eight aspects:

1. Leadership of management
2. Assignment of responsibility
3. Safe working conditions
4. Safety training of all personnel
5. Accident and injury records
6. Analysis of accidents and research in safety measures
7. Employee acceptance of responsibility for safety
8. First aid and medical services

Industry has recognized and developed safety experts who are usually designated as safety engineers. This concept could well be applied to other povinces of human activity where injuries play an even more important role than in industry.

School environment

For school-age youngsters, accidents loom as a greater threat to life and limb than do diseases. In the age group 5 to 14 years accidents other than automobile accidents are the leading cause of death in the United States.

School injuries. About 43% of accidental deaths among school children in the United States are connected with school life. Of these accidents about 6% occur when children are on their way to or from school, about 20% in school buildings, and about 17% on school grounds. The highest injury rate is among youngsters between the ages of 7 and 12 years. Their vigor and abandon lead to many of their injuries.

Prevention of school injuries. Leadership, vision, organization, and teamwork are the ingredients of an effective school safety program. A designed program on paper is excellent as a working blueprint, but action is the key to a safety program. Further, the school safety program is properly regarded as one facet of the total community safety program. The school driver education–training program has been adopted as a part of the community safety program, but it must be recognized that the overall school safety program, in the same light, is also a phase of community safety promotion.

A safety council composed of students and faculty is the guiding force of a school safety program. A school safety patrol can have subdivisions such as traffic patrol, building and grounds patrol, and a fire patrol. Student participation under teacher guidance is the working pattern.

Surveys of conditions and practices affecting safety in the school environment point up hazards and indicate preventive measures that must be taken. These surveys properly include conditions and practices going to and from home.

A system for reporting accidents and injuries is of legal significance as well as of preventive value. This is particularly true when a systematic investigation and follow-up is tied in with the reporting system.

Safety education as an integral phase of early health education has been effective in the creation of safety attitudes and the establishment of safe practices. It is in the early formative years of life that safety attitudes and habits are most readily acquired.

Schools can prevent accidental deaths and injuries among students and faculty, but a systematic, vigorous, and sustained program is necessary.

Recreational environment

The amount of leisure time available to Europeans, Canadians, Australians, Japanese, and Americans has gradually increased over the years as increased vacation time and early retirement have become popular work benefits from business and industry. Accordingly, the population at risk from various recreational activities has steadily increased, but complete figures on recreational morbidity and mortality are not available. As a result, the injuries in recreational pursuits have not been identified specifically as a major problem except in sports medicine.

It would be unrealistic to restrain recreation for the purpose of preventing all accidents. It would be equally unrealistic to think that recreation could be accident-free, but past experience has demonstrated that recreation can continue to expand and safety promotion can go hand in hand with this expansion.

Accidents in recreation. Public accidents, other than those related to motor vehicle, home, and employment accidents, caused approximately 15,800 deaths in the United States during 1978. Most occurred in recreational and leisure settings. Disabling injuries numbered approximately 2 million. Approximately 100,000 sports team injuries in 1976 were serious enough to require a physician's attention.

Drownings accounted for 6,900 deaths in 1978, most of which involved water sports such as swimming and boating. This number has remained relatively constant over 15 years despite the increasing numbers of people participating in water sports. About one third of adults who drown have high levels of alcohol in their blood, and more than 90% of the boating accident drownings involve occupants of small boats.

Approximately 8,100 fatalities were reported under the "other public" category. Hypothermia (exposure) fatalities were included in this category among other causes of death. Although complete figures regarding the incidence of hypothermia are unavailable, the population at risk appears to be increasing with expanded interests in cold weather activities and the increasing numbers of individuals participating in recreational events.

There are some 50.5 million boaters using 10 million boats in the waters of the United States. During 1976 alone there was an increase of 365,000 boats. Recreational boating accounts for approximately 1,400 fatalities each year in the United States. Although few by comparison with the number of motor vehicle deaths, it does represent approximately 44 fatalities per 100 million exposure hours compared to the automobile rate of about 55 fatalities per 100 million exposure hours (Russell, 1977).

As there has been a yearly increase in recreational activities, the yearly death toll in recreation has tended to increase accordingly. Yet when considered in terms of the increased number of participants in recreation, the *rate* of fatal accidents has declined. Not all of these deaths are strictly chargeable to recreation. Flying and railway fatalities can occur in commercial travel as well as in recreational travel.

Most of the people who lose their lives in accidents in recreation are in the prime of life. This is particularly true in sports and water accidents, boating, accidents with firearms, and flying.

Prevention of injuries in recreation. On the community level, organized, supervised recreation is usually safe recreation. Trained personnel, definite responsibilities, established regulations, regular supervision, safety surveys, and safety education have produced results. It is in unsupervised recreation that action is most needed, and here the primary approach is safety education. This is not a simple matter because education in the safe use of firearms does not carry over into safe conduct in swimming or boating.

Part of the safety education in recreation is provided by such organizations as rifle clubs, boating clubs, and camping and sportsman clubs. In the United States the Red Cross, Boy Scouts, Girl Scouts, Y.M.C.A., and similar organizations have contributed greatly to the promotion of safety education for recreation with such activities as swimming instruction and cardiopulmonary resuscitation (CPR) training. Despite these efforts, safety education for recreational needs is inadequate on all levels. Yet to conduct an organized community program of safety education in this sphere of activity is a difficult assignment. The individual efforts of all agencies and individuals promoting safety education in other activities make an indirect contribution to recreational safety.

Regulations governing recreational activities have a considerable effect on the promotion of safety. This is particularly true of regulations designed to prevent the inexperienced from participating in activities for which they are not prepared or qualified. It is the inexperienced or unskillful recreationist who is most likely to be involved in accidents. It is the reckless person who is most likely to involve others in accidents.

Each community can survey the recreational safety needs of its people and formulate a program accordingly. The cooperation of all groups sponsoring recreational activities or programs will add assurance for the success of the safety program. Recreational safety promotion should be coordinated with other safety programs in the community.

COMMUNITY SAFETY PROGRAM

The promotion of community safety poses a problem because safety in a community is the province of many organizations and individuals. Organizations involved in community safety include the health department, fire department, police department, recreation department, schools, industry, chamber of commerce, service clubs, civil defense, medical profession, and news media. The need is to integrate the contributions of all agencies into one unified, effective community safety program.

Organization. The community health department is the most logical agency to bring together the various forces that play on the problem of accident prevention in the community. While the official health department can be the catalyst in the reaction, a basic ingredient is a community safety council with representation from the various groups that have a contribution to make to safety and that have a dynamic interest in safety. This voluntary, nonofficial body is at one and the same time a sounding board, a source of information, an expression of community thinking, and a supporter of the various safety programs operating within the community.

Community safety promotion. Each agency will continue its ongoing program, expanding as conditions and the council indicate. Unnecessary duplication can be eliminated, but it should be recognized that some duplication is highly desirable. Unmet needs will be recognized, and an understanding will be reached on which agency will deal with a recognized need.

A *poison control center* is a valuable segment of the community safety program. It is the place where people can call for help in case of poisoning—accidental or intentional. Properly, a center is open 24 hours of the day and is manned by a person who knows how to use the standard references on poisons and recommended countermeasures. He or she needs to know both the physiology and pathology involved. In small communities a hospital is the logical location for such a center. In larger communities a poison control center may be located elsewhere.

Surveys of safety are sponsored by safety councils or may be initiated by member organizations. The two essential factors are to discover where injuries occur and where hazards exist in the community. Once hazards and the causes of injuries are located, measures can be initiated to reduce or even eliminate them.

Safety education is a province of all agencies concerned with safety in the community, but safety education must be coordinated and integrated to be extensive enough to be fully effective. Safety consciousness in a community can be developed but it takes a clear focus on specific, attainable objectives.

U.S. OBJECTIVES FOR 1990

Objectives for injury control developed by the Public Health Service for the United States reflect the consensus of experts on possible outcomes if communities apply the principles and methods outlined in this and preceding chapters.

Improved health status

- By 1990 the motor vehicle fatality rate should be reduced to no greater than 2.0 per 100,000,000 vehicle miles, or 18.0 per 100,000 population. (In 1979 it was 3.40 per 100,000,000 miles, or 22.9 per 100,000 population.)
- By 1990 the motor vehicle fatality rate for children under 15 should be reduced to no greater than 5.5 per 100,000 children. (In 1978 it was 9.2 per 100,000 children under 15.)

- By 1990 the home accident fatality rate for children under 15 should be no greater than 5.0 per 100,000 children. (In 1978 it was 6.1 per 100,000 children under 15.)
- By 1990 workplace accident deaths should be reduced to less than 11,000 per year. (In 1977 there were approximately 13,000 deaths.)
- By 1990 the rate of work-related disabling injuries should be reduced to 8.3 cases per 100 full-time workers. (In 1976 there were approximately 9.2 cases per 100 workers.)
- By 1990 lost workdays due to injuries should be reduced to 54 per 100 workers annually. (In 1976 approximately 60.5 days per 100 workers were lost.)
- By 1990 mortality from falls should be reduced to no more than 2.0 per 100,000 persons. (In 1979 it was 6.3 per 100,000.)
- By 1990 mortality from drowning should be reduced to no more than 3.0 per 100,000 persons. (In 1979 it was 3.3 per 100,000.)
- By 1990 the number of tap water scald injuries requiring hospital care should be reduced to no more than 2,000 per year. (In 1978 it was 4,000 per year.)
- By 1990 residential fire deaths should be reduced to no more than 4,500 per year. (In 1979 it was 5,000 per year.)
- By 1990 the number of accidental fatalities from firearms should be held to no more than 1,700. (In 1978 there were 1,800.)

Reduced risk factors

- By 1990 the proportion of automobiles containing passive restraint protection should be greater than 75%. (In 1979 the proportion was 1%.)
- By 1990 at least 110 million functional smoke alarm systems should be installed in residential units. (In 1979 there were approximately 30 million systems.)
- By 1985 all firms with more than 1,000 employees should have an approved plan of hazard control for all new processes, new equipment, and new installations. (Baseline data are unavailable.)
- By 1990 all firms with more than 500 employees should have an approved plan of hazard control for all new processes, new equipment, and new installations. (Baseline data are unavailable.)

Increased public-professional awareness

- By 1990 at least 25% of workers should be able to state the nature of their occupational health and safety risks and their potential consequences prior to employment, as well as be informed of changes in these risks while employed. (In 1979 an estimated 5% of workers were fully informed.)
- By 1985 workers should be routinely informed of life-style behaviors that interact with factors in the work environment to increase risks of occupational illness and injuries. (Baseline data are unavailable.)
- By 1990 the proportion of parents of children under age 10 who can identify measures they have specifically taken to address three major risks of injury to their children (i.e., motor vehicle accidents, burns, and poisonings) should be greater than 80%. (Baseline data are unavailable.)
- By 1990 virtually all pediatricians and other primary care providers should include instruction about use of child restraints to prevent injuries from motor vehicle accidents as part of their routine interaction with parents. (In 1979 the proportion of pediatricians who reported that they advised people on automobile safety measures was approximately 20%.)

Improved services-protection

- By 1990 at least 75% of communities with a population of over 10,000 should have the capability for ambulance response and transport within 20 minutes of a call. (In 1979 approximately 20% had this capability.)

- By 1990 virtually all injured persons in need will have access to regionalized systems of trauma centers, burn centers, and spinal cord injury centers. (In 1979 about 25% of the population lived in areas served by regionalized trauma centers.)
- By 1990 at least 90% of the population should be living in areas with access to regionalized or metropolitan area poison control centers that provide information on the clinical management of toxic substance exposures in the home or work environments. (In 1979 about 30% of the population lived in such areas.)

Improved surveillance-evaluation systems

- By 1990 at least 75% of the states will have developed a detailed plan for the uniform reporting of injuries.

COMMUNITY OBJECTIVES

The U.S. objectives for 1990 can be related to community health plans by adjusting the dates and assuring that specific needs and services of the local population are addressed, as suggested by *Model Standards for Community Preventive Health Services,* 1979.

- By 19___ the incidence of (insert name of specific type of injury or accident) will not exceed _____ .
- By 19___ mortality associated with (insert name of specific type of injury or accident) will not exceed _____ .
- By 19___ the community will be served by an injury surveillance system that determines baseline injury rates and categorizes the occurrence of each type of injury by age, sex, socioeconomic status, time, place of occurrence, seriousness, and other pertinent epidemiological data deemed necessary according to the particular community environment.
- By 19___ the surveillance system will routinely monitor and analyze data from the appropriate community sources, including

emergency rooms, schools, prisons, nursing homes, vital statistics section of the official health agency, private physicians and dentists, fire and police department reports, workplace illness and injury reports, park and recreation departments, and special interest groups such as consumer safety organizations.

- By 19___ the community will have a public information program for injury control that places special emphasis on high-risk groups, such as young children and the aged, and that has the following components: (1) injury control in the home setting and (2) injury control in nonhome settings, the types of which are to be determined by injury patterns in the community.
- By 19___ community schools will offer students instruction about injury control.
- By 19___ the community will have a system for identifying and correcting problems and preventing the occurrence of these and future problems. Such a system will include (1) investigation of clustering of major injuries and recommendation for correction of the precursors to these injuries, (2) ongoing review of the adequacy of community codes and their enforcement, and timely updating of codes as necessary, and (3) implementation of appropriate environmental controls to prevent injuries.

QUESTIONS AND EXERCISES

1. Evaluate this statement: "Even if all accidents cannot be eliminated, the promotion of injury control could reduce accidental deaths."
2. If you were to study the epidemiology of accidents in your community, what factors would receive your attention?
3. A certain community (M) has a much better safety program than another community (N), yet community M has a higher accident rate, a higher accidental death rate, and a higher injury rate per 100,000 population. What factors would account for this paradox?
4. The accidental death rate in the United States has declined since the turn of the century, yet accidents as a

cause of death now rank fourth. In 1900 accidents ranked seventh. How do you explain this apparent contradiction?

5. How is your state or provincial highway safety program organized and administered?

6. Make proposals to improve your state or provincial highway safety program.

7. Why in the United States is the state industrial safety program generally more effective than the state traffic safety program?

8. On the state or provincial level, who has responsibility for the promotion of home safety?

9. What agencies in your locality promote farm safety?

10. Why have the people of the United States failed to go all out in halting the slaughter on our highways?

11. Make some proposal for controlling the unsafe driver.

12. If a car travelling 55 mph crashes into a fixed concrete abutment, with how much force will a person of 160 pounds be thrown forward? Use the equation MV = Ft, in which M = mass, V = velocity, F = force, and t = time (1 second).

13. Set up an organizational chart for a model motor vehicle safety program for some community.

14. Design a model community home safety program.

15. Who in your county is engaged in the promotion of farm safety?

16. Evaluate the safety record and safety program of one of the industrial firms in your community or in some other community.

17. How effectively have the schools of your community taken advantage of their opportunity to promote safety, particularly safety education?

18. What are some obstacles to the promotion of recreational safety?

19. If you were to set up a safety council for your community, who would be on the council and what would be the specific provinces of the council's program?

20. What is the greatest safety need in your community?

BIBLIOGRAPHY

Bergner, L.: Falls from heights: a childhood epidemic in an urban area, Am. J. Public Health 61:90, 1971.

Blumenthal, M.: Traffic safety research review, Natl. Safety Council 12(1):1968.

Centers for Disease Control: Morbidity and Mortality Weekly Reports 27:124, April 14, 1978a.

Centers for Disease Control: Morbidity and Mortality Weekly Reports 27:192, June 9, 1978b.

Chisholm, J.J.: Lead poisoning, Sci. Am. 224:15, Feb., 1971.

Dietz, P.E., and Baker, S.P.: Drowning, epidemiology and prevention, Am. J. Public Health 64:303, April, 1974.

Florio, A.E., and Stafford, G.T.: Safety education, ed. 3, New York, 1969, McGraw-Hill Book Co.

Green, L.W.: The oversimplification of policy in prevention, Am. J. Public Health 68:953, 1978.

Green, L.W.: To educate or not to educate: is that the question? Am. J. Public Health 70:625, 1980.

Haddon, W.: A logical framework for categorizing highway safety phenomena and activity, J. Trauma 12(3):193, 1972.

Haddon, W., Jr.: Strategy in preventive medicine: passive versus active approaches to reducing human wastage, J. Trauma 14:353, 1974.

Haddon, W., Jr., and Baker, S.P.: Injury control. In Sartwell, P. et al., editors: Preventive medicine, ed. 2, Boston, 1978, Little, Brown and Co.

Healthy People: The Surgeon General's report on health promotion and disease prevention, Washington, D.C., 1979, Office of the Assistant Secretary for Health, Public Health Service.

Iskraut, A.P.: The epidemiological approach to accident causation, Am. J. Public Health 57:1708, 1967.

Model standards for community preventive health services, Washington, D.C., 1979, Office of the Assistant Secretary for Health and Surgeon General, Public Health Service.

National Safety Council: Accident facts—1979 edition, Chicago, 1980, The Council.

National Safety Council: Accident facts, 1979 preliminary condensed edition, Chicago, 1979, The Council.

Promoting health, preventing disease: Objectives for the nation, Washington, D.C., 1980, Office of the Assistant Secretary for Health and Surgeon General, Public Health Service.

Russell, W.J.: Emergency procedures for untrained persons, Public Safety, Chicago, National Safety Congress Transactions, vol. 27, 1977.

Seaton, D.C., et al.: Administration and supervision of safety, New York, 1968, Macmillan Publishing Co., Inc.

U.S. Department of Commerce, National Fire Prevention and Control Administration: Highlights of fire in the United States, Washington, D.C., 1978, U.S. Government Printing Office.

U.S. Department of Commerce, Statistical Abstract of the United States, 1979, Washington, D.C., 1979, U.S. Government Printing Office.

12

LIFE-STYLE AND COMMUNITY HEALTH PROMOTION

Both in importance and in time, health precedes disease, so we ought to consider first how health may be preserved, and then, how one may best cure disease.

Galen (AD 200)

Four habits will be considered in this chapter—alcohol misuse, cigarette smoking, eating patterns, and drug misuse. All share a compulsive and dependent component in behavior and result in major increases in mortality, morbidity, and social pathology in the community. Together with physical activity, stress management, and safety behavior, they constitute the set of personal health actions referred to as life-style.

Chapter 2 introduced the health field concept with four elements contributing to health or premature mortality. Of these four (the health care system, life-style, the environment, and human biology), the one that today contributes most (over half) of the years of life lost is life-style, as seen in Table 12-1. To put this revealing statistic in more positive terms, the greatest gains in preventing premature death are to be gained today through changes in life-style. These behavioral changes, of course, will depend on organizational supports in the health care system and environmental supports for behavior in the community. The interaction of the organizational, environmental, and behavioral factors defines health promotion, but most of the contribution of the health care sys-

tem and the environment to health in the decade ahead will be through behavior.

The objectives for improving the health status of the community presented in previous chapters can be summarized in broad goals with associated life-styles as shown in Table 12-2. The most frequently appearing behavioral risk factors are those addressed in this chapter.

ALCOHOL MISUSE

Alcohol is the second most important known cause of mortality and morbidity in most Western countries, second only to tobacco. Epidemiological, clinical, and laboratory evidence have made it clear that cirrhosis of the liver is caused primarily by alcohol consumption. Other diseases and conditions associated with alcohol include acute and chronic intoxication; toxic psychoses; gastritis; pancreatitis; fetal alcohol syndrome; cardiomyopathy; peripheral neuropathy; automobile, home, and occupational fires and accidents; suicide; homicide; injuries; and cancer of the mouth, pharynx, larynx, esophagus, and liver. Alcohol contributes to ill health, crime, poverty, broken homes, unintended pregnancy, divorce, social conflicts, loss of earning power, social

TABLE 12-1. The majority of years of lost life before age 65 and after infancy are attributable to life-style*

Ten leading causes of death among the total population 1+ years of age, ranked by number of years of life lost before age 65, United States, 1975		Estimated percentages of lost life attributed to each of the four elements of the health field concept†			
Ten leading causes of death	Years of life <65 lost	Health care system	Life-style	Environment	Human biology
Cancer	1,802,820	10	37	24	29
Heart disease	1,769,180	12	54	9	28
Motor vehicle accidents	1,424,823	12	69	18	1
All other accidents	1,166,793	14	51	31	4
Homicide	621,846	0	65	40	5
Suicide	583,751	3	60	35	2
Cerebrovascular disease	352,524	7	50	22	21
Cirrhosis of the liver	320,457	3	70	9	18
Influenza and pneumonia	206,673	18	23	20	39
Diabetes	118,119	6	26	0	68

*Adapted from Centers for Disease Control, Public Health Service, 1978.
†These estimates are based on professional judgment rather than on death certificate data, but they reflect consensus approximations of the relative importance of the four contributing factors in premature mortality. For another view of the total contribution of the four elements of the health field concept to the combined mortality for the 10 leading causes of death, see Fig. 4-1.

TABLE 12-2. Health status goals and their contributing life-style risk factors*

Health status goals	Life-style risk factors
1. Reduce the incidence and severity of premature cardiovascular morbidity and mortality	Smoking Nutritional practices Alcohol use Exercise Risk management Stress management
2. Reduce emotional impairment and its physical sequelae (alcohol misuse, drug misuse, mental health, suicide, etc.)	Alcohol use Habituating drug use Human sexuality–contraceptive use Stress management Coping-adaptation
3. Reduce the incidence of mental retardation	Smoking (pregnant women) Nutritional practices Alcohol use Risk management

*From Healthy People, Appendices: Task force report on disease prevention and health promotion, U.S. Department of Health and Human Services, Office of Disease Prevention and Health Promotion, Washington, D.C., 1978, unpublished.

TABLE 12-2. Health status goals and their contributing life-style risk factors—cont'd

Health status goals	Life-style risk factors
4. Reduce the incidence of morbidity and mortality in mothers and infants	Smoking Nutritional practices Alcohol use Habituating drug use Human sexuality–contraceptive use Family development
5. Reduce the incidence of morbidity and mortality from malignancy	Smoking Nutritional practices Alcohol use Risk management
6. Reduce the incidence of traumatic injury and death (homicide, poisoning, motor vehicle, and other accidents)	Alcohol use Risk management Stress management
7. Reduce the incidence of morbidity and mortality from respiratory disease	Smoking Exercise Risk management Stress management Coping-adaptation
8. Reduce the incidence and complications of other disabling conditions (diabetes, arthritis)	Smoking Nutritional practices Alcohol use Exercise Risk management Coping-adaptation
9. Reduce the incidence of communicable diseases (vaccine preventable diseases, sexually transmitted diseases, etc.)	Human sexuality–contraceptive use Risk management
10. Promote dental health	Nutritional practices Risk management
11. Protect vision and hearing	Risk management
12. Protect the integrity of other body systems (skeletal, nervous, etc.)	Nutritional practices Habituating drug use Exercise Risk management Stress management
13. Promote personal control over environmental hazards	Smoking Nutritional practices Alcohol use Driving Risk exposure Stress management

Continued.

TABLE 12-2. Health status goals and their contributing life-style risk factors—cont'd

Health status goals	Life-style risk factors
14. Improve, preserve, and enhance the individual's general physical well-being	Smoking Nutritional practices Alcohol use Habituating drug use Exercise Risk management
15. Improve, preserve, and enhance the individual's general, emotional well-being	Habituating drug use Risk management Stress management Coping-adaptation
16. Enhance optimum development of children, adolescents, and adults, including the development of relationships	Risk management Family development Enhanced self-esteem

TABLE 12-3. Estimates of alcohol-related mortality and morbidity, United States, 1975*

Cause of death	Percent related to alcohol	Cause of morbidity or disability	Percent related to alcohol
Alcohol as a direct cause		Burns	87
Alcoholism	100	Digestive tract	
Alcoholic psychosis	100	Esophageal varices	27
Cirrhosis	41–95	Pancreatitis	68
Liver cancer	90	Ulcers	8
Alcohol as an indirect cause		Nutritional deficiencies	
Accidents	50	Avitaminosis	60
Motor vehicle	30–50	Cancer	
Falls	44.4	Oral cancers with smoking in males	75
Fires	25–87	Esophageal cancer cases	76
Drownings	20–78		
Other†	11.1		
Pneumonia	5–10		
Homicides	49–87		
Suicides	25–84		
Total mortality	29–40		

*Data from Day, Nancy: Alcohol and mortality. Paper prepared for National Institute on Alcohol Abuse and Alcoholism under Contract No. NIA-76–10(P), Jan., 1977. As cited in Third special report to the U.S. Congress on alcohol and health, June, 1978, Table 8, p.19, National Institute on Alcohol Abuse and Alcoholism, U.S. Department of Health, Education, and Welfare; and data on morbidity, cancer deaths, and pneumonia deaths from a briefing for the Surgeon General, Public Health Service, by the National Institute on Alcohol Abuse and Alcoholism, March 11, 1980.
†Includes all accidents not listed above, but excludes accidents incurred in medical and surgical procedures.

degradation, and other social pathology (Table 12-3).

Epidemiology of alcohol misuse

Alcohol is undoubtedly the most abused drug in North America, Europe, Australia, and New Zealand today. Four to six million Americans have been diagnosed as alcoholics, and 10% of the U.S. adult population are believed to have a serious drinking problem. It is estimated that 50% of traffic fatalities are alcohol related. Employees suffering from alcoholism are estimated to cost the United States $20 billion in lost productivity costs.

Cirrhosis of the liver was the eighth leading cause of death in the United States in 1979. Cirrhosis is prevalent in both sexes and all races, but the rates are higher in males and blacks.

Low socioeconomic groups have a higher prevalence of cirrhosis than do high socioeconomic groups. There is a relationship to occupation—those handling alcohol show increased rates of hepatic cirrhosis. Mortality from hepatic disease drops suddenly if alcohol is removed from the community.

Prevention of alcohol misuse

Prevention of alcoholism may again be considered intervention on agent, host, and environment levels. Alcohol is the agent, an anesthetic that is toxic in overdose. The healthy adult liver can oxidize about $1/4$ ounce of absolute alcohol per hour. The alcohol content is half the proofage, so $1/4$ ounce is equal to 0.6 ounce of 86% proof alcohol. The absorption of alcohol into the bloodstream is delayed by food in the stomach, thus peak blood levels are not reached so quickly after eating. It is alleged that there is a safe level of drinking in terms of dosage and that 45 milliliters per day of absolute alcohol may not harm the liver if the alcohol is taken diluted and is spread throughout the day. This is equivalent to $3^{1}/_{2}$ ounces of 86% proof alcohol daily. The effects of alcohol

are strictly dose related, regardless of the form (whisky, wine, beer, etc.) in which the alcohol is taken. It does not seem possible to detoxify alcohol, and dosage must be regulated.

Altering behavior of the host is the most popular way of intervening, and exhortation, coupled with deprivation, is usually tried. Group therapy using behavioral modification techniques is most likely to succeed, and in the United States, Alcoholics Anonymous is the leading exponent of this approach. Counselors are frequently former alcoholics, who are better able to appreciate the difficulties of abstinence than are those who have never overcome such a problem. A nonjudgmental, supportive, understanding relationship must be established. Medical treatment employing aversion therapy using disulfiram (Antabuse) is most effective. This therapy must be restricted to the motivated alcoholic and used in conjunction with the supportive group therapy described.

Most medical treatment merely results in rendering the alcoholic fit enough to resume drinking. Survivorship in cirrhosis depends on cessation of alcohol consumption. If, in the alcoholic, consumption persists, all medical and surgical measures are to no avail. All social networks to help alcoholics, such as Alcoholics Anonymous and the support of family and friends, should be employed.

The communication of effective alcohol-related health messages is particularly challenging and difficult. Few products can match alcohol in its ability to evoke strong sentiments—both positive and negative. Most people already have firm opinions concerning the appropriate role of alcoholic beverages in their personal lives, and such perceptions, whether based on accurate information or not, are highly resistant to change.

These perceptions may be acquired through personal experience with alcoholic beverages or through the experiences and influence of associates, friends, and family members. Perceptions may also be acquired vicariously through the depiction of alcohol use in publications and films, radio, and television dramatizations. Unfortunately, some of the perceptions are incorrect. A Gallup poll in July 1978 found that about 1 person in 12 believed there are no risks involved with regular use of alcohol. Other perceptions are incomplete. Many people do not know how alcohol is metabolized in the body and have incomplete knowledge about the effect that food or time can have on this process; they also assume, incorrectly, that coffee can have a mitigating effect. People are insufficiently aware that consumption of large amounts of alcohol in a short period of time, such as may occur in a drinking contest, can cause death. They are also unaware that drinking can cause or contribute to the various health hazards described earlier in this chapter.

An important source of perceptions is alcoholic beverage advertising, particularly for young people. For example, the favorable image alcohol users are given in television advertising and programming creates a barrier to be overcome in alcohol education efforts. The alcoholic beverage industry commits hundreds of millions of dollars annually to an extensive array of product advertising, print, and broadcast.

Professor Lambert of the University of Washington in Seattle analyzed 504 copies of 42 popular magazines issued in 1978, finding 3,131 alcoholic beverage advertisements. The greatest number of advertisements of alcohol (1,060) appeared in *Playboy, Psychology Today, Cosmopolitan,* and *Penthouse*. In 1977 network television in the United States carried about 5,000 beer and wine ads, mostly during evening prime time shows and weekend sports programs. These advertisements, particularly the beer advertisements, associate the use of the product with attractive individuals, enjoyable activities, and pleasant surroundings, without communicating any of the potential negative consequences.

Considering the pervasiveness of positive images concerning alcohol use, communication techniques that could be effective in carrying appropriate health-related messages about alcohol use to current or potential users must include mass media and product labeling to inform, to raise awareness levels, or to reinforce old knowledge, and to change potentially harmful responses to social situations in which alcohol use is encouraged.

Altering the environment is the most effective way of reducing alcoholism in the community. The social environment of schools, colleges, worksites, and public gathering places creates unfortunate pressures for drinking in many instances. Education should be used to inform people of the methods of advertising of alcohol. Social ambience must be altered so that alcohol is not regarded as a reward, as a status symbol, or as something that is glamorous.

The cost of alcohol can be greatly increased by taxation, so that a significant part of discretionary income must be expended to buy alcohol, and competing needs considered. This economic approach tends to penalize the poor. It has an effect on overall community consumption, but not on the most addicted and heaviest drinkers.

CIGARETTE SMOKING

Cigarette smoking is the greatest community health hazard, a self-imposed risk. Mortality and morbidity is greatly increased in smokers versus nonsmokers, especially in respiratory and cardiovascular diseases.

Epidemiology of smoking

Although cigarette smokers suffer the highest relative risk with respect to the cancers listed in Fig. 12-2, the community impact of smoking is greatest in cardiovascular disease because the latter is so prevalent.

Cigarette smoking accounts for 19% of cancers among all persons and 32% among males.

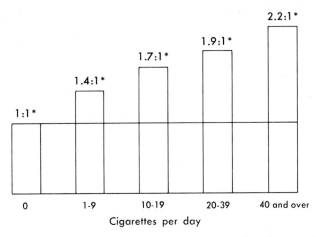

FIG. 12-1. Daily cigarette consumption and death rates. Asterisk indicates relative risk ratio in death rates from all causes.

From Progress against cancer 1970, a report by the National Advisory Cancer Council, p. 40.

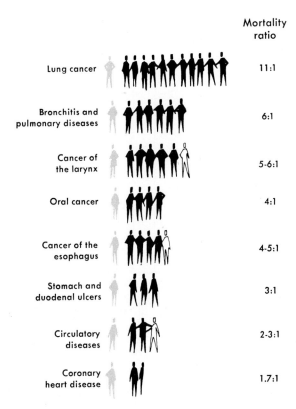

FIG. 12-2. Mortality ratio of smokers to nonsmokers for several diseases. A mortality ratio of 11:1 means that the death rate for smokers is 11 times that for nonsmokers.

From Progress against cancer 1970, a report by the National Advisory Cancer Council, p. 41.

TABLE 12-4. Sites of high attributable risk of cancer from cigarette smoking*

Site	Attributable risk (smoking)	No. of cases† (incidence)	No. of deaths† (mortality)
Lung	85%	98,000	89,000
Bladder	52%	29,900	9,800
Pancreas	48%	21,800	11,800
Buccal cavity	67%	17,300	4,650
Larynx	82%	9,200	3,350
Esophagus	76%	7,600	6,900
Pharynx	86%	6,600	3,800

*From American Cancer Society: CA—A Cancer Journal for Clinicians **27**(1):34, Jan.-Feb., 1977.
†Estimates for 1977—American Cancer Society.

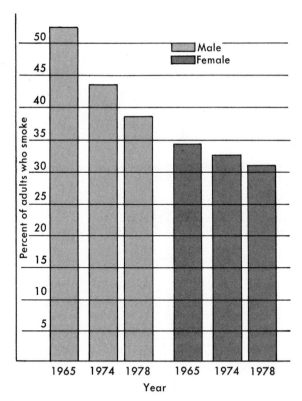

FIG. 12-3. Percent of adults who smoke, by sex, 1965, 1974, and 1978, United States.
From National Center for Health Statistics, U.S. Department of Health and Human Services, 1979.

Selected sites, where the attributable risk (AR) caused by smoking is high, are listed in descending order of incidence in Table 12-4.

AR is the percentage of total cases that can be ascribed to the particular risk factor, in this case cigarette smoking. It is computed by using the relative risk of smokers and the prevalence of smoking in the community.

Although the trend in smoking in the United States was upward for the first 65 years of the century, from 1965 to 1971 there was a sharp decline, presumably resulting from the impact of antismoking campaigns. The annual rate of decline was even greater between 1974 and 1978 (Fig. 12-3).

Cigarette smoking is a social class habit. It is also a city dwellers' habit. Cigarette smoking began and first spread in cities. The cities have remained ahead of the rest of the country both in the numbers of smokers and in the average number of cigarettes smoked each day. Studies in this country have shown that the prevalence of cigarette smoking increases as the socioeconomic status (SES) decreases. The habit starts at an earlier age the lower the socioeconomic status.

Although females used to feel safe from lung cancer because their death rate was low compared with that for males, this picture is beginning to change alarmingly. The female lung

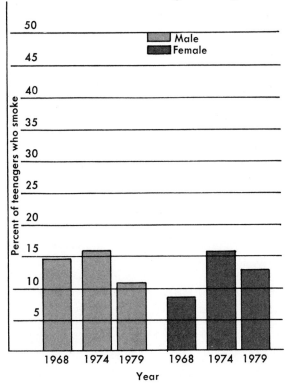

FIG. 12-4. Percent of teenagers who smoke, by sex, 1968, 1974, and 1979, United States.

From National Clearinghouse for Smoking and Health, U.S. Department of Health and Human Services, 1980.

cancer death rate has doubled in the past 10 years in the United States. Female death rates from lung cancer are now approaching the death rate for males and are increasing more rapidly.

The recent upsurge in the lung cancer death rate for females can be attributed to the fact that females began to smoke in much greater numbers about 30 years ago and the trend had increased since then, possibly as a result of advertising.

Smoking habits established in the teens, in the great majority of cases, will persist into adulthood. Teenage girls, who never smoked to the extent that teenage boys did, have now caught up. In 1968 only about half as many teenage girls smoked as boys. But by 1974 15.3% of girls between ages 12 and 18 years were smoking, only slightly less than the boys' 15.8%. In 1979 girls had surpassed boys in teenage smoking (Fig. 12-4).

Smoking parents set the example for children. Studies show that youngsters whose parents smoke are more likely to adopt the habit than are children of nonsmoking parents.

Women seem to find smoking more difficult to give up. Of women smoking in 1966, 25% had quit by 1970. Men, in the same period, had a quitting rate of 39%. One woman in nine who was an exsmoker in 1966 had returned to the habit by 1970.

The rise in the number of women smokers has not been lost to the attention of cigarette manufacturers, who have stepped up advertising campaigns for new brands of cigarettes designed expressly for women.

Prevention of smoking

Reducing the toxicity of the agent is possible. Most American adults who continue to smoke are smoking cigarettes with lower tar and nicotine levels. In 1975 only 20% of smokers said they used cigarettes with 20 milligrams or more of tar, down from 55% in 1970. The proportion of persons smoking cigarettes with nicotine levels of 1.4 milligrams and above declined from 45% to 18%. The average tar content of cigarettes sold in the United States dropped from 23 milligrams in 1954 to 17 milligrams in 1977. Nicotine levels went from 2.0 milligrams to 1.1 milligrams. Dosage can be reduced by smoking fewer cigarettes, inhaling less, leaving a longer stub, taking fewer puffs from each cigarette, and taking the cigarette out of the mouth between puffs.

Economics. Tobacco has been a major economic factor in the first 200 years of the development of the United States. The profitability of its industry has been legendary and has resulted in lavish promotional efforts, particularly during the last 100 years. With the invention of automatic manufacturing equipment, the use of cigarettes has increased dramatically during that period, aided by astute advertising through the press, the movies, and later through the electronic media. The two major wars and the several minor wars of this century also contributed to the diffusion of cigarettes and to their image as cultural symbols of sophistication.

From a few hundred cigarettes per adult citizen at the turn of the century, annual consumption has skyrocketed to about 4,000 per adult at the present. If one considers smokers only, individual average annual consumption now approaches 12,000 cigarettes. Cigarettes have indeed reached an unprecedented position in the mythology of Western culture, a condition that is rapidly spreading to other cultures as well.

Governments, of course, have not been indifferent to this potential source of revenue. Today local jurisdictions in the United States derive over $5 billion annually in taxes from tobacco, and the federal treasury similarly obtains over $2.5 billion.

The tobacco industry contributes, from the tobacco field to the vending machine, some $18 billion to the gross national product of the United States and gives livelihood to a well-publicized segment of the population in several states. Naturally, these economic activities are protected and fostered by the U.S. Department of Agriculture and the Department of Commerce and add some billion dollars annually to a precarious balance of payments. As the U.S. and European markets for tobacco products decline, U.S. and European manufacturers of cigarettes are advertising and selling more aggressively in the less-developed nations where smoking is regarded as a symbol of modern living.

It is estimated that in the United States alone over 37 million, or 17.5%, of the present population may be expected to die prematurely because of smoking, as analyzed in Table 12-5. It is against this historical background that community efforts against smoking must be planned. The following listing of the major constraints to community or national action in the United States may be useful.

- Government action is likely to be ambivalent, and it is not surprising that adversary positions are taken by different departments, considering their differing constituencies and purposes.
- The habituating, hedonistic, and cultural aspects of smoking are not likely to be stamped out for many years to come in the current social climate of generally permissive attitudes, although recent progress is notable.
- Fifteen years of public education may have prevented a large number of new smokers and provided support for many who wanted to quit, but the absolute number of smokers has been increasing steadily until recently. The proportion of smokers in the population and the per capita consumption have decreased to the lowest levels in 20 years. Yet about 54 million Americans still smoked in 1980, consuming more than 615 billion cigarettes each year. (Smoking in Third World countries has been increasing.)
- Research and action must be continued to

TABLE 12-5. Projected distribution of deaths, by cause, to current U.S. population, estimated assuming that there will be no major changes in recent mortality statistics during the lifetimes of persons now living in the United States*

Cause of death	Ultimate no. of deaths within present population		Premature deaths having tobacco-related causes within present population	
	No.	As percent of present population	No.	As percent of present population
Diseases of the heart	81,700,000	38.0	24,510,000	11.4
Bronchitis/emphysema	2,150,000	1.0	1,828,000	0.9
Arteriosclerosis	3,655,000	1.7	1,206,000	0.6
Cancer of the oral cavity	667,000	0.3	467,000	0.2
Cancer of the esophagus	731,000	0.3	219,000	0.1
Cancer of the pancreas	2,150,000	1.0	753,000	0.4
Cancer of the larynx	366,000	0.2	183,000	0.1
Cancer of the lung	9,009,000	4.2	7,837,000	3.6
Cancer of the kidney	789,000	0.4	158,000	0.1
Cancer of the bladder	1,045,000	0.5	418,000	0.2
Other diseases	112,738,000	52.4	—	—
TOTAL	215,000,000	100.0	37,579,000	17.5

*From National Cancer Institute, U.S. Department of Health and Human Services, 1977.

educate the public against smoking, but at least an equal effort should be directed at reducing the hazardous and habituating properties of cigarettes.

- The tort law in the United States would expose a manufacturer to class action suits if he or she were to express doubt on the safety of his or her products. Thus the cigarette industry can be expected to continue to deny any association of tobacco and disease, even to the point of not engaging in research toward less hazardous products; indeed, this would presume an admission of hazard. Moreover, the cigarette industry has little incentive to develop products that are less habit-forming and therefore more likely to allow habit cessation in the smoker. Because of this situation, it is clear that the demonstration of the feasibility of less hazardous cigarettes should be the responsibility of public health agencies.
- Traditionally, legislatures have been more sensitive to the immediacy of economic issues, and their attention to funding public health needs in smoking has been a token one. The situation is not likely to change in the foreseeable future, and it is necessary to analyze the cost-effectiveness of the various antismoking initiatives so that feasible

and promising ones are given preferred attention.

- The eventual demise of smoking as a socially acceptable habit will be achieved by persistent action and a variety of concerted approaches. Realistic achievement of goals should be expected in a time frame of several years, perhaps of decades.

The economics of a successful national program of smoking prevention becoming fully effective by the year 2000 can be seen in Table 12-6. The estimates are based on increased longevity of slightly less than 1 year for 80-year-old individuals, between 1 and 2 years for those 60 to 79 years old, and increases of slightly more than 2 years for those under 60. The model does, of course, take into account risks to other diseases for those who are assumed to become at lower risk to adverse tobacco effects.

Increased life expectancies and concomitant changes in health statistics concerning tobacco usage can lead to changes in various economic indicators, as shown in Table 12-6. For example, the gross national product for the United States would be projected to increase by 0.6%, or almost $15 billion in constant dollars greater than otherwise projected, by the year 2000. Private housing starts are projected to increase by 4%, and unemployment would decrease by

TABLE 12-6. Projected changes in selected economic indicators, assuming a gradual reduction (fully effective by the year 2000) in disease incidence attributed to tobacco usage*

Economic indicator	Percent difference for projected program†		
	1990	1995	2000
Gross national product	0.3	0.8	0.6
Private housing starts	2.3	6.2	4.0
Multiple unit housing starts	2.0	3.1	2.1
Civilian labor force	0.1	0.3	0.6
Unemployment	−0.6	−4.6	−3.9
Government receipts	0.3	0.9	1.1
Supplemental unemployment insurance benefits paid out	−0.7	−5.5	−4.8

*Based on data from National Cancer Institute, U.S. Department of Health and Human Services, 1977.
†Based on standard Wharton forecast.

nearly 4% with the reductions in smoking. These estimates assume that efforts to eliminate the adverse health effects of tobacco usage will gradually become fully effective by the year 2000. Even if this is a realistic goal, the fact remains that millions still smoke and will continue to do so, at least for the immediate future. The percentage improvements in economic indicators shown in Table 12-6 could be used to justify local government support for smoking prevention programs in communities.

Health education. Communities can mount antismoking campaigns, and local groups can reinforce national leadership on this issue. People must be made aware of the hazards of cigarette smoking. This awareness results in (1) individuals being motivated not to smoke, and (2) smoking becoming less socially acceptable, which will reinforce their decisions not to smoke. This is very important in the young. Advertising presently directed at youth estab-

lishes that smoking is socially acceptable and desirable.

In the young, it is also necessary to negate peer influence. Risk taking is part of peer group culture. During the socialization process, nonsmoking must be instilled. Role models—persons teenagers admire—may prove effective. The difficulty is that not smoking is a "nonaction" and not a dynamic force, thus associations cannot be made with hero figures. Smoking may also be a symbol of independence and rebellion to teenagers against the norms of the family or group to which they belong.

The primary objective of the community smoking prevention program is to reduce the morbidity and mortality associated with smoking. To accomplish this, three approaches can be used in support of the community health educational component, as illustrated in Fig. 12-5.

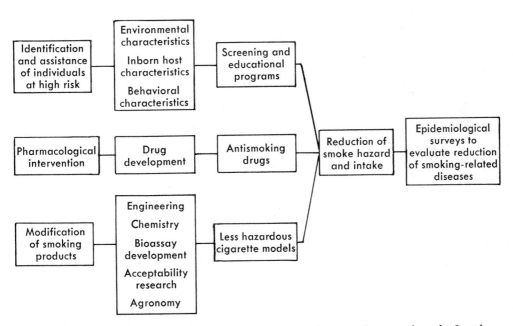

FIG. 12-5. U.S. national plan in support of community programs to decrease the risk of smoking-related diseases.

From National Cancer Institute, 1977.

The educational approach requires identification of, and provision for assistance to, those individuals at an increased risk of tobacco-related diseases. Epidemiological surveys are conducted to determine the environmental, biological, and psychological characteristics of the population at risk. The main thrust in this component of smoking education has been in the development of epidemiological methods for identifying groups at high risk of tobacco-related disease; the analysis of smoking patterns and behavior; research in smoking cessation techniques; and evaluation of smoking education programs.

Pharmacological approaches (host). The third part of a national strategy, in addition to economics and health education, is based on the hypothesis that cigarette smoking is a form of drug dependence on nicotine. Nicotine is recognized as a potent drug eliciting pharmacological effects on the central nervous system and playing an important role in controlling smoking behavior. Consequently, pharmacological intervention is a possible method for controlling smoking behavior. Several pharmacological agents have been tried by other researchers, but with mixed success, and no one seems to have had clear-cut success. Pharmacological activities are directed at reducing relapse in smoking cessation programs through combined pharmacological, physiological, and psychological approaches; improving and maintaining initial quitting rates; improving people's understanding of the physicochemical properties of nicotine and its metabolites; and identifying substances that taste, smell, or react like nicotine to use as pharmacological substitutes for cigarette smoking.

Less hazardous cigarettes (agent). In the pharmacological approach the characteristics of the agent may be altered. The genetics and agronomical practices of tobacco growing and curing are analyzed to reduce precursors of tobacco smoke toxicity. This entails the following sequence of events: (1) tobacco blends are ana-

lyzed to determine their chemical constituents, (2) cigarette smoke condensate, whole smoke, and chemical constituents are bioassayed by use of several animal models, (3) flavor components are identified, (4) bioassays are conducted to assess whether toxicity results from the reintroduction of flavor components, and (5) chemical, bioassay, and flavor results are correlated to identify the characteristics of less hazardous cigarettes. Average tar and nicotine content of cigarettes sold in the United States have declined by 50% since 1954 as a result of these efforts, although a truly "safe" cigarette does not exist.

Schools and worksites (environment). The foregoing approaches are addressed to the host and the agent of cigarette-induced diseases. The environment in which smoking occurs or is encouraged is the other essential point of intervention in the social history and personal histories of smoking. The school classroom is most frequently regarded as the setting in which antismoking education should take place. This curriculum focus on schools often ignores the even greater problems and opportunities outside the classroom where children and youth gather, observe, and are exposed to smoking influences. Some of the most promising health education programs in relation to smoking are those addressing the school environment and "inoculating" pupils against the social pressures they may encounter in that environment. Role playing and rehearsing in the classroom as to how to decline a cigarette offer from a peer has proved effective in delaying the uptake of smoking.

Worksites represent the other environment where people gather, observe, and are influenced by their social and physical surroundings for the largest part of their waking hours. In 1980 a survey conducted by the National Interagency Council on Smoking and Health indicated that about 15% of businesses in the United States have programs to help their employees stop smoking and one third of businesses are interested in such programs. The survey, which went out to the top 1,000 companies in the United States, plus 1,000 medium-size companies and 1,000 small companies, indicated that a significant number had policies to restrict or prohibit smoking in the workplace, most frequently in blue-collar areas where smoking might be a health hazard. Antismoking programs were the third most common health education program sponsored by companies, after hypertension control and diet-weight management.

Smoking causes about $5 billion to $8 billion in health care costs each year and about $12 billion to $18 billion in lost productivity, wages, and absenteeism in the United States. So business and industry have a substantial stake in controlling smoking.

OBESITY AND NUTRITIONAL PRACTICES

Over the last 80 years, the mean body weight of Americans has steadily increased. Between 1963 and 1973 mean body weight of men increased 6 pounds (2.7 kg), and of women 3 pounds (1.4 kg). Height did not play an appreciable role in this trend. For people 20 to 74 years of age, 14% of men and 24% of women are significantly overweight (i.e., 120% of ideal weight for their height and age). There is little difference between the rates of significant overweight between black men and white men, but black women are about a third more likely to be obese than white women. Forty-six percent of American adults feel themselves to be overweight, yet only a third of all adults actually know the recommended weight for their own height and age.

Epidemiology of nutrition

The United States appears to be a nation of dieters: a Harris survey in 1978 reported that 16% of all adults said they were currently on a diet, and 31% reported that they had dieted in the past. Nevertheless, of the 53% who had never dieted, 44% were at least to some extent overweight. In 1978 one out of every four adults said they were watching their calorie intake more carefully than in 1977; among people of lower socioeconomic status, one out of every four did so.

Status and trends. People of the developed countries appear to be increasingly concerned not only about the amounts of food they eat but with its content. In 1978 30% of American women and one of every four adults reported that they were eating more nutritious food than in 1977. For clues as to dietary practices and foods that are presently being avoided, the same survey showed that more than 80% of the adult population believe that cholesterol and fat pose a great degree or some degree of threat to health. A little less than 70% thought that salt posed some threat. The recent shift from foods high in cholesterol, fat, and sugar is confirmed by the food consumption trends in Table 12-7, but there is still some distance to

TABLE 12-7. Per capita consumption of selected foods, in pounds, United States, 1969 and 1979*

Food item	1969	1979	Percent change
Beef and veal	84.7	81.3	−4.0%
Pork	60.6	64.8	+6.9
Fish	11.2	13.7	+22.0
Poultry	46.7	62.0	+32.8
Eggs	39.3	35.8	−8.9
Milk and cream	301.0	284.2	−5.6
Cheese	11.0	18.1	+64.5
Fats and oils	51.9	57.6	+11.0
Fresh fruit	79.5	83.2	+4.7
Processed fruit	55.8	56.0	+0.4
Fresh vegetables	98.7	104.5	+5.9
Canned vegetables	53.7	55.0	+2.4
Frozen vegetables	9.1	11.1	+22.0
Wheat flour	112.0	112.0	0
Coffee	11.9	9.7	−18.5
Sugar	101.0	91.6	−9.3

*From U.S. Department of Agriculture, 1980.

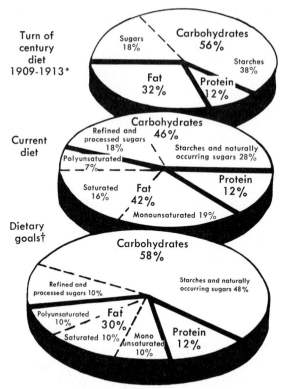

Turn of century diet 1909-1913*

Current diet

Dietary goals†

*From U.S. Dept. of Agriculture
†Developed by the McGovern committee

FIG. 12-6. Trends in consumption of carbohydrates, fats, and protein require a return to the balance struck in the U.S. diet of the early twentieth century.

From U.S. Congress, Senate Select Committee on Nutrition and Human Needs, 1979.

go toward the balance of carbohydrates and fats that prevailed 70 years ago and reflect the dietary goals (Fig. 12-6).

The increasing consumer attention to diet is undoubtedly responsible for the fact that average cholesterol levels in the U.S. population have declined nearly 10% in the past 20 years. Most of this decrease has occurred in higher educational and occupational groups, but it does reflect the potential for change in the populations reachable through community health programs.

Nutrition and food consumption involve complex interactions among social, cultural, economic, behavioral, and physiological factors. Adequate intakes of sources of energy and of essential nutrients are necessary for satisfactory rates of growth and development, reproduction, lactation, and maintenance of health. Deficits of essential nutrients or energy sources can lead to several specific diseases or disabilities and increased susceptibility to others. Excessive or inappropriate consumption of some nutrients may contribute to adverse conditions, such as obesity, or may increase the risk for certain diseases (e.g., heart disease, adult-onset diabetes, high blood pressure, dental caries, and possibly some types of cancer). Such chronic diseases are clearly of complex cause, with substantial variation in individual susceptibility to the several risk factors. While the role of nutrients in these diseases is not definitively established, epidemiological and laboratory studies offer important insights that may help people in making food choices that will enhance their prospects of maintaining health.

Health implications. Frequent consumption of highly cariogenic (decay-producing) foods (those containing fermentable or orally retentive carbohydrates), especially between meals, can nullify some of the caries preventive benefits of adequate fluoride intake and can cause rampant caries in children with a fluoride deficiency. No consistent or independent relationship has been shown, however, between sugar consumption and the onset of heart disease or diabetes. Once diagnosed, of course, a diabetic person must control sugar intake.

Inadequate nutrition may be associated with poor pregnancy outcome, including some fraction of low birth weight deliveries and suboptimum mental and physical development. Excessive sodium intake has been associated with high blood pressure in susceptible individuals. Dietary fat, saturated fat, and cholesterol may influence risk factors for heart disease, along with smoking and high blood pressure.

Eating more foods high in fiber may reduce the symptoms of chronic constipation, diverticulosis, and some types of "irritable bowel" in some individuals. Dietary fat has been associated epidemiologically with some cancers, but better understanding of the strength of the relationship must await the outcome of ongoing studies. Finally, poor nutrition may increase susceptibility to infections, fatigue, and stress.

Overweight infants become obese adults (Charney, et al., 1976); and during adolescence they are obese children. Prevention must begin early, before learned patterns of overeating are established. Obesity is associated with increased rates of coronary heart disease, adult-onset diabetes, hypertension, stroke, and accidents, and the combined toll on community health is very large.

Prevention and nutrition promotion measures

Education. A variety of nutrition education measures directed at the community can include increasing awareness of safe weight reduction strategies based on energy balance concepts; increasing awareness of the science base and areas of scientific controversy about the relation of diet to heart disease, high blood pressure, certain cancers, diabetes, dental caries, and other conditions; providing information and behavioral skills to enable people to select and prepare more healthful diets; developing more effective means of communicating nutrition information to people in different age and ethnic groups; and providing nutrition information and education about healthy food choices imparted in the home (via the media), in schools, at the worksite, by and to health care providers, at the point of purchase, as a part of government food service programs (such as Project Head Start, school lunch, and Woman, Infant, and Child programs in the United States), and by appropriate advertising of food products.

Service measures. The provision of food and counseling services in the community should include nutritious breakfast and lunch programs for school children and meals for senior citizens in congregate nutrition sites; food stamps for low-income populations; food supplements for low-income women, infants, and children; nutritious food offered in business and institutional settings; counseling related to dietary practices routinely offered to high-risk individuals by health care providers, schools, and employers; and psychosocial support groups focused on weight control and weight maintenance.

Technological measures. Most of the technological means of improving nutrition must be exercised at a national or state or provincial level, but some community action is possible in assuring nutritional quality and content of manufactured foodstuffs, from production through consumption; changing livestock practices to produce leaner meat; fortifying certain foodstuffs (e.g., bread); developing and making readily available new products lower in fat, saturated fat, cholesterol, sodium, and sugar; positioning products in supermarkets so that key information on caloric, cholesterol, sodium, and sugar contents of products is readily apparent.

Legislative and regulatory measures. Again, national or state or provincial action is often required to obtain legislation or regulatory changes. Communities can assist by promulgating guidelines to maintain or improve the nutritional quality of the food supply; requiring nutrition labeling on foods about which nutrition claims are made or to which nutrients are added; including information on calories, fat, carbohydrate, protein, cholesterol, sugars, sodium, and other nutrients of public health concern; providing explicit discretionary authority to control fortification of foods when this control is of public health significance; controlling food vending practices in schools to reduce or eliminate highly cariogenic foods and snacks; grading standards to give greater emphasis to lower fat products; and regulating televised advertisements directed at young children that promote cariogenic and nonnutritious foods and snacks.

Economic measures. The prospect for economic incentives or sanctions include possibilities for adjusting insurance premiums, in relation to relative risk, for corporations offering employee health promotion programs with a nutrition component; assessing feasibility and cost benefits of reimbursement by third party payers of counseling services that meet appropriate standards; and decreasing local sales taxes on staple foods.

Appraisal of the measures. Service programs are likely to be effective in improving the nu-

tritional status of pregnant women and children and in reducing the incidence of low birth weight infants. Certain segments of the public in the United States have responded to educational messages about fats and cholesterol by reducing their intakes. On the other hand, some government messages have been mixed and contradictory, leaving the public confused. Technological measures hold real promise, particularly if governmental policies could be generated in support of such measures and if resultant products are acceptable to consumers. With the exception of food sanitation, regulation and economic incentives have not been employed and are therefore of uncertain potential.

World hunger and nutrition

While the developed countries are preoccupied with the problems of obesity and nutritional content, the Third World countries and some populations within the developed countries have a more compelling problem of malnutrition and hunger. The developed nations have a special capability and special responsibility to lead the campaign against world hunger. The United States is by far the most powerful member of the world's increasingly interdependent food system. It harvests more than half the grain that crosses international borders. Its grain reserves are the world's largest. Because of its agricultural productivity, its advanced food technology, and its market power, the United States automatically exerts a major influence, intended or not, on all aspects of the international food system. Together with the other developed nations, these resources must be deployed to address nutrition and health on a global scale.

The nature and extent of world hunger today. The major world hunger problem today is not periodic famine, but the less dramatic one of chronic undernutrition. Chronic undernutrition results when people consume fewer calories and less protein than their bodies require to lead active, healthy lives. Although chronic or repeated shortages of calories may appear less newsworthy than outright starvation, they steadily take a greater toll in human lives. The Food and Agriculture Organization of the United Nations estimates that as of 1975 approximately 450 million people were severely malnourished in the developing world. More than three quarters of the world's inadequately nourished people live on the Indian subcontinent, in Southeast Asia, and in sub-Saharan Africa. Many also live in parts of Latin America and the Middle East, and pockets of the poorly nourished persist in the United States and other rich countries as well.

In the United States hunger is particularly common among migrant and seasonal farmworkers, native Americans, the elderly, and those with incomes below the poverty level. Federal programs to alleviate hunger were greatly expanded during the 1960s, and there is evidence that the nutrition of the American poor participating in the programs has improved. Yet participants remain poor and dependent on federal assistance, and only a small percentage of eligible people actually participate in the programs. Life-style and priorities of poor people do play a role in program participation rates. Health education can help to offset these problems.

Children under 5 make up over half of the world's malnourished population, and significantly more women are affected than men. Despite the magnitude, moral aspects, and high social and economic costs, world hunger seldom captures widespread public attention except in times of catastrophe and dire emergency. World hunger is at least as much a political, economic, educational, and social challenge as it is a scientific, technical, or logistical one.

Public education on world hunger. The broad-based plan of action recommended by the Presidential Commission on World Hunger (1980) calls for a major reordering of national priorities. For such a marked shift in established policies and practices to occur, public support must be mobilized. The public is only dimly aware of what Western as well as Third World nations could gain if people in all nations could afford to feed themselves. A successful effort to end hunger will require long-term economic and political support, and this support can only exist if the North American and European publics understand the realities of world hunger. The Presidential Commission on World Hunger recommended that the U.S. Congress provide funds to establish an organization to educate and inform the American public about world hunger.

In the end, like so many issues in community health, especially those related to life-style, the issue of ending world hunger comes down to a question of political choice—a factor that is no more predictable than the weather, but far more susceptible to human control. The quantities of food and money needed to eliminate hunger are very small in relation to available global resources. Political will is the missing ingredient and will be required in abundance at community as well as national levels.

Hunger is the floor on nutrition. Nutrition is the foundation on which other aspects of health and life-style depend for their development. Without attending first to issues of hunger, community health programs may gain the attention of the affluent at the expense of the poor and disadvantaged populations who have the most to gain from health promotion.

DRUG MISUSE

As recently as the close of World War II, the term "problem drugs" generally meant only morphine or its derivative, heroin. This limited concept of problem drugs has now been expanded to a point where morphine represents one of the lesser drug problems. As more and more people become dependent on drugs, there has arisen an alarming misuse of stimulants, depressants, hallucinogens, and narcot-

TABLE 12-8. List of drugs—medical uses, symptoms produced, and their dependency potentials*

Name	Slang name	Chemical or trade name	Classification	Medical use
Heroin	H, horse, scat, junk, smack, scag, stuff, Harry	Diacetyl-morphine	Narcotic	Pain relief
Morphine	White stuff, M	Morphine sulfate	Narcotic	Pain relief
Codeine	Schoolboy	Methylmorphine	Narcotic	Ease pain and coughing
Methadone	Dolly	Dolophine, Amidon	Narcotic	Pain relief
Cocaine	Corrine, gold dust, coke, Bernice, flake, star dust, snow	Methylester of benzoyl ecgonine	Stimulant, local anesthesic	Local anesthesic
Marijuana	Pot, grass, tea, gage, reefers	*Cannabis sativa*	Relaxant, euphoriant in high doses, hallucinogen	None in U.S.
Barbiturates	Barbs, blue devils, yellow jackets, phennies, peanuts, blue heavens	Phenobarbital, Nembutal, Seconal, Amytal	Sedative-hypnotic	Sedative, relieve high blood pressure, epilepsy, hyperthyroidism
Amphetamines	Bennies, dexies, speed, wake-ups, lid poppers, hearts, pep pills	Benzedrine, Dexedrine, Desoxyn, methamphetamine, Methedrine	Sympathomimetic	Relieve mild depression, control appetite and narcolepsy
LSD	Acid, sugar, big D, cubes, trips	d-Lysergic acid diethylamide	Hallucinogen	Experimental study of mental function, alcoholism
DMT	AMT, businessman's high	*N,N*-Dimethyl-tryptamine	Hallucinogen	None

*From Ray, O.S.: Drugs, society, and human behavior, St. Louis, 1974, The C.V. Mosby Co.
†Question marks indicate conflicts of opinion.

How taken	Usual dose	Effects sought	Long-term symptoms	Physical dependence potential	Mental dependence potential
Injected or sniffed	Varies	Euphoria, prevent withdrawal discomfort (4 hr)	Addiction, constipation, loss of appetite	Yes	Yes
Swallowed or injected	15 milligrams	Euphoria, prevent withdrawal discomfort (6 hr)	Addiction, constipation, loss of appetite	Yes	Yes
Swallowed	30 milligrams	Euphoria, prevent withdrawal discomfort (4 hr)	Addiction, constipation, loss of appetite	Yes	Yes
Swallowed or injected	10 milligrams	Prevent withdrawal discomfort (4 to 6 hr)	Addiction, constipation, loss of appetite	Yes	Yes
Sniffed, injected, or swallowed	Varies	Excitation, talkativeness (varies, short)	Depression, convulsions	No	Yes
Smoked, swallowed, or sniffed	1 to 2 cigarettes	Relaxation, increased euphoria, perceptions, sociability (4 hr)	Usually none	No	Yes?†
Swallowed or injected	50 to 100 milligrams	Anxiety reduction, euphoria (4 hr)	Addiction with severe withdrawal symptoms, possible convulsions, toxic psychosis	Yes	Yes
Swallowed or injected	2.5 to 5.0 milligrams	Alertness, activeness (4 hr)	Loss of appetite, delusions, hallucinations, toxic psychosis	Yes?	Yes
Swallowed	100 to 500 micrograms	Insightful experiences, exhilaration, distortion of senses (10 hr)	May intensify existing psychosis, panic reactions	No	No?
Injected	60 to 70 milligrams	Insightful experiences, exhilaration, distortion of senses (less than 1 hr)	?	No	No?

Continued.

TABLE 12-8. List of drugs—medical uses, symptoms produced, and their dependency potentials—cont'd

Name	Slang name	Chemical or trade name	Classification	Medical use
Mescaline	Mesc	3,4,5-Trimeth-oxyphenethylamine	Hallucinogen	None
Psilocybin		3-[2-(dimethylamino) ethyl]indol-4-ol dihydrogen phosphate	Hallucinogen	None
Alcohol	Booze, juice, etc.	Ethanol, ethyl alcohol	Sedative-hypnotic	Solvent, antiseptic
Tobacco	Fag, coffin nail, etc.	*Nicotiana tabacum*	Stimulant-sedative	Sedative, emetic (nicotine)

ics, cutting across all social strata. (A list of drugs, their medical uses, symptoms produced, and their dependency potentials are in Table 12-8.)

Adverse drug reactions

In addition to purposeful misuse, the uninformed or misguided mixing of prescription drugs, over-the-counter drugs, alcohol, and certain foods leads to adverse reactions, including hormonal imbalances, digestive disturbances, mood alterations, and other problems that interfere with normal functioning, productivity, and safety. To say that we are a "pill happy" society is not an exaggeration, and reliance on pills is the genesis of much drug misuse.

The elderly, who make up 10% of the U.S. population, spend an estimated 20% of the national total for drugs. The per capita expenditure by the elderly for prescribed drugs exceeds that for other age groups. The average elderly person spends almost $100 for prescribed and over-the-counter drugs annually and averages more than 13 prescriptions (including renewals) a year.

It is now well recognized that older patients are more likely to have adverse drug reactions than younger patients. In a study of 700 hospitalized patients at the Johns Hopkins Hospital, 25% of those over age 80 had adverse drug reactions compared with 12% in the 41- to 50-year-old age group. A recent report from the University of Florida indicated that 3% (177) of 6,063 consecutive admissions were due to drug-induced illness. Of those 177 patients, 41% were over the age of 60. Similar data have been obtained in England.

In the United States recent hearings in the House Select Committee on Aging revealed that patients in the country's 23,000 nursing homes take an average of 7 to 10 different drugs a day, drugs often administered by unlicensed, untrained personnel. As a result, there

How taken	Usual dose	Effects sought	Long-term symptoms	Physical dependence potential	Mental dependence potential
Swallowed	350 milligrams	Insightful experiences, exhilaration, disortion of senses (12 hr)	?	No	No?
Swallowed	25 milligrams	Insightful experiences, exhilaration, distortion of senses (6 to 8 hr)	?	No	No?
Swallowed	Varies	Sense alteration, anxiety reduction, sociability (1 to 4 hr)	Cirrhosis, toxic psychosis, neurological damage, addiction	Yes	Yes
Smoked, sniffed, chewed	Varies	Calmness, sociability (time varies)	Emphysema, lung cancer, mouth and throat cancer, cardiovascular damage, loss of appetite	Yes?	Yes

have been reports of adverse reactions and serious side effects. The hearings were prompted by a recent report from the Congressional General Accounting Office that said that although the Department of Health and Human Services has, for 6 years, required that medication given to Medicaid nursing home patients be reviewed monthly, there is still no definition of what that review should entail.

There is no readily accessible, single source of information on drugs, their uses, and monitoring. The most frequently used source is the labeling on each drug approved by the Food and Drug Administration.

Among the top 10 threats to health identified by the U.S. public from a list of 30 possible health threats, diet pills and tranquilizers were ranked number 6 and number 9, respectively. Marijuana was ranked third, cigarettes fourth, crash diets fifth, being overweight seventh, and liquor eleventh.

Drugs can be variously classified, but four classes of primary concern in drug misuse, habituation, and addiction are narcotics, stimulants, hallucinogens, and depressants. These are based on the effects produced.

Drug misuse is a complex social and health problem. Its solution must come through education and social change, not punishment. Perhaps there is a place for a "crash" program based on education, but the problems of drug misuse call for a long-term, continuing program of education and related organizational, economic, and environmental change.

Addiction and habituation

Drug addiction is a psychosomatic entity in which a derangement of cellular metabolism occurs causing a physiological alteration and having psychological effects. The altered state of the body tissue produces a physical dependence that becomes known only after discontinuation of the drug. This dependence is masked while the drug is being taken.

Physical effects of dependence exhibited on withdrawal include body aches, hot flashes, fever, perspiration, nausea, nasal discharge, muscle cramps, body jerks, tremors, and irritability. All of these effects produce anxiety, restlessness, and insecurity. The drug is sought to obtain relief from the distress. Thus a drug can be a danger to the individual and to the community if it produces drug dependence that can result in impaired judgment, physical damage, and psychotic reactions. Morphine, heroin, and alcohol produce physical and psychological dependence.

In the United States, the National Commission on Marihuana and Drug Abuse has divided the entire spectrum of drug-using behavior into the following five patterns:

1. Experimental. The most common type of drug-using behavior—a short, nonpatterned trial of one or more drugs, motivated primarily by curiosity or desire to experience an altered mood state

2. Recreational. Voluntary or patterned use of a drug, usually in social settings; behavior is not sustained by virtue of the dependence of the user on the drug

3. Circumstantial. Behavior generally motivated by the user's perceived need or desire to achieve a new and anticipated effect to cope with a specific problem or situation (for example, students preparing for examinations; long-distance truckers)

4. Intensified drug-using behavior. Drug use that occurs at least daily and is motivated by an individual's problem or stressful situation or a desire to maintain a certain self-prescribed level of performance (for example, housewives who regularly consume barbiturates or other sedatives, business executives who regularly consume tranquilizers, youths who have turned to drugs as sources of excitement or meaning); the salient feature of this group is that the individual still remains integrated within the larger social and economic structure

5. Compulsive use. Patterned behavior at a high frequency and high level of interest, characterized by a high degree of psychological dependence and perhaps physical dependence as well. This category encompasses the smallest number of drug users. The distinguishing feature of this behavior is that drug use dominates the individual's existence, and preoccupation with drug-taking precludes other social functioning (for example, chronic alcoholics, heroin-dependent persons)

Personality and its relation to drug misuse and abuse is difficult to categorize because one can identify a wide spectrum of personalities misusing and abusing alcohol and, to some degree, morphine and heroin. The misuse of marijuana and lysergic acid diethylamide (LSD) involves unique social behavior; perhaps some degree of personality identity is discernible.

While a vast range of personality structure may be found among drug addicts, it is possible to identify certain personality traits that indicate persons more likely than others to resort to drugs. For example, the psychopathic personality type of individual uses drugs to gain a certain mental state or emotional thrill, while the neurotic person turns to drugs to relieve tensions and anxieties. A person who is psychopathic will seek to suppress delusions or relieve depression through drugs. Morphine users seek to escape from or avoid situations that they find distressing. Alcoholic persons may have been depressed, hostile, dependent, or otherwise socially inadequate, to their own way of thinking.

In any consideration of the relationship of personality to drug use is the social environment in which persons find themselves. Social conditioning is extremely important, especially when chance, accessibility, and curiosity combine with a social background weak in personal responsibility and community standards of self-esteem.

Habituation has the connotation of the customary use of a practice of one kind or another that a person finds pleasurable, either as relaxation or activation. Habituation to a drug means that the drug has not produced a physical or psychological dependence because the individual can easily terminate the use of the drug without discernible side effects. Habituation to coffee, tea, and cola drinks is widespread, but no evidence exists that addiction occurs.

Heroin addiction. In the United States the heroin addiction problem is actually not as great as that of several other drug problems such as alcoholism and the use of hallucinogens and depressants. The number of reported deaths from heroin overdoses decreased from approximately 1,800 in 1976 to less than 800 in 1977 and 1978. More than half of known addicts live in four cities—New York, Washington, D.C., Chicago, and Los Angeles.

That addiction to heroin or morphine is a phenomenon predominantly of early adulthood is revealed by the age distribution of known addicts.

Age (years)	Percentage
17 and under	0.2
18 to 20	3.1
21 to 30	47.4
31 to 40	38.1
Over 40	11.2

While studies show that young adults constitute a disproportionate part of the addict population, it has been difficult to identify a particular personality vulnerability or pattern. While some addicts are dullards, many are above normal in intelligence. Some are loafers, some are hard workers, some are physicians.

People who become addicted generally tend to be noncompetitive people who prefer to avoid difficulties rather than face them. They tend to be people who will look for the easiest, least painful solution to their problems. It is true that most people who become addicted had personality problems, but most people with the same problems do not turn to narcotics as a solution.

It takes three things to produce an addict—a poorly adjusted person, an available drug, and the means for bringing the person and drug together. Usually bringing the person and drug together is neither premeditated nor planned but sheerly accidental. Associates usually introduce the drug to the person.

Blighted areas in the large cities are the breeding grounds for narcotics addiction. Where social and economic deprivation exists, drug addiction flourishes. Before World War II a high proportion of addicts was among the foreign-born and first generation of Americans with parents of European ancestry. Today blacks have replaced the foreign-born and account for a disproportionately high percentage of drug addiction.

Boys and girls with a delinquent orientation toward life are most likely to experiment with drugs. Juveniles are prime targets for addiction when they come from homes in which there exists hostility, divorce, separation, personality clashes, low ambitions, distrust, or little opportunity for identity. Association with a delinquent group can then lead the way to drug addiction.

The mere fact of narcotics addiction does not turn addicts into criminals unless they find it necessary to commit crime to obtain drugs. Addicts are usually arrested for possession or selling drugs, not for using drugs.

An epidemiological model of drug misuse

If drug misuse is seen as a practice that is transmitted from one person to another, it may be considered for operational purposes as a contagious illness. This approach makes it possible to apply to its study the methods and terminology used in the epidemiology of infectious disease. (See Chapter 3.)

In the epidemiological model the infectious *agent* is the drug, the *host* and reservoir are both the human, and the *vector* is the drug-using peer. The conventional notion of the "pusher" as the vector is effectively dispelled by a careful review of those studies in which an effort was made to trace the spread of heroin use from person to person. In these studies it is clear that, in the vast majority of instances, an addict was introduced to the use of heroin by a well-meaning friend, usually in the setting of previously established peer group activity. Beginners must learn intravenous injection techniques from other addicts.

The disease presents all the well-known characteristics of epidemics, including rapid spread, clear geographic bounds, and certain age groups and strata of the population being more affected than others.

Treatment of addiction. The physician may not legally dispense heroin to an addict without attempting to cure the addict. This usually means treating the addict in a hospital or referring him or her to a facility where effective treatment can be received. Voluntary patients compose about half the hospital population and pay a nominal fee if they are financially able. While treatment has been excellent, there have been difficulties in providing posthospital care and rehabilitation service. In the United States, as a replacement for federal hospitals, subsidies support state and community centers that can provide local posthospital care and rehabilitation service.

State and community centers have been established to provide care for narcotics. New York City and Los Angeles have such centers, through which highly effective programs have been developed. Physicians, psychologists, nurses, social workers, and other personnel work out effective treatment and posthospital programs to fit the needs and situation of each specific patient. This can be duplicated in the moderate-size communities of the nation. Certainly, every state should provide a complete narcotics control and treatment program.

Drugs are now available to help the narcotics addict through the withdrawal phase. The drugs used temporarily replace heroin and can be withdrawn gradually without the physiological distress created by withdrawing heroin. Successful treatment requires further psycho-

logical, sociological, and personal supervision in the hospital, the home, and the community. A guidance center is not adequate. Posthospital care must go with patients, especially if they go back to their old environment.

The methadone maintenance approach is the most widely used treatment for heroin addiction. Methadone, a synthetic substitute for heroin, can be made available legally. It is administered in a fluid, and heroin addicts stop at the treatment center only long enough to take the drink containing methadone. It appears that methadone induces a cross-tolerance to heroin so there is no craving for heroin. Because methadone treatment in fact substitutes methadone addiction for heroin addiction the treatment leaves something to be desired, but until something better is developed methadone programs are valuable, being used on an ambulatory basis is a community.

In California any addicted person may voluntarily seek treatment in the California Rehabilitation Center, a hospital to which an addict may also be committed by a court. All admissions must stay at least 6 months. On release some patients may be transferred to a halfway house to prepare for entrance to the outside world. Patients are released on parole from the hospital and remain on parole until they have remained drug-free for at least 3 consecutive years.

To deal in the community with the narcotics addict, Great Britain decrees that a physician may administer drugs to an addict if withdrawal would be harmful to the patient or if he or she would not be capable of continuing a normal, useful life without the drug. This removes the profit incentive from illicit drug sales. Responsibility for the control of the addicts rests with their physicians, and the plan has been highly successful. This program might well be tried in the United States, but it must be recognized that conditions in the United States differ from conditions in Britain, and modifications of the plan would doubtless be necessary.

Prevention of addiction. Legal control of nar-

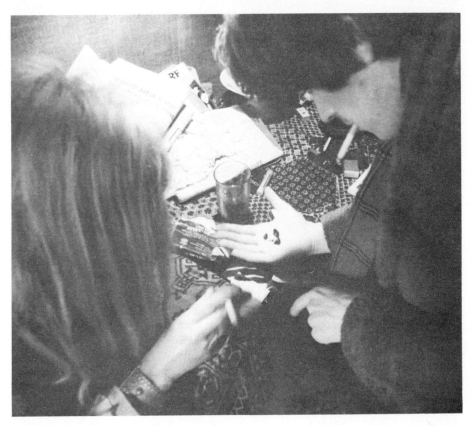

FIG. 12-7. Drug use in the Netherlands. Some take drugs for the mind-altering effects, others to symbolize their membership in a special group.

Courtesy World Health Organization.

cotics traffic is essential at all times. The federal Harrison Narcotic Act and its enforcement by the Bureau of Narcotics has been effective in control in the United States, although the law does have some deficiencies. On the local level, communities generally have not carried their end of the program to control narcotics.

Upgrading of social conditions that spawn drug addiction is the great preventive. Better housing, better neighborhoods, better recreation and jobs, participation in community affairs, better health promotion, and respect for every human being are the foundations on which rests the prevention of narcotics addiction. Education to supplement and complement social and economic development com-

pletes the foundation of any community program to prevent drug addiction.

Misuse of other drugs

Rebellion, boredom, curiosity, seeking new experiences, fun, kicks, pressures, feelings of being trapped, rejection of society, the impersonal nature of our complex society, peer group conformity, revolt against the older population that has created the present state of the world, depression, escape, quest for identity—the possible reasons why people take drugs are legion. Heavy users of drugs are frequently people with inner conflicts who rarely look to external experiences or what is happening about them. They seek change in their inner

TABLE 12-9. Projected estimates of the numbers of people who reported having used drugs nonmedically, U.S. young adults and the total population over the age of 12, 1979*

	Young adults 18-25 yr (population, 31,985,000)				Total population over age 12 (179,358,000)			
	Ever used†		Current user‡		Ever used†		Current user‡	
	%	No.§	%	No.§	%	No.§	%	No.§
Marijuana and hashish	68	21,700,000	35	11,200,000	30	54,800,000	13	22,600,000
Inhalants	17	5,400,000	1	300,000	7	12,700,000	1	1,400,000
Hallucinogens	25	8,000,000	4	1,300,000	9	15,800,000	1	1,800,000
Phencyclidine (PCP)	15	4,800,000	‖	=	5	8,200,000	‖	=
Cocaine	28	9,000,000	9	2,900,000	8	15,100,000	2	4,400,000
Heroin	4	1,300,000	¶	¶		2,600,000	¶	¶
Stimulants	18	5,800,000	4	1,300,000	8	13,900,000	1	2,100,000
Sedatives	17	5,400,000	3	1,000,000	6	13,900,000	1	2,100,000
Tranquilizers	16	5,100,000	2	600,000	5	9,800,000	¶	¶
Analgesics	12	3,800,000	1	300,000	5	8,200,000	¶	¶
Alcohol	95	30,400,000	76	24,300,000	90	160,800,000	61	108,600,000
Cigarettes	83	26,500,000	43	13,800,000	79	142,100,000	36	62,400,000

*Estimates from National Institute on Drug Abuse: National survey on drug abuse: main findings, 1979, The Institute.

†Used one or more times in a person's life.

‡Used at least once in the 30 days prior to the survey.

§The numbers of users are estimated by multiplying the percentages obtained from the national survey sample by the total population of the United States in the corresponding age group. The same procedure (called synthetic estimates) can be used to estimate the number of users in any community or college by multiplying the percentage by the population (divided by 100).

‖Not included in the survey.

¶Amounts of less than 0.5% are not listed.

thoughts to relieve pain they feel or to obtain a more pleasing mental state. Many are psychotic, and a greater number are neurotic.

Prevalence of nonmedical drug use. The most comprehensive estimates of various drugs used without prescriptions in the United States come from national household surveys sponsored by the National Institute on Drug Abuse (1979). Despite the increased use for some "hard drugs" and marijuana, the 1979 survey shows that alcohol is still the drug of choice for most people. Table 12-9 shows that 76% of young adults were current alcohol drinkers in 1979 (compared to 69% in 1976). Current drinkers are more likely to also have used psychotherapeutic pills, marijuana, and "stronger" drugs. Further, 55% of young people, ages 16 to 17, were current drinkers in 1979 compared to 35% in 1972.

The survey likely underestimated the real level of drug use. The interviews were done only in households and did not include people who are transients or who live on military bases, in college dormitories, or prisons. All of these populations probably have higher rates of use. Much of the survey concentrated on marijuana, which is the third most frequently used drug in the United States, after alcohol and tobacco.

Marijuana. Marijuana, a hallucinogen, is obtained from the dried flowering tops of the pistillate (female) plant *Cannabis sativa*. The plant grows in all of the 50 states in the United States, and the dried, crushed leaves and flowering top are smoked as a cigarette. Some smokers develop a certain psychological dependency on marijuana, but there is no hangover.

Marijuana is neither as good nor as bad as has been claimed. The federal marijuana law is far too severe in terms of the drug's danger. State laws against use generally are also too severe. The sale of marijuana should be the focus of the law, and penalties imposed for trafficking in the drug should receive more attention.

LSD. In its pure form LSD cannot be distinguished from water, being tasteless and odorless. It can be transported via sugar cubes, liquor, gum, and virtually any food.

LSD produces hallucinations, delusions, distortions, anxieties, and even psychoses. Under the influence of LSD, some users take their own lives, and some take the lives of others. The drug can produce damage to the brain, to bone marrow, and to chromosomes. The consequences of chromosome damage can be awesome in terms of genetic and other effects that are the concern of the community and its present and future welfare.

Many who experiment with LSD could be classed as normal individuals. Fortunately for these people, one "trip" may not cause permanent damage, although the danger is always present. Repeat trips insidiously produce long-term deleterious effects.

Prevention of LSD use must be directed toward education of the public and the prevention and correction of conditions that lead a person to turn to LSD as an escape from the present environment.

Barbiturates. Americans consume more than 3 billion sleeping pills in a year. Most of these are barbiturates in some form and are used for producing sleep or for purposes of sedation. Barbiturates are beneficial when properly used. It is in the indiscriminate misuse of barbiturates that the problem lies, and the extent of barbiturate addiction may be exceeded only by alcohol addiction.

The person intoxicated with barbiturates is drowsy, confused, depressed, morose, irritable, and quarrelsome. Withdrawal results in severe physiological disturbances and may be fatal. The drug should be withdrawn only under medical supervision.

While some people deliberately take an overdose of barbiturates, some deaths regarded as suicides resulting from an overdose of sleeping pills are accidental. Barbiturates produce a twilight zone in some people, causing individuals to forget that they have taken a pill, so they take one pill after another.

In the United States barbiturate deaths have

declined by 10% to 20% per year since 1970. Barbiturates have a role in medical practice, but the misuse of the drug will continue.

Amphetamines. Pep pills such as Benzedrine and Dexedrine are prescription drugs, yet their misuse appears to be on the increase. Amphetamines are used to reduce the appetite in the medical treatment of obesity. These drugs reduce the feeling of fatigue and are used as rejuvenators by people who burn both ends of the candle.

Fad drugs. In setting health promotion targets in drug misuse prevention, communities must recognize that it is impossible to predict which drugs will achieve popularity between now and 1990. Individual drugs can become widely popular within very short periods of time. A community drug misuse prevention strategy must be able to react to such drug problems rapidly and effectively. By their unpredictable nature, fad drugs are difficult to incorporate into long-range health promotion objectives; nevertheless, their health impact can be profound, and it is important to understand how their popularity can be influenced by prevention efforts.

PCP. A good example of a drug whose popularity increased rapidly during a short period of time is PCP. Fig. 12-8 depicts the trend in emergency room cases in the United States in which PCP was reported as a contributing factor. The data come from a special panel of hospital emergency rooms that consistently reported to the Drug Abuse Warning Network between April 1976 and September 1978. While some of the increase may have been

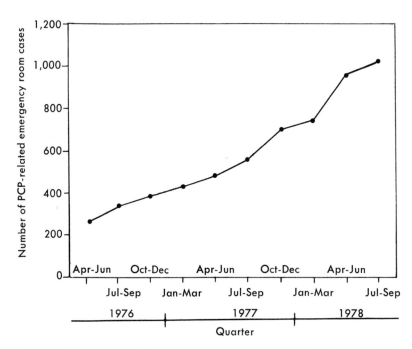

FIG. 12-8. Number of PCP-related emergency room cases reported by 677 consistently reporting hospital emergency rooms, 1976-1978, United States.

From Forecasting Branch, National Institute on Drug Abuse, 1979.

caused by increased awareness of PCP toxicity on the part of emergency room personnel (due in part to official warnings issued in late 1977), such increased sensitivity is unlikely to account entirely for the almost fourfold increase shown in Fig. 12-8. Much of the increase is believed to have resulted directly from increased levels of use.

Known on the street as "angel dust" and by a variety of other names, PCP can be synthesized rather easily from widely available precursor chemicals. The many industrial uses of these chemicals reduce the effectiveness of law enforcement measures in controlling availability of the drug. As a result, PCP is widely and readily available at a price young people can afford.

The sudden popularity of PCP is paradoxical. Although positive reactions ranging from heightened sensitivity through euphoria are reported by users, the effects of PCP are unpredictable, and chronic use in particular is associated with a variety of negative consequences. The range of potential negative outcomes associated with PCP use makes it difficult to understand the drug's popularity. In part, PCP has become popular precisely because its attractions and dangers have been publicized so widely. Risk itself can be a powerful incentive, especially to youth. Widespread publicity of an emerging drug problem may have the unintended effect of stimulating further interest in the drug, interest that fosters additional use, more medical accidents, and more publicity.

This vicious circle can be interrrupted. New drugs develop "street" reputations very quickly. Although not always scientifically accurate, these reputations are important determinants of drug use. PCP is a good example of how a drug's street reputation can influence patterns of use. It first appeared as a recreational drug on the West Coast in the mid-1960s. At that time the drug's negative effects became rapidly known and it had only limited popularity. Although PCP use has subse-

quently increased in other parts of the United States, medical emergencies related to the drug have fallen in some areas after users became aware of the hazards associated with its use.

APPLICATION OF THE COMMUNITY HEALTH PROMOTION MODEL

Misuse of drugs, like smoking, alcohol abuse, obesity, and stress management, is an intertwined social and health problem. Any program to deal with the problem must encompass the social, environmental, economic, psychological, and physiological factors encompassed by the life-style in question. Communities and health officials alike recognize the importance of the drug misuse problem, yet only sporadic attempts have been made by communities to deal with it.

Health education, traditionally, has been called on to alert the public to such complex community health problems, but health education by itself can hardly be expected to solve such problems. The life-styles in question are too embedded in organizational, economic, and environmental circumstances for people to be able to change their own behavior without concomitant changes in these circumstances. Health *promotion* combines health education with these organizational, economic, and environmental supports for behavior conducive to health.

In the United States limitations of the federal program are apparent in the 1966 Drug Abuse Control Law, which was not aimed at the user but at the trafficker. The program of the federal agencies has been important and should be expanded, but the solution to the problem must come on the community level with support from a state or provincial program.

The legal approach to drug misuse must be supplemented by a broad, constructive program of prevention and control. While the legal approach to manufacture and sale of drugs must be continued, the use of drugs must be placed in the category of health, and the individual concerned must be regarded as a person with a behavioral problem. An effective community program for the prevention and control of drug misuse should include the following five aspects:

1. Improvement of conditions in the deprived neighborhoods, where addiction is most common
2. Promotion of mental health programs for the normal individual and clinical and other services for disturbed persons
3. Public health education on the use and misuse of drugs
4. Increased measures to reduce the availability of drugs
5. Providing treatment for people with addictions, including the necessary follow-up and guidance in rehabilitation

As this chapter concludes Part Two of this book, the models and concepts introduced in Part One can be reviewed as they apply to community health promotion, and more specifically to the difficult problems of life-style exemplified by drug misuse and drug misuse prevention. In Chapter 4 a model of health education was introduced and applied to problems of maternal and child health. That model will now be expanded to include the additional elements of economic, organizational, and environmental supports for behavior conducive to health, and applied as a model of health *promotion* for drug misuse prevention (based on Iverson and Green, 1981).

Public health and drug misuse prevention

Most public health professionals employ a taxonomy of three levels of prevention: primary, secondary, and tertiary. Primary prevention is accomplished by activities that promote optimum health and provide specific protection against a health problem (e.g., proper nutrition, genetic counseling, fluoridation, disease inoculation). In drug misuse prevention, the goal of primary prevention activities is to decrease the rate at which new cases of drug misuse appear in a population by counteracting circumstances conducive to the development of drug misuse before they have a chance to produce drug misuse behavior. Secondary prevention refers to activities concerned with the early diagnosis and prompt treatment of health problems (e.g., Papanicolaou [Pap] smear, troubled employee programs, regular physical examination, neonatal metabolic screening). The goal of secondary drug misuse prevention activities is to reduce the disability rate caused by drug misuse by lowering the number of drug misuse cases in the community. Tertiary prevention refers to minimizing the disability from existing illness through treatment and rehabilitation efforts (e.g., treatment for persons with lung cancer, alcoholism rehabilitation, treatment of sexually transmitted diseases). The goal of tertiary drug misuse prevention efforts is to reduce the complications and social pathology in the affected population by reducing or eliminating the misuse of drugs.

Prevention strategies. Three types of strategies can be used in each of the three prevention levels to accomplish the desired goals (Mullen, 1981):

- Educational strategies—including strategies to inform and educate the public about the dangers of drug misuse, the benefits of automobile restraints, or the relationship of maternal alcohol consumption to the occurrence of the fetal alcohol syndrome.
- Automatic-protective strategies—including public health measures directed at environmental variables such as milk pasteurization, fluoridation, infant immunizations, and burning or chemical killing of marijuana crops.
- Coercive strategies—including strategies that employ legal and other formal sanctions to control individual behavior such as requiring up-to-date immunizations for school entry, tuberculosis testing of hospi-

TABLE 12-10. Levels of prevention with examples of strategies in prevention of health problems, including those associated with drug misuse

| | Levels of prevention | | |
	Primary	Secondary	Tertiary
Educational	Genetic counseling School health education Public education about drugs	Community hypertension screening–education programs Teacher training in recognition of drug problems	Drug education programs for patients in coronary care
Automatic- protective	Fluoridation of community drinking water systems Legal control of prescription drugs	Neonatal metabolic screening Requiring medical prescription for drug refills	Referral to community mental health center for counseling following discharge from drug treatment centers
Coercive	Immunization requirements for school children Arrests of drug traffickers	Mandatory classes for persons convicted of drinking while intoxicated or using illicit drugs	Mandatory treatment for persons having a sexually transmitted disease or addiction

tal employees, and compulsory use of child automobile restraints, and arrests for drug possession or use.

A matrix of examples of community health programs directed at each of the three levels of prevention using the three categories of prevention strategies is presented in Table 12-10. Examples are included to illustrate both the traditional public health strategies and the new strategies in community health promotion and drug misuse prevention.

Preventive programs in public health can also be classified by the site where the program occurs. While the community has been the primary site for most prevention programs, increasingly, programs can be found in the work, school, and medical care settings.

Health education methods and theories. Regardless of the setting in which the community health promotion program occurs, the promotional methods used in the program can be classified into several broad categories, three of them essentially concerning education:

- Direct communications with the people whose behavior is in question to *predispose* behavior conducive to health. These include lecture-discussion, individual counseling or instruction, mass media, audiovisual aids, educational television, and programmed learning.
- Training methods to *enable* or *reinforce* behavior conducive to health, including skills development, simulations and games, inquiry learning, small group discussion, modeling, and behavior modification.
- Organizational methods to *support* behavior conducive to health, including community development, social action, social planning, and economic and organizational development. These methods go beyond health education in supporting behavior.

Table 12-11 presents an overview of the appropriate use of the various educational strategies according to characteristics of the health behavior addressed by the program.

One of the most noticeable changes in pre-

TABLE 12-11. Educational strategies according to characteristics of the health behavior*

Diagnostic criterion	Prevalent category	Audiovisual aids	Lecture	Individual instruction	Mass media	Programmed learning	Educational television	Skill development	Simulations and games	Inquiry learning	Peer-group discussion	Modeling	Behavior modification	Community development	Social action	Social planning and organizational change	No recommendations
Educational outcome desired	Cognitive: knowledge comprehension	X	X	X	X	X	X		X	X	X						
	Cognitive: application, analysis, synthesis, and evaluation								X	X	X						
	Affective								X	X	X	X					
	Psychomotor							X	X				X	X	X	X	
Complexity of the health information	Simple				X	X	X										
	Complex								X	X	X						
Complexity of the health behavior	Simple	X			X												
	Complex			X									X	X	X	X	
Duration of the health behavior	Short term	X	X		X												
	Long term							X	X	X	X	X	X	X	X	X	
Frequency of the health behavior	Infrequent		X		X												
	Frequent							X		X	X	X					
Extent of the health behavior	Rare																X
	Widespread								X			X					
Additive vs. substitutive nature of the health behavior	Additive			X									X				
	Substitutive								X		X		X				
Promptness vs. delay of the health behavior	No delay				X												
	Delay															X	X

*Adapted from Green, L.W., et al.: Health education planning: a diagnostic approach, Palo Alto, Calif., 1980, Mayfield Publishing Co., with thanks to Edward Bartlett.

vention and health promotion programs in community health in recent years has been the increasing integration of behavioral theory into health education and other phases of program development. Insofar as health behavior is only partially understood (the level of understanding varies with the complexity of the health behavior), multiple theories have been used in planning for prevention programs. The model presented in Chapter 4, for example, combines theories and concepts from the Health Belief Model (Becker, 1974), cognitive consistency theory (Aronson, 1968), behavioral intention theory (Fishbein and Ajzen, 1975), developmental theory (Piaget, 1972), social learning theory (Bandura, 1971), psychological-inoculation theory (McGuire, 1963), and diffusion theory (Rogers and Shoemaker, 1971). The most successful programs consult relevant theory in their planning to clarify the assumptions about the causes of behavior on the basis of which the strategies are selected or developed.

The prevention approach of public health has differed from that frequently found in past drug misuse prevention efforts, but the two fields are converging. The National Institute on Drug Abuse now refers to four modalities of prevention: information, education, alternatives, and intervention (Bukowski, 1979). Similar to the public health approach, drug misuse prevention programs are targeted at populations (e.g., demographically defined groups, families, peer groups) and settings (community, school, workplace) and usually employ multiple educational methods.

Drug misuse programs have differed from traditional public health programs, with the educational and behavioral theories and models increasingly incorporating principles from developmental and social learning theories. The bases of earlier drug misuse programs were drawn primarily from personality, cognitive, and sociological theories.

Another important distinction between the theoretical underpinning of program development efforts in the two fields is the level of understanding of the target behaviors. Many of the target behaviors of traditional public health programs were relatively simple and easily understood (e.g., immunization behavior, infant feeding), whereas drug misuse behavior was far more complex, but recently has been more thoroughly studied (Austin, Macari, and Lettieri, 1979; Bloom, 1977; Lindblad, 1977). For example, studies on the continuing reinforcers of drug misuse (Crawley, 1972) as well as reinforcers related to the initiation of drug use (Blachly, 1974) have allowed programs to match prevention strategies to target populations.

A third distinction is in the role of ethnicity and racial background in influencing health behavior. Public health programs have always been cognizant of the ethnic and racial influences in health behaviors, such as public use of health practitioners, and have designed prevention programs to account for these influences. People in the drug misuse field have taken increasing notice of ethnicity and racial background as powerful influences on the causes of drug misuse, so much as to alter the nature of the problem and subsequently the prevention techniques that may be effective. The information on drug misuse among black populations has indicated that prevention efforts must focus on social and environmental factors rather than an individual factors, as they often do with white populations.

Whatever differences that may have existed in the program planning approaches between the drug misuse field and the more traditional public health field, the two have increasingly converged, as both address social problems involving life-style. Strategies for intervention differ; but there are some common elements. They include prevention through education that starts early and extends throughout life; altering the social climate of acceptability; reducing individual and social stress factors; and legal enforcement.

Lengthy and detailed examinations of the public health problems currently facing the United States, Great Britain, Canada, and Australia were initiated by their respective legislatures and national administrations in the 1970s. Canada was first with the publication of *A New Perspective on the Health of Canadians* (Canadian Ministry of Health and Welfare, 1974). Agencies within the U.S. Department of Health, Education, and Welfare (DHEW, now the Department of Health and Human Services [DHHS]) analyzed departmental activities in disease prevention and health promotion, identified health problems of the highest priority as well as measures to address the problems, and assembled them in the documents *Disease Prevention and Health Promotion: Federal Programs and Prospects,* (U.S. Department of Health, Education, and Welfare, 1978) and *Healthy People: The Surgeon General's Report on Health Promotion and Disease Prevention,* (U.S. Department of Health, Education, and Welfare, 1979a). A framework similar to the Health Field Concept from Canada, described in Chapter 2, was useful in devising strategy to affect public health problems. The framework included three points of intervention:

1. Human life-style—recognizing that the choices an individual makes about personal life-style can increase risk of health problems in a variety of behaviors
2. Human environment—recognizing that settings and other external sources of hazards can increase health problems
3. Human services—recognizing that preventive services can influence the incidence or course of preventable diseases and conditions for any individual

It is the thesis of both the Canadian and the American initiatives in disease prevention and health promotion that programs or interventions in all three areas—life-style, environment, and services—are required to address the leading causes of death. A drug misuse prevention program would include program components, as in Table 12-12, intended to affect individual behavior (life-style), to provide medical treatment of drug misuse and drug dependence as early as possible to prevent permanant damage (human services), and to modify the environmental factors influencing the misuse of drugs (economics and the human environment). The balance of these areas in a community drug misuse prevention program has seldom, if ever, been attained.

The next step in the American initiative in disease prevention and health promotion was the development of the consensus on specific measurable objectives for each of the 15 activities identified in *Healthy People* (U.S. Department of Health, Education, and Welfare, 1979a). A national panel of experts was convened for each of the 15 priorities to formulate measurable objectives. Background papers were prepared by government agencies for use by the experts. The background paper on drug misuse prevention, prepared by the Alcohol, Drug Abuse, and Mental Health Administration, included a number of factors to consider when planning drug misuse prevention programs. Some of the factors discussed in the

TABLE 12-12. Priorities for drug misuse prevention activities

Framework areas from the health field concept	Goals-activities
Life-style	Inclusion of drug misuse prevention as a major component of a comprehensive school health education program
	Public and physician education programs to reduce the number of sleeping pill prescriptions, emphasizing problems of crossaddiction
Services	Education of providers on the taking of a drug history for adolescents and preadolescents
	Promotion of involvement of national and local youth-serving agencies in drug misuse prevention
	Strengthened drug misuse prevention research
Environment	Encouragement of parent groups to provide supportive networks to resist drug misuse among youth
	Improved enforcement of legal and economic regulations of drug market

background paper *Preventing Disease/Promoting Health Objectives for the Nation: Alcohol and Drug Abuse* (U.S. Department of Health, Education, and Welfare, 1979c) were the following:

- Drug abuse is a social problem having both health and legal aspects. To prevent drug abuse, society applies legal sanctions and promotes positive behavioral alternatives (p. 1).
- Despite the heavy social cost generated by drug abuse, the use of most illegal drugs (with the important exception of marijuana) remains a relatively rare event (p. 2).
- Current public policy for some drugs (e.g., heroin and cocaine) has used law enforcement mechanisms to keep the price of drugs as high as possible. The desired effects of this policy is to motivate current users to stop using the drug and to make it difficult for nonusers to initiate use of the drug (p. 2).
- Treatment (especially for heroin use) is offered as an alternative to continued use of a drug. This helps to reduce the level of active drug use in the community at large. Treatment also has the effect of reducing the risk of future medical drug-related dysfunction (p. 2).
- Some drugs have gained popularity because their attractions and dangers have been widely publicized. Risk itself can be a powerful incentive, especially to youth (p. 4).
- There is good evidence that drug use among young people develops in predictable stages and that marijuana use is a key "gateway" through which those who become involved in serious drug abuse usually pass (p. 6).
- Current drug abuse prevention strategies focus on enhancing an individual's personal and social development as a way to prevent the adverse consequences of drug use. Given current levels of drug use, it is important that prevention activities attempt to reduce the negative consequences of drug use rather than, unrealistically, attempt to prevent all use of drugs (p. 9).
- A strategy particularly applicable to preventing the misuse of prescription drugs is to encourage more appropriate use of drugs (p. 14).

Given the complexities, only two achievable objectives were identified in the background papers: (1) to reduce current marijuana use among youth ages 12 to 17 years and (2) to reduce the number of deaths in which barbiturates are a direct contributing factor.

The U.S. expert panel reviewed information on the status and trends of drug use, the health implications of drug use, and the potential drug-related prevention-promotion measures available, including the strength and feasibility of the measure. The panel then identified two major objectives and 11 measurable objectives that were to be achieved by 1990. These objectives were circulated to more than 3,000 organizations and additional experts for comment and review. This process has resulted in the closest that one can expect to come to consensus on U.S. national objectives to be achieved by 1990. The objectives for drug misuse in the final document of *Promoting Health/Preventing Disease: Objectives for the Nation* (U.S. Department of Health and Human Services, 1980) included the following:

- Drug-related mortality (other than alcohol) will be reduced to 2.0 per 100,000 per year. (In 1978 the rate was 2.8 per 100,000.)
- Adverse reactions from medical use of drugs sufficiently severe to require hospital admission should be reduced to 25% fewer such admissions per year. (In 1979 estimates ranged from approximately 105,000 to 350,000 admissions per year.)
- The proportion of 12- to 17-year-olds who abstain from using alcohol or other drugs should equal or exceed 1977 levels. (In 1977 the proportion of abstainers was 46% for alcohol; and for other drugs, the proportion ranged from 89% for marijuana to 99.9% for heroin.)
- The proportion of young adults and youths reporting frequent use of other drugs (excluding alcohol) should be limited to 1977 levels. (In 1977 it was less than 1% for drugs other than marijuana and 19% for marijuana.) (*Frequent use* refers to the nonmedical use of any specific drug on 5 or

more days during the previous month.)
- Eighty percent of high school seniors should state (in response to survey questions) that they perceive great risk associated with frequent marijuana and cigarette smoking, barbiturate use, or alcohol intoxication. (In 1979 63% perceived great risk to be associated with one or two packs of cigarettes smoked daily, 42% with regular marijuana use, 75% with regular barbiturate use.)
- The proportion of workers in major firms whose employers provide an active substance prevention and referral program should be greater than 70%. (In 1976 50% of the *Fortune 500* firms offered employee assistance programs.)

These measurable objectives, when met, will result in the satisfaction of the two major objectives:
- To minimize the adverse social and health consequences associated with the use of drugs, especially among adolescents and young adults.
- To minimize the number of adolescents who become users of alcohol and other drugs.

The question that remains is, How can communities plan their drug misuse prevention programs to satisfy these major and minor objectives?

The planning framework applied to drug misuse

Drug misuse prevention efforts have too often been based on attitude change and fear-arousal strategies. Although such strategies have valid uses, their applicability to community health programs is limited. To maximize the effectiveness of a community drug misuse prevention program, concurrent efforts should be initiated in the three health field categories described in *A New Perspective on the Health of Canadians* (Canadian Ministry of Health and Welfare, Lalonde, 1974) and in *Healthy People*

(U.S. Department of Health, Education, and Welfare, 1979a)—human life-style, human environment, and human services. In all three, attention must be directed at factors that predispose, enable, and reinforce behavior conducive to health.

Prevention programs, whether they be directed at drug misuse, communicable disease, or teenage pregnancy, have as a base health education activities. Health education is defined in Chapter 4 as any combination of learning opportunities designed to facilitate voluntary adaptations of behavior conducive to health. Well-planned drug education programs have been shown to be effective for some people (Blum, 1976; Goodstadt, 1974; Schaps et al., 1978), but they have not demonstrated an ability to resolve a community drug misuse problem. Perhaps no single effort will be able to resolve such problems totally. But drug misuse prevention programs incorporating educational, organizational, and economic supports for life-style, environment, and services conducive to health have a much greater chance of success than programs directed at only one of these categories. Programs directed at a combination of these categories to support behaviors conducive to health are called health promotion programs.

Health promotion is defined as any combination of health education and related organizational, environmental, and economic supports for behavior conducive to health. With health education as an integral part of all health promotion interventions it follows that the interventions should be directed toward voluntary behavior at all levels—individuals, organizations, and communities. At the community, state or provincial, or national level, additional interventions may be legal, regulatory, political, or economic and therefore potentially coercive. Nevertheless, such interventions must be supported by an informed and consenting public. Such informed consent requires health education. Ideally, the coercive measures are directed at the behavior of those whose actions may affect the health of others, such as the manufacturers, distributors, and advertisers of hazardous products. Even then, public health education may be required to assure the support of an informed public because taxes, prices, availability, and jobs may be affected by such regulations of health- or drug-related industries and sources.

For example, one part of health promotion programs could be targeted toward organizational change. Health education could be combined with various incentives (e.g., free program consultation services) and persuasion techniques (e.g., program promotion by local public leaders) in an attempt to increase the number of schools offering peer counseling programs for those who misuse drugs. If the program were targeted toward political change, community organization techniques could be combined with health education activities to develop "concerned parent groups" in neighborhoods and to apply political pressure to local school and law enforcement officials who are not supportive of drug misuse prevention

efforts, and, of course, to provide support for those officials supportive of existing prevention efforts. If the program were targeted toward economic change, health professionals and others could work with representatives of insurance carriers to initiate changes in existing health insurance reimbursement regulations that preclude payment for counseling and rehabilitation services. The point is simple—when health education activities are combined with appropriate changes in organizations, political systems, and environmental and economic supports for behavior, the end result is more likely to be favorable than is the result achieved by a series of single, uncoordinated changes. Indeed, uncoordinated changes sometimes make things worse by throwing a community system out of balance and forcing an overreaction or overcompensation by the wrong elements in the community.

The relationships of health education and health promotion activities to the three prevention targets and the relationships of these targets to the health or drug misuse objectives set for the community and the nation are de-

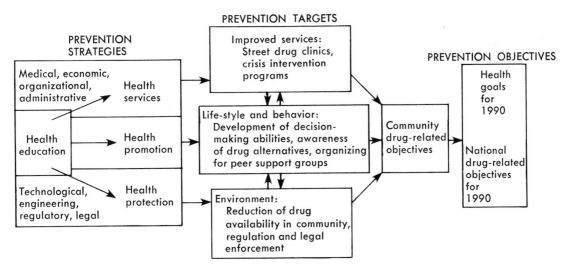

FIG. 12-9. Interventions and processes for drug misuse prevention: relationship of community health education and health promotion activities to national health objectives.

picted in Fig. 12-9. The three prevention targets are not isolated. Life-style is continually affected by the human environment and the organization of services (as seen in Chapter 4). Further, a successful program must effectively integrate and coordinate activities in relation to each of these targets. To facilitate the integration of activities within and between the prevention strategies, a planning framework is needed. The planning framework proposed in Chapter 4 forces an encompassing and systematic analysis of public health problems in the context of social problems or quality of life concerns (see Fig. 4-2).

When using the framework in Fig. 4-2 to plan community drug prevention programs, one starts with the final consequences, namely, social problems usually defined as concerns with the quality of life but not necessarily as health concerns. It works back from there to the original causes, that is, predisposing, enabling, and reinforcing causes of the behavior, which influenced the health problem, which in turn influenced the social problem. The following is an application of the phases in this process to prevention of drug misuse.

Phase I: social diagnosis. The social diagnosis phase involves a consideration of the quality of life in a community by assessing the social problems of concern to the various segments of the population. This has the effect of forcing planners to consider the desirable social outcomes of a program before setting priorities on health or selecting program approaches. It also helps to justify a program to the community. This is especially important in the planning of community drug prevention programs because of the relationship between drug-related health problems and the social problems that a community is encountering. For example, when a community has a large number of drug-dependent persons, it is likely that there will be high rates of violent and nonviolent crime, school truancy, early dropouts from school, juvenile delinquency, and unemploy-

ment (all social problems). Conversely, when a community is experiencing such social problems as high unemployment, inadequate housing, inadequate private and public school programs, or discrimination, a serious drug dependence problem will be present because the use of drugs for some will be the "best available" method of coping with the social problems. By identifying the major social problems of concern to the community, one can select potential outcome evaluation measures and gain an understanding of the community's concerns as they relate to the particular health problem that is the target of the prevention program.

Data on a community's social problems can be generated from analyses of existing records, files, publications, and informal interviews and discussions with leaders, key informants, and representatives of various community populations. This is an important first step that should not be undertaken too hastily, because its outcome may well affect program scope and quality as well as the extent of community support.

Phase II: epidemiological diagnosis. The objective of the epidemiological diagnostic phase is to identify the specific health problems that appear to be contributing to the social problems noted in phase I. By using data from community surveys, hospital admissions, city and county health departments, health systems agencies, and selected state or provincial and national data, the drug-related morbidity, mortality, and disability trends can be identified. For each of the identified health problems, such as serum hepatitis, the incidence, prevalence, distribution, intensity, and duration of the problem should be described (see Chapter 3). These data can be analyzed for various populations to determine the populations most affected by the health problem. This process will often reveal and locate a variety of existing health problems such as drug dependence, drug-related psychoses, drug-related depression or anxiety, and other drug-related problems such as serum hepatitis and endocarditis. The use of spatial maps to depict the distribution of the identified health problems within the city or county is an effective way of presenting data if there is reason to believe that the problems vary by geographical location (King, Muraco, and Vezner, 1974).

By use of the results of epidemiological analyses, program objectives should be developed. The objectives should be stated in epidemiological terms and answer the following: Who will be the recipients of the program? What benefit should they receive? How much of that benefit should they receive? By when or for how long? For example, between January and August 1975 it has been estimated that 1,017 persons died of drug overdose in New York City (Gottschalk, McGuire, Heiser, et al., 1979). Data from other U.S. cities suggest that approximately 55% of the deaths are related to the use of opiates. Therefore a program objective for a drug prevention program in New York City could be stated in the following way: To reduce the number of drug overdose deaths in New York City by 25% within 1 year and an additional 25% within the next year, until the national average is reached. The major health (drug) problem for most communities would not be death or drug overdose, rather it would be physiological or psychological dependence.

Phase III: behavioral diagnosis. The behavioral diagnosis phase requires the systematic identification of health behaviors that appear to be causally linked to each of the health problems identified in the epidemiological diagnosis. The outcome of the behavioral diagnosis is the generation of a ranked list of specific behaviors that will be used as the basis for specifying the behavioral objectives of the program.

The process of identifying the health behaviors linked to the health problems usually relies on the professional literature. The review of the literature can be combined with structured and unstructured interviews of persons familiar with the health problem (e.g., drug treatment personnel), data from observations, and intuition based on personal experiences. When drug dependence is the identified health problem, the behavioral causes leading to the health problem would obviously include the personal patterns of drug use and drug misuse. But these behaviors could be subdivided to include misuse of prescription medications, use of illicit drugs such as marijuana and cocaine, and use of illicit drugs in a manner that predisposes the user to health problems, that is, drug misuse. For example, if the identified health problem was cardiovascular disease, the behavioral problems would include smoking, high intake of saturated fats, heavy alcohol consumption, and a sedentary life-style. In the current example in which the identified health problem is drug dependence, the behavioral causes are drug use and drug misuse. These should not be perceived as distinct behaviors, rather they should be viewed as a continuum of drug use to drug misuse with varying types and amounts of drugs used (e.g., National Commission on Marihuana and Drug Abuse, 1973).

A second part of this phase is the identification of the nonbehavioral causes that contribute to the health problem. Nonbehavioral causes are the organizational and environmental factors that contribute to the health problem but that are not controlled directly by the behavior of the target population. Nonbehavioral causes of drug dependence include such factors as the age and sex of the target population, the housing situation in the community, the school environment, and the law enforcement activity in the community. The identification of these factors is important because it provides the planners with direction for health promotion activity other than educational, such as organizational and economic interventions directed at the regulation of the environment and the availability of services.

Phase IV: educational diagnosis. The educational diagnosis phase assesses the relative in-

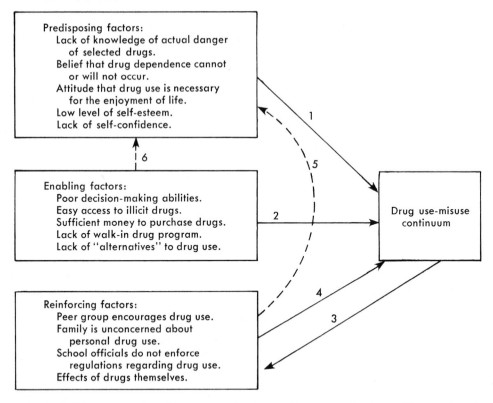

FIG. 12-10. Three categories of factors contributing to drug use and misuse. The numbered arrows indicate the approximate order of cause and effect.

Adapted from Green, L.W., Kreuter, M.W., Deeds, S.G., and Partridge, K.B.: Health education planning: a diagnostic approach, Palo Alto, Calif., 1980, Mayfield Publishing Co.

fluence of various predisposing, enabling, and reinforcing factors on each of the identified behavioral causes of the health problem. Fig. 12-10 focuses attention on the order of causation of behavior, as indicated by the numbered arrows: (1) an initial motivation to act, (2) a deployment of resources and skills to enable the action, (3) a reaction to the behavior from someone else (or in the case of drug use, it can be the drug effects themselves), (4) the reinforcement and strengthening of the behavior or the punishment and discouragement of the behavior, (5) the reinforcement or punishment of the behavior as it affects the predisposing fac-

tors by strengthening or extinguishing the motivation to act, and finally, (6) the increased ability to take certain actions tends to increase the predisposition or motivation to take such actions.

In the process of identifying factors in the three areas, one may include factors that seem to encourage the behavior as well as those that seem to discourage the behavior. On completion of listing the factors, the next step is to select from among the predisposing, enabling, and reinforcing factors those that will be most likely to bring about the behavior desired. The factors that should be selected as targets for the program are those that are most changeable and most important. Importance is determined by the responses to the following questions:

- How widespread or frequent is the factor: (e.g., low self-esteem, use of drugs by peer group members, easy availability of drugs)
- How compelling or urgent is the factor? (e.g., lack of alternatives to drugs, lack of knowledge of effected drugs)
- How close is the connection between the factors and the behavior? (e.g., lack of decision-making skills and drug use, availability of drugs and drug use)

Changeability is assessed from responses to the following questions:

- Does the literature suggest that the factor can be changed? (e.g., Can self-esteem levels be changed? Can decision-making skills be taught? Can school officials be encouraged to enforce regulations?)
- Does the experience of previous programs indicate that a factor can be changed? (e.g., Have programs been successful in changing parental attitudes and behaviors? Have community organization efforts been successful in stimulating development of drug alternatives programs?)

The factors determined to be both important and changeable form the basis of the prevention program. This level of specificity helps to use scarce resources in the most appropriate manner as well as to enhance the chances of the program being successful. Difficult choices will be made in this phase of the planning process, but in the process of making the decisions the level of understanding of the nature of the problem usually increases dramatically.

Phase V: program development. The program development phase selects the right combination of strategies to affect the selected predisposing, enabling, and reinforcing factors. As a general rule, selected communication methods are appropriate in altering predisposing factors; organizing resources and training are effective in altering enabling factors; and strat-

egies such as consultation, training, feedback, and group development are effective in altering the reinforcing factors. Refer to Table 12-10 for an example of considerations in selecting appropriate educational strategies according to characteristics of the problems addressed by the program.

Phase VI: administrative diagnosis. The administrative diagnosis phase assesses the organizational problems likely to be encountered as the program becomes operational. Factors such as interagency cooperation, staffing patterns, and budgeting should be thoroughly discussed. This phase of planning analyzes the potential problems within programs, within organizations, and between organizations. A well-planned program is seldom effective without a properly conceived implementation plan.

SUMMARY

There is obviously no simple solution to the life-style problems of drug misuse, alcohol misuse, obesity, smoking, and sedentary inactivity. Problems as complex as these may defy even well-planned preventive efforts. Nevertheless, the effects of well-planned and systematically implemented preventive efforts are more likely to be successful than the single-focused, uncoordinated efforts that have typified many of the early attempts to address life-style, particularly those at the local level.

The Canadian Ministry of Health and Welfare and the United States Public Health Service have proposed that their prevention efforts focus on three areas: life-style, environment, and services. Specific measurable objectives for the United States have been set, which if met by 1990, will have the effect of substantially reducing the scope and intensity of health problems attributable to life-style, the environment, and inadequate health services. These objectives can serve to concentrate the limited resources of communities where they can be most productive. To illustrate community health programs to affect the objectives, a planning framework that encompasses the three areas of life-style, environment, and services has been presented.

Efforts should be targeted at individuals and environments, as well as at organizational, political, and economic systems. Applying the latest findings from the rapidly developing research and evaluation in designing prevention programs, and assuring the necessary quality and quantity of resources for programs will not guarantee success but will increase the probability of reaching the objectives set for 1990.

QUESTIONS AND EXERCISES

1. Distinguish between addiction and habituation.
2. Why is there no justification for the popular view that drug addicts fit into a common personality pattern?
3. Design an alcoholism control and treatment program for your community.
4. What should the schools teach in alcohol education?
5. Distinguish between stimulant and hallucinogen.
6. Why has there been no recent increase in heroin addiction?
7. Not all poorly adjusted people are drug addicts. Why?
8. What provisions does your state or province make for the treatment and care of heroin addicts?
9. What are the merits and demerits of the British program for dealing with heroin addicts if the program were to be considered for your state or province?
10. To what extent does the tension of the present world enter into the mounting menace of drugs?
11. For a person with personality problems, what does your community have to offer as an alternative to drugs?
12. Why not legalize the use of marijuana in your state or province?
13. Why would you expect a marijuana smoker to be a person who most likely would try PCP?
14. Why do today's youth tend to be attracted to PCP?
15. Under what circumstances should a user of PCP, marijuana, or barbiturates be classed as psychotic?
16. As a part of a community drug control program, what purpose would a suicide prevention center serve?
17. Survey the drug addiction prevention, control, and treatment facilities of your community and recommend an effective program.
18. How does health promotion go beyond health education?

BIBLIOGRAPHY

Abelson, H.I., Fishburne, P.M., and Cisin, I.: National survey on drug abuse: 1977, Washington, D.C., 1977, National Institute on Drug Abuse.

Aronson, E.: Dissonance theory: progress and problems, In Abelson, R.P., editor: Theories of cognitive consistency: a source book, Chicago, 1968, Rand McNally & Co.

Austin, G.A., Macari, M.A., and Lettieri, D.J.: Research issues update, 1978, Washington, D.C., 1979, National Institute on Drug Abuse.

Bandura, A.: Social learning theory, Morristown, N.J., 1971, General Learning Corp.

Becker, M.H.: The health belief model and personal health behavior, Thorofare, N.J., 1974, Charles B. Slack, Inc.

Bennett, B.I.: A model for teaching health education skills to primary care practitioners, Int. J. Health Educ. 20(4):232, 1977.

Bertrand, J.T., and Bertrand, W.E.: Health education among the economically deprived of a Columbian city, Int. J. Health Educ. 22(2):102, 1979.

Blachly, P.H.: How to decrease the self-destructive behaviors that threaten the goals of preventive medicine. In Kane, R.L. editor: The behavioral sciences and preventive medicine, Washington, D.C., 1974, U.S. Government Printing Office.

Blane, H.T., and Chafetz, M.E., editors: Youth, alcohol, and social policy, New York, 1979, Plenum Publishing Corp.

Block, M.A.: Alcohol and alcoholism, Belmont, Calif., 1970, Wadsworth Publishing Co. Inc.

Bloom, E.S., editor: An approach for casual drug users, Washington, D.C., 1977, National Institute on Drug Abuse.

Blum, R.H.: Drug education: results and recommendations, Lexington, Mass., 1976, Lexington Books.

Bukowski, W.J.: Drug abuse prevention evaluation: a meta-evaluation process. Paper presented at the American Public Health Association annual conference, New York, 1979.

Calahan, D., et al.: American drinking practices, New Brunswick, N.J., 1969, Rutgers University Press.

Carney, R.E., editor: Risk-taking behavior: concepts, Springfield, Ill., 1971, Charles C Thomas, Publisher.

Centers for Disease Control: The ten leading causes of death, Atlanta, 1978, Public Health Service, U.S. Department of Health and Human Services.

Charney, E., Goodman, H.C., McBride, et al.: Childhood antecedents of adult obesity: do chubby infants become obese adults? N. Engl. J. Med. 295(1):6, July, 1976.

Claridge, G.: Drugs and human behavior, New York, 1970, Praeger Publishers, Inc.

Crawley, T.J.: The reinforcers of drug abuse: why people take drugs, Compr. Psychiatry 13(1):51, 1972.

Farquar, J.W., Maccoby, N., Wood, P.D., et al.: Community education for cardiovascular health, Lancet 1(8023):1192, 1977.

Feldman, H.W.: Ideological supports to becoming and remaining a heroin addict, J. Health Soc. Behav. 9:133, 1968.

Fielding, J.E.: Successes of prevention, Milbank Memorial Fund Q./Health and Society 56(3):274, 1978.

Fishbein, M., and Ajzen, I.: Belief, attitude, intention, and behavior: an introduction to theory and research, Reading, Mass., 1975, Addison-Wesley Publishing Co., Inc.

Fishburne, P.M., Abelson, H.I., and Cisin, I.: National survey on drug abuse: main findings 1979, Washington, D.C., 1979, National Institute on Drug Abuse.

Fors, S.W.: On the ethics of selective omission and inclusion of relevant information in school drug education programs, J. Drug Educ. 10(2):111, 1980.

Frankle, R.T.: It's never too early for nutrition education, J. Sch. Health 50:387, 1980.

Gellman, J.P.: The sober alcoholic: an organizational analysis of Alcoholics Anonymous, New Haven, Conn., 1967, College & University Press.

Goodstadt, M.J.: Myths and methodology in drug education: a critical review of the research evidence. In Goodstadt, M.: Research on methods and programs of drug education, Toronto, 1974, Addiction Research Foundation.

Gottschalk, L.A., McGuire, F.L., Heiser, J.F., et al.: Drug abuse deaths in nine cities: a survey report, Research Monograph Series #29, Rockville, Md., 1979, National Institute on Drug Abuse.

Green, L.W., Heit, P., Iverson, D.C., et al.: The school health curriculum project: its theory, practice and measurement experience, Health Educ. Q. 7(1):14, 1980.

Green, L.W., Kreuter, M.W., Deeds, S.G., and Partridge, K.B.: Health education planning: a diagnostic approach, Palo Alto, Calif., 1980, Mayfield Publishing Co.

Green, L.W., Rimer, B., and Elwood, T.W.: Public education. In Shottenfeld, D., and Fraumeni, J., editors: Cancer epidemiology and prevention, Philadelphia, 1981, W.B. Saunders Co.

Harris, R.T., et al.: Drug dependence, Austin, Tex., 1971, University of Texas Press.

Health Education Center: Strategies for health education in local health departments, Baltimore, Md., 1977, State Department of Health and Mental Hygiene.

Iverson, D.C.: Utilizing a health behavior model to design drug education/prevention programs, J. Drug Educ. 8:279, 1978.

Iverson, D.C., and Green, L.W.: Prevention theory. In Bukowski, W., editor: A review of prevention theory, program concepts and evaluation results, National Institute on Drug Abuse, Washington, D.C., 1981.

Jessor, R., and Jessor, S.: Problem behavior and psychosocial development, New York, 1977, Academic Press.

Kandel, D.: Stages in adolescent involvement in drug use, Science 190:912, 1975.

Ketcham, F.S.: Alcoholics and the community, J.A.M.A. 202:980, 1967.

King, J.A., Muraco, W.A., and Vezner, K.O.: Adolescent drug use: the problem in perspective, Toledo, Ohio, 1974, The Bridge, Inc.

Lalonde, M.: A new perspective on the health of Canadians, Ottawa, 1974, Government of Canada, Ministry of National Health and Welfare.

Lambert, M.D.: Alcohol advertising in magazines: prevalence and content. Paper presented at the 11th Annual Medical-Scientific Conference of the National Institute on Alcohol Abuse and Alcoholism, Rockville, Md., 1979.

Lettieri, D.J., editor: Predicting adolescent drug abuse: a review of issues, methods and correlates, Washington, D.C., 1975, U.S. Government Printing Office.

Lewis, C.E.: The study of a strategy to improve decision-making related to health and illness among children (Actions for Health). Unpublished annual report, Los Angeles, 1979, University of California Center for Health Services Research.

Lindblad, R.A.: Self-concept and drug addiction: a controlled study of white middle socioeconomic status addicts, Washington, D.C., 1977, National Institute on Drug Abuse.

Maril, R.L., and Zavaleta, A.N.: Drinking patterns of low-income Mexican-Americans, J. Stud. Alcohol. 40:480, 1979.

McGuire, W.J.: Immunization against persuasion, New York, 1963, Columbia University Press.

Meyer, A.J., Nash, J.D., McAlister, A.L., et al.: Skills training in a cardiovascular health education campaign, J. Consult. Clin. Psychol. 48(2):129, 1980.

Mullen, P.D.: Behavioral aspects of maternal and child health: natural influences and educational intervention. In the report of the Select Panel for the Promotion of Child Health, to the United States Congress and the Secretary of Health and Human Services, vol. 4, Background Papers, Washington, D.C., 1981, Public Health Service.

National Cancer Institute: Smoking and health: a program to reduce the risk of disease in smoking, Bethesda, Md., 1977, National Institutes of Health.

National Commission on Marihuana and Drug Abuse: Drug use in America: problems in perspective, second report, Washington, D.C., 1973, U.S. Government Printing Office.

National Institute on Drug Abuse: National survey on drug abuse: main findings 1979, The Institute, P.O. Box 1909, Rockville, Md. 20852.

Piaget, J.: Intellectual evaluation from adolescence to adulthood, Hum. Dev. **15:**1, 1972.

Portnoy, B.: Effects of a controlled-usage alcohol education program based on the health belief model, J. Drug Educ. **10:**181, 1980.

Presidential Commission on World Hunger: Overcoming world hunger: the challenge ahead, Washington, D.C., 1980, The Commisssion.

Puska, P., Koskela, K., McAlister, A., et al.: A comprehensive television smoking programme in Finland, Int. J. Health Educ. **24**(suppl.):1, 1979.

Quelch, J.A.: Resource-allocation process in nutrition policy planning, Am. J. Clin. Nutr. **32:**1058, 1979.

Redican, K.J., Olsen, L.K., Stone, D.B., and Wilson, R.W.: Cigarette-smoking attitudes of lower socioeconomic sixth grade students, J. Drug Educ. **9:**55, 1979.

Rogers, E.M., and Shoemaker, F.F.: Communication of innovations: A cross-cultural approach, New York, 1971, The Free Press.

Schaps, E., DiBartolo, R., Palley, C.S., and Churgin, S.: Primary prevention evaluation research: a review of 127 program evaluations. Unpublished paper, Walnut Creek, Calif., 1978, Pyramid Project.

U.S. Department of Health, Education, and Welfare: Adult use of tobacco, Washington, D.C., 1975, U.S. Government Printing Office.

U.S. Department of Health, Education, and Welfare: Disease prevention and health promotion: federal programs and prospects, Washington, D.C., 1978, U.S. Government Printing Office.

U.S. Department of Health, Education, and Welfare: Healthy people: the Surgeon General's report on health promotion and disease prevention, Washington, D.C., 1979a, U.S. Government Printing Office.

U.S. Department of Health, Education, and Welfare: Healthy people: the Surgeon General's report on health promotion and disease prevention, background papers, Washington, D.C., 1979b, U.S. Government Printing Office.

U.S. Department of Health, Education, and Welfare: Preventing disease/promtoing health/objectives for the nation: alcohol and drug abuse, Washington, D.C., 1979c, U.S. Government Printing Office.

U.S. Department of Health and Human Services: Promoting health/preventing disease: objectives for the nation, Washington, D.C., 1980, Office of the Assistant Secretary for Health.

Yetley, E.A., and Roderuck, C.: Nutritional knowledge and health goals of young spouses, J. Am. Diet. Assoc. **77**(1):31, 1980.

PART THREE

Environmental health

13

COMMUNITY WATER RESOURCES

All water has been through living systems
and must be used over and over again,
so man is required to regenerate the environment.

Anonymous

Environment in the modern, complex community, presents more and more threats to health and life. Water, air, land, waste, shelter, and food represent what is regarded as the inanimate environment; but other people—individually, in the family, in groups, and in masses—represent an important and formidable aspect of the environment in which one operates. From the earliest times society has been striving to control the environment, but society itself makes the environment a greater and greater threat to health and life, as seen in the interface of natural history and social history in Chapter 2. Greater congestion of people in metropolitan areas, the concentration of industry, population mobility, and sheer increase in numbers have made control of the environment more imperative and equally more challenging.

INFECTIOUS AND TOXIC AGENT CONTROL

Health problems attributed to infectious and toxic agents include acute effects such as infection and poisoning; teratogenic (damage to fetus during pregnancy) and developmental abnormalities; mutagenesis (damage to genes); oncogenesis (including cancer); neurological and behavioral impairment; immunological

damage; and chronic degenerative diseases involving the lungs, joints, digestive and vascular systems, kidneys, liver, and endocrine organs.

Infectious and toxic agents affect people differently, depending on their sex, age, history of past exposures, and possible genetically predisposing conditions. Similarly, the genetic effects of infectious toxic agents may be manifested differently in future generations. For these reasons, and because it takes many years before some of the resulting chronic diseases are revealed, the current incidence rates of diseases associated with infectious and toxic agents do not accurately measure either their true potency or the effectiveness of existing control and prevention efforts. This makes the tasks of risk identification and of risk reduction enormously difficult, particularly since more than 60,000 chemical compounds are produced commercially, and approximately 1,000 new compounds are introduced each year. Over 13,000 toxic substances currently in commercial use in the United States have been identified. Most of the infectious agents of greatest concern have been addressed in previous chapters. Their control in the physical environment will be covered in this chapter and in Chapters 14 to 16.

Current evidence builds a convincing case

for the carcinogenicity in humans of 20 chemicals and compounds; over 2,300 specific chemicals are suspected carcinogens. Also, more than 20 agents are known to be associated with birth defects in humans; many times this number are associated with birth defects in animals.

The principal sources of environmental health hazards presently subject to federal regulation in the United States include air and water emissions or effluents, hazardous waste disposal, transportation of hazardous materials, and occupational exposures. Standards have been established in the United States for air quality, for safe drinking water, and for certain types of occupational exposure. Standards are being developed for hazardous waste disposal and for transportation of toxic materials. These are addressed in Chapter 14. Standards and objectives for housing and food protection in the community are presented in Chapters 15 and 16.

Ionizing radiation can produce skin burns, gastrointestinal disturbances, bone marrow depression, and cancer. Most man-made sources of ionizing radiation derive from diagnostic and therapeutic medical applications; the remainder, so far a small percent, derive from fallout from nuclear power. These and various occupational hazards are covered in Chapter 17.

Environmental objectives for the United States for 1990 include eliminating miscarriages and birth defects associated with toxic agent exposures; reducing health risks to the general population from the contamination of groundwater, surface water, or the soil from industrial toxins associated with wastewater; and assuring that the population has good air to breathe and safe water to drink.

No one knows the extent of the current contamination of water and soil. In 1980, however, the Environmental Protection Agency (EPA) in the United States started a series of programs to prevent new contamination. By 1990 there should be almost no preventable contamination of water associated with wastewater management, if this program is maintained. A related objective is to develop a plan to protect communities from the consequences of toxic agents in existing sites of toxic solid waste disposal, as from the Love Canal in upstate New York. Approximately 30,000 solid waste disposal sites may be involved.

While there are serious inadequacies in the reporting of data about the presence of toxic agents and exposure to low-level ionizing radiation in the United States, considerable experience with infectious agents and some crude baseline data on toxic agents are available to use in tracking future progress toward risk reduction objectives, such as the following:

- By 1990 100% of the population should be living in communities that experience no more than 1 day per year when air quality exceeds an individual ambient air quality standard.
- By 1990 95% to 100% of the population should be living in communities served by water systems that meet national and state or provincial standards for safe drinking water.

Today only about 50% of the U.S. population live in communities that meet the 1990 air quality objective, and only 85% to 90% of the population is served by water systems that meet safe drinking water standards.

Exposures to ionizing radiation can be reduced by gradually eliminating the 30% of x-ray film taking (medical and dental) that are estimated to be unnecessary. By 1990 the total number of diagnostic x-ray examinations should be reduced by approximately some 50 million. Also, by 1990 hazards from inhalation of fumes from toxic materials during transportation should have been eliminated.

No pesticide for sale in 1990 should contain carcinogens, and individuals purchasing a potentially toxic product of any kind should be protected by clear labeling of contents and directions for the product's use and disposal. Also by 1990 80% of communities should experience an incidence rate of lead toxicity among children 1 to 5 years of age less than 500 per 100,000 population, and 90% of that age group identified with lead toxicity will have been brought into medical and environmental management. Finally, and most broadly, by 1990 all citizens should be protected through standards and regulations for each class of substances known to be hazardous to human health.

Better access to information about hazardous exposures is an important goal. Objectives include informing managers of industrial firms; educating consumers and health professionals about how to detect, control, and deal with the effects of hazardous exposures; and increasing the capabilities of community health agencies and hospitals to respond appropriately.

There is as yet no comprehensive surveillance system in any country to monitor new or continuing environmental threats to health. Thus one other objective for reducing the risks from infectious and toxic agent exposures is especially important:

- By 1990 a fully appropriate and broad-scale surveillance and monitoring system should be operating to discern and measure environmental hazards of a continuing nature as well as those resulting from isolated incidents. Such activities should be continuously carried out at both national and state or provincial levels.

WATER CONSUMPTION

Communities need water for recreation, irrigation, industry, and domestic use. The population increases, industry expands, and other water uses multiply, yet the quantity of water remains fixed. Water must be reused in most places in the world. Humankind's ingenuity is economically and technically challenged by the task of retaining the quality of water.

At the turn of the present century, communities used water of a quality so poor that people today would refuse to use such water. It is sad but true that many citizens assumed that if water was clear it was safe for household purposes. Not until residents recognized that water was a vehicle for disease transmission was action taken to prevent the transmission of diseases via water. It took years of community education before citizens understood what had to be done to protect the people in the community. In some communities officials took the lead in providing the people with a safe and adequate water supply. In some cities it was the people who had to push the officials to take the necessary action to provide the citizens with a safe and ample supply of water.

Today the concern is as much with toxic agents in the water as with infectious agents. Chemicals and nuclear wastes threaten community water supplies in ways that worry citizens now as much as organic pollution ever worried their parents and grandparents.

From over 2,200 contaminants of all kinds identified in water, 765 have been identified in drinking water. Of these, 12 chemical pollutants were recognized carcinogens, 31 were suspected carcinogens, 18 were carcinogenic promoters, and 59 were mutagens. It is not known what the additive effects of these chemicals will be on the total cancer burden. As water resources become in shorter supply, more and more surface water used for drinking water will be recycled or reprocessed, continuing the recycling of pollutants.

Water is the most important commodity humans consume, and the consumption of water goes steadily up, so that today in the United States the average daily use for domestic purposes is 150 gallons per person. Communities with industries requiring vast amounts of water may have a total use that reaches 2,000 gallons per person per day. Community leaders tend to be too conservative in estimating future water requirements. Many areas in the United States will experience an increasing shortage for the rest of this century unless low-cost desalinization is employed or the harnessing of runoff from glaciers is successful.

The price of water to the consumer is reasonable but, with the supply becoming inadequate, new costly procedures such as desalinization of sea water will double and even triple the cost of water for the nation.

WATERBORNE DISEASES

Pathogens of humans do not normally multiply in water, yet they can survive in water and remain virulent enough to set up an infection in a new host. Water serves as a vehicle of transfer of diseases of the alimentary canal and of transfer of certain worms, notably the schistosomes. No evidence exists that the respiratory diseases of humans are conveyed via water. However, toxic chemicals may be carried to human communities through water.

Evidence is conclusive that four infectious diseases—typhoid, paratyphoid, cholera, and bacillary dysentery—are transmitted by water. The contention that viral hepatitis, amebic dysentery, and poliomyelitis are transmitted by water is not substantiated.

CHARACTERISTICS OF WATER

For community purposes, water must be in sufficient supply and free from contamination, pollution, and turbidity. Water that may be suitable for household purposes may not be satisfactory for individual use if it is high in mineral content.

The primary source of water is rainfall, whether it is surface water impounded in a lake, pond, river, or reservoir created by a dam, or whether it is groundwater that has percolated through the ground to a stratum of gravel. In nature there is no pure water. Water contains dissolved gases, minerals, and organic matter from the decay of such forms as algae and fungi.

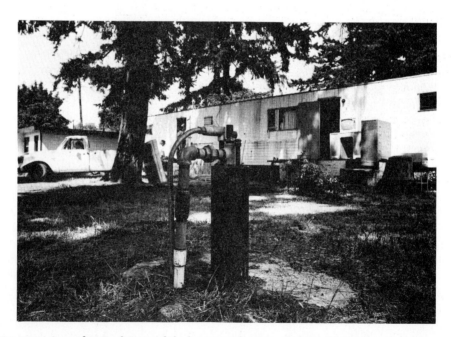

FIG. 13-1. Groundwater for a mobile home settlement of about 15 living units. Water is obtained by driving pipe down to a gravel bed holding water. Pumping power is from electricity and is controlled automatically by a float.

Hardness of water is caused by the presence of calcium and magnesium salts. Hardness of 100 parts per million (ppm) or less, expressed as calcium carbonate, is soft enough for household use. Softening can be done at the time of filtration by adding lime and soda, and the calcium carbonate formed will precipitate out and leave a residual hardness of less than 100 ppm. To reduce alkalinity, the effluent from the softening process may be carbonated with carbon dioxide.

Drinking water containing too much sulfate (2,000 ppm), chloride (1,000 ppm), or calcium carbonate (300 ppm) will cause digestive disturbances in most people. Osmotic balance in the human colon can be upset by water high in mineral content, and severe diarrhea can result.

GROUNDWATER SUPPLIES

Groundwater is usually the preferred source for communities under 50,000 population. Rarely will a larger city locate sufficient groundwater for its needs, although San Antonio, Texas, with more than one million people, has a groundwater supply. Groundwater has certain merits. It is free from contamination, pollution, turbidity, and color. Its disadvantages are its scarcity, the threat of sinking property when groundwater levels are lowered by overuse, and the highly mineralized state of groundwater.

As a community supply, groundwater is usually safe, and the low capital funds and operating costs make groundwater an economical source. The first requirement is to locate an adequate supply. This means locating a gravel bed that serves as a natural reservoir. Test wells are drilled to outline the reservoir. The object is to locate a yard-thick gravel bed below an impervious layer 60 feet or more beneath the surface. At least one more gravel stratum should be located to assure an uninterrupted flow of water by having a second and even a third source. The rate of underground flow can

be measured by putting dye into one hole and timing the interval required for the dye to get to another hole that is being pumped. An electrical conductor can also be used for this purpose. When the conductor put down into one hole reaches the next hole, the electrical circuit is completed and is recorded on a dial.

Producing wells are cased with pipe that is 6 to 24 inches in diameter and that has a brass intake screen where the pipe is embedded in the gravel. Spacing of wells depends on the underground flow and community needs. Electrically operated centrifugal pumps raise the water into a receiving reservoir of concrete construction. A second set of pumps forces the water up into a large storage or pressure tank.

Bacteria attach to sand grains and secrete a sticky covering that causes other bacteria to stick to this biological film. As water percolates into the ground, bacteria are filtered out by the sticky film. Groundwater may be contaminated by seepage along the well casing, by limestone, by other previous material above the groundwater supply that does not intercept bacteria, and by direct surface contamination into the groundwater stratum.

Well water is normally free from turbidity and can be chlorinated without filtration. Frequently, it is unnecessary to chlorinate groundwater, although it may be done as an extra precaution. Many communities do not chlorinate their groundwater but have a chlorination unit standing by in the event the water should become contaminated.

SURFACE WATER SUPPLIES

New York City requires about 1 billion gallons of water a day. Multiply this by 365 and one gets some concept of the task that city has supplying its citizens with water. Consider what would happen if the city were without water for 48 hours. New York gets 10% of its water from wells. The remainder comes from surface water and necessitates a number of protected storage reservoirs and flumes. Cities like

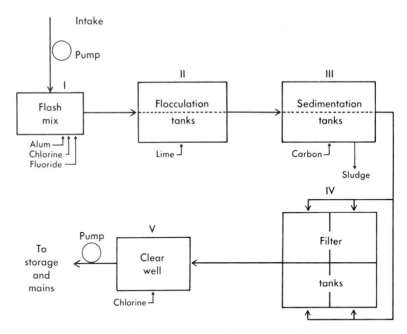

FIG. 13-2. Schematic diagram of water treatment, beginning with the introduction of floc material, then through flocculation, sedimentation, and filter tanks. After this process, the water is clear and ready for final chlorination to assure potability of the water.

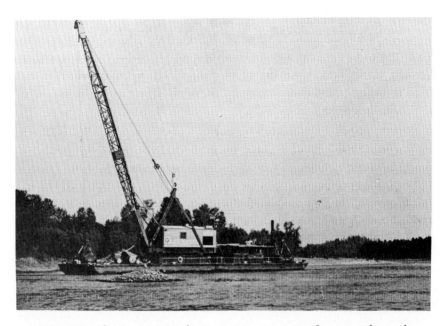

FIG. 13-3. Dredging a river to obtain a greater quantity of water at the intake.

Chicago and Milwaukee are fortunate in having Lake Michigan as an excellent water source. The Mississippi River serves as both a water source and a sewage disposal receptacle for a long string of cities, including Minneapolis, St. Louis, and New Orleans. Surface water has certain merits. It is more abundant, more easily measured, and softer than groundwater. However, it is frequently polluted by shore wash, transportation waste, industrial waste, and human waste. It is usually contaminated, is highly colored, and is often turbid.

With the increasing population and the high mobility of people today, virtually all surface water must be treated before it is safe for human consumption. Some lakes and streams have clear water, so no filtration is necessary, however, chlorination may be required. Most surface water is so turbid, polluted, and contaminated that both filtration and chlorination are necessary.

Rapid sand filtration was developed in the United States and is designed to filter out particles and bacteria. If the water contains considerable sediment, a preliminary settling chamber may be used to precede the treatment process. Otherwise, the water is pumped directly from the intake in the river or lake into the series of tanks comprising the treatment plant. These tanks are usually of concrete construction and, frequently, more than a sufficient number of tanks will be constructed so that some tanks may be shut off and cleaned or repaired while the rest of the tanks carry on the treatment process.

The treatment usually consists of five steps: flash mix, flocculation, sedimentation, filtration, and chlorination, as shown in Fig. 13-2.

Flash mix is done in a relatively small tank. Aluminum sulfate is fed into the incoming water and forms a flaky hydrate or floc. At the same time, chlorine is added.

Flocculation consists of trapping particles of turbidity by the mechanical process of adsorption of suspended solids. Because flocculation causes an increase in the density and size of coagulated particles, floc particles settle at a fast rate. Flocculation tanks are fitted with slowly rotating wooden paddles to ensure an even and continuous water-chemical mixture.

Sedimentation is the settling of the flocculation and is carried out in sedimentation tanks connected directly to the flocculation tanks. Water is retained here for about 2 hours to allow the floc to settle to the bottom of the tanks. From the bottom of the tanks floc will be scraped into troughs. Other troughs around the top of the tanks collect the upper layer of water, which is relatively free of floc.

If the water has an odor, activated carbon may be added to the water in the sedimentation tank, although the carbon may be added at some other stage of treatment. The activated carbon is effective in removing odor and objectionable taste.

Filtration is necessary to remove whatever turbidity may remain after the flocculation and settling. At the bottom of a filtration tank is a layer of gravel, topped by either sand or anthracite coal. Water percolates through this medium and goes out via drains at the bottom of the tank. To clean floc that accumulates on the anthracite coal or sand, the water level is lowered to the top of the troughs just above the coal level. The water flow is then reversed so that the accumulated floc is flushed into the troughs and carried off as waste.

Chlorination, the final step, decontaminates the water and is a simple, effective method for destroying bacteria. Postchlorination is designed to bring the residual chlorine to a level between 0.25 and 0.7 ppm. The chlorine residual property is determined for water in the distribution system as well as at the plant of origin. Two samples a day at the plant and one from the system are recommended. A chlorine residual between 0.2 and 0.3 ppm will destroy all bacterial pathogens of humans and, at this concentration, the chlorine cannot be detected by either taste or smell. In emergencies a chlorine residual of 0.7 ppm may be maintained. Although chlorine can be detected at this con-

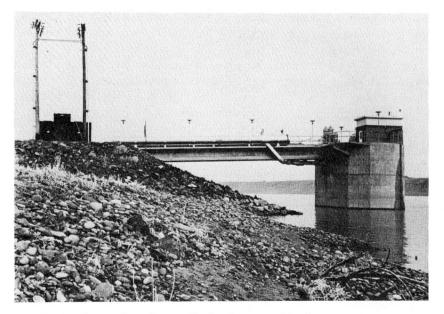

FIG. 13-4. Intake of water from filtration bed and conveyed to the community water system.

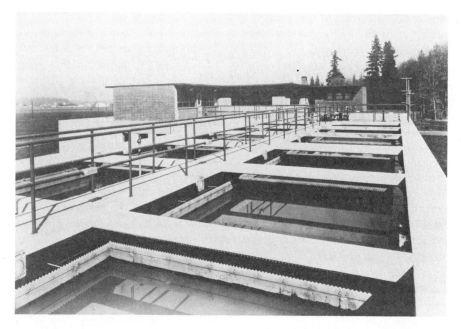

FIG. 13-5. Flocculation tanks in a series. The advantage of this arrangement is that not all tanks need to be in use at the same time, thus providing a favorable situation for cleaning or otherwise servicing the tanks.

Courtesy CH₂M-Hill, Corvallis, Oregon.

centration, it is not harmful to humans.

The slow sand (European) method of filtration is similar to the rapid sand method except that instead of an artificial gelatinous layer, a film produced by bacteria is the interceptive medium. The rapid sand method is 40 times faster and generally more reliable. Thus the rapid sand method is preferred in most communities establishing new water systems.

Addition of fluorides

Based on available knowledge, the most effective, inexpensive, and simple method of preventing dental caries is the fluoridation of the public water supply. Beginning with studies of local areas where people had a low incidence of dental caries, scientists discovered that these areas had water that naturally contained about 1ppm of fluorides. Where the fluoride content of water was much lower than this, the incidence of caries was high.

On the recommendation of dentists and public health scientists, U.S. municipalities began adding fluorides to water supplies as a preventive measure against dental caries. Most water supplies contain a small amount of fluorides and the need is simply that of adding enough fluorides to bring the concentration up to 1 ppm. Northern cities in the United States raise the fluoride content slightly above this level, and southern cities hold the fluoride content just a little below 1 ppm. This is an adjustment to the difference in water consumption.

In 1980 more than 10,000,000 people in the United States were drinking water with a natural fluoride concentration between 0.7 and 3.0 ppm. Another 132 million people were drinking water to which fluoride had been added. People in more than 5,860 communities had public water supplies containing an adequate concentration of fluorides. It has been the history of public health that the small communities are the last to adopt new health measures, and this has held true for fluoridation. New York City, San Francisco, Baltimore, Chicago, Philadelphia, Pittsburgh, Milwaukee, St.

Louis, and Washington, D.C. have fluoridated water supplies. Only about 40% of cities with populations between 2,500 and 10,000 have adopted fluoridation, and less than 20% of communities under 2,500 now fluoridate. Sweden, the Netherlands, West Germany, Japan, and many other nations are making fluoridation available to their populations.

Public health people are not surprised by the opposition to fluoridation, because health innovations have always been opposed. Vaccination, pasteurization of milk, chlorination of water supplies, and even indoor plumbing were, in turn, opposed by the easily frightened, those who resist change, the uninformed, people with aggressions, and others. Fortunately, fluoridation is gradually gaining acceptance, and this is repeating public health history. Unless effective means are used to reduce dental caries in the United States there will not be enough dentists to provide the necessary dental service for the more than 220 million people. Courts in the United States have ruled that fluoridation is a reasonable legal exercise of the local police power in the interest of the public health and not a violation of individual rights. One state after another is requiring fluoridation of community water supplies.

Some communities have water supplies with a high natural fluoride content of 8 ppm. This concentration prevents caries but causes mottling of the teeth. The only other harm to the human body that has been suspected is possible orthopedic problems for the elderly. These communities add phosphate to the water to reduce fluorides to a level of 1 ppm. In communities having a water supply with a natural fluoride content of 2 ppm, people have health histories showing no deviation from that of the population at large.

In communities that do not fluoridate their municipal water supply, some citizens have their family dentist or physician brush their children's teeth with a covering of fluoride whenever the child visits them. Some elementary schools have their children retain fluoridated water in their mouths for about 40 to 60 seconds.

Objectives related to fluoridation include the following:

- By 1990 at least 95% of the population should be on community water systems that have fluoridated water. (In 1975 in the United States it was 60%.)
- By 1990 at least 50% of school children living in fluoride-deficient areas should be served by an optimally fluoridated school water supply. (In 1977 in the United States it was about 6%.)

TESTING OF WATER

Quality of community water is usually a health concern. Thus bacteriological and chemical examination of a municipal water supply can be of great importance to industry and of significant importance to the general public as well. Radiological examination of water is of more recent vintage and not generally a concern, but in specific instances the possibility of radioactive contaminants in water can be significant. Bioassays are necessary to evaluate toxicity in fish, and biological examinations are used to determine the extent of plankton and other life forms.

Bacteriological examination of water is necessary to ascertain possible contamination. Samples are collected at representative locations throughout the community water system. Frequency of collection is adjusted to the likelihood of contamination. A groundwater supply may be so safe that a sample once a month may be adequate. The size of a community, as well as possible contamination, may require more frequent sample collections. For routine purposes, the usual minimum is as follows:

Population	Minimum samples per month
Under 2,500	1
25,000	25
100,000	100
1,000,000	300

Pathogens are not routinely isolated in the water. The coliform group of bacteria has been used as the index of contamination. U.S. Public Health Service standards set a maximum monthly density of coliform organisms at 1 per 100 milliliters of water tested.

A sample is collected under sterile conditions so that any contamination discovered would have to be in the water. A milliliter is spread over an agar medium. A colony will form from each of the *Escherichia coli* in the sample, and thus a bacteria count can be made.

Water may have *E. coli* and be safe. The contamination may come from lower animals. Citizens do not relish the idea of drinking water from the discharges of either lower animals or humans. The test is merely an indicator of contamination. Investigation is necessary to determine the source of contamination before the discharges of a typhoid carrier or of a patient with cholera get into the water. Every precaution should be taken to prevent the community water supply from being a vehicle of disease transmission.

Chemical examination of water varies, depending on the specific chemical one wishes to detect. Tests for hardness are most frequent. A test for chlorine residual is used to determine the decontamination effect of chlorination. Nitrite and nitrate determinations indicate recent and old pollution of water. Iodine, iron, phosphate, and sulfate content are of interest. Dissolved oxygen and carbon dioxide indicate water quality before treatment. Most community water supplies in the United States are tested routinely for chlorine residual and this may constitute the only chemical examination unless some special problem arises.

REGULATION OF U.S. PUBLIC WATER SUPPLIES

Providing water to a community is a recognized function of local government in the United States. The city government usually constructs and operates the water system as a corporate function. This is not a responsibility of the health department, but a special water department or the department of public works usually operates the water system. A few communities grant a franchise to a private corporation to sell water as a commodity to the public.

Providing water to the community is a local government function, but the regulation of public water supplies is the responsibility of the state, which usually delegates this authority to the state department of health. A public water system is one that provides piped water for human consumption that has at least 15 service connections or that regularly serves at least 25 people. If a city wishes to erect a water plant, the plans must be approved by engineers from the state department of health. In practice, these engineers actually serve as advisors for the city in developing the plans. This advisory service is without cost to the city. Even though the city pays to have plans drawn and the water system constructed, it is the state that passes on the adequacy of the plans and the construction.

Once the plant is in operation, the state continues its supervisory authority. Plant operators must be certified by the state. Regular reports on water analysis must be submitted to the state as the state department of health decrees. The state representative serves as a consultant if the community should encounter a problem in the operation of its water system. This consulting service is given without cost to the community.

Safe Drinking Water Act of 1974

Drinking water supplied to most U.S. homes is usually recognized as being safe. Yet the National Community Water Supply Study of 1970 revealed that the quality of household water was declining. Part of this decline is attributed to the careless use of various chemical substances and other toxic wastes. As an outgrowth of this study by the U.S. Environmental Protection Agency (EPA), Congress enacted the Safe Drinking Water Act of 1974.

This act provides for the establishment of water standards. Congress also authorized the EPA to support state and local community

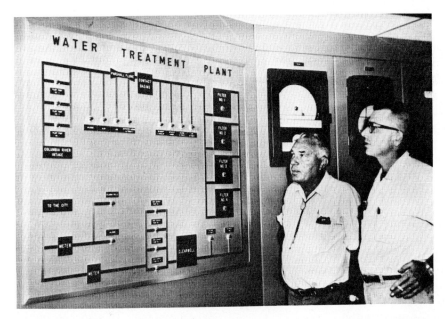

FIG. 13-6. Electronic controls of all operations providing water for a community.

drinking water programs by providing financial and technical assistance. It is recognized that the federal government—through the EPA—has the authority and responsibility for enforcing standards and otherwise supervising public water systems.

The major provisions of this act provide for an extended list of guidelines and responsibilities such as the following:

1. Establishment of primary regulations for the protection of the public health
2. Establishment of secondary regulations relating to the taste, odor, and appearance of drinking water
3. Measures to protect underground drinking water sources
4. Research and studies regarding health, economical, and technological problems of drinking water supplies; specifically required are studies of viruses in drinking water and contamination by cancer-causing chemicals
5. A survey of the quality and availability of rural water supplies
6. Aid to the states to improve drinking water programs through technical assistance, training of personnel, and grant support; a loan guarantee is provided to assist small water systems in meeting regulations if other means of financing cannot reasonably be found
7. Citizen suits against any party believed to be in violation of the act
8. Record-keeping, inspections, issuance of regulations, and judicial reviews
9. A 15-member National Drinking Water Advisory Council to advise the EPA Administrator on scientific and other responsibilities under this act
10. A requirement that the Secretary of Health and Human Services ensure that the standards for bottled drinking water conform to the primary regulations established under the act or publish reasons for not doing so

Thus a vigorous, organized program was au-thorized by Congress to assure the people of the nation safe drinking water. Standards ultimately will include maximum contaminant levels and general criteria for operation, maintenance, and intake water quality. Secondary standards have also been prescribed relating only to taste, odor, and appearance of drinking water. These standards will be enforced only when the individual states want to enforce them. Conservative administrations tend to put less pressure on states and industries to implement federal guidelines.

A state can continue to enforce its own laws and regulations governing drinking water supplies if they meet certain requirements such as the following:

1. Adoption of regulations at least equal to federal regulations
2. Adoption and implementation of adequate enforcement preocedures
3. Provision for emergency circumstances
4. Keeping adequate records and provide reports for the EPA

Supporting the water needs of communities

Indispensable as water is, many communities resist proposals to improve and increase the municipal water supply. The resistance is based primarily on cost. With the importance of a safe and ample water supply, it is difficult to understand why citizens will resist investing in this indispensable commodity. With population increases, communities should anticipate a commensurate increase in demands for water. The cost usually is the hurdle, but after some time a proposal is submitted to the citizens.

Several measures are considered for financing improvements and enlargements. Few communities have funds immediately available. Revenue bonds are repaid by increases in city water rates. General obligation bonds are repaid by an increase in property taxes. Such rate increases and taxes are resisted in an inflationary economy. This makes public services in general highly vulnerable, and capital investments in new public facilities requiring expensive construction are particularly hard to pass at the local level. Intensive community health education efforts are required in advance of public debates or votes on bonds to assure public awareness and understanding of the health issues related to water and other environmental decisions by the community.

Appraisal. Next to oxygen, water is most indispensable for human existence. Yet despite its importance, water can be a medium for the transmission of disease. It is commendable that lawmakers on the federal and state levels have provided the leadership in establishing safe drinking water programs. Human relations have been a key factor in the advancement in this program despite the fact that human relationships may well be humankind's greatest unsolved problem. The admonition of perpetual vigilance applies critically to community water safety.

SAFE DRINKING WATER OBJECTIVES

The overall health goal for community water supplies is that residents of a community will have access to drinking water that is free from contaminants. Specific objectives, to be further specified for a given community, would include the following:

- By 19___ there will be zero confirmed outbreaks of waterborne illness from those water systems serving more than 15 connections or 25 or more persons more than 60 days a year.
- By 19___ There will be no more than two confirmed outbreaks every _____ years from waterborne illness from water systems serving two or more households or systems where drinking water is regularly available to the public.
- By 19___ there will be no more than ____ confirmed outbreaks of waterborne illness per 100,000 population from water supplies serving individual families.
- By 19___, excluding emergency situations, there will be no more than one valid con-

sumer complaint per 1,000 population per year based on water quality, pressure, volume, or system operations.

Safe, reliable, and acceptable public water supplies

- By 19___ each community water system will be served by a program of crossconnection control, maintenance of interconnection with adjacent water supplies, and provision of sufficient auxiliary power to operate minimum water supply facilities during power outages.
- By 19___ the community public water system will meet national and state or provincial bacteriological and chemical standards.
- By 19___ the public water system serving more than 15 connections or 25 persons will have bacteriological and chemical water quality monitoring.
- By 19___ the public water system will have a written policy for identifying technical quality standards and procedures for correcting deficiencies that occur.

Problem identification and correction: public water systems

- By 19___ all public water systems will be covered by a program for surveillance, control, and technical assistance.
- By 19___ 100% of complaints received by the regulatory agency regarding water quality, pressure, volume, or system operations will be investigated, and where problems are verified, corrections will be made.
- By 19___ a public water system with 15 connections or serving 25 persons will have a mechanism to identify problems and initiate improvements. All smaller systems will have such a mechanism by 19___.
- By 19___ the review and approval of each new public water supply project by a governmental agency will be required and performed.

- By 19___ water utility operators, consulting engineers, and local agencies will have access to necessary technical consultation and assistance.
- By 19___ each public water system will collect and make available to the appropriate review agency information necessary to track compliance of regulations.
- By 19___ each public water system will have a written policy for responding to emergency situations.

Problem identification and correction: private water supplies

- By 19___ a system of required monitoring and assistance shall be available to all citizens with private water supplies.
- By 19___ no more than 25% of private supplies inspected will be found unsatisfactory.
- By 19___ appropriate bacteriological and chemical tests will be made on 100% of samples submitted by persons with individual water supplies.
- By 19___ appropriate response will be given to 100% of requests for help by persons with individual water supplies.

Well construction

- By 19___ the community will have a program to assure adequacy of location and construction of new private wells.
- By 19___ location and construction standards will be established.
- By 19___ technical consultation regarding location, selection, and well design and construction will be available.
- By 19___ assistance in water quality monitoring will be available to potential users of new wells.
- By 19___ the private well construction quality assurance program will have in place a construction permit system for monitoring purposes.
- By 19___ all commercial well drillers serving the community will be registered or licensed.

Bulk ice

- By 19___ the community will be served by a program to assure the safety and purity of commercial bulk ice manufacture and distribution systems.

• • •

All water quality analyses performed for public and nonpublic systems should be done by laboratories approved for such analyses by the state or provincial and national governments. (See U.S. federal standards that have been established by the EPA under authority of the Safe Drinking Water Act, P.L. 93-523.)

QUESTIONS AND EXERCISES

1. To what extent are humans creating a more hazardous environment at a more rapid rate than the development of their knowledge on how to control the environment?
2. If water is more important to a human being's health than any drug, why should not water cost more than any drug?
3. The total water supply in the world remains the same. What then is the task of society?
4. It is important to determine that a certain source of water is the vehicle for the transmission of typhoid fever, but why is it more important to determine who put the typhoid bacilli in the water?
5. Why do public health officials favor groundwater as a community supply?
6. From your observations and other data, who has the safest water supply, urban dwellers or rural people?
7. What is the source of your community's water supply, and what are the merits and demerits of the water?
8. In one area groundwater less than 30 feet below the surface is a safe water supply. In another area groundwater more than 60 feet below the surface is an unsafe supply. Why the difference?
9. What is the authority of a state or provincial government to order a municipality to cease using its public water supply?
10. Locate some community where the fluoridation of the community water supply is a controversial issue, and analyze the basic factors underlying the controversy.
11. Analyze the statement that all groundwater is safe for human consumption, and no surface water is safe for potable use.
12. Examine the contention that a community has the right to remove fluoride from water but no community has the right to add fluoride to water.

13. If the water in all the wells in a rural area is known to be contaminated, what is the responsibility of the local health department and health officials?
14. Appraise the potential value of the U.S. Safe Drinking Water Act of 1974.
15. How is it possible for water to be contaminated and still be safe?
16. Why is the bacteriological examination of water not directed at finding the typhoid bacillus?
17. Why do most citizens in a large city give little attention to their municipal water supply?
18. Why should local government regulate community water supplies?
19. What is the responsibility of the federal government in providing safe and ample water for all citizens in the United States?
20. Propose a program of health education to interest people in the safety of their community water supply.

BIBLIOGRAPHY

Ackerman, B.A., et al.: The uncertain search for environmental quality, Riverside, N.J., 1974, The Free Press.

American Public Health Association: Standard methods for the examination of water and wastewater, ed. 13, New York, 1971, The Association.

American Water Works Association: Officers and committee directory, Washington, D.C. 1970-1980, The Association.

Aylesworth, T.J.: This vital air; this vital water: man's environmental crisis, rev. ed., Chicago, 1974, Rand McNally & Co.

Berger, M.: The new water book, New York, 1973, Thomas Y. Crowell Co., Inc.

Blake, R.: Water treatment for HVAC and potable water systems, New York, 1979, McGraw-Hill Book Co.

Bloome, E.P.: Water we drink, Garden City, N.Y., 1971, Doubleday & Co., Inc.

Cairns, J., Jr., and Dickson, K.L., editors: Biological methods for the assessment of water quality, Philadelphia, 1973, American Society for Testing Materials.

Ciaccio, L.: Water and water pollution handbook, vol. 3, New York, 1972, Marcel Dekker, Inc.

Cross, F.L., Jr., editor: Water pollution monitoring, the Environmental Monograph, Westport, Conn., 1976, Technomic Publishing Co., Inc.

Culp, R.L., and Culp, G.L.: New concepts in water purification, New York, 1974, Van Nostrand Reinhold Co.

Dieterich, H.B., and Henderson, M.J.: Urban water supply conditions and needs in seventy-five developing countries, Public Health Papers No. 23, Geneva, Irvington-on-Hudson, 1963, WHO International Document Service, Columbia University Press.

Dunne, T., and Leopold, L.B.: Water in environmental planning, San Francisco, 1978, W.H. Freeman and Co. Publishers.

Elliot, S.M.: Our dirty water, New York, 1973, Julian Messner.

Foerstner, U., et al.: Metal pollution in the aquatic environment, New York, 1979, Springer-Verlag New York Inc.

Fried, J.J.: Groundwater pollution (developments in water science, vol. 4), New York, 1976, American Elsevier Publishing Co., Inc.

Gehm, H.W., and Bregman, J.I., editors: Handbook of water resources and pollution control, New York, 1976, Van Nostrand Reinhold Co.

Giefer, G.J., and Todd, D.K.: Water publications of state agencies, Port Washington, N.Y., 1972, Water Information Center, Inc.

Gloya, E.F., and Eckenfieldor, W.W., Jr., editors: Advances in water quality improvement, Austin, Tex., 1967, (Water resources symposium, no. 1), University of Texas Press.

Holden, W.S., editor: Water treatment and examination, ed. 8, Baltimore, 1970, The Williams & Wilkins Co.

Hopkins, E.S., and Bean, E.L.: Water purification control, ed. 4, Baltimore, 1975, The Williams & Wilkins Co.

Hopkins, E.S., Bingley, W.M., and Schucker, G.W.: The practice of sanitation, ed. 4, Baltimore, 1970, The Williams & Wilkins Co.

Hynes, H.B.: Biology of polluted waters, Toronto, 1970, University of Toronto Press.

James, A.: Mathematical models in water control, New York, 1978, John Wiley & Sons, Inc.

Johns Hopkins University, Department of International Health: The functional analysis of health needs and services, Baltimore, 1976, The Johns Hopkins University Press.

Kerns, F.R.: Simplicity of water purification, Ardmore, Penn., 1972, Dorrance and Co., Inc.

Maier, F.J.: Manual of water fluoridation practice, ed. 2, New York, 1972, McGraw-Hill Book Co.

McCaull, J., and Croseland, J.: Water pollution (Commoner, B., editor), New York, 1974, text ed., Harcourt Brace Jovanovich, Inc.

Warner, D., and Dajani, J.S.: Water and sewer development in rural America, Lexington, Mo., 1975, Lexington Books.

World Health: European standards for drinking waters, ed. 2, Albany, N.Y., 1970, World Health Organization, Q Corporation.

Wrigley, D.: Water (Raintree editions), Milwaukee, 1976, Raintree Publishers, Ltd.

14

COMMUNITY WASTE DISPOSAL

The soil is the great organ
in which toxic substances of all kinds
are neutralized or destroyed.

Milton J. Rosenau

The task of community waste disposal has become increasingly more difficult with the rapid increase in population, the movement of people to the metropolitan areas, the mobility of modern life, the increase in outdoor recreation, the expansion of industry, and the general use of nuclear and toxic chemicals.

COMMUNITY WASTES

Household wastes, commercial wastes, recreational wastes, and industrial wastes are the general sources of community wastes. These wastes are in the form of garbage, refuse, street cleanings, human discharges, kitchen wastes, scavenger wastes, commercial wastes, and wastes from manufacturing and processing plants. The sheer volume in a year would run into millions of tons and would make a mountainous stockpile. If each year's wastes accumulated, in a period of 20 years a community would be buried by its own waste products. Fortunately, the lowly bacteria, by decomposing animal proteins, not only reduce the great mass of wastes to a negligible volume but also make the invaluable nitrogen available for reuse. This process is customarily referred to as the nitrogen cycle, as shown in Fig. 14-1.

Nitrogen cycle. Animal proteins begin de-composing by the action of bacteria that converts the proteins to amino acids. Another set of bacteria next converts the amino acids to ammonia. The ammonia combines with carbon dioxide to form ammonium carbonate, which in turn is converted to nitrites by a third type of bacteria. Nitrites combine with sodium and potassium, and the resulting nitrites are converted into nitrates by yet another group of organisms known as the *Nitrobacters*. Nitrates dissolved in soil water diffuse into the root hairs of plants, where they combine with carbon dioxide and water to form plant proteins. The plant proteins are consumed by animals and are converted into animal proteins, thus completing the nitrogen cycle.

Communities aid nature in this process of waste disposal by providing the beneficial bacteria with a favorable environment and by dilution, chemical treatment, and the burning of wastes. The task of disposing of wastes is a continual one that is both important and costly. Processes involved in getting rid of human wastes are also processes for destroying or removing pathogens that can cause disease and death. In this category perhaps the most important of these processes is sewage disposal.

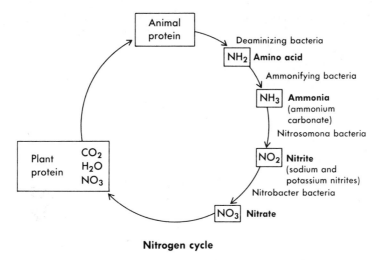

Nitrogen cycle

FIG. 14-1. Nitrogen cycle. The decomposition of organic material goes on continuously, thanks to bacteria that save communities from being buried by their own wastes.

SEWAGE DISPOSAL

"Sewage" consists of the liquid wastes from household effluents, commercial effluents, and industrial liquid wastes. It is carried in a system of pipes and other means of conveyance called a "sewerage system." In some communities storm water is carried in the sewerage system, and in other communities a separate system of pipes carries off storm water.

Generally, community sewage will be about 99% water containing animal, plant, and mineral matter in solution and in suspension. Bacteria of many types, mostly nonpathogenic, are always present. Paper, sticks, grease, and other materials are in suspension.

The strength of sewage is measured by its biochemical oxygen demand (BOD), which is the quantity of oxygen required in a given time to satisfy the chemical and biological oxidation demands of the sewage. A high BOD means that an excessive quantity of oxygen is being used up by the biochemical action in the sewage, indicating a high sewage concentration.

While the primary purpose of sewage treat-
ment is to prevent the spread of disease among human beings, for additional reasons the proper disposal of sewage is imperative in any community or nation, particularly one with a high population concentration. Sewage treatment protects water supplies, protects fish and other aquatic life, protects food by preventing soil pollution, protects livestock, and renders water fit for industrial use. Thus, in addition to the prevention of disease spread, sewage treatment returns water to such a condition that it can be reused with safety and with its general condition unimpaired.

SEWAGE TREATMENT

Treatment of community sewage is directed toward five factors: solids in suspension, organic matters in suspension, inorganic matters in suspension, organic matters in solution, and bacteria. A properly designed and efficiently operated sewage disposal plant will eliminate all five of these undesirable factors and leave an end product of clear, uncontaminated water that can be safely consumed.

A community sewage disposal plant that does

the complete job of treatment involves the following five steps or processes:

1. Preliminary treatment to remove solids such as sand, sticks, paper, and other floating objects, and metal and plastic objects
2. Primary treatment to clarify the sewage by employing sedimentation to settle suspended particles and provide an environment devoid of free oxygen, so that anaerobic bacteria can digest the organic materials settling to the bottom of the clarifying tank
3. Secondary treatment to provide an environment in which the effluent comes in contact with air so that aerobic bacteria can oxidize putrescible material and thus reduce the oxygen demand of the sewage

4. Chlorination to decontaminate the effluent by destroying any bacteria that may remain
5. Final disposal of the liquid end product into a lake, river, canal, or other body of water, and the solids into landfills or incinerators

Sewage from about one third of the population in the United States is treated before final disposal, but only about 40% of this sewage is completely treated. Some communities have only preliminary and primary treatment, which could be acceptable. Other communities follow primary treatment with chlorination and, depending on conditions, the result may be acceptable to state sanitary authorities. Method of treatment depends on conditions. If the final effluent is to be discharged into a large body of

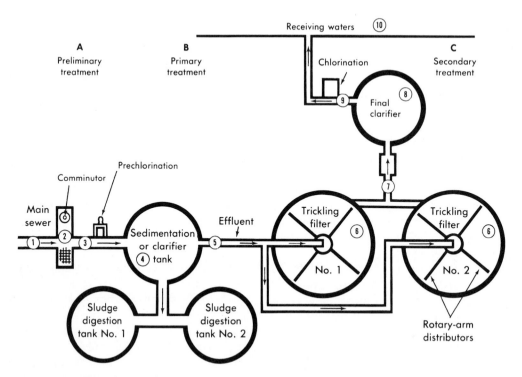

FIG. 14-2. Plan of a complete sewage treatment plant. After preliminary treatment, the sewage goes through primary (anaerobic) treatment, secondary (aerobic) treatment, and chlorination before being emptied into the receiving stream or lake.

water, less complete treatment may be necessary than if the discharge is into a small body of water. Complete treatment is the ideal, and more and more communities will be compelled to complete sewage treatment to protect human life and prevent stream pollution.

Preliminary treatment. Screens consisting of a series of parallel bars set at an angle permit sewage to flow through but intercept large suspended objects. Mechanically or manually operated rakes clean the debris and dump it into receptacles, where it is burned. This raking process may be continuous or intermittent. Some plants use shredders or comminutors, which cut coarse material into fine enough particles to pass through with the effluent.

Grit chambers for preliminary treatment are tanks or basins in which sewage flow is re-

duced, causing gravel, sand, and other heavy materials to settle to the bottom. Two or more grit chambers are necessary so that one can be in operation while the other is being cleaned.

Primary treatment. Sedimentation or clarifier tanks are either rectangular or circular and are about 10 feet deep. A concrete circular tank has many advantages and has become the prevailing choice. The effluent comes into the center of the circular tank through a pipe coming up from the bottom. This prevents agitation of the effluent in the tank and assures that the effluent is quiet, so that particles will settle to the bottom. To aid this sedimentation, chemicals are added to form a gelatinous floc that settles, carries suspended solids to the bottom, and forms sludge.

In some plants digestion of the sludge by an-

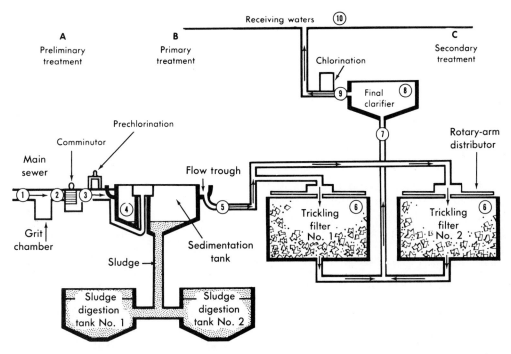

FIG. 14-3. Diagrammatic cross-section of a complete sewage treatment plant. Succession of numbers is used to show direction of flow. Tanks, pipes, and other segments are not necessarily in proper proportion as presented here.

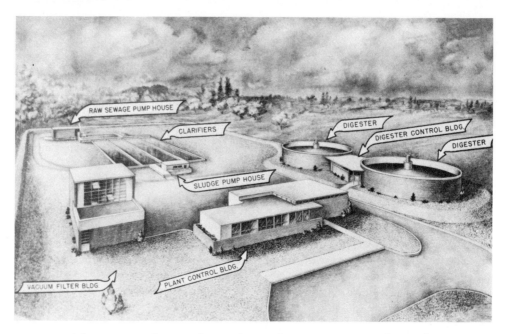

FIG. 14-4. Schematic reproduction of a complete preliminary, primary, and secondary sewage treatment plant. The plan here is similar to that shown in Figs. 14-2 and 14-3.

Courtesy CH₂M-Hill, Corvallis, Oregon.

aerobic bacteria takes place in the sedimentation tank. A better procedure is to pump the sludge from the bottom of the settling tank into concrete sludge tanks and permit the anaerobic bacteria to act there. Not all sludge will be digested. Undigested sludge will be pumped out and hauled away to be used as fertilizer because it is high in nitrogen content. Sludge-drying beds will dehydrate the sludge. Fresh sludge is contaminated and is not safe for truck garden plots.

Because bacterial action is slow, scientists have been experimenting with chemicals as a replacement for bacteria. Their efforts have been fruitful and, while some expense is involved and the precipitate has to be disposed of, chemical disgestion is fast-acting and will become the standard method of primary treatment.

Secondary treatment. To reduce the oxygen demand of the sewage, the secondary treatment requires aeration so that organisms can convert the organic matter in the effluent into stable nitrogenous products. Trickling filters serve admirably. Walls of the filters are constructed of concrete, brick, tile, or other building material. Underdrains of tile leading to central drainage channels are laid on the filter floor. Over this is laid a bed of gravel, crushed stone, or similar material, which provides good ventilation of the bed.

Effluent comes from the clarifier, or primary tanks, in pipes. Connected to these pipes is a series of equally spaced nozzles or rotary spray heads, 1 or 2 feet above the surface of the stone bed. Automatic dosing devices permit one set of nozzles to spray effluent while the other is not operating.

A gelatinous film that intercepts bacteria, algae, protozoa, worms, molds, and other forms of life forms on the stones as the effluent sprays over the stone bed. The organisms in this film convert dissolved, suspended, and colloidal materials into stable nitrogenous material.

Intermittent sand filters are also used for secondary treatment. The underdrains are similar to those in the trickling filters. Surface distributing channels flood the effluent over the surface of the sand bed. Sand grains become coated with a gelatinous film, as do the stones in the trickling filters. In many respects, this is the slow sand filtration method used in water treatment; it is highly effective but rather slow-acting.

Sand filtration beds are alternated—one flooded, one idle. The surface of the sand bed must be cleaned and thus requires constant attention. The dry sludge is an effective fertilizer.

A new process that expands on the present trickling filter system uses a deeper secondary tank and gently stirs the wastewater to further separate out the solids. At that point, air is bubbled through the wastewater, which is piped back through the clarifying tanks one more time, resulting in a cleaner end product. Known as a trickling filter solids contact process, the modifier system saves money for a community when an existing plant needs upgrading. This type of operation can cut energy requirements from 30% to 50%.

Tertiary treatment. Some community sewage treatment plants have used a third process to remove or reduce certain chemicals such as phosphates, nitrogen, and even carbon. Removal of these chemicals is desirable and even necessary because they can lead to eutrophication, a process that occurs in nature but normally requires thousands of years. However, the process is accelerated when excessive nutrients (such as nitrates and phosphates) stimulate marked growth of algae and other aquatic plants. The flourishing plants consume the oxygen essential to marine life and to the natural purification of wastes. This essentially has been the condition in Lake Erie in the United States.

Phosphorus compounds enter streams, lakes, and other bodies of water through synthetic detergents, domestic wastes, and precipitation from farm and other land runoff. Detergents are not the major source of phosphorus in the effluent of sewage treatment plants, and this phosphorus is no more difficult to remove than that of other sources. In community sewage more than half of the total phosphorus comes from domestic wastes, detergents account for about 35% of phosphates, and the remainder comes from fertilizers used in farming and lawn care.

Removal of phosphorus is not too difficult. It can even be done as a phase of the usual primary treatment process. It involves the conversion of soluble phosphorus into insoluble forms and then precipitation of the insoluble forms, which is usually done by adding metal salts, for example, aluminum sulfate or ferrous chloride. When settled out, the phosphorus compounds are removed with the sludge, which is disposed of where it will not enter a body of water.

Nitrogen removal is not so simple. In the first place, the dose of metal salts used in phosphorus removal raises the effluent pH, and with a high pH, ammonia is present as dissolved gas. Lowering the pH is accomplished by recarbonating the effluent through the addition of calcium carbonate.

One method for removing nitrogen uses a stripping tower from 25 to 50 feet high. The inside of the tower is laced with wooden slats. Effluent is pumped to the top of the tower and is distributed uniformly from a horizontal tray across the top of the latticework. As the falling water strikes a slat, droplets are formed. Droplet surface films are of minimum thinness, which favors the escape of ammonia gas from the droplet. Air in the tower enters through side louvers and, by completely surrounding the droplets, promotes a maximum transfer of ammonia from water to the air. The process of water falling and forming new droplets is repeated at least 200 times. This tertiary treatment vastly improves the efficiency of chlorination.

It becomes quite clear that tertiary treatment of most community sewage is imperative if the United States is to save its streams, lakes, and ponds. Ecology makes clear that all life on earth (human life included) depends on good quality water. The cost of complete sewage treatment will be high, but compared with the alternative, it will be essential.

Chlorination. Primary treatment of sewage may be all that is necessary when the effluent from community sewage is emptied into receiving waters that provide extreme dilution. In some instances, dilution is sufficiently great so that after secondary treatment it is safe to empty the effluent into the final disposal lake,

river, or sea. However, when great population concentrations exist and available bodies of water are not great, a good safety measure is to chlorinate the effluent coming from the primary or secondary treatment unit. In some instances chlorination is necessary only during the summer months when available stream flow is low. Two-stage chlorination, in which chlorine is added to the grit chamber at the beginning of treatment and again to the final effluent, provides added safety.

Besides destroying organisms, chlorine reduces the BOD and odor of effluents. The chlorine injection mechanism is similar to that used in water treatment plants.

Final disposal. The receiving waters into which the final effluent is emptied are usually public waters and, as such, are under the jurisdiction and supervision of a state agency. Other

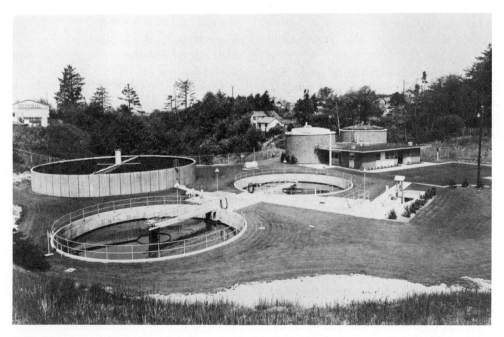

FIG. 14-5. A relatively complete sewage disposal plant. Controls are in the building near upper right of the picture, near the two sludge digestion tanks. The two tanks with catwalks are the sedimentation or clarifier tanks. A single trickling filter is identified by the rotary arms.

Courtesy CH₂M-Hill, Corvallis, Oregon.

communities and citizens have a claim to the use of the waters. The larger the body of receiving water, the greater the safety factor. While the supervising state agency recognizes practical considerations, no community has the right to jeopardize the health of anyone. If a community is to be granted the privilege of disposing its wastes, it must take reasonable precautions to assure that its sewage effluent is not a threat to human life and welfare.

Lagoon treatment. Cost of a typical sewage treatment plant can be beyond the financial means of a small community. Raw sewage lagoons can provide economical and satisfactory treatment of community sewage. A lagoon is a shallow pond in which natural processes produce an acceptable purification.

A lagoon is usually located at least a quarter of a mile from residential areas, where seepage will not pollute groundwaters that may be used for domestic purposes. A lagoon is a rectangular excavation, at least half an acre in area and from 3 to 5 feet in depth. The soil at the bot-

tom of the lagoon should be relatively impervious to prevent excess loss of effluent by seepage. Embankments prevent outside surface drainage from entering the lagoon. The inlet from the sewerage system should be near the center of the lagoon. Grinding objects in raw sewage will provide a desirable dispersal of the solids, prevent an accumulation of sludge deposits, assure better treatment, and help prevent odors.

Organic material that settles to the bottom of the lagoon is decomposed by bacteria and is converted into ammonia, carbon dioxide, and water. Algae feed on these soluble nutrients and, in the presence of sunlight, produce oxygen and thus maintain aerobic conditions and help prevent odor. If the lagoon freezes over, the ice shuts out sunlight and interferes with the treatment process. In addition, a low temperature slows down bacterial action.

Decontamination of sewage effluents may be necessary if they are being discharged into public waters, especially during the summer

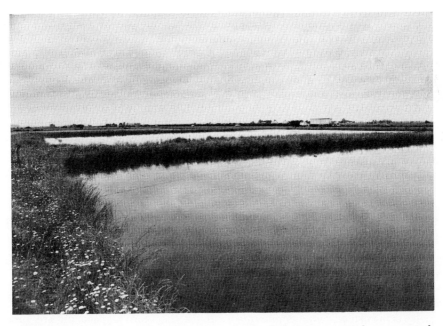

FIG. 14-6. Lagoon treatment of sewage. Raw sewage lagoons can provide economical and satisfactory treatment of community sewage.

months. Raw sewage lagoon effluents are generally not discharged into public waters with less than 20 to 1 dilution.

Lagoon treatment may not be the equivalent of the standard methods of treatment, but it can be highly acceptable. It serves when the community concerned is not able to finance the more costly, more elaborate standard primary and secondary treatment plants.

Financing sewage treatment

Sewage treatment plants are costly but are a necessary community investment in protecting health, in maintaining an esthetic environment, and in disposing community wastes. No fully equitable method has been developed for paying the costs of treatment plant construction and maintenance. Virtually all payment methods are based on the volume of water citizens use from the community's water supply.

Most communities in the United States find it necessary to issue bonds for the construction of a treatment plant. The security for the bonds is the community's ability to collect fees and levy taxes to redeem the bonds when due. All establishments connected to the public sewerage system are charged a monthly sewer fee that is based on the amount of water the establishment used during the month. The practice is based on the assumption that the amount of water a household uses is a reasonable index of the extent to which the household uses the sewer service. During winter months the sewer fee is usually a higher percentage of water used than during summer, when the sewer rate is low to adjust to the fact that much of the water going through the meter is used for lawn sprinkling and does not go into the sewer lines.

What of the landlord whose property value is enhanced by having sewage treatment? He may pay nothing toward the construction and maintenance of a sewage treatment plant if his tenant pays all of the fee. This is an inequity that has been hard to correct. Some communities have a property tax to help defray the cost

of the sewage treatment plant, and this equalizes the cost somewhat.

Regulation of sewage disposal

In the United States construction and operation of sewage treatment facilities and disposal of the final effluent is the responsibility of the community, but the regulation of the community sewage treatment plants and disposal of final effluents is the province of the state. This authority may be vested in the sanitary engineering division of the state department of health or in a special state sanitary authority. There are advantages in having a special authority to regulate sewage disposal, largely because water pollution is increasing as a problem. In addition, a separate authority can deal with air pollution and other problem of the total environment.

The state can order a community to treat its sewage before emptying the final effluent into public waters. Courts have held this to be a proper function of the state and have ordered communities to raise the necessary funds to provide for proper sewage disposal. Plans for a community sewage disposal plant must be approved by state engineers, who also work with communities in an advisory role. Sewage disposal plant operators must pass state examinations to be certified operators. The operation of the sewage plant must meet state requirements and satisfy state sanitary authorities.

Septic tanks

A serious community health problem may exist when a residential area is not served by sewers. A septic tank for each domicile is the means used for sewage disposal in such areas. The fringes of a city or the outlying area just beyond the city limits are the usual sources of these problems.

A septic tank can be satisfactory for the disposal of household liquid wastes if the tank, drain tile, and seepage pit are properly constructed. When improperly installed, a septic tank can constitute a hazard to health and, esthetically, can be a severe nuisance. Sewage sporadically coming to the surface or, during flooding, washing over a neighborhood can constitute a hazard to the well-being of everyone in the vicinity. There is a pattern that usually exists in such situations—first, a long-time toleration of the situation; then, protests to the health officials or others; then, perhaps, court action. The final solution is usually the installation of sewers as a part of the community sewerage system. When at all feasible, even at considerable cost, sewer lines rather than septic tanks should be the choice.

Cities without sewer systems

Many cities in the United States have inadequate sewerage systems, and the general public is concerned about the possible danger to health and life resulting from negligence. As a consequence, pressures are exerted on officials and on voters to provide the necessary finances and plans for an adequate sewerage system for their community. Federal and state funding

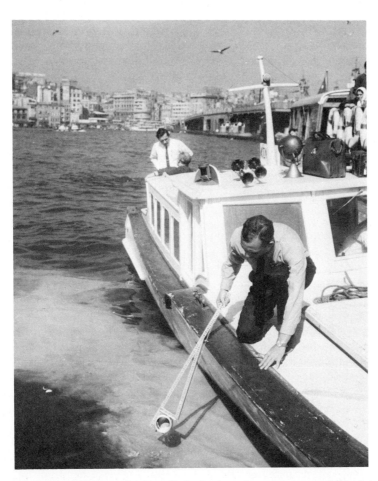

FIG. 14-7. Water pollution. Checking drift of submarine sewerage outfall in Istanbul.
Courtesy World Health Organization.

adds to the incentive to provide the community with an approved, safe means for the disposal of the community's wastes.

Throughout the world one can find cities of more than 1 million inhabitants without a sewer system. Tokyo, Japan, (with more than 10 million people) has the largest population of any city in the world. Yet Tokyo does not have a sewer system but depends on collection tanks and tanker trucks to collect and dispose of sewage.

Hiroshima was leveled by a nuclear bomb, which necessitated a complete rebuilding of the city. Environmentalists assumed that Hiroshima would begin by putting in a complete sewer system before erecting structures above the ground. The situation was ideal for this sequence. But no sewer system was built. The tank system apparently is the system of choice. This event could well cause Western countries to ask themselves whether they have overemphasized the necessity for all of the sewerage systems they have built. But experience justifies their concern for the protection of the health of their people.

STREAM POLLUTION

Stream pollution is the creation of objectionable conditions through the discharge of sewage or industrial wastes into natural waters. With the growth of cities and the expansion of industry, stream pollution has become a major concern.

A single river may have many uses—navigation, power, swimming, boating, fishing, industrial waste disposal, domestic sewage disposal, industrial water supply, community water supply, and irrigation. Control of all conditions affecting a stream is as essential as it is demanding.

While stream pollution is generally thought of only in terms of a threat to human health, water pollution actually affects many factors of economic and other significance. It affects ag-

riculture by altering the taste of milk from cows drinking polluted water. Polluted irrigation water represents possible dangers. Water fowl and other animals are exposed to botulism and cyanide poisoning. Turbidity of 6,000 parts per million (ppm) is lethal for fish. Thermal pollution can destroy marine life. Decomposition of nitrogen wastes forms nitrates and, because all of the oxygen is consumed, green plants die and anaerobic bacteria survive. Farther down the stream where little or no pollution exists, green plant life may be profuse and give off oxygen. Pollution may render water unsuitable for industrial use. Pollution with acids may cause dock deterioration. Pollution from such industries as mining and quarrying may interfere with navigation and thus require dredging of the stream.

It is apparent that stream pollution affects many factors, but its effect on use for domestic purposes is the most important. This holds priority for the public sector over all other considerations. To reduce pollution to a point where streams are as clear as they were in their natural state would be an unrealistic ideal. If we can hold our own so that streams do not become more polluted, we will be doing very well.

Criteria of stream pollution

In the final analysis, the most reliable single index of stream pollution can be the BOD, expressed as the quantity of oxygen required for oxidation of organic matter (expressed in pounds). The capacity of any body of water to oxidize wastes depends on the water's oxygen, oxygen resulting from photosynthesis in algae and other green plants, and the dissolved oxygen already in the water. If the oxygen utilization exceeds oxygen production, a negative oxygen balance occurs and an anaerobic condition results that provides for undesirable bacterial action. A stream need not be in a state of negative oxygen balance to be badly polluted. If the total oxygen demand exceeds the standard per capita demand from domestic sewage of 0.168 pounds of oxygen per day, the stream is likely loaded with excessive pollution.

Other criteria of pollution are also employed. Plankton are used as an index because pollution destroys the normal fauna and flora of a stream. By determining the populations of various species of plankton, it is possible to get an index of the degree of pollution. Other biological forms can also be used as indicators of pollution. A marked reduction in clean water species of life can be used as a criterion of severe pollution.

In the United States classification of streams was established by the first state stream regulating agency, the Pennsylvania Sanitary Water Board, created in 1923. This board established standards for three classes of streams. Class A streams are those in their natural state, probably subject to chance contamination by human beings but unpolluted or uncontaminated from any artificial source. They are generally fit for domestic water supply after chlorination, will support fish life, and may be safely used for recreational purposes. Class B streams are those that are more or less polluted. The extent of regulation, control, or elimination of pollution from these streams will be determined by a consideration of (1) the present and probable future use and condition of the stream, (2) the practicability of remedial measures for abatement, and (3) the general interest of the public through the protection of the public health, the health of animals, fish, and aquatic life, and the use of the stream for recreational purposes. Class C streams are so polluted that they cannot be used as sources of public water supplies, will not support fish life, and are not used for recreational purposes. From the standpoint of the public interests and practicability, it is not necessary, economical, or advisable to attempt to restore them to a clean condition.

Other standards have been established by other stream pollution control boards. Some boards zone rivers. From the practical standpoint, perhaps, standards must be developed for each stream.

Control of stream pollution in the United States

The long-established principle of riparian rights holds that landowners have the right to have a stream come down to them with its quality unimpaired and its quantity undiminished. Most people agree that there should be an equitable distribution of water, particularly between states and between communities. Obtaining some degree of equitable distribution and protecting natural waters is a formidable assignment.

Control of pollution of interstate waters is a recognized function of the U.S. federal government, and Congress passed the Federal Water Pollution Control Law, which went into effect in 1948. This act declared the pollution of interstate waters to be a public nuisance that must be abated. It protected the rights of the states in controlling water pollution. It also provided funds for surveys, investigations, and research. With the expiration of this law in 1956, the act was replaced by PL 660, which delegated to the U.S. Public Health Service responsibility for administration of the law.

The essence of the law is cooperation with all federal, state, and community agencies engaged in efforts to reduce or eliminate pollution of interstate waters and tributaries. As a supplement to the specifications of the law, provisions are made for personnel training programs, research, and grants to states and interstate agencies for administration purposes. Funds are made available for the construction of community sewage treatment facilities. PL 660 also provides for public hearings, conferences, and even abatement proceedings. This legal action may be taken on the request of any state affected by interstate pollution.

The 1965 Water Pollution Act passed by Congress provided that each state determine the uses of its lakes and rivers. This water quality approach has much to recommend it but from the practical standpoint is difficult to administer. After 10 years, many states had not established water quality standards, and other states were unable to reconcile the relationship between pollutants and water use.

In 1971 the Federal Water Pollution Control Act shifted from water quality standards to direct effluent limits with the theoretical goal to be zero discharge. This act requires polluters to apply for a discharge permit from the Environmental Protection Agency (EPA). The first phase of this program ended in 1976, by which time all firms and agencies were obligated to use the best available knowledge to control water pollution. The goal of the second phase, ending in 1981, is to achieve water clean enough for swimming and fish propagation. The goal for 1985 is the elimination of all effluents.

Both communities and industries find costs of effluent elimination to be the main hurdle. The National Council on Environmental Quality acknowledges that costs rise exponentially with the degree of cleanliness sought so that the last 1% of treatment could cost as much as the previous 99%. Because of prohibitive costs even with federal subsidies, zero discharge may be an unattainable goal. Zero discharge may not be necessary and something less can be satisfactory.

Some communities have developed land disposal systems in which wastes are routed through a simple treatment, then stored in lagoons, and finally sprayed over a wide acreage of land. Ecologists favor this approach because it returns invaluable nutrients to the soil. This type of simple approach may provide an acceptable, if not satisfactory, answer to the problem of effluent discharge.

Two or more states set up compacts when a stream is contiguous to more than one state.

Some of these agreements are formal, others are informal. Usually, an interstate commission or water control council is created. Cooperation is the purpose for and the key to these programs for pollution control.

Within a state, pollution control may be vested in the state department of health; or some other agency will be responsible for general environmental health problems, including air pollution. The state agency may set up districts or drainage areas to provide control measures best suited to particular problems in specific sections of the state. The state sanitary authority may establish standards of pollution, conduct surveys, and take action to abate a pollution nuisance. However, cooperation is the reasonable approach, and only after all other measures have failed will the state agency resort to legal measures. There is a need for waste disposal and a need for water protection. To reconcile the two is the task that faces every community and every country.

GARBAGE AND REFUSE

Community wastes consist of garbage, ashes, rubbish (boxes, papers, other scraps), street sweepings, trade wastes, and occasionally such things as dead animals. Leaves, grass, and shrub cuttings will often be considered wastes that must be disposed of. That communities vary in particular wastes is a common observation. Industrial wastes are normally not a community problem, because industries usually dispose of their own wastes.

Of the solid wastes of a community, garbage poses the most significant health menace because it provides feed for stray dogs, rats, and insects. In some sectors of a country this may be a minor factor in health, but in some geographical areas dogs, rats, and mosquitoes are hosts of serious diseases and thus constitute a significant threat to health. Rubbish can also harbor rats and insects, but the removal of rubbish is more an esthetic matter and one of convenience rather than health.

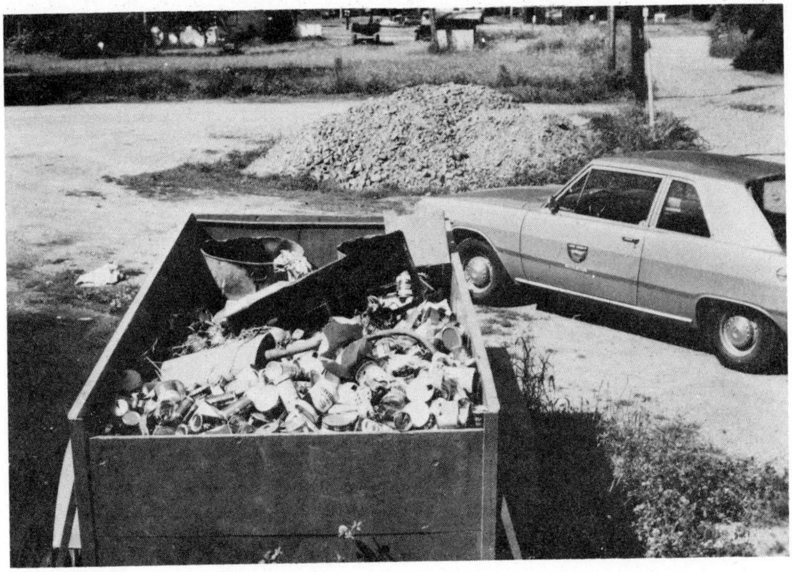

FIG. 14-8. An available container for disposal of household wastes is a first step, but a fly-tight covering is necessary to complete the operation.

Courtesy Environmental Health Division, Lane County, Oregon.

Collection. Both the collection and the disposal of garbage and refuse are accepted government functions in the United States. Some communities collect household and commercial garbage and rubbish without charge, the cost being met through general tax funds. Some have charges for garbage and rubbish collections. The responsibility for collection usually rests with the department of public works or some other comparable department, and responsibility for proper sanitation relating to garbage and rubbish usually rests with the health authorities of the community.

Some communities in the United States contract with private firms to collect garbage and rubbish. Specifications for collections are set up by the city council and bids are called for. The successful bidder is then granted a franchise for a period of about 5 years, when bids are again called for. The city council specifies what the charges will be and stipulates the frequency of collections. Each householder pays the disposal company for hauling garbage and refuse. The garbage is usually collected at regular intervals, and the rubbish is hauled away only on the special request of the householder. Some cities have a can-exchange arrangement, in which the city provides a can, picks up the filled can, and leaves a clean, empty one at each collection. Garbage collections in residential areas vary from weekly to every other day. When ashes are kept separate, a weekly collection of ashes is frequently the pattern. Collections from commercial districts are made six times a week.

A 30-gallon container for garbage is usually adequate for a typical family. Community regulations specify that the containers must be of metal, be rubberized, or be of other special composition. The containers must be watertight, fly-tight, and easily cleaned. A tightly fitting lid is required. The householder is responsible for cleaning out the container and occasionally decontaminating it with some strong

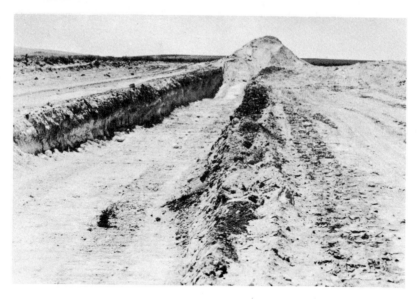

FIG. 14-9. Sanitary landfill. Excavated trench 6 feet deep and 20 feet wide provides an approved method for disposing of solid wastes. When filled almost to the top, a covering of dirt is scraped over the fill.

Courtesy Idaho Department of Health.

germicide such as Lysol. Some communities require that garbage and ashes be separated when incineration is the method of disposal. This may also be required when reduction or hog feeding is the method of disposal.

Some communities require that garbage cans be lined with paper. Others require that garbage be wrapped either in ordinary paper or in wet-strength paper bags. Again, wrapped garbage is not desirable when hog feeding or reduction is the method of disposal.

Enclosed trucks with hydraulic hoists for loading, compressing, and unloading are both sanitary and economical. At least once a week the trucks are steamed and cleaned with detergents.

Disposal. Open dumps, sanitary landfills, incineration, hog feeding, reduction, and grinding are the recognized methods of garbage disposal. Most communities use dumps for the disposal of garbage and refuse. Burning at the dump creates a fire hazard and obnoxious smoke and odor. In addition, dumps are breeding grounds for rats and vermin. When the dump is in an isolated area and properly supervised, it could be an acceptable method of disposal.

Sanitary landfills require a land depression or excavating a trench into which garbage is dumped and then covering the fill with dirt. This method serves to reclaim wastelands, does not require separation of ashes and garbage, can be virtually odorless, and can be free of rats and vermin. Availability of an acceptable area may be a problem.

Incineration is an expensive disposal method but is regarded as the most acceptable. Garbage and rubbish need not be separated. Ashes are excluded and, usually, magnetic separators remove cans and other metal objects. Incinerators are composed of a receiving bin, from which refuse is carried by conveyor to a hopper that feeds the refuse into a furnace. Oil, coal, or gas may be used as supplementary fuel for maximum combustion in the furnace. The final ash is removed from the bottom of the furnace and hauled to a dump or a landfill.

Hog feeding is an old method of garbage disposal still in use but not approved by health authorities. It requires both a separation of garbage from other wastes and a sorting of the garbage. An area of 2 acres and a ton of garbage per day for 100 hogs is the accepted standard. Even if the piggery is far removed from the community and even if it is well operated, feeding garbage to hogs is objectionable. Spreading garbage, raw and cooked, creates an environment where stench, flies, rats, and other objectionable factors exist. As a source of human trichinosis, garbage-fed hogs must always be regarded as a primary threat, even when an informed public cooks pork adequately before it is placed on the table.

Grinding of garbage and disposal of it in the community sewage is both effective and practical. A large grinding plant receives garbage from the collection trucks and empties the ground garbage into the trunk sewer. Experience indicates that ground garbage causes no serious interference with sewage treatment. Oxygen demand of the sewage is increased, but not to a degree that would have an adverse effect on the effluent of the treatment or on the terminal waters into which the sewage effluent is emptied.

Domestic garbage grinders attached to kitchen sinks are highly satisfactory although bones and other objects must be separated out. The individual householder can purchase his or her own grinder from a commercial firm, the city may install home grinder units on a city-wide basis and resell to the householder on an installment plan, or the city may retain ownership and charge a monthly rental fee. The municipal sewage treatment plant can handle the ground garbage if the biochemical oxygen demand is in a controllable range. To take care of household garbage in this manner, the community rightfully makes a regular monthly charge.

Recycling certain combustible and noncombustible solid wastes is receiving increased attention by research agencies and community officials. In the United States some states have passed legislation making mandatory a deposit on containers made of glass or metal. Whether this will reduce littering is still a matter of conjecture, but certainly recycling merits further study and trial. Up to the present time recycling has not been financially self-sustaining, but the question remains whether recycling should not be continued even at some cost. In the meantime, further research may make recycling financially feasible and the chosen disposal method for certain solid wastes.

Reducing litter

However ugly litter may or may not be, it serves as a signal of a blight on the community that disregards the common good. It would indeed be difficult to establish a relationship between litter and physical health, but the effect of litter on mental health could be appraised although not in precise data.

A great deal is involved in litter reduction and any program to be effective must be based on organization of resources and professional leadership. In the United States the principal voluntary organization for the prevention of litter is *Keep America Beautiful, Inc.* (KAB).

Oregon, Vermont, and recently Massachusetts have passed "bottle bill" legislation emphasizing the return of certain containers and responsibility for preventing and controlling litter. Total litter in Oregon has been reduced 10.6%. In Vermont total litter has been reduced by 14.6%. Both states report that although their programs are not perfect, results thus far have been highly satisfactory.

EVALUATION

Disposal of human wastes will become a spiraling problem demanding greater and greater investment in disposal plants and greater and greater expense in the process. It is a price that must be paid for progress. Humankind must conduct research to improve methods of waste disposal.

While the individual citizen has a personal responsibility in disposing of wastes, the very nature of waste disposal in a highly urbanized, highly populated nation makes it a community responsibility. It is through a cooperative community approach that this problem will be solved. Citizens must be willing to make the necessary investment for the protection of their health and for the creation and maintenance of an attractive, pleasant environment.

WASTEWATER MANAGEMENT OBJECTIVES

The overall goal of community wastewater management programs is that residents of the community will not experience disease or adverse health effects from the substances associated with the management of wastewater. Specific objectives to be further refined for a given community should include the following.

Outcome

- By 19 __ there will be no common source toxic effects or disease outbreaks from waterborne sources.
- By 19 __ there will be no preventable contamination of groundwater, surface water, or the soil from (insert name of specific contaminant, for example, industrial toxins–arsenic) associated with wastewater management.

Process

System compliance. By 19 __ the community wastewater system (wastewater collection, transmission, treatment, and discharge) will provide information to the proper review agency to track compliance with relevant wastewater regulations.

System development and maintenance. By 19 __ the community wastewater system will

meet applicable national and local construction and operation requirements. By 19 __ all wastewater system construction projects will conform to a community sewage plan.

Individual systems. By 19 __ the community will be served by a program of subsurface sewage disposal–septic tank drainfield approval in areas where sanitary sewers are not available or economically feasible. (No drainfield will be permitted without adequate demonstration of drainage and adequate protection of drinking water and surface recreational waters.)

Industrial wastewater. By 19 __ no industrial wastewater may be discharged into surface waters without a waste discharge permit or license specifying the conditions, class of effluent, and impact, *or* adequate pretreatment processing. (Discharge of wastewater into community sewerage systems will be permitted only if those wastes can be handled appropriately and safely by the system and effectively processed at the treatment plant.) By 19 __ special requirements will be applied to the treatment and disposal of toxic substances (solid or liquid).

Water quality maintenance. By 19 __ the community will be served by a program to assure water quality maintenance and to provide early problem identification and corrective action to avoid potential contamination.

Surface waters. By 19 __ the community will be served by a program to control degradation of surface waters.

SOLID WASTE MANAGEMENT OBJECTIVES

The overall goal of community solid waste management programs is that residents of the community will not experience disease, including adverse health effects from toxic substances or physical injury associated with the management of solid waste materials. Specific objectives to be completed for a given community should include the following.

Outcomes

- By 19 ___ the number of common source toxic effects, disease outbreaks, or physical injury associated with the management—collection, storage, processing, disposal—of (insert name of specific solid waste material or contaminant) will not exceed _____ .
- By 19 ___ there will be no preventable contamination of groundwater, surface water, soil, or the atmosphere from the collection, storage, processing, or disposal of solid waste.
- By 19 ___ there will be no breeding of insects or rodents that is stimulated by the collection, storage, processing, or disposal of solid waste materials.

Process

Governmental surveillance. By 19 ___ solid waste collection, treatment, and disposal services and facilities will be under governmental surveillance and control.

Technical requirements. By 19 ___ all solid waste collection systems and disposal facilities will meet applicable national and local technical requirements.

Hazardous waste management. By 19 ___ all hazardous waste management systems and facilities will meet national and local technical requirements relating to hazardous materials.

Technical assistance. By 19 ___ technical assistance to facilitate compliance with technical requirements will be provided to managers and staff of solid waste collection, treatment, and disposal services.

Public information. By 19 ___ a continuing public education program will be conducted to advise individuals of procedures and community services for handling and disposing of hazardous solid wastes.

Incentives. By 19 ___ an incentive program will be available in the community to encourage entities collecting and processing solid

waste to recover materials and energy when it is technically and economically feasible and safe.

• • •

U.S. federal standards with applications to wastewater, water pollution, and solid waste management have been established by the EPA under authority of the Safe Drinking Water Act, PL 95-190; the Federal Water Pollution Control Act (The "Clean Water Act"), PL 95-217; and the Resource Conservation and Recovery Act, PL 94-580.

QUESTIONS AND EXERCISES

1. What problems of waste disposal have been created by the development of suburban areas?
2. What is the relation of sewage disposal and a clean, attractive city?
3. The Tokyo system for dealing with sewage appears to be effective. Why should not U.S. cities adopt the Tokyo system?
4. What are the merits of having voluntary organizations initiate and support programs to keep communities clean and attractive?
5. How would you initiate a program to make your community more attractive?
6. Under what circumstances would you agree that community sewage need not be treated?
7. A community of 6,000 people has installed a complete sewerage system and has ordered all establishments to connect into the system, but one family has installed a septic tank and refuses to connect into the community system. What is your viewpoint and suggestions for resolving the conflict?
8. Appraise the so-called bottle bill as a measure for reducing litter.
9. A community of 10,000 people is considering a bond issue of $1,000,000 to construct a sewage disposal plant. What case would you present to justify the investment?
10. Why, under U.S. law, is a court justified in ordering a community to build and operate a community sewage disposal plant?
11. Locate a community that should construct a lagoon-type sewage disposal unit and explain the basis for your recommendation.
12. What is the most equitable method of charging for sewer service?
13. If communities are responsible for the erection and

operation of their own sewage disposal plants, why should the state be the regulating agency?

14. We have had stream pollution with us for 50 years, so why all the concern now about it?

15. If brown scum appears on the surface of a large pond inside a large community, what would be your interpretation and recommendation for action?

16. It has been proposed that certain streams and lakes be abandoned for all purposes except as receiving waters for community sewage. What is your reaction?

17. What governmental agencies should contribute finances for the prevention and correction of stream pollution?

18. Why are garbage collection and disposal not regarded as functions of the health department?

19. Some communities permit householders to burn rubbish in metal incinerators in backyards. What are the pros and cons of such a practice, and what is your recommendation for the matter?

20. What type of garbage and refuse disposal do you recommend for your community, and what is your rationale?

BIBLIOGRAPHY

American Public Health Association: Standard methods for the examination of water and wastewater, ed. 14, New York, 1976, The Association.

Bartlett, R.E.: Surface water sewage, New York, 1976, Halsted Press.

Brenniman, G.R., Rosenberg, S.H., and Northrop, R.L.: Microbial sampling variables and recreational water quality standards, Am. J. Public Health **71:**283, 1981.

Cargo, D.B.: Solid wastes: factors influencing generation rates (Research Papers Series No. 174), Chicago, 1977, University of Chicago Press.

Davies, J.: Politics of pollution, Indianapolis, 1970, Pegasus.

Fair, G.M., et al.: Elements of water supply and waste-water disposal, ed. 2, New York, 1971, John Wiley & Sons, Inc.

Fried, J.J.: Groundwater pollution, New York, 1976, American Elsevier Publishing Co., Inc.

Hopkins, E.J., Bingley, W.M., and Schucker, G.W.: The practice of sanitation, ed. 4, Baltimore, 1970, The Williams & Wilkins Co.

Imhoff, K., et al.: Disposal of sewage and other waterborne wastes, rev. ed., Ann Arbor, Mich., 1971, Ann Arbor Science Publishers, Inc.

James, R.W.: Sewage sludge treatment, Park Ridge, N.J., 1972, Noyes Data Corporation.

Johns Hopkins University, Department of International Health: The functional analysis of health needs and services, Baltimore, 1976, The Johns Hopkins University Press.

Mara, D.: Sewage treatment in hot climates, vol. 2, New York, 1976, John Wiley & Sons, Inc.

Marx, W.: Man and his environment: waste, New York, 1971, Harper & Row, Publishers, Inc.

Mayall, K., editor: Advances in sewage treatment, Forest Grove, Ore., 1974, International Scholarly Book Service, Inc.

Prichard, H.M., Gesell, T.F., and Davis, E.: Iodine-131 levels in sludge and treated municipal wastewaters near a large medical complex, Am. J. Public Health **71:**47, 1981.

Sinks, R.L., and Asano, T., editors: Land treatment and disposal of municipal and industrial wastewater, Ann Arbor, Mich., 1976, Ann Arbor Science Publishers, Inc.

Small, W.E.: Third pollution: the national problem of solid waste disposal, New York, 1971, Praeger Publishers, Inc.

Tchobanoglons, G., et al., editors: Waste water management, a guide to information sources, vol. 2, Detroit, 1976, Gale Research Co.

Velz, C.J.: Applied stream sanitation, New York, 1970, John Wiley & Sons, Inc.

15

HOUSING

A comfortable house is a great source of happiness. It ranks immediately after health and a good conscience.

Sydney Smith

There is a growing recognition that in the modern complex social structure the public has a responsibility and must have an interest in providing, or making available by some means, acceptable housing for all citizens. This has cast a different light on the role of government in housing, yet it is a logical development, since government has always had an interest in the environment affecting its citizens.

Housing is a private concern, a public health responsibility, a matter of economics, and a measure of personal and family status. Housing is important in terms of physical, mental, and social health, but it also has implications for all phases of human existence.

RELATION OF HOUSING TO HEALTH

It is difficult to isolate the impact of housing on health because many factors other than housing have a simultaneous effect on the people involved. Where there is top-level housing there is usually a top-level income, a high level of intelligence and education, availability of the best in medical care and hospital services, an excellent nutritional level, beneficial personal health practices, proper dental care, and a host of other factors related to health promotion and protection. Conversely, in poor housing there tends to be other factors that threaten health and life. Yet it is valid to point out those factors in housing that are directly and indirectly related to human health.

Physical health. Crowded living conditions increase the transmission of communicable diseases, as revealed by studies on the occurrence of infectious diseases in slum districts. The common communicable diseases occur earlier in slum childhood and the incidence is typically higher than is customary for the child in the general population. The incidence of tuberculosis rises with increased crowding. Communicable diseases may begin in a slum district but can spread to all strata of society.

Inadequate toilet facilities can be a constant threat to health. Lack of sunshine, inadequate artificial lighting, and deficient ventilation and heating can have an adverse effect on general physical well-being.

Defective heating units produce hazards of carbon monoxide and fire. Defective floors, stairs, railings and other structures account for a high accident rate.

Lead in paint has long been recognized as a danger to children, but this concern has increased in recent years as more children become seriously ill or die from eating or sucking on a chip of paint containing lead. Early symptoms and signs of lead poisoning are the skin appearing pasty, sallow, and pale, foul breath, anorexia, indigestion, abdominal pains, joint pains, malaise, fatigue, and weakness.

A program of prevention begins with the firms that produce paints. The industry has accepted its responsibility by producing lead-free

393

paint, but paint 30 years old, which may contain lead, can be peeled off by youngsters and put into their mouths. Health education directed to parents must be a continual operation. Owners of rented property should be urged and even encouraged to scrape off or otherwise remove the paint containing lead and replace that paint with nonlead paint. Official inspections of rental property can be used as educational programs. Cooperation between tenants, landlords, and health officials is the formula for an effective program to protect children from the dangers of lead poisoning.

Mental health. Poor housing conditions promote a decline in pride and motivation, both of which are essential to optimum mental health. There frequently follows a carelessness in living practices, in personal grooming, and in self-growth. Social and esthetic decline results from the uncleanliness and disorder often associated with substandard housing. Confusion, noise, and a lack of privacy are not conducive to a feeling of self-esteem. Poor housing conditions can be depressing. A person living in substandard housing conditions very easily acquires a feeling of being a second-class citizen. From the standpoint of positive mental health, perhaps the lone contribution of poor housing is that it does challenge some individuals to rise above it.

CRITERIA OF SUBSTANDARD HOUSING

In the United States the Committee on the Hygiene of Housing of the American Public Health Association (1952) conducted an extensive study of the relationship of housing to health. Its findings and recommendations have been the standard for people in the health field. The committee declared that if *any four* of the following criteria existed, the term "slum" applied:

1. Contaminated water
2. Water supply outside
3. Shared toilet or outside toilet
4. Shared bath or outside bath
5. More than 1.5 persons per room
6. Overcrowding of sleeping quarters
7. Less than 40 square feet of sleeping room per person
8. Lack of dual egress
9. Installed heating lacking in three fourths of the rooms
10. Lack of electricity
11. Lack of windows
12. Deterioration

Substandard housing is to be found particularly in the blighted areas of cities, that deteriorating section between the business center and the residential section of the community. This is the area on the fringes of the business section, where people live in retail store buildings that are no longer acceptable for commercial purposes. Owners put nothing back into the buildings in the way of maintenance. As a consequence, deterioration, rubbish, garbage, flies, vermin, rats, and fire hazards prevail.

BASIC PRINCIPLES OF HEALTHFUL HOUSING

The U.S. Committee on the Hygiene of Housing proposed minimum standards of housing based on fundamental human needs and necessary protection against hazards to health and life.

Fundamental physiological needs

Maintenance of a thermal environment that will avoid undue heat loss from the human body

Maintenance of a thermal environment that will permit adequate heat loss from the human body

Provision of an atmosphere of reasonable chemical purity

Provision of adequate daylight illumination and avoidance of undue daylight glare

Provision of admission of direct sunlight

Provision of adequate artificial illumination and avoidance of glare

Protection against excessive noise

Provision of adequate space for exercise and for the play of children

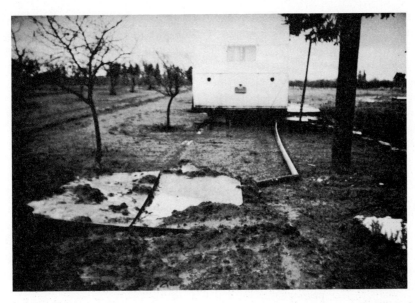

FIG. 15-1. New dangers from new modes of living. The recent trend toward mobile homes poses special health problems, particularly in sanitation. Sewage disposal of the type shown here is a community health hazard.

Fundamental psychological needs

Provision of adequate privacy for the individual

Provision of opportunities for normal family life

Provision of opportunities for normal community life

Provision of facilities that make possible the performance of the tasks of the household without undue physical and mental fatigue

Provision of facilities for maintenance of cleanliness of the dwelling and of the person

Provision of possibilities for esthetic satisfaction in the home and its surroundings

Concordance with prevailing social standards of the local community

Protection against communicable disease

Provision of a water supply of safe, sanitary quality, available to the dwelling

Protection of the water supply system against pollution within the dwelling

Provision of toilet facilities of such character as to minimize the danger of transmitting disease

Protection against sewage contamination of the interior surfaces of the dwelling

Avoidance of insanitary conditions in the vicinity of the dwelling

Exclusion from the dwelling of vermin, which may play a part in the transmission of disease

Provision of facilities for keeping milk and food from decomposing

Provision of sufficient space in sleeping rooms to minimize the danger of contact infection

Protection against accidents

Erection of the dwelling with such materials and methods of construction as to minimize danger of accidents due to collapse of any part of the structure

Control of conditions likely to cause fire or to promote their spread

Provision of adequate facilities for escape in case of fire

Protection against danger of electric shocks and burns

Protection against gas poisonings

Protection against falls and other mechanical injuries in the home

Protection of the neighborhood against the hazards of automobile traffic

These are the minimum basic requirements of good housing considered from the standpoint of health but also significant in economic, esthetic, and social terms. These basic housing needs may vary from one geographical location to another, from one community to another, and even from on section of a community to another. Housing in the center of a metropolitan area may best be served by high-rise apartments, in the periphery by single unit dwellings. The criteria of housing requirements as set forth by the Committee on the Hygiene of Housing of the American Public Health Association (1952) can still serve as a guide wherever needed, regardless of the circumstances.

BUILDING REGULATIONS AND CODES

Regulations of the construction of housing has long been a recognized governmental function in the United States. In the community this authority is exercised through ordinances providing for building zones and for codes governing construction. Zoning is designed to control the type of building to be erected in a given section of a community. One zone may provide only for single-family structures. Another zone may provide for single- or two-family dwellings. Another zone may provide for single, double, or multiple dwelling structures. Another area may be zoned commercial, and another one may be zoned industrial. Zoning protects the interests of those people owning houses or other structures in an area against having their mode of life jeopardized and the value of their property reduced. Zoning provides a degree of uniformity in planning. In some communities a special planning commission considers matters of zoning and makes recommendations to the city council, which alone has the legal authority to enact local zoning ordinances.

Community building codes specify the type and quality of materials that may be used, standards of construction, quality and proper installation of plumbing fixtures, wiring specifications, and other provisions that will give the prospective dweller, the neighborhood, and the community assurance that the building will

meet the needs of the inhabitants in terms of safe and secure living. Communities can enforce building codes by requiring a permit to build. The fee for the permit may be nominal, but in granting the permit the issuing community authority specifies that the permit is issued on the provisions of the building code. Plans for the building must meet zoning and code standards and must be followed in the construction.

The Committee on the Hygiene of Housing of the American Public Health Association has developed a model housing ordinance regulating supplied facilities, maintenance, and occupancy of dwellings and dwelling units. The International Conference of Building Officials has also developed a Uniform Housing Code. Both of these instruments can serve as excellent guides for health personnel and community authorities in developing ordinances or codes.

A building already erected before a building code was in effect will be bound by the requirements of the code if remodeling is to be done. Requiring a permit to remodel provides community officials with a means for requiring that the completed structure conform to code standards.

The housing problem of greatest general concern to the community and of particular concern to the health department is the house that was constructed years before a code existed but that now has deteriorated to a subminimal standard and will continue to decline. All of the objectionable aspects of deterioration will become progressively more apparent. It is doubtful that provisions of the building code can be enforced. Thus the avenue for relief may be closed. However, it is in this type of situation that health departments can play a vital role.

When, in the judgment of health officials, a particular dwelling is a threat to the health of the public, health officials can take necessary steps to abate the condition by negotiation and advisement with the owner or, as a last resort, court action to declare the condition a public nuisance. This approach is also extended to an area where inspections are made, hazards and other unsatisfactory conditions are reported, and a notice is issued to correct the unsatisfactory condition. Diplomacy and reasonable restraint are usually exercised by health officials. Legal measures are taken only as a last resort. Public support, always essential to the health department, is not something that just happens. It is developed by a continuing program of public education, respect for the health staff earned by its exemplary professional conduct, and high quality of service to the public.

COMMUNITY RESPONSIBILITY

People living in substandard housing sometimes become so discouraged that they do not recognize the deterioration going on about them. Tragically, children growing up under these circumstances can become so conditioned that they know nothing else, expect nothing else, and care for nothing else. Many people in substandard housing would like to get into something better, but their economic situation

has them enslaved. A rising social consciousness has brought the United States to the realization that society has a responsibility to help these people to help themselves in obtaining acceptable housing. For decades housing was left to the individual or to private enterprise, but it has been recognized that this was inadequate. A new partner has come into the picture—the governmental agencies. These are but a logical development if government exists to serve the public in fulfilling its needs. Certainly, one of the primary human needs is that of adequate housing—adequate in terms of today's standards. Today there is individual initiative, business enterprise, and governmental agencies participating in the prodigious program of providing appropriate housing for all people.

U.S. FEDERAL GOVERNMENT HOUSING

In 1937 the U.S. federal government instituted a slum clearance and low-rent housing program by creating local housing authorities

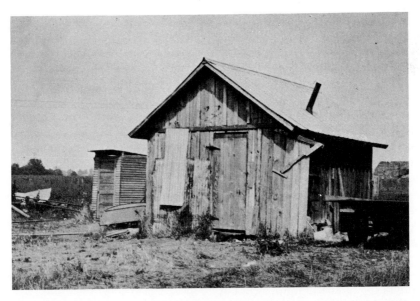

FIG. 15-2. Social engineering needed. Migrant workers living in substandard housing need more than better housing to attain an optimum level of health.

committed to slum clearance and to the construction of low-rent housing. Projects were initiated by community agencies, which also constructed and operated the housing. Federal funds made up 90% of the financing, with remainder from municipal or private sources. Loans of federal funds at low interest rates were available. A community was obligated to eliminate a slum dwelling unit for each new low-cost dwelling unit.

The Housing Act of 1949 further extended federal aid to housing by authorizing financial assistance to communities for the elimination of blighted areas and slums and for redevelopment sites. Federal financial assistance for housing was also given to private enterprise through local agencies. The Housing Act of 1949 also made provisions for area redevelopment. Funds were provided for clearing slums and blighted areas. The work to be done by the community that possessed the right of eminent domain and could thus appropriate these properties at a fair price. Communities, in turn, could build on the sites or could interest private capital in purchasing the sites from the city and in building approved dwellings or other structures. Certain tax benefits have been granted to private purchasers and developers.

Urban renewal was established by the Housing Act of 1954 as a combination of federal, community, and private resources to replace slum and blighted areas with adequate residential business facilities. To qualify for federal aid, the community must agree to certain requisites, such as a comprehensive plan of development, and administrative organization, financial adequacy, citizen participation, and responsibility for adequately relocating persons displaced by urban renewal. Not all urban renewal leads to better housing, but the business and other structures that are erected are truly in harmony with the concept of urban renewal and contribute to the physical improvement of the community.

INSTITUTION LOW-COST HOUSING

Institutions with great financial reserves have moved into the housing field and have financed and established many housing developments. Insurance companies are classic examples of firms that have provided housing for low-income families. These have not been philanthropical enterprises but have been soundly financed and soundly operated business promotions. Low-cost apartment houses with low rental rates have been highly successful. Two-, three-, and even ten-story apartment houses have been constructed in these programs and have given support to the contention that adequate low-cost housing is economically not only feasible, but profitable as well.

NEW APPROACH TO HOUSING AND HEALTH

In public health circles it has long been recognized that the existing static programs of housing and health must be replaced by a dynamic program that has a demonstrable effect on the dwellers, their health, and their mode of living. Richter et al. (1973) have come forward with a program modeled after the U.S. agricultural extension approach. This certainly is one of the most forward-looking programs that has been developed in this area of human need.

Richter et al. point out that there has been a breakdown of the environment within the public domain. As a result of the breakdown, severe health and safety burdens are now imposed on people living in buildings that have every conceivable faulty condition. These authors define semipublic domain as the domain falling between the responsibility of the individual household family on one hand (for example, indoor cleanliness, safety) and municipal government on the other (public water supply, public sanitation, sewage disposal, etc.).

These investigators report that during the period of 1965 to 1968 in New York City, owners abandoned 107,000 dwelling units housing

428,000 people. It was estimated that during the same period 10,115 low-rent units housing 40,500 people were constructed. Dr. Richter and his staff pointed out that poor maintenance was the primary problem and that buildings often are structurally sound but poorly maintained. If there is to be preventive maintenance, training of building superintendents is necessary. Building superintendents were poorly paid, with salaries ranging between $2,000 and $4,000 per year. This obviously was one factor in poor maintenance. An upgrading of the role of the tenement superintendent was in order. Dr. Richter and his staff point out that publicly subsidized tenement maintenance is a good health measure.

The East Harlem Environmental Extension Service, Inc. (a nonprofit corporation representing housing groups, owners, tenants, and job-training organizations working with the Department of Community Medicine of the Mount Sinai School of Medicine and New York City's Board of Education), is operating a training, stipend, and field service program for east Harlem residents. The extension service began its training programs in the winter of 1970. The program started three training cycles of 15 men and 10 more added. During training each participant received $80 per week, rising to $100. By the end of August 1971 there were 41 extension agents in the program, but lack of sufficient funding made it necessary to cut back the crew to 25. Subjects taught were boiler maintenance, plastering, painting, electrical work, simple plumbing, carpentry, fire prevention, and rodent and pest control. Red Cross First Aid training was a key part of the training. A field manual on health and safety was put to use. The program was linked with family health workers, public health workers, public health nurses, and community health guides.

A diversity of projects and proposed programs was introduced into the curriculum. For example, consideration was given to the community provision of steam heat, which would assure residents of home heating without air pollution. What the program did for the trainees was to give them assurance that they now had a vocational skill and service that gave them a place in the employment field.

Perhaps not all communities could operate a program such as that in New York City, but this pioneering project shows the way and encourages other communities to take a look at their situation and to develop a program that will provide improved housing for its citizens. Community leadership is offered an opportunity to initiate and develop housing betterment. A similar concept with inner-city youth was demonstrated in Baltimore, Maryland, by Wang et al. (1975), activating the youth enrolled in a community pediatric center to repair broken windows in their neighborhoods.

HOUSING SERVICES OBJECTIVES

The overall goal of community housing services is that residents of the community will live in homes that are dry, warm (or cool), safe, clean, and free from vectors and toxic substances, and will have adequate space, light, water, sanitary facilities, and food storage and preparation facilities. Specific objectives for a given community should include the following.

Outcome

- By 19__ the incidence of health and safety problems associated with residential housing (e.g., lead-based paint poisoning) will be no greater than _____.

Process

Housing code. By 19__ the community will be protected by minimum health and safety standards for residential shelter.

Substandard housing. By 19__ the community will be served by a program that identifies substandard housing and assures that such housing meets applicable codes. By 19__ __% of the community housing units will be inspected annually to identify those that are substandard. By 19__ __% of all identified substandard units will be made to meet applicable codes or be demolished. By 19__ all housing units determined to be uninhabitable will be vacated and either rehabilitated or demolished.

Surveillance. By 19__ the community will be served by a program that identifies residents with health problems associated with residential housing (e.g., children with lead toxicity) to determine the nature and extent of the problem in the community. By 19__ the community will be served by a program to assure that residents identified with health problems associated with residential housing receive appropriate follow-up care and are protected from further exposure to the substandard conditions (e.g., lead-based paint).

QUESTIONS AND EXERCISES

1. In health terms, what can be the contribution of mobile homes and what are some potentially adverse effects?
2. Explain this statement: "The effects of substandard housing on health are subtle effects."
3. Explain how the health conditions in the slum can affect the health of all strata in the community.
4. What financial factors enter into the development of improved housing?
5. Some outstanding men and women have come out of slum areas. What is the explanation and why do not all people in the slums rise above their circumstances?
6. What single deficiency in housing would you regard as the greatest threat to health and why?
7. What is your reaction to this statement: "Blighted areas are entirely a matter of financing."
8. What factors in substandard housing have an adverse effect on mental health?
9. In a substandard house, who in the family is likely to be most affected—the parents, teenagers, or young children?
10. Why would housing tend to be of low quality where tenants move frequently?
11. Poor maintenance is more than poor business, but what other effects does poor maintenance cause?
12. Objections are made to the government providing housing for private citizens, the contention being that this is socialism. What is your reaction?
13. People moving from the center of big cities to the suburbs in many instances create housing problems in the

big city. What is the nature of the problem that is created?
14. Explain this statement: "It is not possible to draw up a universally applicable housing code."
15. If an inhabited house in a well-kept neighborhood becomes dilapidated and an eyesore, what factors and interests must be considered in solving the problems involved?
16. To what extent should governmental agencies become involved in housing problems?
17. If an uninhabited house in a well-kept neighborhood becomes dilapidated and a community liability, what steps should be followed to deal with the problem?
18. Various community organizations sponsor home clean-up and paint-up campaigns. What community health implications are involved and what should be the role of health people in such campaigns?
19. Zoning always creates clashes of different interests. What should be the role of official health agencies in resolving problems that have health significance?
20. Analyze your home community in terms of factors that will affect future housing conditions, and indicate the community health implications.

BIBLIOGRAPHY

American Public Health Association: Appraisal method for measuring the quality of housing; 1, Nature and uses of the method; 2, Dwelling conditions; 3, Appraisal of neighborhood environment, Washington, D.C., 1952, The Association.
American Public Health Association: Committee on the hygiene of housing: planning the neighborhood, rev. ed., Washington, D.C., 1960, The Association.
American Public Health Association: Guide for health administrators in housing hygiene, Washington, D.C., 1967, The Association.
Clinard, M.B.: Slums and community development, New York, 1966, Macmillan Publishing Co., Inc.
Curran, W.J.: Recent Supreme Court decisions on health and housing inspections, Am. J. Public Health 57:1714, 1967.
DeLeeuw, F.: The distribution of housing services, Washington, D.C., 1972, Urban Institute.
Grier, E., and Grier, G.: Privately developed interracial housing, Berkeley, Calif., 1960, University of California Press.
Guomo, M.: The crisis of low-income housing, New York, 1974, Random House, Inc.
Halperin, L.: Cities, New York, 1967, Reinhold Publishing Corp.
Hartman, C.: Housing and social policy, Englewood Cliffs, N.J., 1975, Prentice-Hall, Inc.
Hepler, D.E., and Wallach, P.I.: Housing today, New York, 1965, McGraw-Hill Book Co.

Kaufman, M.: Housing of the working classes and of the poor, Totowa, N.J., 1975, Rowman & Littlefield.

Kleevans, J.W.: Housing and health in a tropical city, Detroit, 1972, International Book Center.

Lansing, J.B.: New homes and poor people, Ann Arbor, Mich., 1969, University of Michigan Press.

Lansing, J.B., et al.: Planned residential environments, Ann Arbor, Mich., 1970, University of Michigan Press.

Mandelker, D.R.: Managing our urban development, Indianapolis, 1971, The Bobbs-Merrill Co., Inc.

Mandelker, D.R.: Housing subsidies in the United States and England, Indianapolis, 1973, The Bobbs-Merrill Co., Inc.

Mandelker, D.R., and Montgomery, R.: Housing in America: problems and perspectives, Indianapolis, 1973, The Bobbs-Merrill Co., Inc.

Mascai, J., et al.: Housing, New York, 1976, John Wiley & Sons, Inc.

Meehan, E.J.: Public housing policy: convention versus reality, Edison, N.J., 1975, Transaction Books.

Paulus, V.: Housing: a bibliography, New Brunswick, N.J., 1975, Center for Urban Policy Research.

Richter, E.D., et al.: Housing and health—a new approach, Am. J. Public Health 63:(10):878, Oct., 1973.

Senn, C., et al.: Housing—basic health principles and recommended ordinances, Washington, D.C., 1970, American Public Health Association.

Smith, W.F.: Housing, the social and economic elements, Berkeley, Calif., 1970, University of California Press.

Starr, R.: Housing and the money market, New York, 1975, Basic Books, Inc., Publishers.

Wang, V.L., et al.: An approach to consumer-patient activation in health maintenance: A report of the Maryland 1-year health education demonstration project, Public Health Reports 90:449, 1975.

Wilner, D.M., et al.: Housing environment and family life, Baltimore, 1962, The Johns Hopkins University Press.

Wolman, H.L.: Housing policy in the United States and the United Kingdom, Lexington, Mass., 1975, Lexington Books.

16

COMMUNITY FOOD PROTECTION

I aimed for the public's heart and hit it in the stomach.

Upton Sinclair

Dr. Harvey W. Wiley, leader in pure food and drug legislation in the United States, carried on a long battle to have the first Pure Food and Drug Act passed by Congress in 1906. The act was directed primarily at food adulteration and was supplemented by the Copeland-Tugwell Act of 1938, which aimed at proper sanitation in processing and handling of foods. The final act was considerably watered down from the original proposal as the result of lobbying by manufacturers with vested interests. Yet the Food and Drug Administration (FDA) has ample authority to protect the interests of the U.S. public. In addition, other agencies and persons have responsibility for the sanitation and safety of foods.

Legally, in the United States the producer, processor, or manufacturer of foods is responsible for sanitary and safe food, which means food that is clean and safe for human consumption. This has long been referred to in common law as the implied warranty or guarantee that the product is safe. Ignorance of the fact that food is contaminated or otherwise objectionable is not a valid defense. Regulatory control of foods sold to the public is still necessary, and the closer this control is to the consumer, the more effective the control. On the state level, the department of agriculture as well as the department of health has responsibility in controlling foods. On the community level, the county or city health department has this responsibility.

DISEASE TRANSMISSION BY FOODS

No normal person wants to consume dirty or decomposed food, even though there may be no threat to health. Food must be sanitary and safe in that it is not a vehicle for the transmission of disease. Food can be a source of disease by four different means—inherently harmful characteristics, ptomaine poisoning, toxin transfer, and infection transfer.

Inherently harmful foods. *Food poisoning* is a term so generally used that it encompasses a spectrum of digestive disorders, but distinction should be made between a food that is itself poisonous and a food that merely serves as a vehicle for the transmission of pathogens to humans. Certain types of mushrooms are inherently poisonous to all people. Yet these poisonous plants are not a serious community health problem because the general public is well informed in this regard. Commercial producers of such foods as mushrooms have both the knowledge and the legal responsibility for providing the market with safe foods.

A food may also be classed as poisonous for a person who is allergic to it. By "allergy" is meant a condition of altered tissue reaction, in which reexposure to a substance produces disturbing effects. About 30% of Americans exhibit food allergies. Rarely does a person have an allergy to a single food. From the community health standpoint, it is important that, through public health education, the public know that food allergy may cause rhinitis, asthma, gastrointestinal disturbances, cardio-vascular disturbances, and various skin disorders. The logical corollary is for the informed citizen to seek medical services to determine whether allergies exist.

Ptomaine poisoning. A ptomaine is a toxin formed in the decomposition of protein through bacterial action. Meat that is sufficiently decomposed to possess ptomaines would be totally unpalatable to the human. Even though the meat were this badly decomposed, if it were well cooked before being eaten there would be no harmful results because the heat would break up the protein chains that compose the ptomaines. It is doubtful that anyone in the United States dies of ptomaine poisoning. The public needs education regarding the question of ptomaine.

Toxin transfer by food. Food occasionally serves as the vehicle for transferring toxins to the digestive system of humans. Normal cooking processes usually disintegrate toxins but, because of a lack of understanding, people fail to take precautions necessary to protect themselves against poisoning by toxins carried on food.

Botulism is caused by a toxin produced by the spore-forming organism *Clostridium botulinum,* which is found in alkaline and neutral soils throughout the United States. Raw vegetables have vast numbers of the organism on them but are harmless because the organism is an anaerobe and does not produce toxin in free air. A human being eating raw beans, peas, beets, or other vegetables would not be affected. However, if these vegatables in canning are subjected to an ordinary boiling temperature of 212° F (100° C), the spores withstand that temperature and the organism survives. Placed in the anaerobic conditions of a can or jar, the organism produces toxin. If the vegetables are cooked before they are eaten, the toxin is destroyed. If the vegetables are eaten without being brought to a boil, the toxin can be fatal as it is one of the most potent of known poisons. About 24 hours after the toxin has been ingested, gastrointestinal symptoms may appear. This being a neurotoxin, an acute poisoning of the nervous system becomes apparent and paralysis of the respiratory system occurs or the muscles of swallowing are affected.

Polyvalent antitoxin is given intravenously. Antitoxins are available for two more known types. The important thing is that the antitoxin should be administered as soon as possible to be effective.

Commercial canners using pressure cooking at 248° F (120° C) have the problem solved. The community health problem is that of educating the public of the need to use pressure cookers for canning or to use tyndallization. That means bringing the kettle to a boil (212° F) on 3 consecutive days before canning. The public should know that, regardless of the method of home canning, the best security measure is to bring the vegetables or meat to a boiling temperature before they are eaten.

Infection transfer by food. A food cannot transfer pathogens unless the following favorable conditions exist:

1. The organism must be virile and exist in large numbers.
2. The time interval from reservoir to a new host must be short.
3. The temperature must be favorable (in the neighborhood of 100° F (38° C), which is optimum for pathogens of humans).
4. Moisture must be available.
5. Very little light can be present.

Many pathogens of humans are not transferred by food. Except for a few respiratory diseases transferred via milk, virtually all infectious diseases of humans transferred by food are those of the digestive system—amebic dysentery, salmonellosis, tapeworm, trichinosis, typhoid fever, and viral hepatitis. Because cow's milk can be an excellent medium for pathogens affecting the respiratory and other human systems, a few other diseases also transferred by milk must be mentioned—bovine tuberculosis, brucellosis, diphtheria, human tuberculosis, Q fever, and streptococcal infections. Protection of food is primarily directed toward the prevention of food becoming a vehicle of pathogen transmission, a task that can be accomplished by preventing pathogens from reaching food and by destroying the organisms that have reached food.

CONTROL OF MILK AND MILK PRODUCTS

Pathogens can enter milk from many sources, but there will likely be only two reservoirs—the cow, and human beings who handle the milk. Accordingly, all cows should be tested for tuberculosis, brucellosis, and mastitis, and all reactors should be culled out. Even though pasteurization would destroy the organisms causing these diseases, it would be foolhardy not to use the added safety of preventing pathogens from entering the milk to be consumed by human beings.

Clinical examination of dairy personnel is of questionable value. A history of tuberculosis or typhoid fever would be a significant factor. Most important are knowledgeable personnel who know how disease may be transmitted by milk and who remain off the job during an illness and until a physician has declared the illness to be no longer communicable.

Milk processing. With the use of modern equipment, milk can go from the cow's udder to the bottle without ever being exposed to light. Yet even with the finest equipment, the key factor in milk processing is the quality of the operating personnel. Crews on the farm and in the milk plant who have both know-how and pride are the important link in providing the public with sanitary and safe milk.

Well-constructed stables with cement gutters and outfloors, ample light, and well-maintained ventilation are essential. Fly control should be effective. A separate milking room has merit from the standpoint of sanitation. Whether hand milking or machine milking is used, there should be decontamination of all objects that might conceivably contaminate the milk.

The milk house should preferably be at least 50 feet away from the stable. This applies whether it is merely a producing farm or one that bottles its milk for retail sale. The milk house should be ample in size and should have a cement floor and excellent drainage. Ample ventilation, light, and screening should be provided. An adequate supply of potable water is required and facilities for providing hot water are necessary for sanitizing all equipment and utensils. All equipment must be noncorrodible and in good condition. Producing farms should filter, or strain, all milk and cool it to 50° F (10° C) immediately after milking.

Pasteurization is the best available safeguard against transmission of disease via milk. Pasteurization consists in heating a medium to a certain temperature over a period of time, which will destroy pathogens of humans but will not appreciably affect the quality of the medium. In the "holding" method of pasteurization, the milk is heated to 143° F (62° C) and is held at this level for 30 minutes. This method destroys pathogens but does not affect taste, proteins, fats, sugars, or salts. Vitamin C is reduced, but milk is not relied on as a source, because the vitamin C content of milk is normally low. The "flash" method of pasteurization does the same job by heating the milk to 161° F (72° C) for 15 seconds. Modern pasteurizers with extremely sensitive thermostats hold the temperature stable and thus assure dependable pasteurization.

Underpasteurization can be detected easily, because 96% of the milk enzyme monophosphoesterase is destroyed in pasteurization and the ability of the enzyme to liberate phenol is reduced by that amount.

Cooling and bottling should be done immediately after the pasteurizing. A temperature of 50° F (10° C) should be maintained. Paper containers have advantages and are in wide use.

Regulation of milk supplies. In some states in the United States the regulation of milk supplies is a function of the state agricultural department. In other states the agricultural department regulates economic factors and the health department regulates sanitation of milk supplies. Some states have a milk control board. State regulations are essential, but it is on the local level that the most effective control can exist. Accordingly, on the recommendation of the city health department, cities pass milk ordinances regulating the sale of milk in the community. A county, through its health department, can pass and regulate the sale of milk within its jurisdiction. These regulations can exceed state standards but cannot be lower than state standards.

The U.S. Public Health Service has developed a model ordinance governing the marketing of milk. Communities adopt ordinances that are modifications of the model but that retain the essentials of the model.

Health authorities favor the pasteurization of all milk sold to the public, but in a small village where a milkman may be selling only 20 or 25 quarts a day, the price of a pasteurizer would be prohibitive. However, a milk-borne epidemic of typhoid or dysentery would be far more costly.

The model ordinance recognizes two grades of milk to be sold to the public. In addition to specifications dealing with farm facilities, processing methods, and other essentials, the ordinance sets up laboratory examination criteria of grades of milk (see chart below).

Obviously, pasteurized milk with a bacteria count of 50,000 would be much safer for human consumption than raw milk with the same count. These bacteria are harmless to humans but they are an index of the sanitary handling of milk. The ordinance also recognizes grade C milk for manufacturing purposes only.

Enforcement of regulations is effected through the issuance of a permit to sell milk following approval of the farm, the processing facilities, and other factors. Inspections by sanitarians from time to time will apprise the dairyman of the sanitary quality of his operations. A health department, after reasonable warnings, may order a dairyman to discontinue the sale of milk. He has the right to appeal to the governing health board or to the courts, or the department may refuse to renew the permit when it expires.

The competitive economic system does much to give Americans high-quality milk products. The dairyman who cannot meet the quality standards of competitors soon falls by the wayside.

Milk-borne epidemics are relatively rare in the United States, but they can happen. Knowledge and vigilance will continue to protect the community.

Milk products. Manufacture of milk products has become big business, with processes controlled to a degree where the public is well protected. State regulation in the United States is supplemented by local supervision. Epidemics or endemics originating with milk products are rare but are always a possibility.

| | Maximum bacteria count | |
	Grade A	Grade B
Sold as raw milk	50,000 per milliliter	200,000 per milliliter
Sold as pasteurized milk		
Raw milk	200,000 per milliliter	1,000,000 per milliliter
Pasteurized milk	30,000 per milliliter	50,000 per milliliter

Ice cream mixes are pasteurized. Freezing is usually with chilled brine, and storage is at 10° F (− 12° C). Contamination would come from containers, dippers, and dispensers.

Butter requires pasteurization at higher levels than market milk. Temperatures between 155° and 160° F (68° and 71° C) for 30 minutes are used. The fat is promptly cooled and then held in vats for churning.

Cottage cheese should always be pasteurized and stored at 40° F (4° C); otherwise, this medium could easily transmit pathogens of humans. Most producers of cottage cheese pasteurize their product.

Cheese, because its curing process kills most pathogens, is relatively safe. "Green" cheese (not time-cured) can transmit pathogens such as typhoid bacillus. Some cheese manufacturers take the precaution of pasteurizing the milk they use, but most cheese makers do not deem this necessary.

Frozen desserts processing comes under the same official scrutiny as dairy products, generally. Constant supervision is necessary, although the management of most processing plants take pride in their business and can be relied on to produce a safe product. The relationships between processors and inspectors is usually harmonious. Inspectors serve in an advisory capacity on sanitation as well as in a regulating role. Legal measures to control dairy product sanitary standards are usually employed only after all other means have been exhausted.

MEAT PRODUCTS

Meat products are cured or cooked before being consumed. As both processes destroy the pathogens of humans, it is natural to ask why there should be a need for governmental regulation of meat production. The answer is that the public rebels against eating the meat from diseased animals. Even though cooking may kill pathogens of humans, there is always the possibility that biochemical changes in the animal can give the meat a foul taste and even produce human illness. In addition, how meat is processed after slaughter affects its palatable and nutritional qualities. Improper canning can also be a danger to humans in that pathogens conveyed to the meat can survive and harm humans. In addition, the public should be protected against the adding of cornmeal or other grains to ground meat or other meat products.

Training of personnel, health education, demonstrations, and conferences have been more effective in proper meat processing than has been the use of legal authority. There remains a need for governmental inspection of meat on the national, state or provincial, and local levels, nevertheless.

The Meat Inspection Service of the U.S. Department of Agriculture was inaugurated by the Meat Inspection Act of 1906. The agency responsible for the administration of the law is the Meat Inspection Division of the Department of Agriculture. The purpose of the act was to safeguard the public by eliminating diseased or other bad meat from distribution, to supervise the sanitary preparation of meat and meat products, and to prevent the use of false or misleading names or statements on labels. Technically, the authority of the federal agency extends over meats and meat products shipped in interstate or international commerce. In recent years, however, courts have interpreted "interstate" so broadly that virtually all transported meat is being classed as "interstate." This has caused some conflict between federal and state inspection, particularly in those states with decidedly inadequate meat inspection programs. In general, the large meat plants have been under federal regulation and the local plants have been under state or community regulation.

In 1967 Congress passed the first substantive legislation on meat inspection since the original act of 1906. The new act provides that, within

2 or 3 years, the states must have "at least equal" requirements or the U.S. Secretary of Agriculture is authorized to take over interstate meat inspection in states falling below the federal standards. Title I of the act greatly broadens the scope of the inspection, so that more than 500 additional plants come under federal inspection.

Fresh meats. Some slaughterhouses limit their activities to slaughtering and the necessary cold storage, but many meat packing plants combine slaughtering, cold storage, freezing, smoking, and pickling. In the United States most states supplement the federal meat inspection program by having their own inspection services for those slaughterhouses and packing plants not under federal inspection. However, in many instances the small slaughterhouses are not checked by any agency.

Antemortem inspection of animals before slaughter serves to detect any disease or other adverse conditions. Killing, bleeding, and the care of the hides, organs, and carcasses are observed. Postmortem inspections of the carcasses and organs will detect gross pathology. Tissue examination will further detect disease conditions. Questionable carcasses are condemned, although the meat may be used for some purposes. A "grade" stamp on meat designates the grade quality of the meat, while the "inspection" stamp indicates that the meat has been passed as being safe.

Immediately after slaughter, beef is placed in a cooler at 34° F (1° C), where it will be stored from 4 to 6 weeks. This storage improves flavor and texture because of the autolysis that occurs. Beef frozen at −15° F (−26° C) can be stored for more than a year. Pork, veal, and mutton are usually held for 3 days before being cut. Deep freezing and storing at −15° F will keep these meats for long periods.

Curing of such products as bacon, ham, and frankfurters calls for chilled meat that is moderately moist, pickle and brine, and a covered vat to prevent any possible contamination. Cured meats are not necessarily completely protected against spoilage or deterioration. Proper storage is always necessary.

In today's market, luncheon meats pose the greatest danger of all meats and meat products. The usual processing of luncheon meats does not assure the destruction of all pathogens. Packaging and storage under inadequate refrigeration can provide a medium in which pathogens of humans can readily multiply; once the package is opened, after handling, the remaining meat may be left at room temperature for some time, and then, in many instances, placed in refrigerators with temperatures considerably above 50° F (10° C).

Canned meats. Canned meats are first cooked. High temperatures and pressures are used without seriously affecting the quality of the product. Bacterial contamination can occur, the *C. botulinum* being one of the pathogens that might survive. However, the likelihood is slight with modern methods of meat canning.

Fish is processed much like beef products. Fish can be held at a temperature of 40° F (4° C) for 2 weeks and be in excellent condition. Quick freezing of fish, followed by a dip into clean water, produces an airtight coat of ice around each fish. All equipment used in processing fish should be decontaminated daily.

Poultry should be observed for a few days before killing. Poultry is quick frozen at −30° F (−34° C) and stored at −10° F (−23° C). Canned poultry is processed under steam pressure of about 15 pounds per square inch, which should kill the *Salmonella* organism that fowl may harbor. If cold turkey or chicken is eaten without having been refrigerated since being served hot, salmonellosis transmission might occur.

Because of modern refrigeration and cooking facilities, there is no excuse to transmit disease via meat. Cold meats handled by a person who is an active case or carrier of one of the food-borne diseases is a likely mode of disease transmission via meat. People who know how to prevent the spread of disease via meat can feel secure in their knowledge. The need is public health education to make consumers knowledgeable in disease prevention.

EATING ESTABLISHMENT REGULATIONS

Perhaps no valid proof exists that if dust or other dirt gets on food, persons who eat the food will have their health impaired. Likewise there may be no overwhelming evidence that a person coughing on food will produce illness in a person who eats the food. Yet the public is entitled to sanitary and safe food when it eats in a public eating establishment. *Salmonella* infection and viral hepatitis acquired in public eating places is more common than is generally realized. Amebic dysentery and typhoid fever can also result from eating in restaurants.

A citizen walking into a public eating establishment may be neither qualified nor in a position to judge the sanitation of the place. He has to depend on the expertise and vigilance of the community health staff. Yet a better informed public could be a positive aid to the health staff by looking for restaurant ratings and by insisting that all public places practice sanitation standards set forth by the health department.

Control measures

Licensing of public eating places is the instrument of control. To qualify for a license, the establishment must satisfy the equipment and operating requirements of the health department. Once the license has been issued, health department sanitarians make periodic inspections. Frequency and timing of inspections will depend on the known conditions of the restaurant and the available sanitarians.

Rating the restaurants is usually made following the first inspection. Numerical scores are used for ratings, but sanitarians find such precise rating to be difficult. Some health departments give A, B, or C ratings. Other departments give a rating of "approved." A restaurant that is not approved following an inspection will be given a probationary period in which to correct the deficiencies shown on the inspection form. Renewal of the operating permit will be denied if the establishment has failed to correct its faults. The owner may appeal to the community board of health and, in the event of an adverse decision, may appeal to the courts.

Inspections

Many factors covered in the inspection of eating establishments are inferentially related to health. For example, it would be difficult to show that a restaurant floor had to be constructed of smooth and nonabsorbent material to protect patrons. Yet each item checked in an inspection contributes to the overall image of good construction, good maintenance, and good operating practices.

Clinical examinations of new employees, even accompanied by laboratory tests, are of limited value as a means for preventing spread of disease via the restaurant. A more effective measure is to have employees well informed on the nature of disease spread. They should not come to work when they may have a communicable disease. Workshops for food handlers are held periodically by health departments. This is one of the key factors in protecting the patrons against infectious disease.

A second key factor in the protection of the public is a safe water supply. A third factor is proper toilet and lavatory facilities, with approved methods of waste disposal. Proper refrigeration and storage of food are highly important. Corrosion-proof utensils and equipment should be properly sanitized with detergents, decontaminants, and hot rinse water. All other factors are significant but perhaps not as vital as those enumerated. Many sanitarians

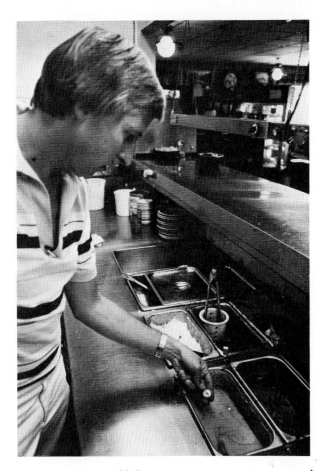

FIG. 16-1. Supervision of eating establishments. In recent years improved techniques and professionally trained personnel have helped in the control of sanitation in public eating places.

contend that rodent control is important.

A meaningful overview of a full inspection can be garnered from the items of inspection of eating and drinking establishments required for its sanitarians by the Oregon State Board of Health. These items are not intended to be listed in the order of importance, but for inspection convenience.

Floors
- [ ] Cleanable, good repair
- [ ] Smooth, nonabsorbent
- [ ] Cleaned properly

Walls and ceilings
- [ ] Clean, good repair
- [ ] Finished, light color
- [ ] Washable to level of splash

Lighting
- [ ] Adequate light: working surfaces, storage rooms, preparation areas
- [ ] Fixtures clean

Ventilation
- [ ] Adequate ventilation
- [ ] Free from odors, condensate
- [ ] Stove hoods and ventilators, adequate design

Toilet facilities
- ☐ Clean, ventilated
- ☐ Convenient, ample number
- ☐ Proper construction, good repair

Water supply
- ☐ Adequate supply and pressure
- ☐ Approved construction
- ☐ Safe, complies with state standards

Lavatory facilities
- ☐ Adequate, convenient to kitchen
- ☐ Hot and cold water
- ☐ Soap, sanitary towels
- ☐ Clean
- ☐ Good repair

Construction—utensils, equipment
- ☐ Cleanable construction
- ☐ Self-draining, no corrosion
- ☐ Free from cracks, chips
- ☐ No open seams
- ☐ No toxic utensils

Cleaning of equipment
- ☐ Clean cases, counters, shelves, tables, meat blocks, refrigerators, stoves, hoods, can openers, freezers, and so on
- ☐ Clean cloths used

Cleaning of utensils
- ☐ Single service used only once
- ☐ Dishwasher, sinks, drainboards, approved and maintained
- ☐ Kitchenware, tableware clean
- ☐ Dishwashing procedures approved

Bacterial treatment—utensils
- ☐ Approved sanitization, time, temperature, chemical concentration
- ☐ Machine properly operated
- ☐ Kitchenware adequately treated
- ☐ Dishtowels not being used

Storage—handling of utensils
- ☐ Protected from contamination
- ☐ No handling of contact surfaces
- ☐ Single serviceware properly handled
- ☐ Dippers kept in running water

Disposal of wastes
- ☐ Approved liquid waste disposal
- ☐ Plumbing complies with state code
- ☐ Approved garbage cans
- ☐ Covered, pending removal
- ☐ Clean and in good repair
- ☐ Garbage storage and removal approved

Food temperatures
- ☐ Cold perishable food below 45° F (7° C)
- ☐ Hot perishable food above 140° F (60° C)
- ☐ Ice storing, handling approved
- ☐ Thermometer in each refrigerator
- ☐ Refrigerators maintained

Wholesomeness of food
- ☐ Clean, no spoilage, safe
- ☐ Approved sources

Wholesome milk products
- ☐ Milk, milk products approved
- ☐ Milk dispensed properly

Wholesomeness of shellfish
- ☐ Approved sources
- ☐ Stored in original containers

Preparation and storage of food
- ☐ No contamination by immersion, leaking, or condensation
- ☐ Neat storage, off floor

Display—serving food, drink
- ☐ Minimum manual contact
- ☐ Food wrapped or covered
- ☐ Cafeteria front protected

Vector control
- ☐ Fly control approved
- ☐ Roaches, insects controlled
- ☐ Rodents under control
- ☐ Structure rat-proof
- ☐ No animals or fowls
- ☐ All poisonous compounds stored away from food, proper use

Cleanliness of employees
- ☐ Clean outer garments
- ☐ Clean hands and nails
- ☐ No spitting, no tobacco used in rooms where food prepared

Housekeeping

- [ ] Site, premises neat and clean
- [ ] No operations in private quarters
- [ ] Adequate clothing lockers and dressing rooms kept clean
- [ ] Storage of soiled clothing, linens, mops, and so on

Control

- [ ] No person at work with any communicable disease, sores, or infected wounds
- [ ] Washing sign posted in all toilets

In the final analysis the integrity of the management and the quality of the employees are the true keys to sanitary and safe food in eating establishments. Restaurant personnel who are aware of their responsibility to the public and who know how to prepare and serve food properly represent the best safeguard the public has when it dines out.

Bakeries and confectionaries. Safeguards in producing bakery and confectionary products are similar to those essential to restaurant operations but somewhat less demanding. Employee exclusion as a communicable disease control measure, safe water supply, proper waste disposal, protection against rodents and insects, refrigeration, and utensil sanitizing are all important. The use of sanitary ingredients and the exercise of sanitary precautions during manufacture are also significant. The use of wrapping and other sanitary provisions are essential in handling and storing the finished product. Cleanliness is the very nature of the bakery and the confectionery and, while sanitary inspections should be made at intervals, these establishments are rarely a source of problems for the sanitarian and even less rarely a vehicle of disease spread.

Retail food stores. Safety of food is a first consideration in protecting the public. Refrigeration and storage are of first importance. Elimination of all spoiled foods should be prompt and complete. Employees who are convalescing from an infection of the digestive tract should not handle uncovered foods, even though it would be difficult for organisms they may put on lettuce or tomatoes to survive the customer's journey home and infect a family member who later eats the vegetable. The risk, though slight, should not be ignored. Safe water should be used for all store purposes.

Cleanliness is a second consideration. Because of modern packaging, the customer is usually assured of clean food, especially because self-service methods give customers an opportunity to do some inspecting themselves. Yet the cleanliness of the whole store is desirable, and store managers know they will not be in business long if their store is not clean.

Community health departments do not find retail food stores a great problem. Occasionally the health department will have complaints against a market. Failure to dispose of discarded produce does pose a problem when employees are lax. A written warning by the health department sanitarian usually produces the necessary results.

APPRAISAL OF FOOD CONTROL MEASURES

Constant vigilance by health officials is essential to protect the public against food-borne diseases. The busy citizen cannot make an inspection of restaurants, dairies, slaughterhouses, or canneries. He must depend on the technical expertise of officials paid from taxes. Yet citizens can aid their own cause by being knowledgeable and by cooperating with public officials who are protecting the public.

From many technical fields humankind has been the recipient of methods and procedures for protection against the transmission of disease and poisons. Freezing as an alternative to canning is both convenient and safe. Chemical additives have been a protection as well as a danger. Legislation has protected consumers against the indiscriminate use of ingredients such as soybeans in hamburgers. Legislation protects the public by requiring sanitation and proper food handling in the retailing business. This has become increasingly important with the growth of food chains and franchise marketing. The "natural food" fads have required some degree of official supervision largely in the area of fair trade rather than as vehicles of disease spread.

Despite all the technical advances in safeguarding the food the public eats, there is always present the need for individual citizens to contribute to their own protection. Such self-supervision requires public health education to be fully effective. Constant, well-formulated health education will be valuable to all health programs.

FOOD PROTECTION OBJECTIVES

The overall goal regarding community food sources will be to protect the community from food-borne illness. Specific objectives for a given community should be elaborated as follows.

Outcome

- By 19__ the incidence of food-borne illness outbreaks will not exceed _____.

Process

Community food protection code. By 19__ the community will be protected by a health code and related system of inspection for protection against food-borne illness. By 19__ all places where foods are produced, processed, transported, stored, sold, commercially prepared, vended, served, or otherwise handled will be identified. By 19__ all places where foods are produced, processed, transported, stored, sold, commercially prepared, vended, served, or otherwise handled will be inspected on the basis of epidemiological risk and their compliance records, but at least annually. By 19__ all places where foods are produced, pro-

cessed, transported, stored, sold, commercially prepared, vended, served, or otherwise handled that violate any provision of the applicable health code will be identified and appropriate follow-up provided to ensure correction of deficiencies. By 19__ provisions of the health code will be enforced and new provisions enacted as necessary. By 19__ a program to identify and restrict distribution of suspect hazardous foods will be established.

Epidemiological surveillance. By 19__ the community will be served by a disease surveillance system that monitors and identifies instances of food-borne disease, detects sources of contamination, establishes factors that contribute to outbreaks, and recommends preventive and control measures. By 19__ a system to stimulate notification of food-borne illness by the community will be established. By 19__ reported outbreaks will be investigated to identify causative factors and agents. By 19__ strategies to prevent food-borne illness will be developed and implemented.

Public education. By 19__ the community will be served by a public information and education program concerning the prevention of food-borne illness. By 19__ there will be an ongoing health education program for the general public that describes the proper ways for storing, preparing, canning, and serving food. By 19__ food hygiene will be taught to children in primary and secondary schools and in technical and appropriate professional schools.

Food service personnel education. By 19__ there will be a program describing the proper ways of storing the prepared food and the necessity for reporting illness, which will be designed especially for food establishment managers and personnel.

Institutional food protection. By 19__ persons in institutional facilities in the community will be provided the same level of protection from food-borne illness as the public being served in restaurants.

QUESTIONS AND EXERCISES

1. Why do manufacturers in the United States lobby against proposed legislation that is designed in the public interest?
2. In terms of health protection, what is the value of home freezers?
3. Why are most cases of food-borne infections to be found in the lowest economic, social, and educational groups?
4. In your community and state or province, is there overregulation of the food industry?
5. To what extent is the prevention of food-borne disease a matter of community health education?
6. In home canning, botulism occurs from improper procedures in storage. How can this be corrected?
7. Why are respiratory diseases not transmitted via solid foods such as vegetables, fruits, and baked goods?
8. If pathogens are destroyed by pasteurization, why are cows with brucellosis, tuberculosis, or mastitis culled out as producers?
9. A dairy inspector once remarked that a certain dairyman could not produce satisfactory milk if he had the best equipment in the world. What was meant and what is the significance?
10. Explain why certain diseases such as smallpox are not transmitted via cow's milk, but other diseases such as typhoid fever are transmitted via cow's milk.
11. Why is more attention given to underpasteurization than overpasteurization of milk?
12. When some cases of disease, such as typhoid, are traced to pasteurized milk, what are some possible breakdowns in the milk processing that account for the disease transmission?
13. Why are knowledgeable dairymen so eager to do everything possible to prevent the spread of disease via the milk they sell?
14. Why is prepackaged meat displayed in open cases an important factor in the sanitary handling of meat?
15. Should governmental officials prohibit adding ingredients to meats or permit adding ingredients under governmental inspection and control?
16. In a certain junior high school, 31 cases of viral hepatitis occurred. Propose a hypothesis on the source and transmission of the disease.
17. Which is more important in restaurant sanitation—what is done in the dining area or what is done in the food preparation area—and why?
18. In restaurant rating, which do you prefer—an A, B, or C rating or an "approved" or "not approved" rating, and why?
19. In a certain bakery one of the bakers was under treatment for syphilis. Appraise the situation and indicate what the community health department should and should not do.
20. In a community health department with 24 professional staff members such as the director, nurses, sanitarians, and other personnel, which staff member in your opinion is most important and why?

BIBLIOGRAPHY

Bigwood, E.I., et al., editors: Food additives tables, New York, 1976, Elsevier Scientific Publishing Co.
Brisco, A.: Your guide to home storage, Bountiful, Utah, 1974, Horizon Publishers.
Centers for Disease Control: Foodborne disease outbreaks annual summary 1978, Atlanta, Ga., 1980, DHHS Pub. No. (CDC)80-8185.
FAO-WHO Expert Committee on Food Additives, Geneva, 1975, World Health Organization.
FAO-WHO Exports on Pesticide Residues, Rome, 1975, Pesticide residues in food, Report, Geneva, World Health Organization.
Food Protection Committee of the Food Nutrition Board: Evaluating the safety of food chemicals, Washington, D.C., 1976, National Academy of Sciences.
Inglett, G.E., editor: Symposium: sweetness: proceedings, Westport, Conn., 1974, Avi Publishing Co.
International Association of Milk, Food, and Environmental Sanitarians, Inc.: Procedures to investigate foodborne illness, ed. 3, Ames, Iowa, 1976, IAMFES.
Jernigen, A., editor: Iowa State Department of Health, Food sanitation study course, Ames, Iowa, 1971, Iowa State University Press.
Longree, K.: Quantity food sanitation, New York, 1967, John Wiley & Sons, Inc.
Mann, J.M.: A prospective study of response error in food history questionnaires: Implications for foodborne outbreak investigation, Amer. Jour. Public Health **71:**1362, 1981.
Marr, J.S.: The food you eat, New York, 1973, M. Evans & Co., Inc.
Roth, J.: Complete book of canning and freezing, New York, 1976, David McKay Co., Inc.
Sullivan, G.: Additives in your food, New York, 1976, Cornerstone Library, Inc.
Verrett, J., and Carper, J.: Eating may be hazardous to your health, Garden City, N.Y., 1975, Anchor Press, Doubleday and Co., Inc.
Whelan, E., and Stare, F.J.: Panic in the pantry, Boro of Totowa, New York, 1975, Atheneum Publishers.

17

OTHER ENVIRONMENTAL AND OCCUPATIONAL HEALTH PROBLEMS

Away, then, with crowded cities, the 30 feet
lots and alleys, the artificial reservoirs of
filth, the hotbeds of atmospheric poison.
Such are our cities. They are great prisons
built with immense labor to breed infection
and hurry men prematurely to the grave.

Noah Webster (1799)

Ecology and general environment are convenient descriptive terms in daily communication but of only theoretical value to the health scientist. Effective community health practice dictates that efforts and actions be directed to specific things in the environment. Health personnel deal with specific conditions in the environment and, while it is practical to speak of air pollution, noise, insect control, and rodent control, specific problems exist within each of these categories. Factors in the environment affecting health, welfare, and life itself must be dealt with as specific entities.

Air pollution, noise, and other aspects of environmental health are not new. These are conditions that have been with society through the centuries. It is a matter of degree and public redefinitions of acceptable conditions that is the concern in dealing with these factors in environmental health.

A minimum criterion for all countries should be the following: both a central clearinghouse for observations of agent-disease relationships and a national environmental data registry to collect and catalogue information on concentrations of hazardous agents in air, food, and water should be fully operational. When safe exposure limits are exceeded, or threaten to be exceeded, prompt action is essential. Two more criteria then come into view: (1) every individual residing in an area with a population density greater than 20 per square mile or in an area of high risk should be protected by an early warning system designed to detect the most serious hazards and (2) every populated area of the country should be reachable within 6 hours by a toxic agent or chemical emergency team in the event of exposure to a serious environmental hazard.

OCCUPATIONAL HEALTH

The objective of occupational health is the personal health of the worker and, logically, also involves environmental health. Modern occupational health promotion has been extended to include nonoccupational as well as occupational factors that affect the health of workers.

Management usually has a legal responsibility for factors affecting the health of workers, but in many instances management goes beyond legal requirements. Indeed, frequently management concerns itself not only with the well-being of workers but with the welfare of their families as well. This policy may be regarded as benevolence by some people and is criticized as paternalism by others. Yet, at times, it is necessary to extend the health program beyond the plant to the home. A classic example is the migratory worker whose home conditions may be a far greater menace to health than is the occupation.

Because many workers are overlooked in the promotion of industrial health, the community must be concerned. This concern extends itself beyond mere legal requirements to the sphere of whatever measures are essential for the protection and promotion of the health of every worker.

In the United States the National Institute for Occupational Safety and Health (NIOSH) estimates that each year 100,000 Americans die from occupational illnesses. Nearly 400,000 new cases of occupational diseases occur annually. (These estimates are controversial, but no better ones are available.) When multiple etiological factors are considered, between 10% and 20% of all cancer cases may be related to carcinogens in the workplace. In 1977 work accidents in the United States resulted in 13,000 deaths and 2.3 million disabling injuries, 80,000 of which were permanently disabling. For every 100 full-time workers there were an average of 9.2 work-related disabling injury cases, and these accounted for approximately 60 workdays lost.

An occupational health program properly goes beyond the prevention of hazards to physical and mental health and extends into the positive promotion of the health of workers. Health education, rest, recreation, treatment of sudden illness, optical services, and even diagnosis of ailments are aspects of modern occupational health promotion. A competent, trained worker is a valuable asset in industry. The same worker possessing a high level of health is an even more valuable asset. Management is interested in the quality of health possessed by its employees for economic reasons, which include concerns with absenteeism, productivity, and satisfaction with working conditions.

Attempts to promote the health of workers should be encouraged as a product of collective bargaining if not as the self-initiating action of management. The protection of workers by preventing hazards of occupations, however, is of such public concern that it must be translated into legal codes recognizing minimum responsibility for reducing hazards in occupations. Most managements accept this responsibility willingly and go beyond legal stipulations, but some are governed entirely by the requirements of the law in dealing with occupational health and safety.

Hazards of occupations

Some hazards to health are always present in any occupation, operation, plant, or industry. It is a matter of degree with which workers deal. Some hazards are so extreme that they must be eliminated or markedly reduced, while others are somewhat innocuous and are of minor concern.

Accidents. Injuries are an immediate concern in virtually all occupations. Industries alert to their responsibilities in injury control, particularly in those hazardous conditions peculiar to their particular industry, and are concerned almost entirely with the safety of their own employees. However, in some industries, such as transportation, the problem is extended to possible injuries to others as well as employees.

Prevention of injuries is an employee, as well as an employer, responsibility. Safe workers carry a certain degree of responsibility for other workers, but such responsibility cannot logically be far-reaching. Because unsafe practices loom so important in occupational accidents, identifiable accident-prone workers must be shifted to jobs that they are qualified to do safely.

Systematic plant inspections are conducted for the detection of hazards that can cause either disease or injury. Safety engineers or other experts carry out these inspections. Rules are formulated to safeguard all employees as well as to promote maximum production. Through their safety committees, workers can participate in the establishment of rules of safety and thus are more responsive to compliance with regulations.

Practices of the workers are most important in industrial safety, but management can supplement their efforts by providing conditions and devices that will afford protection. Guards, goggles, helmets, and other protective clothing may appear to be of little significance but at a particular moment may be the difference between sight and blindness or even between life and death.

First-aid instruction for key employees is a recognized arm of an industrial safety program. On-the-job training in first aid is an investment in the prevention of further harm or even death. The psychological benefits of the first-aid training program can be considerable.

Objectives that should be established in communities for 1990 concern reductions in work-related deaths and injuries, better identification of worksite hazards and illnesses, increased knowledge by workers of their personal worksite hazards and risks, reduction in worksite hazards, and strengthened epidemiological and surveillance capabilities. Once again, the limitations imposed by absence of needed data allow only a few of these objectives to be included in a tracking system. Figs. 17-1 and 17-2, present available U.S. data on work-related illness and injuries. The 1990 objectives for the United States for injury control in occupational settings include the following.

• By 1990 workplace accident deaths should be reduced to less than 11,000 per year.

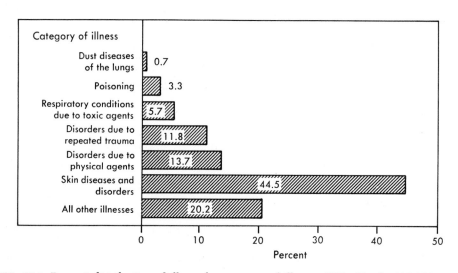

FIG. 17-1. Percent distribution of illness by category of illness, 1973. Nearly 400,000 new cases of occupational illnesses occur annually in the United States. The largest number of reported illnesses was occupational skin disease.

From American Public Health Association, Washington, D.C., 1975; and U.S. Office of Disease Prevention and Health Promotion, 1980.

- By 1990 work-related disabling injuries should be reduced to 8.3 cases per 100 full-time workers.
- By 1990 lost workdays due to injuries should be reduced to 54 per 100 workers annually.

While the reductions to be achieved by 1990 appear modest, They must be made in the face of rising trends during the last years for which data are available.

Dusts, gases, and fumes. Dusts, gases, and fumes can be a hazard to the general public as well as to employees. Fortunately means are available to reduce these hazards to tolerable levels. At conferences of Government Industrial Hygienists in the United States, maximum allowable concentration values for various industrial poisons have been adopted. These standards refer to average concentrations that can be tolerated 8 hours per day continuously without impairment to health immediately or in the future.

Dusts are generally classed as inert, irritating, and toxic. Inert vegetable and animal dusts are present in paper making, weaving, spinning, and other manufacturing processes using wool and similar raw materials, but the dangers are not great. Mineral and metallic dusts are

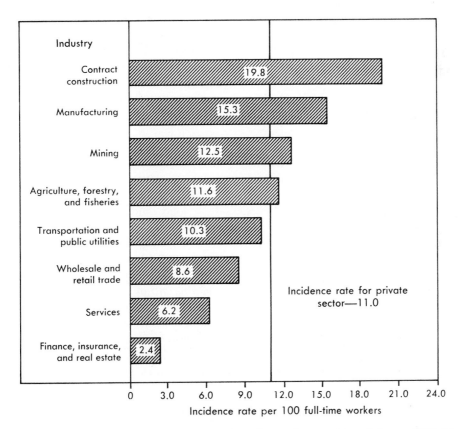

FIG. 17-2. Injury and illness incidence rates, by industry division, United States, 1973. The incidence rates for occupational injuries and illnesses per 100 full-time workers were highest in the contract construction industry.

From Bureau of Labor Statistics, U.S. Department of Labor, unpublished data, 1973; and American Public Health Association, Washington, D.C., 1975.

more dangerous. Stonecutters, drillers, miners, grinders, and polishers encounter respiratory damage resulting from inert dusts. Granite and quartz dust cause damage to the the lungs resulting in a condition termed *silicosis,* which is fatal unless the condition is recognized early and exposure to dust is prevented.

Dusts pose two problems. The first is that of concentration, which can be measured by devices such as the Greenburn-Smith impinger. The second is the important matter of particle size, which can be measured by photographic techniques, microprojectors, filar micrometers, and other devices.

Inert and irritating dusts usually can be reduced and removed. Wet processing reduces the production of dust. Enclosing work that creates dusts, combined with the use of exhaust systems, can reduce dust to a level below the danger point.

Toxic dusts, gases, and fumes such as asbestos, arsenic, mercury, lead, iron oxide, sulfuric acid, carbon monoxide, and manganese pose specific problems of control. Management is usually alert to hazards of this type and is constantly devising procedures to reduce and eliminate these dangers. Research, often with an assist from governmental agencies, is developing measures for the prevention of these industrial hazards. While the immediate concern is for the worker within the plant, management also has a concern for possible effects on the general public. It is generally conceded that no industrial process hazardous to human health is so indispensable to the economy that it could not be eliminated if it cannot be altered sufficiently to protect the health of workers.

Excessive temperature or humidity. Blast furnaces, smelters, kilns, tanneries, textile mills, laundries, and breweries are examples where the industrial process itself makes atmospheric control difficult. Dermatitis, gastrointestinal disturbances, eye inflammations, and even exhaustion result from atmosphere extremes. Air conditioning can bring atmospheric conditions

to tolerable levels. Some workers are physiologically not equipped to tolerate even moderate atmospheric change.

Excessive noise. Industry recognizes that noise is more than a health hazard, as it affects production. Noise is measured in decibels. The lowest sound the human ear can detect is 1 decibel. Loudness is expressed as multiples on a logarithmic scale of the smallest distinguishable sound. Thus a sound of 10 decibels is 10 times louder that 1 decibel. A sound of 20 decibels is 100 times louder than the lowest sound. This logarithmic expression is used as a convenience in avoiding the use of numbers in four or more figures. Long doses of 90 decibels can cause hearing loss. Higher levels can be injurious to hearing, and lesser levels can be disturbing. Annoyance threshold for intermittent sounds is 50 decibels, to 90 decibels, discomfort is at 110 decibels, and pain threshold is in the vicinity of 120 decibels. A short exposure to a noise of 150 decibels can cause permanent hearing loss.

Decibel levels obviously vary: whisper, 10 decibels; quiet street, 50 decibels; normal conversation, 50 to 60 decibels; truck, sports car, 90 decibels; pneumatic jackhammer, 95 decibels; loud outdoor motor, 100 decibels; loud power mower, 105 decibels; siren, 125 decibels; riveting, 130 decibels; jet takeoff, 150 decibels; Rock music bands have adversely affected the hearing of their members, indicating a hazard of that occupation.

Infections. Infections are a latent hazard in all occupations and are a particularly serious hazard in some industries. Slaughterhouse employees, dairymen, and others who handle livestock or hides are exposed to such diseases as brucellosis and anthrax. Other workers handle substances that serve as media for pathogens of humans. The use of disinfectants and sterilizing methods should prevent most infections in these categories. Medical attention to all suspected infection is necessary in industry as well as elsewhere.

Poisons. Harmful substances other than gases

and fumes can be present in industry. Chemicals used in plant operations can cause harm to the skin. Chronic poisoning can occur in workers improperly handling materials in routine operations. Knowledge of the presence of these hazards and proper regulations governing their handling reduces or virtually eliminates the danger. Legal regulations and management alertness combine to make poisoning rather rare in modern industry.

Radiation. Health hazards of radiation are not a new concern. Luminous paints containing radioactive compounds were recognized as a hazard more than 50 years ago.

Today, the use of radioactive products commands special precautions of shielding and the use of personal safety measures such as protective clothing. A necessary safeguard is the use of meters for recording the amount of exposure to radiation. Standards for maximum permissible concentration (MPC) of radiation have been established.

Monitoring, shielding, and other safeguards are practiced constantly. Disposal of radioactive wastes in the United States is in conformity with standards set by the U.S. Atomic Energy Commission. Sufficient knowledge on radiation hazards is now available, and industry is applying this knowledge to prevent any radiation danger to employees or to the general public.

The current opposition to reactors is partially the usual clamor when new developments are introduced, according to those who work with radioactive materials. But the concerns are related to environmental effects as much as to health effects.

Sanitation. Proper sanitation measures have long been a concern and accepted responsibility of industry. Industrial sanitation programs are designed to provide conditions that will safeguard the health of employees as well as provide for maximum production.

A safe and adequate water supply is a first requisite. Industries usually obtain their water from an approved municipal supply. If a private source is used, it should be free from turbidity and contamination and should be tested regularly. A daily test would be called for when a threat of contamination is present. Once a week can be ample at other times. About 20 gallons per worker per day is necessary for all purposes, although the amount varies with the kind of industry involved. Approved-type drinking fountains are placed in convenient locations, the number depending on the number of workers and the nature of their work.

When an auxiliary water supply is used for fire protection, flushing, and other such purposes this second supply should be safe for human consumption or so controlled that there will be no possibility that workers will use the unsafe water for drinking or handwashing purposes. Using red or other color on faucets or fixtures is a common safeguard.

An approved type of sewerage system for liquid wastes is an indispensable sanitation need. If the plant sewerage system cannot be connected to a community system, then provisions must be made for plant sewerage disposal.

Toilets and washrooms must be of good construction with adequate toilets and washbasins. The number of toilet units varies from 1 per 10 workers to 1 for 30 workers. When urinals are installed, only two thirds as many units are needed.

Washing faucets may be preferred over washbasins because they are less likely to be a means of infection spread. Automatic control of temperatures at 125° F (52° C) is possible with the mixtures of hot and cold water running from the same faucet. Liquid soap is preferred merely because bar soap too easily finds its way to the floor. Shower-bath heads are attached to the wall usually just below average worker chin level.

Illumination. Lighting meeting recommended standards reduces accidents and eyestrain and improves efficiency and productive output. Where high detail and speed of vision is required, as much as 100 footcandles are recommended. Illumination of 50 footcandles is required. Along hallways, or where no great visual discrimination is called for, from 10 to 20 footcandles can be adequate. It is always important to avoid great contrasts in degree of illumination. A ratio of 5 to 1 is preferred with 10 to 1 the outside limit.

Ventilation. Properly, ventilation of industrial plants is designed to provide physical comfort by controlling the temperature, humidity, and movement of air. Either natural or artifical means are employed. Removing body heat and moisture in the summer and providing circulation and moderate temperature in the winter are the customary goals. Temperature between 66° and 72° F (19° and 22° C) with a relative humidity of 50, combined with movement of air, provides for physical comfort.

Some industries have the problem of removing dusts, gases, vapors, and fumes, for which exhaust systems are employed. If air is recirculated, the ventilation system must be operating efficiently at all times. This requires competent maintenance.

Responsibility for occupational health. Management, workers, unions, local government, and the national government all have responsibilities in occupational health. Local health departments are rarely equipped to provide the highly technical professional services that occupational health problems command. Whether the local health department can provide extensive or decidedly limited service, the whole approach must be that of cooperation between all persons concerned with a particular occupational health situation. Health departments do not enter these situations as a police force but as public servants ready to assist with health problems that exist. Only when industrial management fails to live up to established and accepted standards will the force of legal authority be exercised.

The identification of occupational worksite hazards and illnesses calls for the development of generic standards for major common health hazards for injury and toxic exposures, increased numbers of health hazard evaluations,

and routine questioning about occupational health risks by physicians and other health providers as part of their patients' medical history. National objectives should also relate to increasing worker's knowledge of personal worksite risks. For example, 25% of workers should be able to state the nature of their occupational health and safety risks and their potential consequences prior to employment, as well as being informed of changes in these risks while employed. In 1979 less than 5% of workers in the United States were fully informed. Educational objectives to increase workers' knowledge of risks at work include informing workers routinely of their personal exposure measurements, of the results of their health examinations, and about life-style behaviors that interact with factors in the work environment to increase their personal risks.

A state or provincial occupational health division may be in the department of health or the department of labor. In either arrangement, the purpose of the occupational health staff is to assist all industry with health problems unique to the industry, to conduct surveys, and to enforce regulations relating to occupational health. Teamwork between industry, workers, and official occupational health personnel is the key to effective programs for the promotion of occupational health.

On the national level in the United States the National Institute for Occupational Safety and Health (NIOSH) was created by the Occupational Safety and Health Act of 1970 (PL 91-596). The Occupational Safety and Health Administration (OSHA) was created to implement most of the regulatory provisions of the Act. Congress declared as its purpose and policy in this act "to assure as far as possible every working man and woman in the Nation safe and healthful working conditions and to preserve our human resources"

1. By encouraging employers and employees in their efforts to reduce the number of occupational safety and health hazards at their places of employment, and to stimulate employers

and employees to institute new and to perfect existing programs for providing safe and healthful working conditions

2. By providing that employers and employees have separate but dependent responsibilities and rights with respect to achieving safe and healthful working conditions
3. By authorizing the Secretary of Labor to set mandatory occupational safety and health standards applicable to business affecting interstate commerce and by creating an Occupational Safety and Health Review Commission for carrying out adjudicatory functions under the Act
4. By building upon advances already made through employer and employee initiative for providing safe and healthful working conditions
5. By providing for research in the field of occupational safety and health, including the psychological factors involved, and by developing innovative methods, techniques, and approaches for dealing with occupational safety and health problems
6. By exploring ways to discover latent diseases, establishing causal connections between diseases and work in environmental conditions, and conducting other research relating to health problems, in recognition of the fact that occupational health standards present problems often different from those involved in occupational safety
7. By providing medical criteria which will assure insofar as practicable that no employee will suffer diminished health, functional capacity, or life expectancy as a result of his work experience
8. By providing for training programs to increase the number and competence of personnel engaged in the field of occupational safety and health
9. By providing for the development and promulgation of occupational safety and health standards
10. By providing an effective enforcement program which shall include a prohibition against giving advance notice of any inspection and sanctions for any individual violating this prohibition
11. By encouraging the States to assume the full-est responsibility for the administration and enforcement of their occupational safety and health laws by providing grants to the States to assist in identifying their needs and responsibilities in the area of occupational safety and health, to develop plans in accordance with the provisions of this Act, to improve the administration and enforcement of State occupational safety and health laws, and to conduct experimental and demonstration projects
12. By providing for appropriate reporting procedures to help achieve the objectives of this Act and accurately describe the nature of the occupational safety and health problem
13. By encouraging joint labor-management efforts to reduce injuries and disease arising out of employment

Prevention and promotion for occupational health

Education and information measures. Measures that communities and employers or unions can take to support behavior and to increase awareness include the following.

- Reviewing, recommending, initiating, and publicizing occupational health and safety standards and practices necessary for monitoring and surveillance of on-the-job health and safety standards, including environmental health requirements
- Initiating by management, in concert with workers and their representatives, experimental and innovative educational programs relevant to their occupational health and safety needs
- Initiating and expanding methods designed to motivate labor and management responsibility for the development and maintenance of a safe and healthful work and community environment
- Developing awareness of the potential interactions between occupational health hazards and life-style habits and behavior and their effects on health
- Developing worker awareness through electronic and print media, vocational

training programs, health care providers, campaigns aimed at high-risk worker groups (e.g., asbestos workers, newly employed and elderly workers), and organized labor programs

- Developing professional occupational health and safety personnel, including occupational health physicians and nurses, industrial hygienists, toxicologists, and epidemiologists, and including occupational health education in the curricula of medical and nursing schools and continuing education
- Developing awareness in other groups that either interact with workers or the workplace, including engineers, managers, teachers, social workers, and health care workers
- Developing public awareness of occupational disease and injuries and their high cost to the nation
- Labeling in simple language to inform workers, employers, health professionals, and the public of the hazards, associated risks, and symptoms as appropriate
- Including occupational health as part of the comprehensive health education curricula in high schools

Service measures. The organizational supports for behavior conducive to worker health include the following.

- Well-designed corporate occupational health programs that include preventive and treatment services directed at nonoccupational as well as occupational health
- Consultation services of governmental agencies to assist small businesses to identify problems and to establish suitable programs to eliminate or control them
- Encouraging small businesses to form cooperative groups to seek occupational health expertise
- Developing a personal health service delivery system in which the diagnosis and treatment of occupational illnesses and injuries will be coordinated and integrated

with all other health services that are provided the worker and his or her family
- Upgrading capabilities of state or provincial and local health departments to participate in occupational health and safety services, including monitoring, surveillance, and consultation to small businesses

Technological measures. Ways to improve the physical environment of the workplace to make it more conducive to health include

- Improved architectural and engineering design of worksites to prevent injuries
- Control technology to protect workers, including development of safe substitutes for toxic substances, design or process units that eliminate worker exposure, design of safe maintenance procedures, and design jobs to eliminate harmful physical and mental stress
- Measurement technology to enable quick, accurate, and economical assessment of hazard levels in the workplace by workers, employers, or health professionals

Legislative and regulatory measures. Some of the political and legal maneuvers possible include

- Fully implementing laws related to workers' health as well as product control provisions
- Recommending, initiating, and evaluating measures designed to improve and expand occupational health and safety legislation, paying particular attention to possibilities of standardizing benefits through a national system of worker's compensation
- Developing criteria documents recommending standards
- Promulgating new health standards on hazardous substances
- Annual inspections by industrial hygienist compliance officers
- Conducting mandated industry-wide studies and health hazard evaluations for carcinogenicity and reproductive effects that could lead to emergency temporary standards

- Changing worker's compensation laws to provide stronger economic pressures on employers to reduce hazardous conditions at the worksite

Economic measures. Government agencies can further support improvements through fines and negative publicity for poorly controlled health and safety conditions and tax deductions for capital investment in control technology or occupational health programs.

Relative strength of the measures. Given the broad nature and scope of occupational safety and health problems, the relative strength of the measures varies with the problem at hand, with the nature and adequacy of enforcement effort, and with research capacity. Most occupational health problems require the simultaneous or consecutive application of several types of measures as a total strategy to comprehensive hazard eradication. For example, eradication of the asbestos hazard might be achieved by

- Banning all nonessential uses of asbestos
- Substitution of other materials found to be nonhazardous
- Research to determine all human exposure during the "life cycle" of the fiber
- Worker information to minimize exposure that may still occur during demolition and repair work
- Rigid enforcement of asbestos standards wherever and while use remains necessary
- Professional education for physicians to assure proper medical help for exposed individuals

This type of eradication program focuses public attention on the problem and goes beyond establishing a standard for permissible exposure levels.

Finally, better data and better surveillance systems are required if occupational safety and health are to be measurably improved. National objectives for monitoring and surveillance include the following.

- By 1985 an ongoing occupational health hazard/illness/injury survey and surveillance capability should be developed. It should include identification of cancer and coronary risk factors.
- By 1985 at least one question about lifetime work history and known exposures to hazardous substances should be added to all appropriate existing health data reporting systems (e.g., hospital discharge abstracts and death certificates).
- By 1990, by use of the above as well as existing records and demonstrated associations, the extent and distribution of occupational cancer and other possibly occupationally related illness, including heart disease and injuries, will be systematically and continuously assessed.

OCCUPATIONAL HEALTH OBJECTIVES

The overall goal of community occupational health programs is to reduce factors in occupational environments that cause death, disease, or disability; minimize further personal damage from existing occupationally related illness; and promote good health and well-being among workers. Specific objectives for a given community should include the following.

Outcomes

- By 19__ sick leave absences for ____*____ will not exceed X days per 100 employees.
- By 19__ occupationally related disability for _____*_____will not exceed X injuries per 100 employees.
- By 19__ occupationally related injuries for _____*_____will not exceed X days per 100 employees.
- By 19__ occupationally related deaths for _____*_____will not exceed X per 100 employees.
- By 19__ the incidence of _____†_____

---

*Insert name of specific industry.
†Insert name of specific occupationally related disease-condition.

will not exceed _____ among workers and their family members.*
- By 19__ worker exposure to _____†_____ will not exceed _____.

Process

Surveillance. By 19__ the community will be served by a system to assess the nature and extent of its occupational health problems on a continuing basis and to establish priorities for community intervention.

Case detection. By 19__ the community will be served by a system that identifies and brings to treatment employees with detectable undiagnosed or asymptomatic occupational disease. By 19__ the community will be served by a system that ensures that all of its industries and businesses employing over 50 individuals participate in a standardized occupational health reporting program. By 19__ the community will be served by a mechanism for the early detection of occupationally related injuries and illnesses, and their precursors, in workers and their exposed family members.

Worker protection. By 19__ employees will be protected by occupational health and safety requirements appropriate to their industry (e.g., in the United States, OSHA, state occupational health program, Department of Agriculture), with particular emphasis on vulnerable populations (e.g., farm workers, pregnant women, and children).

Program development. By 19__ industry in the community will have access to technical support in the development of an occupational health and safety program.

Medical services. By 19__ the official health

---

*This objective is intended for selected problems in communities with populations large enough to develop meaningful data.
†Insert name of specific occupational hazard or substance (e.g., asbestos). Threshold Limit Values (TLVs) for a variety of occupational exposures exist in standards developed under the U.S. Occupational Safety and Health Act.

agency or other appropriate governmental agency will provide directly or make available through contractual agreement health-related services needed in some industries (e.g., inspection and consultation, health education and promotion, part-time nursing, and cooperative programs with community physicians). By 19__ employees will have ready access to selected health promotion and disease prevention services (e.g., hypertension screening, tetanus immunization).

Public and employer-employee education. By 19__ a program will be implemented to educate the public, labor unions, employers, and employees concerning occupational health hazards. By 19__ there will be a periodic cataloging and assessment of occupational health programs available to employees of community industry. By 19__ there will be employee health promotion and risk appraisal programs available in all companies and government agencies with 50 or more employees.

AIR POLLUTION

Community air pollution is generally regarded as the presence in the ambient (surrounding) atmosphere of substances put there by the activities of humans in concentrations sufficient to interfere directly or indirectly with one's comfort, safety, or health, or with the full use of one's property. In general, it does not refer to the atmospheric pollution incident to employment in areas where workers are employed, nor is it concerned with air-borne agents of communicable disease, nor with overt or covert acts or war. It does not deal with natural air pollution such as dust from deserts or barren areas, gases from volcanoes or geysers, sea spray, or pollution from other sources to which humans have been exposed. From the earliest of times man-made pollution has been the concern and the problem.

Man-made pollution comes from industrial exhausts, home heating, incineration, open fires, open dumps, dust from roads such as blacktop roads, engine exhaust, crop spraying, construction debris, and other sources. Pollutants may be in the form of solids, liquids (vapors), and gases. The atmosphere of a representative industrial area will have about 22% of its pollutants from industrial sources, about 10% from commercial sources, and the remaining 68% from public sources. It must be pointed out that pollution is not a problem unless there is a receptor—essentially, human beings adversely affected by the pollution.

Smog is the result of the photochemical reaction of hydrocarbons and sulfur oxides produced by sunlight. Nitrogen dioxide acts as a photoreceptor and is decomposed to nitrogen oxide and atomic oxygen. This reactive form of oxygen attacks hydrocarbons, and a further chain of reactions results in a complex mixture of toxic substances. Smog thus tends to have both an irritating and a direct toxic effect on human beings.

As a threat to human well-being, the most devastating effect of air pollution results when a temperature inversion occurs. The Los Angeles area in the United States is particularly plagued by this problem. Warm air normally rises, but a layer of warm air resting on top of relatively cool air pins the cool air down much like a lid on a kettle. The topography formed by the mountains to the east prevents winds from driving off the immense amounts of smoke, fumes, and other pollution.

Health aspects. More research is necessary before precise statements can be made on the specific effects of pollution on human health. Sufficient empirical evidence does exist to alert

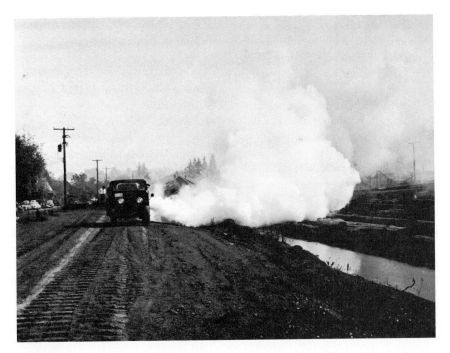

FIG. 17-3. Insect eradication. Solving one problem can create another problem. Eliminating mosquitoes by spraying can create air pollution. Solving the energy crisis may create additional pollution.

Courtesy Lane County, Oregon, Department of Health and Sanitation.

communities to the possible dangers of air pollution. Some effects are acute and can be fatal, while some effects are delayed and may be apparent only after years of exposure.

Three cities have experienced air pollution disasters. In the Meuse Valley, Belgium, in 1930, 60 people died as the result of heavy air pollution. In Donora, Pennsylvania, in 1940, a reported 20 people died from pollution. In London in 1952, during a 2-week period of air pollution, about 4,000 more people died than normally. In all of these cities a heavy fog settled over the area and did not lift, but retained the air pollutants. In all three cities most of those patients who died had had chronic respiratory or circulatory diseases. A large portion were the elderly.

People with asthma and other respiratory diseases have their condition aggravated by air pollutants. Eye, nose, and throat irritation may be mild, moderate, or severe, depending on sensitivity and specific air pollutants. Irritation of the lungs may make individuals more susceptible to lung infections. Carbon monoxide poisoning may affect heart action adversely and have delayed advers effects on a person. Gastrointestinal disturbances, especially in children, appear to be more prevalent during periods of heavy air pollution.

Economic and esthetic aspects. Air pollution can damage trees, shrubs, and flowers and ruin crops. Cattle become ill from air pollutants. Air pollution causes damage to residences and other structures. It can soil and damage clothing. It can interfere with the enjoyment of an otherwise attractive environment. Air pollution properly can be declared a nuisance on esthetic as well as health grounds. Economic damage has been adjudicated on a monetary basis. Persons who believe that they have been harmed or inconvenienced or have suffered monetary loss can obtain redress in court. A suit for damages against the firm or persons creating the objectionable air pollution can result in a judgment of monetary compensation for the damage to the plaintiff's person or property. Courts have awarded compensation for harm to cattle resulting from air pollution caused by industrial plants producing aluminum products.

Volcanic ash. Volcanic ash is a relatively new hazard, although the United States and other nations have had similar attacks before the recent Mount St. Helens volcanic activity occurred in the southwestern part of the state of Washington in the United States. As experienced in Washington, relatively few people were affected, largely because of advance warnings.

Volcanic ash is not "ash" at all. It is pulverized rock. One inch of dry ash weighs 10 pounds per square foot as it lands. It often contains small pieces of light, expanded lava called pumice. Because a volcano gives advance warning, the immediate neighborhood can be moved to a safer area perhaps 20 or 30 miles away by officials. Long before this is necessary, local and national personnel should have conducted classes and used other means to inform the residents near-by of what actions should be taken at the first warning of a volcanic ashfall.

Intermittent ashfalls may continue over several years. They may cause people to move away from the area, but some of the residents apparently accept that pattern of life as a challenge. When residents of a volcanic area refuse to leave a threatened area, officials may order residents to move. If some families need assistance, help is provided by officials. All in all, this is a localized problem with relatively low loss of life and serious injuries. It is a problem in which governmental agencies assume a major responsibility, but citizen cooperation is important.

Pollution control

In the absence of precise air quality criteria, the *usual* approach has been to control the *sources* of pollution even though such control measures must rely on empirical methods. To control and regulate air pollution by solid particles is not difficult. Various smoke-inspection devices are available for measuring the density of smoke and other particles in the air.

With established means for measuring smoke pollution, cities have passed ordinances limiting the emission of smoke to periods of 6 minutes in 1 hour for industrial plants. Proper firing and design of coal furnaces eliminates 90% of smoke from industrial plants.

Control of pollution by smoke is relatively easy. Unfortunately, most serious air pollutants are sulfur oxide, nitrogen oxide, and motor vehicle pollution, and these are more difficult to measure.

Sulfur oxide pollution arises principally from the combustion of sulfur-containing coal and fuel oil and is highly injurious to human health, to property, and to vegetation. The increased use of sulfur-containing fuels threatens a fourfold increase in sulfur oxide pollution by the end of this century. Use of low-sulfur fuels or removing sulfur from fuels before they are burned will reduce pollution. Natural gas is somewhat free of sulfur and is preferable to other fuels in terms of reduction of air pollution. Coal is still the nemesis, because only a fraction of its sulfur content can be removed before burning. Efforts are now directed toward removing the sulfur oxides from the combustion gases before they escape into the air.

Nitrogen oxides are a by-product of all combustion processes, including those from automobiles. At present, nitrogen oxide pollution is not as serious a problem as sulfur oxide pollution; but, as fuel combustion increases, the nitrogen oxide pollution problem will increase proportionately unless control methods are discovered.

Motor vehicle air pollution is more extensive than sulfur oxide and nitrogen oxide pollution, but motor vehicle air pollution is yielding to newly developed control techniques. Among the methods effective in reducing tailpipe emissions are the modification of motors to achieve more complete combustion, the injec-

tion of air into the exhaust system to oxidize the gases before they reach the tailpipe, and the passage of exhaust gases through afterburners before they are released into the air. Some of these methods were applied by U.S. automobile manufacturers in the form of catalytic converters and exhaust gas recirculation to comply with the standards established by the Clean Air Act adopted in 1965.

U.S. legislation. Back in the era when air pollution meant smoke pollution, community ordinances could be enacted to control the problem because the smoke constituted an obvious nuisance. In addition, the degree of smoke pollution could be measured with some precision. Today, air pollution is more subtle and can no longer be regarded as a localized, strictly community concern. Air pollution is a national problem that recognizes no geographical or political boundaries. Pollution originating in one state can affect people in an adjoining state. It thus becomes evident that air pollution must be regarded as a national problem dealt with on a national scale in which cooooperation and mutual assistance rather than coercion is the approach. Regional and local planning are essential, but such planning must be coordinated with all related programs.

The first identifiable federal air pollution control program was established in 1955 as a consequence of the action of Congress, which passed PL 84-159 "to provide research and technical assistance relating to air pollution control." With the adoption of the Clean Air Act in 1965, Congress acknowledged that federal financial assistance is essential for the development of programs to control air pollution. Matching funds encouraged state and local governments to initiate air pollution control programs. The act encouraged area-wide interjurisdictional control of air pollution on a regional basis.

In 1967 Congress passed and the President signed the Air Quality Act, authorizing the federal government to step in to control air

TABLE 17-1. The seven air pollutants for which U.S. standards exist, their main sources, their health effects, and recent trends in their emission.*

Pollutant	Description	Main sources	Health effects	Trends in the U.S.
Ozone	Main component of smog, formed in air when sunlight "cooks" hydrocarbons (like gasoline vapors) and nitrogen oxides from automobiles	Not directly emitted but formed from emissions of automobiles, etc.	Irritation of eyes, nose, throat; impairment of normal lung functioning	Levels measured at 230 urban sites remained the same 1974-1979, despite strong control efforts
Carbon monoxide	By-product of combustion	Cars and trucks	Weakens heart contractions; reduces oxygen available to body; affects mental function, visual acuity and alertness	Levels measured at 223 urban sites dropped 36% 1972-1979; vehicle emissions dropped 5% 1970-1979, despite 35% increase in vehicle-miles traveled
Particles	Soot, dust, smoke, fumes, ash, mists, sprays, aerosols, etc.	Power plants, factories incinerators, open burning, construction, road dust	Respiratory and lung damage, in some cases cancer; hastens death	Emissions declined 50% 1970-1979
Sulfur dioxide	By-product of burning coal and oil, and of some industrial processes; reacts in air to form sulfuric acid which can return to earth as "acid rain"	Power plants, factories, space heating boilers	Increases acute and chronic respiratory disease, hastens death	Emissions declined 7% 1970-1979

Nitrogen dioxide	By-product of combustion, is "cooked" in the air with hydrocarbons to form ozone (smog); on its own, gives smog its yellow-brown color	Cars, trucks, power plants, factories	Pulmonary swelling; may aggravate chronic bronchitis and emphysema	Levels measured at 180 sites increased 15% in a recent 5-year period
Hydrocarbons	Incompletely burned and evaporated petroleum products; is "cooked" with nitrogen dioxide to form ozone (smog)	Cars, trucks, power plants, space heating boilers; vapors from gasoline stations	Negligible	Emissions decreased 4% from 1970-1979
Lead	A chemical element	Leaded gasoline	Brain and kidney damage; emotional disorders; death	Levels decreasing rapidly

*From U.S. Environmental Protection Agency.

pollution when the state fails to act. No national emission standards for specific pollutants were set up, but provisions were made to study the problem of standards.

The Clean Air Act of 1970 was the most ambitious and costly environmental legislation in history. It led to a vast national cleanup. The most deadly emissions—sulfur oxides and toxic particles from industry—declined sharply enough to increase the life of the average American by a full year, although the less dangerous smog caused by car emissions remains a problem.

The Clean Air Act was an aggressive piece of legislation that grew out of an era when polls showed that Americans were rating pollution above crime as a serious problem. It was the year of Earth Day 1970, a time when Girl Scouts wearing gas masks crowded into congressional air quality hearing rooms in support of irate citizens demanding cleaner air. Declaring air "our most vital resource" and seizing the political initiative to the dismay of Democrats, President Richard Nixon asked Congress in 1970 for sweeping and stringent new clean-air legislation.

The resulting Clean Air Act was in the form of amendments to earlier laws. It ordered the automobile industry to cut emissions 90% by 1975—a deadline that was pushed back to 1981. Specific emission allowances were set for various industries. National standards were set for allowable levels for seven air pollutants—sulfur dioxide, particles, hydrocarbons, nitrogen oxide, carbon monoxide, ozone, and lead—and states were ordered to meet them or to forfeit federal highway and sewer money (Table 17-1).

After further amendments in 1977, however, the initiative began to lose momentum. By 1978 the Carter administration was singling out federal clean air rules as a chief cause of inflation. Today, polls show people are only about half as concerned about air pollution as they were in 1970. The Reagan administration has promised to ease the standards.

Table 17-2. Ranking of 40 metropolitan areas of the United States by their air quality standards in 1980*

No. of days with pollution at the "unhealthy" level	Area	Total unhealthy days		Days when air is bad enough to be termed "hazardous"	
		3-yr average	Min/max annual	3-yr average	Min/max annual
More than 150	Los Angeles	242	206-268	118	95-142
	New York	224	174-273	51	14-87
	Pittsburgh	168	168	31	168
	San Bernardino-Riverside-Ontario	167	145-182	88	68-108
100-150	Cleveland	145	60-230	35	17-52
	St. Louis	136	119-164	29	17-44
	Chicago	124	81-150	21	14-31
	Louisville	119	94-160	12	8-14
50-99	Washington, D.C.	97	70-147	8	3-15
	Phoenix	84	75-93	10	5-14
	Philadelphia	82	79-87	9	7-10
	Seattle	82	62-95	4	2-5
	Salt Lake City	81	61-110	18	9-25
	Birmingham	75	50-100	19	8-29
	Portland	75	70-81	3	2-5
	Houston	69	50-94	16	11-24
	Detroit	65	62-68	4	2-5
	Jersey City	65	56-74	4	0-8
	Baltimore	60	32-79	12	2-25
	San Diego	52	38-74	6	4-9
25-49	Cincinnati	45	30-63	2	1-4
	Dayton	45	32-66	2	1-2
	Gary-Hammond-East Chicago	36	27-50	8	1-16
	Indianapolis	36	17-49	2	1-3
	Milwaukee	33	32-34	6	3-8
	Buffalo	31	23-40	5	3-8
	San Francisco	30	22-45	1	0-1
	Kansas City	29	7-56	6	1-9
	Memphis	28	22-37	2	0-3
	Sacramento	28	19-38	2	0-3
	Allentown	27	27	1	27
0-24	Toledo	24	15-32	2	1-5
	Dallas	22	6-35	1	1-2
	Tampa	12	5-19	1	0-2
	Akron	10	5-14	0	0-0
	Norfolk	9	9-9	0	0-0
	Syracuse	9	7-12	1	0-2
	Rochester	6	4-8	0	0-0
	Grand Rapids	5	2-8	0	0-1

*From Council on Environmental Quality, Executive Office of the White House, Annual Report, 1980.

There are other difficulties with the act in the political and economic climate of the 1980s. Some cities, for instance Los Angeles, will never meet today's air pollution standards unless people there are kept out of their cars by force (Table 17-2.) Relatively clean areas of the nation must meet even tougher standards designed to prevent them from developing air pollution, causing industrialists to complain that development is being hindered in the West and South. There are different standards for different industries and tougher standards for newer plants. Industrialists say these standards tend to encourage the retention of old, inefficient factories. The slowdown in capital investment and the lagging efficiency of American industry are major culprits blamed for inflation.

When pollution was a major public issue and a high priority item on the national agenda, complaints from the public flooded in to local officials; today, other issues have outpaced pollution, but complaints still come in. After a decade of experience, researchers are now able to make estimates of the number of lives saved by the control of the most dangerous air pollutants, sulfur oxides, and particles. Emission restrictions and requirements to burn low-sulfur coal that were imposed on power plants and factories cut the U.S. mortality rate 7%, increasing the average life of Americans by a year.

The problem in determining the effects of pollution on health quantities do their damage over long periods of time. Congress dealt with such uncertainties by ordering national standards set low enough to protect the most sensitive people with "an adequate margin of safety" and without regard for what this might cost industry and consumers. That principle was supported by the National Commission on Air Quality, an independent group that studied the act in preparation for the congressional debate. It was supported more recently by the Supreme Court in its rejection of the Environ-

mental Protection Agency's (EPA) proposal to use cost-benefit analysis in setting new (less restrictive) standards. Both the commission and the Supreme Court concluded that government must act to control potentially harmful pollutants despite scientific uncertainty about the precise harm they cause, the levels of exposure that cause that harm, and the cost. This was the congressional mandate in its "adequate margin of safety" principle.

The principle is being challenged by U.S. industry and the Reagan administration, who seek to replace it with a less demanding one that would define a health hazard in terms of "significant risk of adverse effects." The argument is that the air has already been cleaned enough to save most lives that can be saved, so further expenditures should be limited, with cost to industry and consumers as a consideration.

Scientists now believe that for certain dangerous pollutants there is no threshold below which nobody is affected. If this is true, then to meet the congressional mandate could require the closing of many industries. The law will be amended again before that happens. Industry, in the meantime, must continue to seek alternative production methods and pollution control devices, because even if the direct harm to human life is granted, there are indirect damages to health and the quality of life. Acid rain, for example, is related to the sulfur oxide pollutants carried in rain clouds to remote forests where they may affect marine and plant life, thereby interfering with food chains.

Programs in the United States. While states were slow to initiate pollution control programs, the stimulation of federal legislation and funding had changed this picture. The recognized minimum per capita expenditure for an adequate state program is set at $0.25, and few states have reached this level, indicating that most state programs are not yet in that stage where effective control measures can be taken.

An effective state air pollution control program requires the following basic factors:

1. A sanitary authority with status, funds, and research including field studies
2. Regional approach to air pollution control
3. Calculated program to reduce pollution each year
4. Licensing of new industries and new operations based on realistic appraisal of all factors involved
5. Industrial zoning based on an intensive study of all factors involved, including the economic benefits to be gained for each proposed industrial installation
6. Impartial application of regulations, but with a policy permitting changes in regulations, as dictated by experience

U.S. community programs. Local and regional air pollution control programs in few cities or counties are spending the recognized standard of $0.40 per capita on air pollution control.

On all levels—federal, state, and local—programs are being developed, but many communities have a more serious pollution problem today than they had 5 or 10 years ago. It must be conceded that not until reliable and valid standards of pollution are established can there be fully realistic enforcement of pollution control. To wait for such measures would be foolhardy. Even though present empirical source emission standards for pollution control are not totally adequate, they do have merit and should be applied until new and more precise standards are developed.

Table 17-1 identifies the seven widespread pollutants for which EPA has set standards. All but ozone and nitrogen dioxide have shown reduced emissions in recent years. The standard for particles is inadequate because there is now evidence that only the tiniest ones, those that penetrate deep into the lungs, are dangerous. The standard as now written measures particles of all sizes, including large ones that are trapped in the nose and cause no damage.

In addition to the seven widespread pollutants for which it has standards, the EPA has identified a group of cancer-causing pollutants that it labels hazardous: asbestos, mercury, beryllium, vinyl chloride, benzene, radionuclides, and arsenic. Of 700 atmospheric contaminants, 47 have been identified as recognized carcinogens (adequate evidence), 42 as suspected carcinogens (limited evidence), 22 chemicals as promoters, and 128 as mutagens. These are emitted in small quantities, but the potential adverse health effects from them are "likely to be far more severe than those of the widespread pollutants," according to the commission report. The EPA is studying them and has set emission limits for some.

Concern about carcinogenic pollutants also is beginning to focus on the growing popularity of diesel automobile engines because, while they emit less carbon monoxide and hydrocarbons, they emit more nitrogen oxides and 30 to 100 times more particles, which contain some carcinogenic compounds. The National Academy of Sciences found no conclusive evidence that breathing diesel exhaust causes cancer, birth defects, or lung disease, even though diesel materials painted on or fed to rats may cause cancer in them. Studies of workers regularly breathing diesel exhaust found no excess cancers.

Indoor air pollution is another problem that is just beginning to be assessed as buildings are being sealed tighter to conserve energy, thereby sealing in dangerous pollutants. The usual warning, however, whenever there is a pollution alert is to stay inside, as shown in Fig. 17-4. Tighter insulation prevents the infiltration of outdoor pollutants, but most ventilation systems for smaller and older buildings result in inert gases (such as carbon monoxide) and smaller particles in the same concentration inside as outside. Reactive gases such as sulfur dioxide and oxidants are reduced during infiltration by their interaction with structural elements of the building and the ventilation system. Indoor concentrations of such pollutants are usually one third to one half of those found

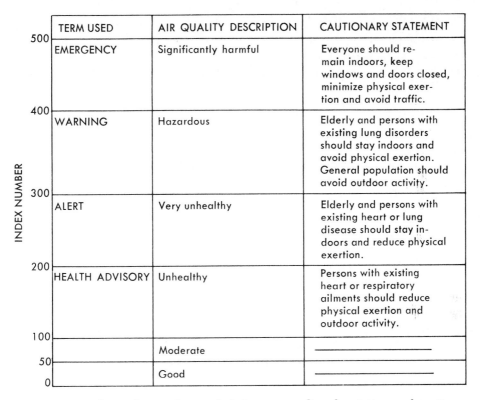

	TERM USED	AIR QUALITY DESCRIPTION	CAUTIONARY STATEMENT
500	EMERGENCY	Significantly harmful	Everyone should remain indoors, keep windows and doors closed, minimize physical exertion and avoid traffic.
400	WARNING	Hazardous	Elderly and persons with existing lung disorders should stay indoors and avoid physical exertion. General population should avoid outdoor activity.
300	ALERT	Very unhealthy	Elderly and persons with existing heart or lung disease should stay indoors and reduce physical exertion.
200	HEALTH ADVISORY	Unhealthy	Persons with existing heart or respiratory ailments should reduce physical exertion and outdoor activity.
100		Moderate	———————
50		Good	———————
0			

(INDEX NUMBER — vertical axis)

FIG. 17-4. Air quality index numbers and their corresponding descriptions and cautionary statements.

From U.S. Environmental Protection Agency: Measuring air quality: the new pollutant standards index, July, 1978.

outside. With forced air ventilation in new, large buildings, pollutants can be greatly reduced, but faulty design, operation, or maintenance can cause pollutant increases or additions.

AIR QUALITY OBJECTIVES

The overall goal of community air quality control programs is to achieve and maintain adequate air quality to avoid adverse effects on human health and welfare and to minimize material and vegetation damage, visibility reduction, odor, and other nuisance effects or esthetic insults to the population. Specific objectives for a given community should be adapted from the following.

Outcome

- By 19__ the community will experience no more than _____ days in any 1 year when (insert the name of the specific pollutant) exceeds acceptable levels (no less stringent than the established primary and secondary U.S. National Ambient Air Quality Standards).

Process

Data base. By 19__ a state, provincial, or local air monitoring station network and a national air monitoring station network will be established as required by national regulation. By 19__ a system will be in place for air quality data validation and quality assurance for all data collected. By 19__ special purpose monitoring and specialized analysis will be conducted as needed to assist in identifying sources of emissions.

Public education and participation. By 19__ a population exposure trend display model employing air quality, emission, and meteorological data will be available to the community. By 19__ all air quality, emission, and meteorological data collected will be routinely reviewed and displayed in such a manner that the data is readily available to support program planning and decision making.

Inspection. By 19__ all mobile and stationary sources of air pollution will be in compliance with applicable regulation. By 19__ all major stationary sources will be thoroughly inspected at least annually. By 19__ all minor stationary sources of air pollution will be inspected annually. By 19__ all stationary sources will be required to meet applicable requirements for continuous source monitoring. By 19__ all stationary sources of air pollution will be routinely observed for obvious violations of applicable regulations. By 19__ the community will have access to a system for filing complaints about air quality. By 19__ all complaints received regarding air pollution will be investigated, validated, and corrected where appropriate. By 19__ all violations observed will be documented and corrected or referred to legal counsel as necessary. By 19__ __% of all mobile sources of air pollution will be in compliance with applicable regulations.

Prevention of air quality deterioration. By 19__ all strategies for potential new sources of air pollution will be reviewed for compliance with applicable national, state or provincial, and local requirements, and approval-disapproval responses will be given for all such strategies.

Control strategy. By 19__ the community will adopt a strategy to control and reduce air pollutants, including episode planning, that is reviewed and periodically updated. By 19__ control strategies will be developed and adopted for suspended particulates and sulfur dioxide that will lead to attainment and maintenance of the national ambient air quality standards by 19__. By 19__ strategies will be developed for achieving the national ambient air quality standard for carbon monoxide and photochemical oxidants by 19__. By 19__ reasonably available control measures to control hydrocarbon emissions in all nonattainment areas will be developed and enforced. By 19__ the community will be covered by a strategy for the implementation of a motor vehicle air pollution control device inspection and maintenance program.

• • •

Larger communities should consider the development of a monitoring system based on appropriate sentinel reporting that tracks the health effects associated with air pollution. For more specific and detailed information, see U.S. federal guidelines issued by the EPA pursuant to P.L. 91-604, the Clean Air Act Amendments of 1970, and subsequent amending legislation.

RADIOACTIVE POLLUTION

Humans have always been exposed to natural sources of chemical activity and cosmic radiation. This is referred to as background radiation. All people are exposed to a harmless amount of about 0.1 R (roentgens) per year. Not until the split of the atom did radioactive atmospheric pollution become a problem.

The use of radioactive materials for treatment, research, and other purposes must always be regarded as a potential hazard, but these possible sources of radioactivity are usually well controlled and are not a danger to the general public. The immediate danger is to those people working with radioactive materials, and they have the necessary knowledge to take proper shielding and other precautions to protect themselves.

When nuclear weapons are tested, explo-

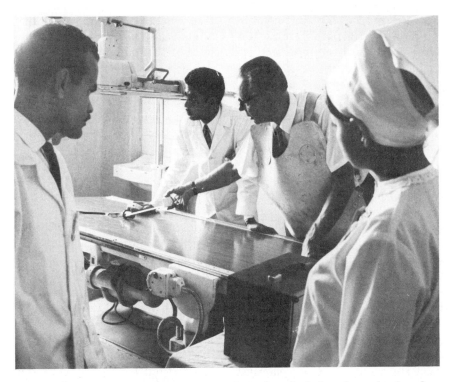

FIG. 17-5. Radiation protection demonstration. Special methods have been developed to assure radiation safety of patients and medical and auxiliary personnel exposed to ionizing radiation in the course of diagnosis and therapeutic procedures.

Courtesy World Health Organization.

sions spray the atmosphere with radioactive particles. These particles, such as strontium[90] and cesium[137] with half-lives of 28 years, settle to the earth. This represents a threat to human life, because penetration of body cells by radioactive particles causes ionization of the atoms of cells, particularly cells undergoing division. The extent of damage depends on the dose received and whether the dose is received externally or internally. For doses received or applied externally, the unit of radiation is known as a roentgen, which means radiation that causes two ionizations per cubic micron. An adult exposed to 1 R would receive about 10^{17} ionizations over the whole body. A dose of less than 100 R produces no symptoms or signs in a person, but 500 R in one dose will be fatal.

The U.S. Atomic Energy Commission reports that the average external dose from fallout is from 0.001 to 0.005 R per year, less than 5% of the background radiation. Internal dosage is expressed by the Sunshine Unit (SU), which is equivalent to 0.003 R per year to bone tissue. Internal doses result from ingesting radioactive water, milk, and other foods. Internal effect of radioactivity is a greater health concern than is external exposure. Strontium[90] is chemically similar to calcium and thus is deposited in bone. In young children, strontium[90] is distributed throughout the bones. Localized high doses may cause malignancies. In adults the cancellous (spongy) bone is usually affected, causing acute poisoning.

Maximum permissible concentration (MPC)

has not been established to the satisfaction of scientists in the field of radiation. The U.S. National Academy of Sciences has proposed 50 SU as the MPC, but the U.S. National Committee on Radiation sets the standard 25% higher.

Fallout is greater in the United States than anywhere else, yet the U.S. Public Health Service, with monitoring stations distributed throughout the nation, keeps a close surveillance of atmospheric radiation and takes all possible action to control sources of radiation. On the state and community level, detection and correction of radiation "leaks" in x-ray machines, fluoroscopic equipment, and other sources of radiation is a continuous effort by health officials and special agencies set up to safeguard the public. At present, the general public is relatively safe from radiation hazards, but constant vigilance is imperative.

Energy needs of the nation are increasing at a rate faster than the rate of population growth, and it is apparent that fossil sources are inadequate to meet rising energy needs. The next available source is nuclear energy, which can be converted to electrical energy. To obtain this additional electrical power the U.S. federal government and public utility companies have developed nuclear reactors. Protesters have raised objections to the proposed plant sites and even to the construction of such plants. The objections are that there may be constant emissions from the reactors, thermopollution from heated water emptied into streams, unsafe disposal or radioactive wastes and, foremost of all, accidents that would saturate the atmosphere with lethal radioactive ions. The "Three-Mile Island" incident in Pennsylvania confirmed the validity of some of these concerns.

Emissions are controlled by shielding and the use of other proved controls. Water is cooled before being discharged into streams, and wastes are buried, disposed of in the ocean, or otherwise rendered distant or relatively harmless to human beings. Accidents that would threaten communities have probabilities close to the order of zero. Those who work at these nuclear plants are the most exposed to any possible danger and the most knowledgeable. These experts who understand the situation tend to minimize any reason for fear. When solar energy is tapped, the need for nuclear reactors and fear of some of the public will be reduced.

Nuclear arms proliferation is a greater threat and could become a by-product of nuclear energy technology if the technology is converted to arms by terrorists. The Europeans have been the most vociferous in objecting to nuclear arms on their territory, but health professionals elsewhere have become increasingly concerned with the health implications of a world faced with the possibility of "the ultimate epidemic." The 1981 annual convention of the American Public Health Association, for example, was devoted to this theme.

RADIOLOGICAL HEALTH OBJECTIVES

The overall goal of community radiological health programs is that residents of the community will not experience preventable adverse health effects from radiation. Specific objectives for a given community should include the following.

Outcome

- By 19___ no residents of the community will experience radiation exposures from _____*_____ sources that exceed a level consonant with the ALARA (As Low As Is Reasonably Achievable) principle.

Process

Control of man-made sources. By 19___ significant man-made sources of radiation exposure will be registered or licensed and will

*Insert specific source (i.e., natural, medical, nuclear energy, nonnuclear energy, weapons related, consumer products, and other).

meet applicable national or state or provincial radiation standards. By 19__ all registered or licensed radiation sources will be inspected periodically on a schedule reflecting the degree of hazard, and appropriate corrective action will be taken where indicated. By 19__ an enforcement mechanism will be established to maintain compliance with the regulations.

Public education. By 19__ the community will be served by an education program that provides enough information to residents to discuss minimum, essential, and necessary levels of radiation with their health care providers.

Provider education. By 19__ the community's physicians, dentists, radiation technicians, and other health professionals will be served by an educational program informing them of the risks and benefits of such radiation to themselves and their patients.

Surveillance. By 19__ the community will be served by a monitoring system to identify radiation exposure from natural and man-made sources and to evaluate the exposure of the population.

• • •

Problems with toxic agents are not only attributable to industry but also to medical care (x-rays), agriculture (pesticides), government (biological and chemical agents), and consumers (incorrect use of consumer products that contain toxic substances). Low levels of ionizing radiation can produce delayed effects, such as cancer and genetic anomalies, after a latent period of many years. Fifty percent of the current U.S. population dose comes from naturally occurring background radiation, radioactive materials in the water, soil and air, and cosmic radiation; 45% results from diagnostic and therapeutic medical applications. Fallout, industrial use, production of nuclear power, and consumer products account for the remaining 5%. Thus roughly half the exposure to the population at large comes from man-made sources.

The synergistic effects of exposures to ionizing radiation and toxic agents may greatly increase carcinogenic risks.

AEROSOL SPRAY

For some time health scientists have recognized that fluorocarbon propellants can produce atmospheric effects harmful to human health. Some American investigators have done research in this field, but Russian and German scientists have been doing a major share of the on-going research.

Fluorocarbon propellants from spray containers do not decompose chemically in the lower atmosphere because they do not react with any other gases. Rainwater does not remove these propellants from the air. Fluorocarbons drift slowly into the upper regions of the stratosphere and release chlorine after being subjected to ultraviolet rays. Released chlorine atoms react with ozone molecules to produce chlorine oxide and oxygen. This in turn reduces the amount of ozone, eventually reducing the ozone equilibrium concentration by as much as 4%. Recovery to normal levels of ozone may take more than 100 years even if the fluorocarbon release were stopped this year.

When the ozone level is lowered, more ultraviolet rays reach the earth, which could result in such effects as cancer, particularly of the skin. In addition, it must be recognized that the human respiratory tract can be directly affected by fluorocarbons. In the nonciliated part of the nasal junction, fluorocarbon particles move slowly. Particles deposited in the ciliated tissue move more rapidly. Thus there can be an immediate threat to the health of exposed citizens as well as possible long-term effects from atmospheric changes created by fluorocarbons.

Fortunately, from the public health standpoint the elimination of this hazard in the environment is relatively easy. At least 44 products on the market in the United States use

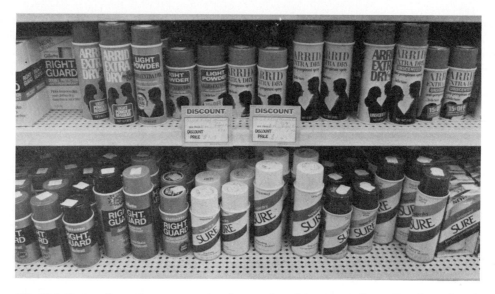

FIG. 17-6. Types of containers once using fluorocarbon-driven propellants. Retailers phased out existing stocks on their own initiative, and producers converted to safe containers. Here is an example of solving a health problem without resorting to legal means.

Photograph by Paul Colvin.

fluorocarbon-driven propellants in spray cans. These propellants can be replaced by different types of spray cans such as pump or water-driven sprays. The U.S. government could require that industry either label containers as being dangerous to human health or completely ban these propellants.

Some states have taken action through legislation that bans the sale of containers using fluorocarbon propellants. The state of Oregon law provides that violation of the propellants ban is a class "A" misdemeanor, a criminal violation punishable by fines up to $1000 and 1 year in prison.

However, members of the public health profession readily see that this problem is primarily a matter of health education, rather than legal measures. When people understand the problem, they will take the steps necessary to ban the use of fluorocarbon. Manufactures will use other sprays, retailers will refuse to sell products using fluorocarbons, and consumers will refuse to purchase spray cans containing the objectionable propellants. Health educa-

tors have an opportunity to serve the public through an education program if it is designed and implemented immediately. Within a relatively short time this hazard to health can be eliminated.

NOISE

Noise is increasing in significance as a public concern. The increasing magnitude and complexity of society has brought with it increases in noises to a degree that calls for programs to relieve people of distress. Not all sound is objectionable, nor is all sound classed as noise. Technically, noise is any disturbing sound that interferes with work, comfort, or rest. It is doubtful that death has ever been caused by noise, yet noise can have an adverse effect on health, particularly mental health. Objectionable noise is not protested on health grounds, but because the noise disrupts and interferes with the normal enjoyment of tranquility.

The urgency of the problem created by noise depends on the frequency of the occurrence, the absolute as well as the relative loudness, and whether the noise is necessary or unnecessary. The honking of an automobile horn may be objectionable, but the siren of a fire truck may not be. A sound may be objectionable but nevertheless must be accepted. As much as the public objects to the boom when jet planes break the sound barrier, citizens in certain locations have had to learn to live with this noise.

Industry noise control. In many industries noise represents a problem of some significance. Exposure to high noise levels can cause deafness. Noises of lower levels can affect workers' efficiency and be otherwise objectionable. Industry usually makes surveys of noise intensities and takes necessary corrective measures. Segregation of noisy operations, insulating for sound, redesigning machinery, and changing operations are among corrective measures. Where noise intensity cannot be avoided, providing workers with ear protectors will safeguard their hearing.

Community noise control. Certain noises in the modern community such as the noise of traffic, street work, construction work, locomotives, and certain industries may be ever-present. The public generally accepts a certain noise intensity from these sources, but, when these sources rise above a certain level of intensity, complaints will be lodged.

City planning, including restricting industrial or commercial operations to particular zones, is a first measure. Cooperation resulting from communication between all parties concerned is the key to dealing with noise problems that arise and that are not covered by existing ordinances. Community organization efforts should precede court action, but if all other efforts fail, court action resulting in an injunction will prohibit the offender from continuing the noise nuisance or will command the offender to reduce the noise to a defined, tolerable level.

NOISE CONTROL OBJECTIVES

The overall goal of community noise control programs is that residents of the community will have an environment free from noise that jeopardizes their physical and mental health. Specific objectives for a given community should include the following.

Outcome

- By 19__ the residents of the community will not be exposed to noise levels in the _____*_____ environment exceeding _____ decibels for _____ period of time, nor to an instantaneous decibel level of _____.

Process

Program services. By 19__ the community will be protected by programs to provide an environment free from noise that jeopardizes its health and welfare. By 19__ criteria will be adopted and disseminated with respect to levels of noise requisite to protect the public health and welfare with an adequate margin of safety. These criteria may be more stringent than the criteria issued in 1974 by the EPA. (At a minimum, the maximum permissible noise levels should be established for residential and industrial areas, with differentiation between allowable daytime and nighttime levels. Criteria should also be developed for special categories of noise-intensive activity, such as construction or recreation. See U.S. Environmental Protection Agency, 1973, 1974.)

By 19__ provisions will be established to review and revise criteria regularly in light of epidemiological advances with respect to the health effects of noise and technological advances with respect to noise control. By 19__ enforcement mechanisms will be established in the community, including penalties for failure to abate violations. By 19__ a protocol identifying noise control responsibilities will be established among different governmental agencies responsible for regulating various elements that may contribute to noise pollution.

---

*Insert specific environment (e.g., residential, recreational, occupational).

Noise control strategy. By 19__ the community will be protected by a strategy for noise abatement throughout the community environment, including residential, transportation, occupational, and recreational environments. By 19__ there will be a mechanism in the community to identify and monitor locations at which people are exposed to excessive noise. By 19__ all complaints about excessive noise will be investigated. By 19__ abatement action will be taken against 100% of persistent violators. By 19__ technical assistance will be available about noise reduction techniques, protection equipment for employees, and protection of the public. By 19__ the community will have available a program to educate employees at risk about health effects of long-term exposure to excessive noise.

Hazard assessment. By 19__ the community will assess potential noise hazards and take measures to avoid these hazards. By 19__ the community will have a mechanism to require review and comment from the local control authority on all proposed noise generating construction projects (factories, shopping centers, sports arenas, truck depots, etc.). By 19__ the community will have a mechanism to protect the population from infrequent high decibel occurrences, including, where applicable, using environmental acoustical controls such as planting shrubs.

Screening. By 19__ a screening program will be operating to identify employees with hearing loss as a result of excess exposure to noise, and to prevent further hearing loss. (See U.S. federal guidlines issued by the EPA pursusant to the Noise Control Act of 1971, PL 92-574.)

SWIMMING FACILITIES

Recent developments in swimming pool construction and natural bathing areas have caused health officials to extend their programs for regulating public swimming facilities. This regulatory function of state, provincial, and community health departments is directed to those facilities that serve the public. This authority extends to pools and natural bathing areas of motels, hotels, resorts, parks and other enterprises serving the public.

Health aspects of swimming facilities. On the positive side, swimming can promote both physical and mental well-being. On the negative side, accidents represent the greatest threat to health and life. In recent years, unsupervised motel pools have taken a frightful toll of lives by drowning. Slipping on slick walkways and in shower and locker rooms has been a source of serious injuries. Accidents related to diving have also taken lives and have been a source of injuries.

Disease spread via swimming facilities is always a possibility, but the general public harbors many misconceptions about the role of swimming facilities in disease spread. It is extremely doubtful that respiratory diseases are ever spread by water in a pool or other swimming facility. No tangible evidence exists that such diseases as the common cold, influenza, tuberculosis, or poliomyelitis are spread via pool water. The close social contact of swimmers themselves may be a factor in the spread of respiratory diseases, but the pool itself is not a vehicle of spread. Pinkeye (conjunctivitis) is not spread by pool water, but swimmers using the same towel or other article may thus communicate it.

Diseases of the intestinal tract are most likely to be transmitted via water in swimming facilities. Typhoid fever and bacillary dysentery may be conveyed by water, but it is doubtful that salmonellosis is thus ever transmitted to an individual. However, if water in a swimming pool is chlorinated properly, the danger of typhoid fever and dysentery spread is zero.

Certain skin infections are transmitted from swimmer to swimmer by physical contact associated with activities at the pool, the locker room, or the shower room, or by handling common objects. Athlete's foot (tinea pedis), boils (furunculosis), and impetigo contagiosa can be transmitted through contacts associated with swimming activities. Swimmer's itch may develop in lakes. Schistosomiasis can be a threat in natural swimming waters harboring schistosomes. However, dragging a bag of copper sulfate around a lake behind a boat will rid the waters of schistosomes.

Swimming pools. The presence of competitive pools, diving tanks, instructional pools, recreational pools, and pools for other purposes indicates that many types of pools are being built. Yet, as specified by the American Public Health Association (1970), there are certain common construction needs—materials impervious and permanent for walls, bottom, vertical ends and sides, inlets submerged in a safe place, outlets synchronized with inlets, overflow gutters all around to allow slight overflow, and nonslip walkways at least 5 feet wide all around the pool. Showers and locker rooms should be well lighted, well ventilated, and clean.

Artificial pools are classified on a basis of quality control.

1. Fill-draw means the pool is filled and emptied at regular intervals. Timing is determined by the physical appearance of the water and the bathing load. This type of pool can be acceptable when properly operated. However, whether this type is used depends on the cost of water and the nature of pool use. Fill-draw pools are acceptable where limited bathing use occurs but are used very little today.

2. Flow-through means there is a continuous passage of water in and out of the pool and the chlorine content is controlled. This type of pool is highly acceptable, but the cost of water makes this class of pool highly uneconomical.

3. Recirculating means that pumps remove the water from one part of the pool; after being filtered and decontaminated by chlorination, the water is returned to the pool. Using the water over and over again

is economical. In addition, the water quality is excellent. For these two reasons, this type of pool is most frequently constructed.

Decontamination of water in swimming pools is usually attained by chlorination, although bromine and ozone are also used. Bromine is more stable and tenacious than chlorine, but bromine fumes are highly irritating to the eyes and respiratory tract. Ozone is extremely expensive and little used, except for pools on ships, on estates, or at clubs.

When chlorine is used, a chlorine residual from 0.4 to 0.6 ppm should be maintained. This chlorine level may be irritating to the eyes of some swimmers. An alkalinity of the water should be maintained at a pH between 7.2 and 8.2. Not more than 15% of water samples should contain more than 200 bacteria per milliliter, as determined by the standard agar plate count, or show more than 1.0 coliform organism per 50 milliliters of sample.

Wading pools. Much less sanitary than swimming pools, wading pools are frequently little more than cesspools. The usual practice is to add water constantly, using a standard of 0.5 ppm chlorine residual for decontamination purposes. Under moderate or heavy use, a wading pool should be drained and refilled at least twice a day.

Natural bathing areas. Lakes, rivers, and ponds used for swimming purposes are frequently dangerously polluted. Sewage, cesspool drainage, and other effluents pollute and contaminate the lake or river water. Many public swimming areas are unsupervised, but even those that are supervised are not always safe.

Supervision of natural bathing areas consists of identifying and preventing all possible sources of pollution and then keeping a close check on the degree of contamination. A permissible maximum coliform count of 1,000 per 100 milliliters is standard. Areas are also classified by the following average coliform index:

Class	Coliforms per 100 milliliters
A	0-50
B	50-500
C	500-1,000
D	Over 1,000 (unacceptable)

Because of the danger of typhoid, dysentery, and staphylococcus infections, even a relatively low coliform index does not make the swimming area safe. For this reason, health officials, using other data, close down swimming areas that may have been used for many years without any apparent mishaps.

Regulations. All public swimming pools are subject to official regulation. A pool is classed as a public pool if it is used by others than the owners or their families. Whether a charge is made for the use of the pool is not a consideration in classifying a pool as public. In the United States authority to regulate public swimming facilities rests with the state. However, if the state legistlature has granted home

rule to a county or city, the county or city thus has authority to regulate public swimming pools within its territorial jurisdiction.

State regulation of public swimming facilities is usually vested in the state department of health. Permits to operate a public swimming facility are issued annually to those individuals or organizations having pools that meet all state specifications relating to construction and maintenance. A nominal fee is charged for the permit. Annual renewal is contingent on the operation and the maintenance of conditions acceptable to the state inspectors, who make periodic inspections.

Community regulation of public swimming pools is based on an ordinance and related regulations. Many communities use as a guide the *Suggested ordinance and regulations covering public swimming pools,* a model developed by the Joint Committee on Swimming Pools of the American Public Health Association in cooperation with the U.S. Public Health Service. This

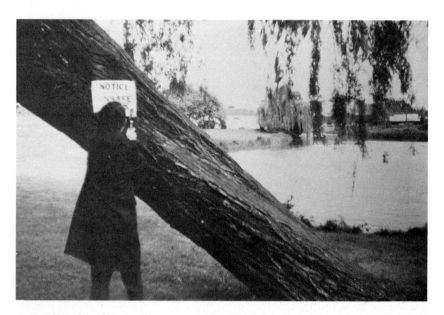

FIG. 17-7. Polluted pools in parks. Even in the apparently unpolluted water of family picnic grounds, contamination is possible.

Courtesy Environmental Health Division, Lane County, Oregon.

model ordinance is a guide to be used in the design, construction, operation, and maintenance of public swimming pools. Provisions are reasonable and are not restrictive or punitive. The ordinance begins by requiring submission of plans and specifications and specifies acceptable materials and construction. This includes specifications for dressing rooms, showers, and toilet facilities. Suggestions for supervision of bathers and pools, including safety requirements and lifesaving equipment, are included. In all respects, this proposed ordinance is a model that can be adapted to all situations and can serve admirably for communities accepting their responsibilities in regulating public swimming pools.

The community health department is customarily charged with responsibility for enforcement of the swimming pool ordinance. This would mean either the county or city health department. Health department sanitarians include this function in their regular responsibilities. In addition, sanitarians provide a consulting service for citizens requesting information or advice relating to private residential pools. Sanitarians also make regular inspections of conditions involving natural bathing areas and take such action as is necessary to protect the public against hazards. Much of the work in swimming facilities regulation goes unnoticed, yet is becoming a progressively more significant public health function as the population and its recreational activities expand.

VECTOR CONTROL

In community health practice the term *vector* is not limited strictly to forms of the class *Insecta* but includes allied arthropods such as ticks and mites. The health interest in these forms is in their role as vectors of organisms pathogenic to humans. Virtually all of these are bilogical vectors in that the pathogen passes through part of its life cycle in the intermediate invertebrate host. The common housefly is strictly a mechanical vector. Some biological

vectors, under certain circumstances, can be mechanical vectors and transfer pathogens on their wings, feet, or body.

In some geographical areas, vectors are not a great community health concern. This is particularly true in some of the northern states and countries. Yet the tick and the common housefly may transfer pathogens of humans even in the northern climes. Humans everywhere do have to contend with the annoyance of mosquitoes, flies, lice, and other arthropods, but the significant health problem is in their role as vectors of disease.

Transmission of disease by vectors can be visualized in these patterns:

Humans—vector—humans
Humans—vector—lower vertebrate—vector—humans
Lower vertebrate—vector—humans

In epidemiology all three of these patterns must be considered as possible routes over which the disease is transmitted.

Vector-disease relationships. Known vector-disease relationships indicate that a specific pathogen is transmitted via a specific vector. To say that the mosquito transmits yellow fever is not a complete statement. Only the specific *Aedes aegypti* mosquito serves as the intermediate host for the pathogen causing yellow fever. For present purposes, however, a list will serve that identifies the type of vector with the disease or diseases it tramsmits to humans.

Mosquitoes—yellow fever, malaria, encephalitis, filariasis
Fleas—bubonic plague, murine typhus
Ticks and mites—Rocky Mountain spotted fever, tularemia
Biting flies—tularemia
Lice—epidemic typhus, relapsing fever
House flies—salmonellosis

Roaches have been suspected of transmitting enteric diseases, and bedbugs have been suspected of conveying relapsing fever.

Control measures. The first principle of vector control is to identify the specific vector and plan control measures accordingly. When the tick is the known vector, control measures will differ from measures taken when a mosquito is the intermediate host. Yet, three factors must always be considered—elimination of breeding places, destruction of the insect or its larva, and protection of possible human hosts by preventing the vector from reaching human beings.

Mosquito control presents the classic example of insect control. whether the particular species is a vector or simply represents a general annoyance. In either event three factors must be considered:

1. Elimination of breeding places
   a. Destroying and emptying containers holding water
   b. Filling water holes
   c. Draining ponds, marshes, and swamps

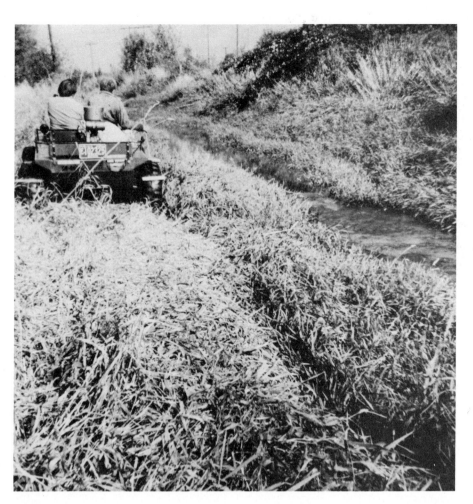

FIG. 17-8. With a bit of ingenuity virtually all places concealing vectors can be cleaned out.

Courtesy Environmental Health Division, Lane County, Oregon.

d. Rendering bodies of water unsuitable for breeding by use of larvicides, releasing water at high velocities, and flunctuating the water level

e. Diverting stream flow

f. Trimming the banks of ponds, lakes, and streams to prevent swamps

g. Introducing natural antagonists of mosquito larvae, such as fish (*Gambusia*)

2. Destroying adult insects
   a. Insecticide sprays in areas inhabited by mosquitoes
   b. Insecticide-impregnated sawdust spread on surface of flowing streams
   c. Oil solution insecticide over rain barrels and other water containers

3. Protecting human beings against contact by mosquito
   a. Screening
   b. Clothing
   c. Nets
   d. Repellents

It must be recognized that insecticides can have harmful as well as beneficial effects. Humans, lower vertebrates (wildlife especially), and vegetation (food) can be harmed if the insecticide solution is too highly concentrated. The controlled use of insecticides is imperative. While *Silent Spring*, by Rachel Carson, overstated the case, there is considerable support for the theme the book presented—overuse of insecticides is destroying wildlife. Because insecticide effects at best are temporary, it is necessary to spray or otherwise apply the insecticide about once a week. A certain degree of air pollution can be created by insecticides.

The community has a responsibility to reduce vector populations in its area. In the United States this is usually a function of the community health department and is carried out in cooperation with state agencies. Community authorities also have a responsibility in regulating the use of insecticides by private citizens. This is primarily a problem of public ed-

ucation directed to specific groups or individuals. Research on insecticides is being carried on by federal agencies and by scientists in universities and colleges throughout the United States. Permissible concentration of insecticides is the immediate problem but the long-range objective is that of developing insecticides that destroy insect life but are harmless to humans, other animals and vegetation.

RODENT CONTROL

Strictly speaking, the term *rodents* encompasses all animals belonging to the order Rodentia and includes squirrels and other forms as well as rats and mice. The ground squirrel can harbor the pathogens that cause Rocky Mountain spotted fever and tularemia in humans and can transmit rabies directly. A vector must transmit most pathogens from rodent to human—the tick for Rocky Mountain spotted fever and the horsefly for tularemia. In the United States control of squirrels is essentially a state and federal problem, and both the federal and state governments have extensive programs to eliminate ground squirrels. Field teams using guns, traps, and poisons carry on a constant campaign to eliminate ground squirrels in regions with endemic Rocky Mountain spotted fever and tularemia.

In communities the rodent problem is essentially confined to rats and mice. These rodents are responsible for economic loss, create esthetic problems, and transmit disease. Rats and mice destroy and eat poultry and eggs grains and sprouts, and corn. They also destroy merchandise. Despite the enormity of this economic loss, it is as a carrier of disease that the rodent poses the greatest threat to humans.

Rat-borne diseases. Rodents harbor several pathogens of humans. In many instances the rat dies of the disease. In other instances the rat remains a carrier of the disease over a considerable period of time. Although many misconceptions exist regarding the relationship of rats to human disease, at least six diseases of humans are definitely known in which the rat serves as a reservoir of infection.

> Murine typhus: rat—rat fleas—humans
> Bubonic plague: rat—rat fleas—humans
> Weil's disease (infectious jaundice): urine of rat
> Salmonellosis: feces of rat and house mouse
> Rat-bite fever: bacteria via bite
> Rickettsial pox: house mouse—mite—humans

Obviously, not all rats harbor pathogens of humans, but the greater the rat population, the greater the potential reservoir.

Varieties of rats in the United States. Three types of rats and the house mouse are of health concern in the United States. The black rat lives in walls and between floors. It has a pointed muzzle, slender body, long tail, and a sooty color. The roof rat is more brown but otherwise resembles the black rat and usually lives off the ground. The brown rat is also called the sewer rat, wharf rat, and Norway rat. It is a large rodent with a blunt head, short ears, and short tail. It burrows and nests in the ground. The house mouse lives in walls, furniture, and other protective places.

Control measures. A community rodent control program must begin with a well thought out plan based on surveys and participation by residents. Education of the public is essential to the success of the control program because an informed public can provide the type of cooperation on which a successful program must be based. When all residents make their premises rat-free, the task of community officials is not a difficult one.

A community program has five aspects: surveys, elimination of food sources, elimination of nesting and breeding places, rat-proofing, and killing of rats. Each aspect involves certain measures.

1. *Surveys*
   Poor sanitation areas
   Slums
   Tenements
   Railroad areas
   Areas near dumps
2. *Elimination of food sources*
   Placing all food in rat-proof containers
   Covering garbage cans
   Prohibiting dumping food wastes in open areas
3. *Elimination of nesting and breeding places*
   Disposing of debris
   Burning trash and rubbish
   Prohibiting piles of building materials
4. *Rat-proofing*
   Closing external openings
   Placing screens and metal over cracks and openings
   Eliminating all possible passages
5. *Killing of rats*
   Trapping
   Use of approved rodenticides with all possible safeguards
   Fumigation with warning signs and other safeguards

Droppings of infected rats and mice on food consumed by humans transmit disease. Keeping all food where rats and mice cannot reach it is of primary importance. Of secondary importance is the practice of all possible safety measures when using rodenticides and fumigation to kill rats. Eliminating mice by trapping is relatively simple.

SANITATION SURVEY

A systematic inventory of environmental conditions in a community can serve to tabulate adequate conditions as well as hazards. It can point up strengths in community health and can place a finger on those conditions that need attention. Such a survey should preferably be conducted by some qualified person not a resident of the community. A qualified citizen of the community can conduct an objective sanitary survey directed toward specific environmental factors such as water supply, sewage disposal refuse disposal milk supply, restaurants and food establishment, public buildings, housing, swimming pools, insect and rodent control, air pollution, health department, and government.

APPRAISAL OF GENERAL SANITATION

As society becomes increasingly complex, the need to control adverse environmental factors becomes more urgent. No one has the right to jeopardize the welfare of one's neighbor by making the environment annoying and even threatening to health. The community must impose requirements on each of us for the best interest of all. Besides the authority of the community represented in legislative requirements, community officials must provide services that will assist citizens in maintaining the best possible environment from the standpoint of health. Equally important each citizen should understand the responsibility for a healthful environment and be motivated to assume responsibility for the quality of the environment the community has. A "blitz" program or clean-up campaign may be justified on occasions but should not be the regular mode of community effort. Constant efforts in promoting environmental health is the effective prescription.

ENVIRONMENTAL PROTECTION AGENCIES IN THE UNITED STATES

With the growing concern about environmental health problems it was logical that special agencies should be created and serve as the responsible agency to safeguard the interests of the general public in the protection and promotion of environmental quality. These agencies are found at all levels of government and basically are regulating agencies. At the federal level is the EPA. State agencies are variously named, but a common designation is Department of Environmental Quality. Some metropolitan areas have environmental control departments, but the nature of environmental quality, being geographically broad rather than localized, dictates that the state agency serve all state needs in matters of environmental control. (See Chapter 20.)

A state department of environmental quality is usually governed by an unpaid lay commission appointed by the governor. The commission appoints a full-time professional director who appoints the professional staff subject to approval by the commission. Usually the state is divided into districts, and members of the professional staff are assigned to the different districts. Responsibilities of the staff in each district usually are as follows:

1. Air quality: investigation of complaints of air pollution and obtain necessary corrections; surveillance of air quality problems in the district; conducting surveys and collecting samples of air; reviewing and preparing permits for air quality emissions.

2. Water quality: investigation of complaints of water pollution and develop necessary controls and enforcement to protect the state's water standards; investigate and review proposed waste treatment plant locations and prepare waste discharge permits for plants; surveillance of existing sewage treatment plants and sewage collection systems and preparation of waste discharge permits for plants; conducting inspections and surveillance of existing industrial treatment facilities and waste discharges with preparation of permits; conducting water quality basin surveys.

3. Solid wastes: investigation of solid waste disposal sites, evaluation of proposed sites, and preparation of solid waste disposal facility permits.

4. Community and interagency responsibilities: provision of technical assistance and advice to local health departments and officials on such matters as sewage disposal, solid waste disposal, industrial waste disposal, water quality surveys; consulting with the public, industry representatives, city, county, state and federal officials, engineers, and others regarding plans and programs related to waste discharge

permits, the design, construction and operation of sewage treatment facilities, industrial waste treatment facilities, air treatment systems, and solid waste disposal systems; providing public information to local groups on all aspects of environmental quality.

While these state environmental quality agencies are separate from the state health departments, cooperation and a close relationship exists. The magnitude of environmental health problems in modern society makes imperative the creation of a self-contained agency to be responsible for environmental quality. Health departments still carry on their traditional functions, perhaps more effectively after being relieved of the many tasks inherent in environmental health programs.

Congress passed a solid waste management bill that created broad new programs to deal with the growing solid waste management problem facing cities and states. The Resource Conservation and Recovery Act called for the establishment of comprehensive hazardous waste regulations, incentives for better state and regional solid waste planning, acceleration of solid waste research and development, and a greater emphasis on materials conservation and resource recovery. Specific provisions included:

1. Grants totaling $70 million in fiscal year 1978-1979 for states initiating solid waste management plans in compliance with the guidelines of the EPA. The EPA is also required to furnish technical assistance when necessary.
2. The authorization of $50 million in fiscal year 1978-1979 for hazardous waste control grants at the state level. The act requires the EPA to establish mandatory federal standards for regulating the generation, transportation, storage, and disposal of hazardous wastes.
3. In fiscal year 1978, $30 million was authorized for grants to states, cities, or regional agencies for research, develop-

ment, and demonstration programs designed to improve methods of extracting reusable materials and energy from waste. The EPA will conduct research in specific areas such as small-scale resource recovery systems for smaller cities.

4. Grants amounting to $30 million in fiscal year 1979 to assist in the planning of solid waste facilities.
5. Over the next 2 years $50 million was authorized in grant assistance to rural communities for solid waste management. Open dumping is banned, with the states administering a 5-year phase-out of this disposal process.
6. The EPA is also required to conduct special studies of solid waste problems including resource conservation, glass and plastic recovery, the composition of the solid waste stream, and the handling of sludge and mineral wastes.

Another important environmental measure was the Toxic Substances Control Act. The purpose of this act is to permit the EPA to test and screen chemicals considered potentially hazardous to public health or to the environment prior to commercial production and distribution. Ninety days before marketing a new chemical or using an old chemical for a significant new use, the manufacturer will be required to supply the EPA with enough information on the substance to allow the EPA to evaluate its safety.

Pesticides represent a special category of toxic substances. Congress has extended the Federal Insecticide, Fungicide and Rodenticide Act (FIFRA), thereby continuing authorizations for the EPA's pesticide programs.

A clean environment cannot be measured only in economic terms or as a function of expended energy resources. Legislation dealing with the environment must weigh the effect of solutions to all problems in the environment.

Voluntary organizations interested in ecology and related health problems have added impetus to the development of official environmental health programs. Voluntary organizations can supplement and complement the work of the official agencies and thus contribute tangibly to the preservation and promotion of environmental quality.

In 1970 a group of young Americans resolved to change some attitudes about the earth and proclaimed the first "Earth Day." The event became an institution. The "throw-away" society has come to realize the cost of waste.

In support of the program, the state legislatures adopted "bottle bill" legislation, which spelled out action that citizens should take. At the federal level other legislation supported the movement. Among these were the Clean Air Act, Federal Water Pollution Control Act, Toxic Substances Control Act, Coastal Zone Management Act, Endangered Species Act, Resources Recovery Act, and laws relating to motor vehicles.

Legislation has been supported by action such as bottle returns, Garbage Day, and recycling of glass, metal, and paper. The "Earth Day" program continues to expand as more people voluntarily join the program and support voluntary organizations such as Keep America Beautiful, Inc., and local recycling campaigns. Much has been done, but much more needs to be done.

QUESTIONS AND EXERCISES

1. Why has there been an increased interest in environmental health despite the great advances in the understanding and control of environmental health conditions?
2. Explain this statement: "Occupational health programs are concerned with more than occupational diseses."
3. Why should not employers alone be responsible for all occupational health promotion?
4. In terms of human health and life, what is the greater hazard, air pollution or vector pollution?
5. Which is the greater threat to human welfare, stream pollution or air pollution?
6. When farmers burn their fields in the fall to destroy parasites, should this be regarded as objectionable air pollution? How can it be controlled?
7. Why must air pollution be regarded as a regional problem?
8. If an industrial firm that will employ 1,000 people wishes to set up in your community a plant that will cause a great deal of air pollution what would be your reply and what would be the rationale of your stand?
9. In the past year, to what radiation dangers have you been exposed?
10. Explain this statement: "What is music to one person may be noise to another person."
11. What requirements would you make of motel and hotel swimming pools to safeguard guests and others?
12. What measures can be taken around a swimming pool to prevent the spread of skin diseases such as athlete's foot"?
13. What are the responsibilities of home owners who permit neighborhood families to use their residential pool?
14. How many different vectors do you have in your neighborhood?
15. How is it possible for an insect to be both a biological vector and a mechanical vector?
16. To what vector-borne disease is your community exposed?
17. Under what circumstances should a person be immunized against vector-borne diseases when such immunization is available?
18. What can be the value of voluntary environmental action groups in your community?
19. What is the significance of the tendency of changing vector types in an urban environment?
20. Will the environment in the future be more hazardous to human welfare than the environment of today?

Bibliography

American Public Health Association: Swimming pools and other bathing places: recommended practices for design, equipment and operation, ed. 10, Washington, D.C., 1970, The Association.

Andrews, W.: Guide to the study of environmental pollution, Englewood Cliffs, N.J., 1973, Prentice-Hall, Inc.

Anerbach, I.L.: The importance of public education in air pollution control, J. Air Pollut. Control Assoc. 17:102, 1967.

Ashford, N.A.: A crisis in the workplace: occupational disease and injury in a report to the Ford Foundation, Cambridge, Mass., 1976, M.I.T. Press.

Berthouex, P.M., and Rudd, D.F.: Strategy of pollution control, New York, 1977, John Wiley & Sons, Inc.

Bragdon, C.R., editor: Noise pollution, a guide to information sources, Detroit, 1976, Gale Research Co.

Brenniman, G.R., Rosenberg, S.H., and Northrop, R.L.: Microbial sampling variables and recreational water quality standards, Am. J. Public Health 71:283, 1981.

Burns, W.: Noise and man, Philadelphia, 1973, J.B. Lippincott Co.

Bush, V.G.: Safety in the construction industry, Englewood Cliffs, N.J., 1975, Prentice-Hall, Inc.

Carpenter, B.H., et al: Health costs of air pollution: a study of hospitalization costs, Am. J. Public Health **69:**1232, 1979.

Catalano R.: Health costs of economic expansion: the case of manufacturing accident injuries, Am. J. Public Health **69:**789, 1979.

Clayton, K.M., editor: Pollution abatement, Pomfret, Vt., 1974, David & Charles, Inc.

Committee on Medical and Biological Effects of Environmental Pollution, Division of Medical Science, National Research Council: Medical and biologic effects of environmental pollution series, Washington, D.C., 1976, National Academy of Science.

Cross, F.L., Jr.: Handbook of swimming pool construction, maintenance and sanitation, Wesport, Conn., 1974, Technomic Publishing Co., Inc.

Curran, W.J., and Boden, I.: Occupational health values in the Supreme Court: cost-benefit analysis, Am. J. Public Health **71:**985, 1981.

Davies, C.M., editor: Aerosol science, New York, 1968, Academic Press, Inc.

Davies, C.M., et al.: Effects of abnormal physical conditions at work, Baltimore, 1967, The Williams & Wilkins Co.

Fletcher, C.M., et al.: The natural history of early chronic bronchitis and emphysema, New York, 1976, Oxford University Press, Inc.

Grey, J.: Noise, noise, noise (Franklin Institute Book), Philadelphia, 1976, The Westminster Press.

Gunningham, N.: Pollution, social interest and the law, South Hackensack, N.J., 1974, Fred B. Rothman & Co.

Hirschborn, H.: All about rats, Neptune, N.J., 1974, T.F.H. Publications.

Hopkins, E.J., Bingley, W.M., and Schucker, G.W.: The practice of sanitation, Baltimore, 1970, The Williams & Wilkins Co.

Kasl, S.V., Chisholm, R.F., and Eskenazi, B.: Impact of the accident at the Three-Mile Island on the behavior and well-being of nuclear workers, Am. J. Public Health **71:**472, 1981.

Kavaler, L.: Noise, the new menace, New York, 1975, John Day Co., Inc.

Klainer, A.S., and Geis, I.: Agents of bacterial disease, New York, 1973, Harper & Row, Publishers, Inc.

Kroeber, F.V.: Public swimming pools: a manual of operation, Cranbury, N.J., 1976, A.S. Barnes ,& Co., Inc.

Kurt, T.L., et al.: Ambient carbon monoxide levels and acute cardiorespiratory complaints, Am. J. Public Health **69:**360, 1979.

Landrigan, P.J. and Gross, R.L.: Chemical wastes—illegal hazards and legal remedies, Am. J. Public Health **71:**985, 1981.

Leh, F.K., and Lak, R.K.: Environment and pollutions: sources, health effects, monitoring and control, Springfield, Ill., 1974, Charles C Thomas, Publisher.

Lipscomb, D.M.: Noise: the unwanted sounds, Chicago, 1974, Nelson-Hall Publishers.

Magrab, E.M.: Environmental noise control, New York, 1975, John Wiley & Sons, Inc.

Miller, R.K.: Handbook of industrial noise management, Atlanta, 1976, Fairmont Press.

National Safety Council Staff: Accident prevention manual for industrial operations, ed. 7, Chicago, 1974, National Safety Council.

National Safety Council Staff, McElroy, F.E., editor: Handbook of occupational safety and health series, Chicago, 1975, National Safety Council.

Olishifski, J.B., and McElroy, F.E., editors: Fundamentals of industrial hygiene, Chicago, 1971, National Safety Council.

Prohansky, H.: Environmental psychology: man and his physical setting, New York, 1970, Holt, Rinehart & Winston, Inc.

Shimkins, D.B.: Man, ecology and health, Arch. Environ. Health **20:**111, 1970.

Smith, R.S.: The occupational safety and health act: its goal and its achievements, Washington, D.C., 1976, American Enterprise Institute for Public Policy Research.

Stilley, F.: One hundred thousand dollar rate and other animal heroes for human health, New York, 1975, G.P. Putnam's Sons.

Strobbe, M.A., editor: Understanding environmental pollution, St. Louis, 1971, The C.V. Mosby Co.

Taylor, R.: Noise, ed. 2, New York, 1975, Penguin Books.

Thuman, A., and Miller, R.K.: Secrets of noise control, ed. 2, Atlanta, 1976, Fairmont Press.

U.S. Environmental Protection Agency: Criteria for noise, July, 1973.

U.S. Environmental Protection Agency: Information on levels of environmental noise requisite to protect public health and welfare with an adequate margin of safety, March, 1974.

Waldbott, G.L.: Health effects of environmental pollutants, ed. 2, St. Louis, 1978, The C.V. Mosby Co.

Wilms, H.G., and Moss, C.E.: A bookshelf on radiological health, Am. J. Public Health **65:**1231, 1975.

PART FOUR

Health services

18

PERSONAL HEALTH SERVICES

One of the first duties of the physician is
to educate the masses not to take medicine.

Sir William Osler, M.D.
Johns Hopkins University

The countries that have invested the most in training for physicians, dentists, nurses, pharmacists, medical technologists, and other health personnel, and in clinics, hospitals, and other health facilities, do not necessarily have the greatest life expectancy or the highest level of health. This paradox is largely attributed to two factors. The first is the tendency of people and communities to expose themselves to unnecessary risks in life-style and in the environment, as outlined in Parts Two and Three of this book. The second has been the difficulty in bringing the citizen who needs medical, dental, and other health services together with the necessary service. The people who need help the most are not getting enough help.

EDUCATION OF THE PUBLIC

Knowledge of when and how to use medical, dental, and other services is invaluable to human well-being, but millions of people are victims of ignorance in matters relating to self-care and the use of medical services. Health superstitions, fads, hopelessness, recklessness, and folklore must be replaced by knowledge and responsibility. The gullibility of the public, as represented in the acceptance of drug advertising, extravagant claims, and outright quackery, must be replaced by confidence in scientific fact and personal responsibility. A primary requirement

is a recognition that health does not come in a package or in a clinic. It comes with a style of life, with protective measures in the environment, and with the appropriate use of self-care products and health services.

Quackery

Defrauding and robbing the healthy as well as the sick, quackery is a parasite of society. Quackery can be defined as a false medical claim, fradulently used to prey on the public by professing to cure disease by useless, ineffective procedures, remedies, nostrums, and diagnostic and therapeutic devices. A nostrum is a secret or patented device for which false therapeutic claims are made. Some "patent medicines" or "proprietary drugs," as contrasted with ethical drugs, are examples.

Where a certain segment of the population is inadequately educated in matters of health protection, quacks are able to operate because many people have emotional needs not adequately met by physicians and clinics.

Classifications of quackery are drug and cosmetic, food and nutrition, and electrical and mechanical. Some quacks use all three, but others operate only one form of quackery so long as it is profitable.

Drug and cosmetic quackery. In the United States alone, more than $1 billion a year is

453

spent on patent medicines, many of which are worthless and some of which are actually harmful. Many of these proprietary drugs mask pain and distress and thus delay the time in which the person seeks medical diagnosis. This delay can be critical. Drug quackery exists in many forms—rejuvenation nostrums, blood purifiers, cancer cures, hay fever remedies, cold cures, breast developers, sex vitalizers, nerve tonics, kidney cures, liver cures, and concoctions that "cure" the whole spectrum of ailments. Cosmetic quackery appears as skin "foods," hormone creams, skin restorers, geriatric cosmetics, salves, tablets, and every conceivable potion. These nostrums usually do nothing. They could do harm.

Nutrition quackery. For more than half a century in the United States, "health foods" have been sold in the form of natural foods, organic foods, exotic foods, miracle foods, bee products, and other dietary cure-alls. "Nutrition experts" and "health lecturers" write books on food fads that find ready sales. Somewhere schools have failed in nutrition education when food and nutrition quackery find a clientele ever eager to pay exorbitant prices for foods that can be purchased at regular food markets at one fourth the cost.

Electrical and mechanical nostrums. Fraudulent devices are frequently only leased rather than sold. This can be a clever bit of strategy from the legal standpoint as well as from the sales angle. Charms, "galvanic" belts, amulets, "radionized" water, radioactive ore, electron o-ray, deploray, and other devices with equally mysterious designations are offered to the public and readily purchased or rented by desperate patients and hypochondriacs. It is tragic but true that the more emphasis on the term *electronic*, the more acceptable the device is to the public.

Advertising. Most quacks use advertising and testimonials, but not in reputable scientific journals. The basis of most quack treatment is "secret," the name of a high-sounding foundation is used, and supporters may be actors,

writers, and politicians. Quacks generally refuse inspection, contend that "the medical trust" is persecuting them, and, when challenged, promise to make their methods or drugs available to health authorities—but they seldom follow through on such a promise. Cultists, hypnotists, arthritis specialists, and purveyors of devices use "health lectures," "clinics," and demonstrations that can be highly dramatic. Communication media permit the advertising of products without sufficient regard for consumer interests.

Protection of consumers in the United States

An informed and alert public is the best protection against fraud and quackery. The low-income groups in particular need health education because of their economic vulnerability. The informed citizen will not be a prey of quacks. Yet all citizens are entitled to protection by their governmental agencies so that they are not victims of the fraudulent claims of health charlatans. This protection is afforded by legal agencies and by professional organizations that help set standards and offer mechanisms of "quality control."

In 1906 the U.S. Congress passed the Pure Food and Drugs Act, regulating the interstate exchange of drugs and adulterated food. Additional provisions were enacted in subsequent years, and in 1931 the enforcement agency was given its present name of Food and Drug Administration (FDA). In 1938 the Food, Drug, and Cosmetic Act was passed to further protect the public against hazardous, worthless, and mislabeled drugs and cosmetics and adulterated, misbranded foods.

To be protected, the consumer needs two kinds of information—information for "informed consent" (whether or not to use a product or take a medication), and information for safe and effective use of a medication or product after the initial decision to use a product has been made. At the very minimum, a consumer has the right to information about risks and benefits associated with any product. It is appropriate for governments and institutions to establish some core, or "floor," of information that should be available to their citizens or members. What that information is, how it might be relayed, and what the government's responsibility is regarding that information are issues to be resolved on a case-by-case basis.

Labels and patient package inserts are needed to convey information, but it is impossible to place on one piece of paper everything that consumers need to know. It is generally agreed that the effect of a labeling program depends on information made available to consumers in other ways. A foundation of knowledge is needed for a consumer to be able to use labels effectively and to comprehend other messages available at "point of use" or "point of sale."

Consumer survey approach. One approach to consumer protection asks people what they want to know or need to know. An information campaign is thus not planned on the basis of wrong assumptions. Consumers can be queried at different times to determine different needs. Regarding medication, for example, they can be surveyed before becoming ill, at the point of purchase, while taking a medication, or after completing a therapeutic regimen. The way in which a question is asked can determine the usefulness of a study's results. Business students learn that what people say they want may not be reflected in their behavior; an option to asking people what they want is market testing in which a new method of labeling is added to a product to see if it changes the sales or use of the product. Regulations concerning patient package inserts for medications are currently being developed. The FDA is conducting research on the effectiveness of various components of patient package inserts. Experimental studies are attempting to identify barriers to the readability, acceptability, and usefulness of patient package inserts.

Nutritional labeling of food. Consumer protection laws saw their best times in the U.S.

Congress in the 1970s, but one law that may have particularly important long-range implications for community health is the landmark FDA legislation on nutritional labeling, which was an outgrowth of the White House Conference on Nutrition in 1969. Even if the law survives the antiregulatory orientation of the early 1980s, and even if the food companies comply fully with this law, however, labeling does not stand alone in its current Latin and numerical form. Apart from understanding the language in its present form, there remains the problem of motivation. A survey in 1973 revealed that 80% of U.S. shoppers were aware and said they were familiar with product labeling information, but only 37% said they use nutritional labeling, open dating, or unit pricing in their purchasing decisions. Consumer educational programs are needed.

Generic drugs. Compilation in 1980 of an Approved Drug Products List by the FDA will give American consumers another protection in relation to drugs. Generic drug products are those sold under their established chemical name. They often sell for less than brand name products. Consumers pay excessive prices when they buy prescription drugs under their brand names when therapeutically equivalent drugs are available at lower prices.

The Approved Drug Products List includes over 5,000 prescription drug products approved by the FDA for marketing in the United States. It identifies those that the FDA believes to be therapeutically equivalent to others within a therapeutic category based on criteria proposed for evaluation of therapeutic equivalency. Consumers can save when the pharmacist dispenses an available lower-cost drug product. For example, a patient who needs ampicillin, a common antibiotic, can save money if the pharmacist dispenses a lower-cost generic ampicillin product, knowing that the FDA has approved it as being therapeutically equivalent to higher-priced versions.

The FDA's Approved Drug Products List accounts for about 75% of prescription drug sales in the United States. Omitted are drugs that are still being evaluated for effectiveness by the FDA and those that were marketed before 1938, when requirements for premarketing drug approval were enacted. About one third of the listed drugs are available only from single manufacturers because of patents or because the drug is of little commercial value. For these, no competitive drug product is available at this time.

Of the 3,300 drugs available from more than one manufacturer, more than three quarters (about 2,400) are evaluated as therapeutically equivalent to another on the list. To be regarded as therapeutically equivalent, the drug products must

- Contain the same active ingredient
- Be identical in strength, dosage form, and route of administration (e.g., taken by mouth or injected)
- Be expected to release the same amount of drug into the body at the same rate and to affect the body in the same way

Drug products that are therapeutic equivalents may differ in some characteristics, such as color, taste, tablet shape, and packaging. Two different drugs (e.g., aspirin and codeine) used to treat the same disease or condition are not considered equivalent.

The list is arranged alphabetically by the generic name of each drug, followed by the dosage forms in which it is sold, the manufacturers approved to manufacture the products, and the brand names, if any, used. Products sold by more than one manufacturer are identified by codes so that users of the list can easily determine which products are considered therapeutically equivalent to others.

Of the 200 most frequently prescribed drugs in the United States, 117 are available from only one manufacturer. Fifty-eight of the remaining 83 multisource drugs are considered by the FDA to have therapeutically equivalent generic substitutes. But in the next few years patents on many more prescription drugs will expire and other manufacturers will make generic versions of these drugs; the increased competition should make it possible for consumers to save even more money.

Nonprescription drugs. The pharmaceutical industry in the United States obtains over $4 billion each year from over-the-counter sales of medications that have been determined by the FDA to be largely ineffective. Vitamin pills, mineral supplements, laxatives, sleeping pills, and analgesics (painkillers) are massively promoted in advertising campaigns sponsored by the pharmaceutical industry but ultimately financed by the public that purchases the products. Three fourths of the American public, according to a recent FDA survey, believe that extra vitamins provide more pep and energy. One fifth of the public is convinced that cancer, arthritis, and other such diseases are caused, at least in part, by vitamin and mineral deficiencies.

The Food and Drug Administration (FDA). The FDA conducts over 50,000 inspections and about 1,500 court actions per year in the United States in connection with seizure of harmful products and requests for injunctions restraining persons from continuing a product or practice hazardous to public health. This agency also tests products, sets standards, passes on claims, investigates imports, and cooperates with state and local officials in matters of food and drug production, marketing, adulteration, and contamination.

The Federal Trade Commission (FTC). The FTC has authority over false advertising and deceptive practices in the United States. Following complaints, the commission investigates and may issue orders to the offending person or firm to cease and desist from continuing the practice. Over 37% of Americans accept the validity of advertisements for health products on the belief that they must be factually correct or such agencies as the FDA and FTC would not permit them to appear.

Post office officials in some countries prevent the use of the mail service in promoting the shipment and sale of deceptive, adulterated, contaminated, or fraudulent foods, drugs, cosmetics, or devices. A citizen complaint is sufficient to initiate an investigation, followed by legal action when warranted.

The Consumer Product Safety Commission (CPSC). The CPSC in the United States evaluates the safety of consumer goods. Some systems that assist the CPSC in assessing injury rates include NICE (a computerized compilation of emergency room records), coroners' reports, and 16 consumer hot lines. Depending on the degree of hazard assessed, actions taken by the CPSC include (1) working through voluntary standards organizations, (2) information and education campaigns, (3) mandatory labeling, (4) banning, and (5) recall.

The first two approaches involve some costs and may meet with industry resistance, but the last three are the most expensive and generally meet with the most resistance. These last three approaches are reserved for situations that pose the most serious risks to consumers.

Other professional and voluntary agencies. The American Medical Association (AMA) has a Bureau of Investigation, a Council on Foods and Nutrition, and a Committee on Cosmetics. These agencies work through state medical associations and together carry out the following measures in the public interest:

1. Determination of the nature of treatment
2. Interviewing of participants and reviewing their backgrounds
3. Examination of clinical evidence
4. Examination of experimental evidence
5. Examination of biopsy or autopsy data
6. Securing of some of the drug for analysis
7. Consultation with other investigators
8. Summarizing and reviewing findings

The American Public Health Association, the American Cancer Society, Inc., and the Arthritis Foundation are other agencies that alert the U.S. public to fraudulent health claims. Patients with cancer or arthritis are prime targets of quacks, and special vigilance is essential to protect these patients because of their greater desperation and vulnerability to deceptive claims. The National (and local) Better Business Bureau also is alert to health frauds and provides protection to the public.

All of these official and voluntary agencies are valuable in the public's protection against quackery, but it is the individual citizen who can do most to put quackery out of business. Education concerning recognition of symptoms and self-medication is the first measure. The second need is to select and to use wisely the available medical, dental, and hospital services when necessary, and safe forms of self-care at other times.

MEDICAL, DENTAL, AND HOSPITAL NEEDS

No one should be denied the medical, dental, hospital, and other health services he or she needs, but making these services available is a most formidable problem. People vary in their knowledge of how or when to use medical services, in their economic ability to obtain medical service, and in the quality and quantity of medical and hospital services available to them. To bring together people and the medical services they need is the task of society, health professions, local communities, and individuals.

The medical needs of people, their use of medical services, and their ability to pay for medical services are determined largely by their age, sex, income, and the location of their community. In any year 20% of the population will generate approximately 60% of all medical and hospital costs. The most meaningful data are frequently in comparisons, as shown in Tables 18-1 and 18-2.

These tables show that discharge rates (a measure of hospital use) and the number of days of stay in short-term hospitals for age groups differed markedly, but for males and females were similar in most of the countries

TABLE 18-1. Short-term hospital discharge rates and mean length of stays, according to age: selected developed countries, selected years 1973-1977*

Country and year	Discharges per 1,000 population			Mean length of stay in days		
	14 years and under	15-64 years	65 years and over	14 years and under	15-64 years	65 years and over
Australia (1976-1977)	126	189	309	4.6	6.7	19.4
Canada (1975)†	104	162	339	6.0	8.7	24.9
England and Wales (1975)†	73	95	164	6.6	9.3	30.7
Federal Republic of Germany (1976)	90	115	189	10.4	12.8	19.7
Finland (1977)	85	147	379	7.6	8.2	19.8
Scotland (1976)†	77	125	229	7.5	10.2	34.5
Sweden (1973)	111	134	272	6.4	9.0	16.5
United States (1977)	73	172	374	4.2	6.5	11.1

*Based on data compiled by National Center for Health Statistics, U.S. Department of Health and Human Services, 1980.
†Long-term hospital patients are included.

TABLE 18-2. Discharge rates and mean length of stays in short-term hospitals according to sex: selected developed countries, selected years 1973-1977*

Country and year	Discharges per 1,000 population			Mean length of stay in days		
	Males	Females	Females, excluding maternity care	Males	Females	Females, excluding maternity care
Australia (1976-1977)	149	218	174	8.0	8.4	8.8
Canada (1975)	135	189	144	11.7	10.7	12.4
Denmark (1974-1975)	141	185	144	—	—	—
England and Wales (1975)	83	116	82	12.9	14.4	17.6
Federal Republic of Germany (1977)	137	163	148	16.0	15.7	16.4
Finland (1977)	133	183	143	11.3	11.2	12.6
France (1976)	—	—	—	13.8	14.1	—
Scotland (1976)	110	144	109	13.9	16.9	19.7
Sweden (1973)	135	166	131	10.9	10.4	11.5
United States (1977)	140	196	157	7.8	7.0	7.8

*Based on data compiled by National Center for Health Statistics, U.S. Department of Health and Human Services, 1980.

compared. Male stays were somewhat longer than female stays in five countries, and female stays were longer in four. In England and Wales and Scotland, female stays were several days longer than male stays; if maternity patients were excluded, the difference would be even greater. If maternity patients were excluded in the other countries, the result would be a higher mean stay for females than for males, except in the United States where no sex difference would exist.

National averages such as these can be used in communities to estimate the "expected" use of hospitals and other personal health services. After estimating the expected use by interpolating from community census data on the age

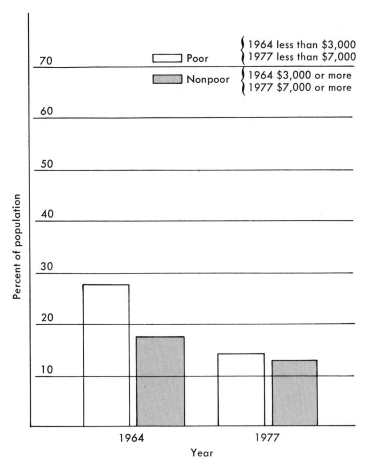

FIG. 18-1. Percent of the population with no physician's visits in the past 2 years by poor and nonpoor status for all ages, United States, 1964 (before Medicaid and Medicare) and 1977 (after Medicaid and Medicare).

From National Center for Health Statistics, U.S. Department of Health and Human Services, 1980.

and sex distributions of the local population, actual rates may be compared from samples of local hospital records or statistics. If the community has exceptionally high or low rates relative to the national averages for its age and sex groups, there may be problems in local hospital policies that can be identified and corrected to save unnecessary hospital expenditures or to educate local physicians who admit patients and keep them unnecessarily long in the hospital.

Families in the lower income brackets gen-

erally have a poorer level of health and a greater need of medical services than do families in the upper income groups. Yet before Medicaid and Medicare were passed in the U.S. Congress, people in the higher income brackets in the United States used most medical services to a greater extent than did people in lower income groups. U.S. data from the National Health Survey show that the utilization differences have been offset by these federal programs (Fig. 18-1), but the differences in health remain.

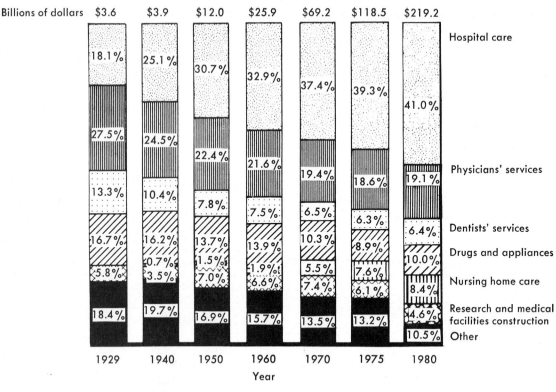

Billions of dollars $3.6 $3.9 $12.0 $25.9 $69.2 $118.5 $219.2

FIG. 18-2. Percent distribution of aggregate national health expenditures by type of expenditure, selected years, United States, 1929-1980.

From Social Security Administration, Office of Research and Statistics; and Health Care Financing Administration, 1980.

The lesson learned from this experience, as in Canada where the installation of a universal health care system also equalized access to medical care without substantially improving health (Lalonde, 1974), has been to recognize the importance of life-style, behavior, and environment. These factors have emerged throughout the preceding chapters as the most effective points of intervention to improve community health. This bears particular emphasis here because the provision of personal health services in the form of medical care alone is an extremely expensive and not very productive way of improving community health. The alternatives of health education, preventive medical services, and environmen- tal health programs have not had proportional investments, as can be seen by the shrinking percentage of "other" expenditures in Fig. 18-2.

PROFESSIONAL PERSONNEL

Reports from the U.S. Public Health Service show that in the United States in 1979 there were 433,600 active physicians. This represents a 34% increase over the 1970 supply. Certainly this would be an adequate number of physicians were it not for two factors. The first is the uneven distribution of physicians. A tendency of physicians to congregate in the metropolitan areas is a problem not unique to the United States. Other nations have the same ex-

TABLE 18-3. Physicians per 10,000 population and percent of active physicians who are specialists: selected developed countries, selected years 1972-1978*

	Physicians			
Country	Year	No. per 10,000 population	Year	Percent who are specialists†
Australia	1972	13.9	1976	48
Canada	1976	17.3	1978	50
Denmark	1976	19.5	1975	61
England and Wales	1974	13.1	1976	54
Federal Republic of Germany	1977	19.9	1977	47
Finland	1977	16.1	1976	50
France	1976	15.3	1976	38
Scotland	1975	16.7	1977	57
Sweden	1976	17.8	1976	88
United States	1977	17.9	1977	85

*Based on data compiled by National Center for Health Statistics, U.S. Department of Health and Human Services, 1980.
†Definitions of specialists vary from country to country.

perience. A second factor lies in the inclination of most physicians to become specialists. In this, the United States is exceeded only by Sweden, as seen in Table 18-3.

With only 39% of U.S. physicians in primary care practice, the result is that preventive services are not available for many citizens. It must be pointed out that in the category of medical specialists, there are internists and pediatricians who in practice are available for primary care service. Having 85% of practitioners in the specialties also creates financial problems. If, in a particular specialization, there are twice as many physicians as necessary in a location, fees likely will be adjusted upward to guarantee specialists an income commensurate with what they think they should have. A new "specialty" of general practitioners, which is called family practice, is developing in response to these needs.

How to make general practice attractive is the problem that must be resolved or the cry will continue that there is a physician shortage, when in fact it is merely a shortage of general practitioners. The new programs in family practice in the United States have at-

tracted some students, and the number of family practice residency programs in hospitals increased rapidly from 62 in 1970 to 219 in 1974 (Stimmel, 1975).

Some communities have been able to attract a physician by building a small but adequate hospital, providing office facilities, and guaranteeing a minimum salary. A second problem is the inefficient use of physician services. Too many physicians are taking too much valuable time doing tasks that others could do or should be trained to do. Others can be trained to take family and personal histories. Nurse practitioners can be trained for further duties. In addition, others can relieve the physician of certain time-consuming tasks. Examples are physicians' assistants, accredited record technicians, medical secretaries, medical transcriptionists, physical therapy aides, inhalation therapists, surgical technicians, and darkroom technicians.

Supply and need

The terms *supply* and *requirements* are used in discussions about the health work force. In addition, the terms *demand* and *need* are used in discussions of requirements. *Sup-*

TABLE 18-4. Estimated numbers of health workers* employed in the United States for selected years, 1970-1978†

Health workers	1970	1978
ALL HEALTH WORKERS	3,820,000	5,412,000
Health care practitioners‡	1,340,000	1,830,000
Allied health personnel	658,000	1,026,000
Dental hygienists	15,000	35,000
Dental assistants	112,000	149,000
Dental laboratory technicians	31,000	47,000
Dietitians	17,000	28,000
Dietetic technicians	2,000	4,000
Medical records administrators	10,000	12,000
Medical records technicians	42,000	68,000
Laboratory workers	135,000	240,000
Medical technologists	(57,000)	(125,000)
Cytotechnologists	(3,000)	(7,000)
Medical laboratory technicians	(1,000)	(12,000)
Other laboratory workers	(74,000)	(96,000)
Occupational therapists	6,000	15,000
Physical therapists	15,000	30,000
Primary care physician's assistants	2,000	6,000
Radiological service workers	87,000	104,000
Respiratory therapy workers	30,000	52,000
Speech pathologist/audiologists	19,000	36,000
Other allied health§	135,000	200,000
Other health personnel	1,822,000	2,556,000
Emergency medical technicians	6,000	269,000
Licensed practical nurses	400,000	504,000
Nurses aides/orderlies	870,000	1,070,000
Psychologists (clinical)	6,000	13,000
Other‖	540,000	700,000

*All numbers are rounded to the nearest 1,000.
†From Division of Associated Health Professions, Health Resources Administration, U.S. Department of Health and Human Services, 1979.
‡Includes dentists, registered nurses, optometrists, pharmacists, physicians, podiatrists, and veterinarians.
§Includes such categories as dietetic assistant, genetic assistant, operating room technician, ophthalmic medical assistant, optometric assistant and technician, orthoptic and prosthetic technologist, pharmacy assistant, occupational and physical therapy assistants, physician assistant, podiatric assistant, vocational rehabilitation counselor, other rehabilitation services, and other social and mental health services.
‖Includes such categories as health services administrators, environmental workers, epidemiologists, health educators, medical secretaries, midwives, nutritionists, health statisticians, and other community and public health workers. (See next chapter.)

ply and *demand* are well-defined concepts in economics. Supply is the number of individuals in a specific occupational category who are seeking employment at the current pay level. Demand is the number of individuals in a specific occupational category that employers will employ at various wages. This is sometimes referred to as "economic demand" or "effective economic demand." Therefore these are different theoretical concepts. What actually happens when demand draws on supply is described in economic theory.

Need is less well defined, and most writers choose for themselves what it is to mean. Need, therefore, is a value judgment that is a completely separate concept from supply and demand. "Need for a specific health occupation" is defined as an adequate minimum quantity and quality of persons in that health occupation which the consensus of a wide variety of persons believes ought to be available to the citizens of a country or community for the purpose of their remaining or becoming reasonably healthy.

Ideally, community planning proceeds with a thorough knowledge of all three of the concepts of supply, demand, and need. Rarely are the data and methods available for a complete analysis. In the next sections a summary of the supply and requirements for the health occupations in the United States will be given as an illustration of health manpower analysis applicable to communities and other countries.

Allied health work force. By 1978 it was estimated that there were more than 5 million workers employed in the health field in the United States (Table 18-4). Approximately 34% are classified as health practitioners (physicians, dentists, optometrists, pharmacists, podiatrists, veterinarians, and registered nurses). The other 66%, or more than 3.5 million workers, could in the broadest sense be classified as allied health workers. Most of these 3.5 million workers are not usually classified as allied health personnel. This term is usually applied to the 1,026,000

workers listed as allied health personnel in Table 18-4. Since 1966 this group of allied health workers has grown from 442,000 to 1,026,000, an increase of 132%, while the total health work force increased by 76%.

Health care practitioners. The number of other professionals in personal health services, including dentistry, nursing, optometry, pharmacy, and podiatry, also have continued to increase in 1978 in the United States, showing substantial gains since the beginning of the 1970s in the supply of personnel for personal health services. Since 1970,

• The supply of active dentists has increased by 19%, to nearly 121,000.
• The number of active optometrists has increased more than 15%, to 21,200.
• The supply of active pharmacists has increased nearly 23%, to 134,600.
• The smallest traditional personal health service profession, podiatry, also had the smallest numerical and percentage increase, rising to 8,100 for an increase of about 14%.
• Nursing, the largest profession, had the greatest increases, more than 43%, from 700,000 to more than 1,020,000.

These increases are helping to ease the problem of availability of personnel for personal health care. Furthermore, projections of physician supply and requirements indicate that the total physician supply will probably be greater than requirements in the years ahead. By 1990 physician requirements are predicted to range between 553,000 and 596,000 physicians, as compared with an anticipated supply of nearly 600,000 physicians in that year. While projections vary somewhat in their estimates of excess physician supply, it appears that the training capacity is adequate for meeting current and future needs of the United States.

Requirements for dentists are expected to be about 148,000 in 1990. This represents a slight oversupply of dentists in the United States in 1990 and reflects a change in estimates presented previously. The projections are based on the expectation that dentists will continue to heighten productivity through the employment of dental auxiliaries and productivity-enhancing equipment. Supply and requirements for optometry are expected to maintain a balance between 1975 and 1990, while the currently perceived shortfall in podiatry may continue into the 1990s. Requirements for pharmacists, on the other hand, almost certainly will be below the available supply throughout the 1980s.

An adequate total supply of personnel, however, does not guarantee accessibility for all people; other barriers—money, education, geography, or language—still keep too many people from needed health care. Many rural and inner-city areas are still experiencing shortages of all health personnel in spite of the increases in supply. The designations of specific areas with shortages of health personnel encompass a broad range of different types of areas, and although a majority of those areas designated are rural (nonmetropolitan) areas, urban areas contain about half of the population who live in shortage areas. Efforts to identify these areas and a number of federal programs, including especially the National Health Service Corps, are dealing with problems of access. Special population groups, such as American Indians, those who are Spanish-speaking, and the medically indigent, have been designated as having health manpower shortages under special provisions, as have special facilities such as state and county jails. Currently, approximately 30 million people in the United States live in designated health manpower shortage areas. By 1990 approximately 16,000 physicians will be needed to address the shortage area needs.

The adequacy of the current and projected total supply also masks the problem of specialty maldistribution. There are too few primary care physicians and related primary care providers while there continues to be a surfeit of other specialists. Recent reports have suggested that at least 50% of the physician supply in the United States should be in primary care practice. By 1990 primary care physicians will constitute only 42% of practicing physicians. The recent shift toward primary care practice among physicians might accelerate if there is continued emphasis on primary care residency training.

Most of the personnel requirements forecasted for 1990 are adjusted for secular trends in per capita use of services, third-party payment sources, and provider fees. However, the estimates generally do not take into account productivity increases through expanded function or task delegation, growth in Health Maintenance Organizations (HMOs), utilization control and cost containment efforts, or National Health Insurance possibilities, all of which will be addressed in subsequent sections in this chapter.

In the past, the more developed countries have relied heavily on foreign medical graduates (FMGs) to fill gaps in supply. FMGs increased from 11% of the physician population in the United States in 1963 to 20% by the end of 1977. The anticipated increase in supply of U.S. trained physicians should lessen reliance on foreign trained physicians. Although the extent to which the FMG entry requirements have had an impact on the number of new FMGs is not certain, by December 1977 there was a 33% decline in the total number of foreign graduate residents from the previous year. The impact of this decline on areas with high concentrations of FMGs (such as New York and New Jersey) and on certain types of medical facilities (such as state mental institutions) will require continued monitoring.

Training health care practitioners. In the past 15 years of increasing enrollments in schools for education of health professions in the United States, educational institutions have seen substantial increases in the numbers of women and minority students attending these institutions. Federal programs of financial assistance, such as the Exceptional Financial Need Scholarship Program, the Guaranteed Student Loan Program, and the Health Professions Educational Assistance Program, have enabled many disadvantaged students to enroll in health professions schools and to enter the health career of their choice. Even with the increases of the past 16 years, however, none of the dominant health professions (medicine, dentistry, optometry, pharmacy, and podiatry) yet has a percentage of practitioners or level of enrollment of minorities and women that reaches parity with their representation in the civilian population. The number of minority students entering medical school in 1978 was somewhat higher than in 1977, although there was a decrease in the number of black students who entered. Less than 3% of physicians and dentists, but over 20% of dietitians, are black. The number of women students entering medical schools continued to climb (Fig. 18-3).

Allied health personnel training. In examining Table 18-4, the reader should be alert to the problem that some manpower changes over time reflect classification changes only. For example, most of the increase in the numbers of emergency medical technicians in the

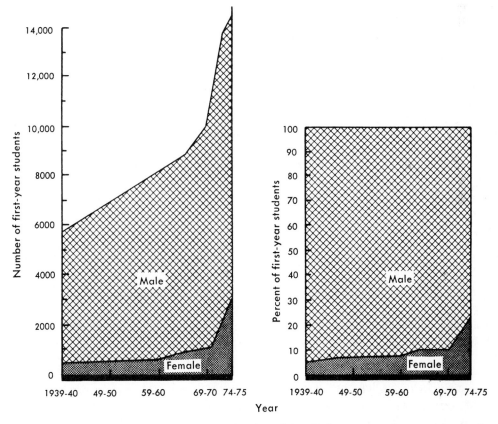

FIG. 18-3. Trend in number and percent of male and female first-year students in schools of medicine in the United States, selected academic years.

From Forward plan for health FY 1978-82, DHEW Pub. No. (OS)76-50046, p. 24.

United States, from 6,000 in 1970 to 269,000 in 1978, is the result of training and certification of large numbers of persons who were already providing emergency services.

Some of these large increases in allied health workers are a result of federal support. Shortages of allied personnel in the United States during the 1950s, 1960s, and early 1970s have been alleviated for all occupations and completely eliminated for some. Significant shortages in the United States are no longer apparent in the fields of clinical laboratory, radiological technology, and medical records. There still may be shortages of dietitians, dietetic technicians, radiation therapists, physical therapists, occupational therapists, and formally trained dental assistants. Shortages are most apparent for respiratory therapists and speech pathologists and audiologists.

New health care provider training. New training programs for nurse practitioners (NPs) and physician assistants (PAs) since 1971 have continued to proliferate in the United States. By 1979 200 NP programs and 51 PA programs existed. Of these, however, 60% of the NP programs and 90% of the PA programs were supported, at least in part, by federal funds. Approximately 27,000 NPs and PAs have been trained. Assuming an average of 10 graduates from each NP program and 50 graduates from each PA program, an additional 2,000 NPs and 1,500 PAs are projected to be trained each year. This will provide a supply of approximately 38,000 to 40,000 NPs and PAs by 1985, and 53,000 to 55,000 by 1990.

Overall, the substantial increases in the U.S. supply of personal health services manpower that have been experienced and that are anticipated in the future could bring about an unprecedented ability to balance supply and demand for health services. Beyond the fact that no severe shortages are foreseen in any personal health manpower category by 1990 in the United States, there is the distinct possibility of provider surpluses arising in a few cat-

egories. Thus the opportunity may present itself for easing or even eliminating many of the problems in personal health services provision, including shortages of primary physician care and the general problem of uneven geographic distribution. Greater attention could then be turned to the neglected personnel shortages in community health services and public health.

Nurses and other allied personnel are assuming expanded roles in personal health services. Their numbers increased faster than the increase in physicians or in population. Nursing aides, orderlies, and attendants have relieved RNs of many direct patient care functions, leaving them more time for supervision, administration, and community and patient education. The ratio of five nurses for every 1,000 people in the average community allows nurses greater time than physicians have with patients. Physicians are less than two per 1,000 population. Nurses have used this time increasingly to help patients cope with emotional and learning aspects of self-care and rehabilitation. The potential for nurses and other allied health workers to bring a humanizing and preventive orientation back into a highly technological health care system gives them a most promising and central role in the future of community health and health promotion. Unfortunately, the growing concern with a "nursing shortage" is concentrated on hospitals and nursing homes. The problem appears to be one not of insufficient supply from nursing schools, but of inability of hospitals and nursing homes to attract and hold their nursing employees.

HOSPITAL FACILITIES

Consideration of community hospital facilities must be centered on short-term general and special hospitals and their bed capacity. It is the bed capacity that is the key factor. Actually, the number of short-term general and special hospitals in many countries was greater 50 years ago than it is today. Half a century ago, because of limited transportation, almost every little hamlet in the United States, for example, had its 15- or 20-bed hospital, poorly equipped, poorly serviced, and poorly administered, but accessible. With modern transportation it is altogether logical to have fewer hospitals and maintain only those hospitals with a large enough bed capacity to warrant extensive equipment and well-trained personnel. There is no longer a need for every town to have a hospital. As a result, large, well-equipped, well-staffed, and well-administered hospitals are erected in the large centers of population. These large hospitals in the United States serve communities for regions as defined and planned by Health Systems Agencies (HSAs).

The standard of four general hospital beds for every 1,000 inhabitants is attained in all 10 of the countries compared in Table 18-5, but there are many communities and countries that have but half this number. The uneven distribution of hospital beds in the United States was partially corrected by the federal Hill-Burton program, which made more than $4.1 billion in grants to hospitals in all of the

states during the 29 years of its existence and added 496,000 beds to the nation's hospital system. These grants were made to local government hospitals, church hospitals, and nonprofit hospitals. Nearly 4,000 communities were aided in the construction of 6,549 public and nonprofit medical facilities.

A short-term general hospital is one in which the average patient stay is 30 days or less. Of these hospitals, about 2% are federal hospitals, 30% are local government hospitals, 14% are church hospitals, 43% are nonprofit hospitals, and 13% are proprietary hospitals. Average occupancy of short-term general and special hospitals should be at least 80%. In the winter months occupancy is high, sometimes exceeding 100%. During the summer months a hospital usually has a low occupancy, which drives up the cost of hospital care with no health benefit.

In 1948, at the time the Hill-Burton program was becoming operational, in the United States, there were 3.4 beds per 1,000 population. There are currently 4.5 nonfederal gen-

TABLE 18-5. Adjusted short-term hospital utilization, according to selected measurements in 10 developed countries, selected years 1973-1978*

Country and year	Utilization measurement (No. per 1,000 population)				
	Beds	Discharges	Bed days	Mean stay in days	Bed occupancy rate in percent
Australia (1976-1977)	6	182	1,376	7.6	59
Canada (1975)	5	163	1,357	8.3	74
Denmark (1977)	6	159	1,622	10.2	77
England and Wales (1975)	5	97	978	10.1	72
Federal Republic of Germany (1976)	8	141	2,317	16.4	83
Finland (1976-1977)	6	154	1,472	9.5	81
France (1976)	6	119	1,568	13.2	76
Scotland (1976-1978)	5	123	1,217	9.9	67
Sweden (1973-1976)	5	145	1,541	10.6	74
United States (1978)	5	168	1,287	7.6	74

*Based on Kozak, L.J., Andersen, R., and Anderson, O.W.: Short-term hospital discharge data in ten countries, a case study in data adjustment. Unpublished document, 1980; and National Center for Health Statistics, U.S. Department of Health and Human Services, 1980.

eral medical and surgical hospital beds per 1,000 population. The distribution over the United States of hospital beds has become more nearly balanced. Mississippi, Alabama, Arkansas, Georgia, and Tennessee had the lowest bed-population ratios in 1948, but now are at the national average or above it. Some of the states with particularly high bed-population ratios in 1948 have actually experienced a decrease. Within states there is also improved balance in hospital facilities between the less affluent and more affluent areas. There has been a shift in recent years from construction and expansion to the modernization of existing hospitals and clinics.

Only one third of all general medical and surgical hospital beds are under governmental ownership in the United States, whereas most psychiatric beds are in hospitals owned by state and local governments. These differences are partly historical, partly economic.

U.S. hospitals offering a full range of special, highly technological services have increased in number over the past decade. Such facilities as intensive care, open-heart surgery, radioisotope, and renal dialysis units have proliferated. This addition of special facilities to a hospital's service capacity has been one of the factors in the rising hospital costs and the general inflation of the medical care dollar.

The number of beds in U.S. nursing homes more than doubled between 1963 and 1973, from 569,000 to 1,328,000. This increase resulted in part from the coverage of the charges for certain types of nursing home care under the Medicare and Medicaid programs which began in 1967. Some of the growth in nursing home use appears to be the result of placement in nursing homes of older patients who in earlier years would have been residents in state and county mental hospitals.

There are 451,000 beds in residential health facilities other than hospitals and nursing homes. These include facilities for the mentally retarded (217,000 beds), orphans and dependent children (49,000 beds), the emotionally disturbed (60,000 beds), alcohol and drug users (33,000 beds), the deaf and blind (24,000 beds), and the physically handicapped (5,000 beds).

Increases in hospital employees, including physicians, nurses, and other personnel, per patient in short-term hospitals have been one of the factors in the rising cost of hospital care in the United States. In 1950 there was a full-time equivalent of 1.78 employees per patient in a nonfederal short-term hospital. By 1973 the number had increased to 3.15 full-time equivalent employees per patient. (Full-time equivalents are calculated by counting two half-time employees as one full-time equivalent employee.)

The availability of home health services is often a factor in determining if a patient must be hospitalized or can remain at home. The number of home health agencies approved for participation in the Medicare program increased appreciably between 1966 and 1970, the first 4 years of the program. Since then the number of approved agencies has remained stable at about 2,200. Most of these agencies are governmental health agencies or visiting nurse associations.

Poison Control Centers in the United States have almost tripled in number since 1960. There are now 594 centers providing emergency and other care for persons who have come in contact with poisonous substances. Other forms of emergency medical services and ambulatory (outpatient) health facilities in general are increasing in number and use.

COST OF PERSONAL HEALTH SERVICES

In the United States in 1979 total expenditure for medical care was $212 billion. Of this, 57% was private expenditure, and $91 billion, or 43%, was public. This would appear to be a monumental sum, but it should be considered in terms of total personal consumption expenditures. In 1977 total personal consumption expenditures in the United States were

$1,206,500,000,000. Medical care expenses constituted 9.8% of this total (Fig. 18-4), but this is a growing proportion of personal consumption and family budgets.

The consumer medical dollar of 1979 was divided, as shown in Fig. 18-5. Hospital costs will continue to rise, despite the decline in the average length of hospital stay resulting from incentives, regulation, advances in medication, surgery, and other procedures. Nursing homes, rest homes, hospices, and home care as adjuncts to the general hospital have reduced the cost of hospitalization during the period of convalescence or dying. Patients who do not require the extensive care available in hospitals can recover as rapidly or die as peacefully in these homes at a lower cost, and at even lower costs with good home health care services and self-care education.

The medical profession has a virtual monopoly in the American economy, but physicians are sensitive of their image as a profession and exercise a supervision and discipline over all members of the profession. Instances of exorbitant medical charges have been substantiated. At the other extreme are the instances in which physicians have donated their professional services. It is not the extremes of overcharging or charity where the problem of the cost of medical care rests, but in the general inflation of prices in this relatively uncontrolled sector of the economy.

The cost of dental care does not vary greatly from year to year for an individual or a family.

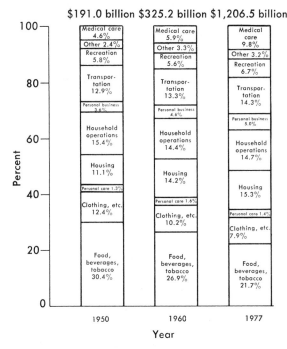

FIG. 18-4. Personal consumption expenditures by product shows medical care taking an increasing share from 1950-1960 and 1977 in the United States.

From U.S. Department of Commerce, Bureau of the Census: Statistical abstract of the United States, 1979, Washington, D.C., 1979, U.S. Government Printing Office, Table 723; and U.S. Department of Commerce, Office of Business Economics: Survey of current business, vol. 59, no. 3, March, 1979.

In 1970 in the United States, consumers paid $8.6 billion for dental services, an average of about $120 per family. Because many Americans have never been in a dental office, the average of $120 does not express actual cost per year for those families who do use dental services.

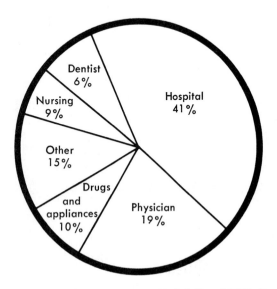

FIG. 18-5. U.S. consumer medical dollar of 1979 divided. Hospital care has become the major cost.

From Health Care Financing Administration, 1981.

But it is neither physician services nor dental services that account for the main increases in health expenditures (Fig. 18-2). The proportion of national health expenditures taken by hospitals and nursing homes has increased more than other categories of health care expenditures. The economics of these trends are beyond the scope of this text, but three major causes and the national policy initiatives to remedy or check these sources of runaway hospital prices are central to community health (see box below).

ABILITY TO PAY FOR PERSONAL HEALTH SERVICES

A considerable proportion of families have an income too low to pay for all of their medical needs. The U.S. Census Bureau defines *poor* as the one fifth of the families in the United States with an annual income of less than $7,000. How much can a family pay for medical care if it has an income of $7,000?

It was acknowledged in 1966 that a family withan annual income of less than $3,000 may be able to pay nothing for medical care. This family would find difficulty in paying monthly premiums on a hospital and medical insurance policy. A medical bill of $600 would be a finan-

SOURCE OF COST INCREASES	RECOMMENDED POLICIES
Physician salaries	Increasing use of paraprofessional, allied health, and "physician-extender" personnel
Unnecessary hospitalization, laboratory tests, length of stay, and elective surgery	Increased incentives for keeping patients out of hospitals by allowing physicians to share in the profits of prepaid medical plans and Health Maintenance Organizations; also, peer review of medical practice and utilization review of hospital practice
Increased use of medical services for conditions that might have been prevented and readmissions for chronic conditions not adequately controlled by patients	Increased emphasis on preventive medicine and health education, including occupational health, patient education, self-care education, health promotion, and environmental health

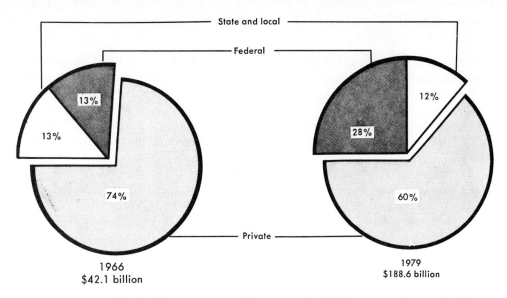

FIG. 18-6. U.S. public funds pay 42¢ out of every medical dollar spent. The medical care dollar is financed both publicly and privately. The private share has always been by far the larger, but in recent years, with the addition of the new programs of Medicare and Medicaid, a shift to more public (especially federal) financing can be seen.

From Health Care Financing Administration, Office of Research, Demonstrations, and Statistics, 1980.

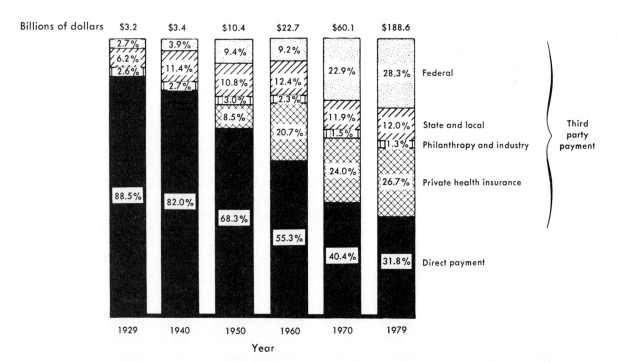

FIG. 18-7. Distribution of personal health care expenditures in the United States, by source of funds, selected fiscal years, 1929-1979.

From Health Care Financing Administration, Office of Research, Demonstrations, and Statistics, 1980.

cial hardship and even a disaster. This family was offered assistance from U.S. governmental agencies that began in 1967 to provide medical insurance or otherwise subsidize medical costs of families in low-income brackets. Families on public welfare increasingly have their medical needs provided by the U.S. government. The low- to average-income family not on welfare also needs assistance and protection against the increasing threat of hospital bills. Fig. 18-7 illustrates the increasing reliance on third-party payment mechanisms.

The problem of making accessible to every citizen the medical care he or she needs involves the economic interests of the public and the professional interests of the medical profession. Access to essential services and freedom from the insecurity of catastrophic medical costs are the concern of communities and the public. Independence in medical practice is the concern of the medical profession.

SOME SUGGESTED PRINCIPLES

Just as the recognition and redefinition of unacceptable conditions must be attributed largely to an increasingly educated and aware public, so too must their further analysis and solution be achieved through the participation of an informed public. No solution imposed on the public by technicians, politicians, or administrators will henceforth be acceptable without such participation in the planning process. We have reached that point in cultural evolution and public sophistication where autocratic, plutocratic, and technocratic solutions, at least in the area of health, are no longer sufficient. Decisions must be reached in close collaboration with informed consumers.

The principle of an educated public arises also in other contexts of personal health services. The proper use of good health services and health insurance mechanisms requires an informed and motivated public. If the *ideal* health care system for some countries were installed tomorrow, it would be highly subject to

disuse, misuse, and abuse by an unprepared public operating under the control of habits, attitudes, and expectations inculcated by a lifetime of coping with the ancient fee-for-service system. Many of the failures or temporary breakdowns in the implementation of new programs in various countries have been traced to problems of communication, knowledge, attitudes, and habits. These educational problems have been diagnosed in both the lay and professional communities.

A third context in which community health and health education is critical to consideration of personal health services is in disease prevention or health maintenance. Any new plan that makes health care more accessible and more acceptable to more people will place pressure on existing resources without a new orientation to prevention and health maintenance. A major criticism of the traditional fee-for-service structure of American medicine is that it provides no incentive for the providers of services to give attention to prevention, health maintenance, and health education. The rewards are tied almost entirely to treatment of the sick. When Americans speak of health care, they mean disease and medical care. There can be little doubt that the primary element in illness prevention and health maintenance is, and will increasingly become, health education.

A fourth principle of community and educational resources is the training and continuing education of existing professionals in concepts of communication, group work, and other methods of patient and community education. The existing pool of health professionals must become better trained to communicate effectively with patients and consumers. These training needs call for the deployment of advanced educational technology and will strain educational resources as much as the health resources themselves. Students too have become more informed consumers in higher education systems and have begun to redefine traditional teaching systems as "unacceptable," forcing an educational crisis within the health crisis. This will call for expansion and upgrading of training programs for educators, educational administrators, and public health educators.

The educational and community health perspective on personnel health services, then, focuses on problems of consumer participation in planning, problems of appropriate use of health care systems, problems of preventive health maintenance, problems of communication with patients, and problems of health manpower training and self-care. The remainder of this chapter comments specifically on national health plans, including those of other countries and some now before the U.S. Congress. In view of the medical, economic, and political perspectives that have dominated the planning and debate surrounding most proposed and existing systems, this text will emphasize the community health and educational perspective outlined previously.

NATIONALIZED MEDICAL SERVICES

A medical program is socialized when it is administered by the government. More than 50 nations have national medical service programs, and virtually all of these are socialized programs. For generations the federal and local governments in the United States have socialized various services—mail service, education, and police and fire protection—but only parts of their medical systems. A city that sells water or electricity to its residents is engaged in the socialization of an economic enterprise.

Personal health services vary from one nation to the next, but three national medical programs in Europe and the Canadian program have been of special interest to Americans. These programs have similarities and dissimilarities and represent basic types of national medical programs.

Germany

The first national medical program was the German Sickness Insurance Plan (Krankenkas-

sen), which was launched in 1883. The Socialists in the Reichstag were planning to present a health and retirement program. To spike the guns of the Socialists, whom he despised, Chancellor von Bismarck instituted his own program. The Krankenkassen is nationalized but not socialized. Supervised by the government, the plan is administered by nonofficial societies or organizations. Practically all workers and their dependents are required to participate in the program. A worker's employer deducts the insurance premium from the worker's pay and adds half that amount as the employer's contribution. This amount is sent to an approved society of the worker's choice. The society may be a social organization, an athletic society, or other civilian organization that has been approved for participation by the central government. If workers or their dependents have any medical service, the attending physician's statement is sent to the worker's society for payment.

Each worker and dependents have a choice of physician, who is paid on a fee basis established by the government. All of the worker's dependents participate in the program, and practically all medical and hospital costs are paid by the insurance program. Fully 95% of Germans are in the program.

England and Wales

England has had a national health program since 1910, but the early plan was inadequate. It provided little more than a medical consultant service for workers and did not include dependents. The plan did not solve the problem of providing medical care for the public, and the cost of medical care that fell unevenly on the people became a burden from which the public demanded relief.

England and Wales instituted the present National Health Service in 1947. It is under the Ministry of Health, with executive councils and regional hospital boards. Approximately 97% of the population are included in the program, and about 98% of the practicing physicians participate. About 75% of the funds for the program come from general taxes and revenue in the National Exchequer, and the premiums paid by the participants and employers provide about a fourth of the funds.

Participating persons and their dependents have a choice of physician, who may accept or refuse a person as a patient. Each physician has a "list" of patients and is limited to 3,500 names. Physicians are paid on a capitation basis, regardless of how often they serve a patient or if the patient is served at all. Physicians receive a flat fee from the government per year for each name on their list. Physicians starting practice must have their location approved by the Ministry of Health to provide a uniform distribution of practitioners. Specialists are salaried and have higher incomes than general practitioners. General practitioners refer patients to the specialists.

All hospital and medical services are without cost to the patient. A minor charge is made for each prescription, spectacles, and filling or other dental treatment.

The British program has been considered successful, despite some shortcomings. Physicians complain that they are underpaid and overworked. Yet England and Wales are satisfied with their National Health Service and no political party would propose that it be terminated.

Sweden

Medical economists generally agree that Sweden has the best structured and administered national health program. Sweden's experience in pension programs, maternal and infant care programs, geriatrics programs, and welfare programs was an excellent preparation for establishing the System of Medical Care and Sickness Benefit insurance, which the Riksdag instituted on January 1, 1955.

All Swedish citizens 16 years of age or over must participate in the program. Children are insured as dependents. The program includes everyone except certain people in institutions. Employees pay a premium not to exceed 2% of their wages, employers pay a tax of 1.1% of their wage total, and the state subsidizes the remainder from general tax revenues.

Sweden's program is administered by the National Social Insurance Institute, but it is highly decentralized. On the local level each county has a county council elected by the local people responsible for local problems. A managing committee composed of a delegate from the county council, a physician, and a supervisory official conducts necessary business between meetings of the county council.

Physicians who are government employees receive a straight salary dependent on rank but irrespective of specialty. Hospitals are operated by the government. All hospital and medical costs were paid when the program first started, but, because people took too much advantage of the program, a change in policy was made. Today the program pays 75% of medical costs, based on outpatient and hospital fees established by the government. When better facilities are requested, the patient pays the cost difference.

Major changes in the Swedish system have resulted recently from the decline in Sweden's basic industries and the increasing cost of medical care. The increasing costs result from a rise in the number of physicians, increased usage, and the demands of people at the local level for more care and more hospitals. The county councils would like to respond to demand by increasing both taxes and expenditures, but the national perspective calls for more industrial production rather than more services. The central government has tried to cut costs, limiting taxation and spending by the county councils, with some resistance; in addition, county council building projects are under careful control by the central government and by local labor-market authorities. The county councils will have to make increasingly difficult decisions, therefore, on allocations and economies. Standing ready to help on a voluntary basis is the national agency for planning and rationalizing health care, which can help train the lay members of the county councils to produce economies through improved organization. A similar strategy has been pursued in the United States with Health Systems Agencies at the local level.

The Swedish program is much like the hospital and medical insurance programs in the United States, except that in Sweden the government is the insurance company and sets physician and hospital fees. In Sweden consumers of medical and hospital services also have a voice in the policies and administration of the program at the community level.

Canada

Because of the similarities between Canada and the United States, Canada is often looked on as a prime laboratory where many of the same basic issues of health care delivery and financing of current concern to the United States are being addressed. Although the average Canadian citizen appears generally satisfied with Canada's national health insurance system, there are critical problems, as there are in the United States, relating to spiraling costs, physician and hospital reimbursement, manpower, and capital expenditures.

As with any system of health care, the Canadian system must be understood in the context of political structure and philosophy. Canadians are traditionally more accepting than their American neighbors of the role of government in social and human services. Canada considers health a right and a national responsibility. While care is provided virtually free to all citizens, the system is a far cry from "socialized medicine" of the British model. Patients have freedom of choice in selecting their health care providers. The medical profession is independent and self-regulating. Physicians are not salaried, but instead are reimbursed on

a fee-for-service basis. Hospitals are not government owned, but are locally controlled, nonprofit organizations. Although the federal government provides approximately half the funding and links some specific requirements to its contribution, the 10 provinces administer their own programs and have the final say about how much is spent and how resources are allocated.

U.S. decision makers see relevance in the Canadian system. Many of its key features such as access, affordability, and comprehensiveness have long been policy goals with bipartisan appeal. Furthermore, in most respects the program does not violate the traditional practice of medicine. The system is decentralized, with considerable autonomy given local governments regarding the scope and provision of health care services. Providers of care are reimbursed in a manner similar to that of the United States and, while some incentives to affect distribution have been adopted, there are no real restraints on specialization or location of practice.

Canada's health insurance program was at least 50 years in the making, growing out of successful voluntary medical service prepayment and municipal plans in several of the provinces. Influenced among other things by the alarmingly poor physical condition of many of the recruits to the armed forces in both World Wars I and II, a 1945 Federal Provincial Conference on Post-War Reconstruction contained an offer by the federal government to underwrite 60% of the estimated costs of provincial medical, hospital, dental, pharmaceutical, and nursing benefit programs. Initially, the concept of a comprehensive national health insurance scheme was widely supported by both the public and the provider community. Hospitals and physicians, concerned about the numbers of uninsured or inadequately insured patients, saw in these proposals an opportunity to stabilize their source of income.

The price tag attached to the program

slowed support; and furthermore, some of the provinces were unhappy at the prospect of having to give up exclusive jurisdiction over certain taxation powers to fund the comprehensive insurance plan. The seed had been planted, however, and several of the provinces started their own insurance schemes, pressuring the government to live up to its commitment. Saskatchewan played a leadership role here and by 1947 implemented a universal compulsory hospital program covering virtually all its residents.

A federal proposal in 1956 offered to pay approximately half the costs of inpatient and outpatient hospitals, and a year later Parliament passed the Hospital Insurance and Diagnostic Services Act. A prepaid service benefit was provided under the program, with federal legislation defining the institutions and services for which costs would be shared. The federal payment formula was characterized by higher proportional payments to those provinces experiencing lower hospital costs and, conversely, a lower proportional share to high-cost areas. By 1958 five provinces had entered the hospital insurance scheme, and by 1961 all provinces were aboard.

In the early 1960s Saskatchewan was once more in the forefront, urging the government to expand its insurance coverage to physician services. At that time, Prime Minister Diefenbaker appointed a Royal commission on Health Services (the Hall Commission), which, after a landmark survey of the Canadian health care system, recommended a universal and government-operated program for medical services to parallel the earlier Hospital Insurance Program. The Medical Care Act (Medicare), which became effective July 1, 1968, embodies four basic principles—universal coverage, comprehensive benefits, portability of benefits, and administration and accountability by government.

Strong opposition came from many sectors of the physician community. Saskatchewan had already witnessed the first physicians' strike in North America as a result of a medical insurance plan implemented in the province in 1962. The Canadian Medical Association's (CMA) motto for government action had now become "supplement, don't supplant," and it pointed to the many hospital- and profession-sponsored plans operating successfully in the provinces. The only role for government, CMA maintained, was to subsidize low-income earners so they could purchase voluntary coverage. To make matters worse, CMA had been instrumental in convening the Hall Commission, never expecting it would result in such far-reaching recommendations.

With more than 2 decades of comprehensive, government-financed health care, it is interesting to note some of the major changes that have taken place and some persisting problems.

Public access. Public access to personal health services improves when economic barriers to care are removed. Canada has seen some shift in resource allocation from rich to poor. Poor people increased their use of physicians, as did the middle- and upper-income groups. Not all problems that are related to access can be solved merely through changes in financing. Certain inequities persist. For example, the poor still use hospital emergency rooms more for primary problems than other income groups, indicating that physician maldistribution may be a persistent problem for primary care.

Use of services. Use of services has not increased at the alarming rate originally projected in some quarters. If Canada's experience is any guide, a national health insurance scheme does not necessarily create a "flood" of people seeking medical care.

Costs. Escalating costs present critical problems. Hospital cost inflation in Canada has less to do with higher use than with increases in earnings of hospital workers and intensity of care. The structure of reimbursement and the organization of medical practice further contribute to the cost crisis. Because hospital insurance was passed 10 years before the Medicare-physician portion, incentives were put in place to hospitalize patients rather than treat them in more cost-effective ambulatory settings.

Hospital reimbursement. Hospitals have their capital budgets as well as their operating budgets approved by provincial authorities. Since it was realized that detailed accounting was no solution and in fact may have aggravated the cost problem, global budgeting is replacing detailed budgetary and control procedures. Global budgets are negotiated in advance for a fiscal year. There is a substantial degree of freedom of expenditures within the budget. If at the end of a financial year, an institution develops an operating surplus, the surplus is not necessarily reclaimed by the government. This provides the hospitals with an incentive to economize.

Financing of the system. Funds for the system are raised through various tax revenues and premiums. Recently, the federal government yielded some tax revenue sources to the provinces in exchange for limiting federal liability. Now the federal share is related to the percentage change in gross national product, rather than the costs of the health services plan.

Health care as a right. Canadians have discovered that granting health care as a "right" has been extremely costly. Consumers have virtually no out-of-pocket expenses for regular hospital and medical care. Some provincial plans have imposed cost-sharing provisions for hospital stays, but the amounts are nominal. At the same time, Canada has an active supplementary insurance market, primarily for drugs, dental care, nonward accommodations, and other services not covered by the program.

In recent years Canada has tried to educate the health care consumer not to overuse services and use the system more effectively.

Great emphasis is being put on individual responsibility and better health habits, reflected in the Lalonde report (1974), as described in Chapters 3 and 12.

Physicians. Medicare payments are based on fee schedules drawn up by each provincial medical association and negotiated with the provincial government. In most provinces the plan's payments are between 85% to 90% of the fee schedules. From the beginning, physicians were given the option of not participating in the health care program. That large numbers of physicians would not participate or would leave Canada has never materialized. In most of the provinces more than 90% of the physicians have chosen to remain in the system.

The question of "extra billing" remains a thorny issue. In Ontario 20% of the physicians have left the plan because they refused to accept assignment. The government, however, feels strongly that the concept of universality would be severely undermined if participating physicians do not accept the negotiated fees or refuse to see certain plan patients unless they can bill extra.

U.S. PROGRAMS

Through the years, various plans to make medical care available have been developed in the United States. For decades industrial firms have provided medical and hospital services for all employees and their dependents. For generations the medical profession has used a sliding scale of fees based on the ability of the patient to pay. The practice is legal, although it has been questioned on ethical or moral grounds. Socialized medicine was selectively in existence in the United States before the turn of the century. The federal government has provided medical and hospital care for members of the Armed Services and their dependents, war veterans, merchant marines, Indians on reservations, foreign service personnel, and various categories of government employees. The federal government, together with the state and local governments, has provided medical and hospital services for families on welfare.

Private health insurance

As shown in Fig. 18-7, America's need to make medical and hospital care available to all at prices people can afford has resulted in the development of extensive programs in medical and hospital insurance. Commercial insurance companies were reluctant to initiate health insurance but began with hospital insurance where actuarial data were available and costs were reasonably stable and predictable. Success with hospital insurance encouraged the companies to expand to medical insurance and, finally, insurance for physician visits. Voluntary, noncommercial organizations, notably the AMA, developed insurance programs for both groups and individuals.

Insurance is a device that substitutes average costs for variable costs. It is not possible to predict the medical and hospital expenses for one person for the next year, but it is possible to predict total medical and hospital expenses for a million people. From such data, insurance premiums are determined and the medical and hospital costs are spread among many rather than falling heavily on a few.

In 1963 68% of all individuals had some form of hospital insurance. In 1978 this figure had risen to over 90%. About 74% of the population has surgical insurance. Hospital and surgical coverage increased with age, family size, education, and income. The surveys by the Public Health Service indicate that those who may have greatest need for hospital and surgical insurance coverage do not have such insurance. One fourth of children in families with incomes below $5,000 per year have no health insurance, public or private.

Commercial insurance companies issue policies covering about 51% of the people with hospital insurance. Of these, about two thirds had group insurance. Blue Cross-Blue Shield issued policies covering about 46% of the people with hospital insurance. The remaining 3% are covered by other programs.

Hospital insurance usually provides for full payment of a bed in a four-bed ward for a period of 70 days for a disability. The policy usually pays half of hospital costs for 5 months beyond the 70 days. Incidental hospital charges are also paid by the policy. Medical insurance policies are written to pay about 75% of all surgery and some of the extended treatment. Policies have a schedule of surgical fees, but the cost of surgery rises at a more rapid rate than the fee schedule. As a result, the policy rarely pays more than half the actual cost of surgery.

Policies to pay physician's services have not been popular. These policies usually pay $15 for each visit to a physician, beginning with the second visit. The problem for most people is not paying $15 for a visit to a physician. It is paying for major surgery and extended medical care.

Catastrophic insurance plans have considerable merit. These are usually group plans that cover both hospital and medical expenses and are designed to cover the major part of heavy hospital and medical costs. A base of $10,000 is usually established for the insured and his or her dependents. The policy pays 80% of medical and surgical expenses after the insured pays the first $100. The policy pays hospital charges for a bed in a four-bed ward. If in a year $4,000 is paid to the beneficiary, the basic fund is reduced to that amount; but each year thereafter another $1,000 is added, until the basic fund is back to $10,000.

It must be recognized that premiums for any insurance policy are based on the benefits to be granted. No insurance firm could continue in business if it paid out more than it took in.

Health maintenance organizations (HMOs)

The most significant American advance in providing prepayment medical care has been the development of Health Maintenance Organizations, sometimes identified merely as prepaid group practice. In recent instances the programs have been subsidized, at least at the outset, but in the main, these have been self-sustaining enterprises. Four principles characterize an HMO. It is (1) an *organized system* of health care that accepts the responsibility to provide or otherwise assure the delivery of (2) an agreed upon set of *comprehensive health maintenance and treatment services* for (3) a voluntarily *enrolled group* of people in a geographical area and (4) is reimbursed through a prenegotiated and fixed periodic payment made by or on behalf of each person or family enrolled in the plan. These four principles of HMO development are further defined and described by Congress in the HMO Assistance Act of 1973.

An organized system. An HMO must be capable of bringing together directly, or arranging for, the services of physicians and other health professionals with the services of inpatient and outpatient facilities for preventive, acute, and other care, as well as any other health services that a defined population might reasonably require. The system is organized in such a way as to assure for the enrollee the most efficient and effective entry into the health care system. It also promises continuity of care for the enrolled population through linkages between the components of organization.

Comprehensive health maintenance and treatment services. The HMO must be capable of providing or arranging for the provision of the health services that a population might require, including primary care, emergency care, acute inpatient hospital care, and inpatient and outpatient care and rehabilitation for chronic and disabling conditions. Primary care, one of the keystones of the HMO, emphasizes those services aimed at preventing the onset of illness or disability, at the maintenance of good health, and at the continuing evaluation and management of early com-

plaints, symptoms, problems, and the chronic aspects of disease. It may be more graphically described as "personal physician care" or the entry point into the system, from which referrals to specialists are made.

An agreed on set of services. The consumers and the HMO will agree on which services will be purchased from the HMO in return for the prepayment figure. Because some HMOs may have groups or enrollees paid for by Medicare, Medicaid, or employer-employee arrangements, the benefit schedule for population groups may differ.

Enrolled group. Members of an HMO are those people who voluntarily join the HMO through a contract arrangement in which the enrollee (or head of household) agrees to pay the fixed monthly or other periodic payment (or have it paid on his or her behalf) to the HMO. Enrollees agree to use the HMO as their principal source of health care if they become ill or need care.

The concept of HMOs grew from the success of a variety of medical foundations and prepaid group practice organizations in various parts of the United States that are now providing health care services for more than 7.4 million people. The Health Insurance Plan of Greater New York cares for three quarters of a million people. The Group Health Cooperative of Puget Sound, of Seattle, Washington; the Group Health Association of Washington, D.C.; and the San Joaquin Medical Care Foundation of California are other major prepaid plans.

These and the 200 other HMOs at the end of 1979 had been started and now operate under a variety of sponsors and financing mechanisms. Their continued effectiveness had led to the conviction that a much greater number of HMO organizations can be created through financial and technical assistance, and that thereby the health services delivery system in the United States will be markedly improved. The U.S. Department of Health and Human

Services expects the number of HMOs to double by 1988.

An HMO can be organized and sponsored by a medical foundation (usually organized by physicians), by community groups who bring together various interested leaders or organizations, by labor unions, by a governmental unit, by a profit or nonprofit group allied with an insurance company or some other financing institution, or by some other arrangement. The HMO may be a hospital-based, medical school–based, or a freestanding outpatient facility.

The Health Maintenance Organization Act (PL 93-222) began offering federal support for HMO development in 1974 if medically underserved populations were enrolled. HMOs applying for federal grants and loans are required also to have provisions for quality assurance and grievance procedures, continuing education for their professional staff, home health services, and preventive services including health education, family planning, and preventive dental care.

The Kaiser Foundation Health Plan. About 3 million members belong to the Kaiser-Permanente Medical Care Program, mainly at various locations in California, Oregon, Washington, and Hawaii. Based on its long experience with prepayment medical care, the Kaiser-Permanente staff is in a better position than most to anticipate some of the problems that medical centers will face if national health insurance is implemented. Garfield (1970) specifically described the problem of overloading "sick-care" services with nonsick patients. The anticipated "entry mix" of patients consists of five groups: the well, the worried well, the early sick, the chronically sick, and the acutely sick. Through the development of a health testing and referral service at the entry point of the system, using paramedical staff and automated history and test analyses, these five groups of patients can be channeled appropriately to one of three centers optimizing the use of special-ized manpower and services. The well and worried well should be referred to a "health-care center" featuring health education, health exhibits, counseling, and special clinics on nutrition, adolescent problems, family planning, and prenatal and well-baby supervision. The acutely sick would be referred to the sick-care center, featuring integrated facilities of clinics and hospitals, special laboratories, radiotherapy, intensive care units, and extended care wards. The early and chronically sick would be referred either to the sick-care center or to a preventive-maintenance service, depending on their symptoms and prior experience. The preventive-maintenance service would have clinics on obesity, diabetes, hypertension, arthritis, back problems, mental health, geriatrics, and rehabilitation.

Patients would be referred from one center to another and in particular could be referred routinely to the health education service on exit from the system. Experience at Kaiser has shown that physicians in various departments are relieved from repetitive and, to them, boring educational tasks by being able to refer patients to health education and health exhibits by prescription. Hence the system proposed by Garfield provides for the efficient use of both clinical and social medicine resources.

The Kaiser program and other HMOs have demonstrated what can be done with organized prepayment medical services. Balanced use of services and facilities, together with efficient administration, is the key to HMO success.

Medicare

The United States launched its first widespread program of socialized medicine on July 1, 1966, when the Medicare program went into operation. It is a combination compulsory hospital and optional medical care program and is available to over 95% of people 65 years of age and older. The program is designed to give the elderly a certain degree of security against overburdening hospital and medical costs and to assure them the essential hospital and medical services. Medicare (PL 89-97) is three plans in one—the basic plan, the voluntary supplement plan, and the extension of the Kerr-Mills plan of medical assistance for the aged, now known as Title XIX or Medicaid.

The basic plan provides hospital care automatically for all people 65 years of age and older except certain federal employees and certain aliens. Whether persons are working or retired they are entitled to the benefits of the basic plan, which is financed by an increase in the Social Security tax but is not limited to those receiving other Social Security benefits.

The basic plan (Title XVIII, Part A) provides for hospitalization up to 90 days for each illness, although the patient must pay the first $92 of the hospital charges (deductible). Hospital care is provided for another 60 days, but the patient must pay a fixed amount (coinsurance) for each of the 40 days of additional hospitalization. Care covers all services usually provided by hospitals for inpatients, such as the following:

1. Semiprivate room and board (two- or four-bed ward) and private room when isolation is necessary
2. Regular duty nursing services
3. Use of operating and recovery rooms
4. Services of anesthesiologists, pathologists, and radiologists
5. Drugs and biologicals
6. Blood transfusions after the first 3 pints
7. Appliances and supplies such as wheelchairs and crutches

Medicare pays the entire cost of home care, up to 100 visits, and posthospital care for 20 days in an "extended care facility" for each illness, plus the additional 80 days for which the patient pays a fixed amount per day. "Extended care facilities" means a special convalescent wing in a hospital or a nursing home with registered nurses. At least 3 days' hospitalization is required before extended care facility services are provided. This last requirement may be dropped to discourage unnecessary hospitalization.

The voluntary supplemental plan (Part B) provides medical care and is subscribed to by over 95% of those covered by Part A. They paid a $6.70 per month premium beginning July 1, 1973. This amount is deducted from the Social Security monthly check if the enrollee is a Social Security recipient. Others are billed for the 3-month premium. The federal government matches this premium, and these are the sources of funds for the medical assistance plan.

Each year the enrollee pays the first $60 of his or her medical expenses (deductible). Thereafter the plan pays 80% of the remaining expenses. Services of a doctor of medicine or a doctor of osteopathy are provided for in the plan. This includes office calls, home calls, consultation, diagnostic tests, surgery, certain types of dental surgery, splints, rental facilities such as oxygen tents, and ambulance services. On a limited basis, treatment outside the hospital for mental disorders is paid up to $250 per year or half of the expenses, whichever is less.

Not covered by the medical plan are such things as eye examinations, eyeglasses, chiropractor services, podiatrist services, private duty nurse service, routine health examinations, drugs and biologicals, and dental services. The government is now considering adding certain preventive services in the hope of controlling costs in the long run.

Commercial insurance companies serve as agents or intermediaries for the Medicare program. Claimants under the program fill out a form and mail it to the designated insurance company serving as agent for the government. Receipts of payments made are attached to the form by the claimant.

The Medicare law specifically prohibits federal interference in the physician-patient relationship, to pacify the medical establishment, but this also precludes monitoring of quality. Freedom of choice is guaranteed—there is no closed panel or prescribed groups of physicians. The use of third-party insurance carriers is a further concession to the private sector.

The $92 deductible would seem to save the government from dealing with petty accounts, but it only adds to the administrative complexity of the financing. Premiums have had to be raised since the program began in order to cover deficits. The payment system has discriminated against federal providers by disallowing payment to certain categories of providers.

The relative isolation of the aged and the lack of an adequate educational program accompanying the introduction of Medicare resulted in low use of benefits during the initial years, but also in the delay of preventive care that might have reduced later use. The Senate Committee on Finance asked the Secretary of Health, Education, and Welfare (now the Department of Health and Human Services) to submit to Congress by 1969 a report on "the possible coverage under Medicare of the cost of comprehensive health screening devices and preventive services designed to contribute to the early detection and prevention of diseases in old age and the feasibility of instituting informational or educational programs designed to reduce illness among Medicare beneficiaries and to aid them in obtaining needed treatment."

The Secretary's Report to Congress (Feasibility Study on Preventive Services and Health Education for Medicare Recipients, December, 1968) recommended that the federal government act to strengthen local community educational activities to reduce illness among Medicare beneficiaries. The Staff and Advisory Committee report submitted to the Secretary originally recommended amending "the conditions for participation in Medicare to require that hospitals, extended care facilities, and home health agencies include qualified educational specialists on their staffs or use qualified

consultants to help insure that educational components of their services are soundly developed." This was apparently too close to "federal interference" from the point of view of the Secretary's office. The Secretary's official report recommended "a national, cooperative, voluntary effort directed at health education for the aged" to be *initiated* by the federal government "in cooperation with medical societies, women's auxiliaries, voluntary agencies, advertising groups, consumer groups, senior citizen's organizations, community hospitals and other providers of services, public health agencies, insurance companies, news media and other groups interested in and capable of providing local leadership, initiative and effective action." To implement this recommendation, the Secretary went on to recommend Congressional appropriations and the establishment of a "focal point for coordination of health education efforts in the Office of the Assistant Secretary for Health." Thus, in effect, the Secretary's recommendation differed from the original in that it placed the responsibility for local educational efforts on a wide range of lay and professional resources at the community level, with consultation and assistance rather than enforcement at the federal level.

This represents a "community organization" and participatory approach to community health and health education and is one that is needed for Medicare as well as for other national health insurance and health care programs. There has been an appointment of a public health educator in the office of the Assistant Secretary for Health, as recommended in the Secretary's report to Congress. The Office of Health Information and Health Promotion is assigned responsibility by Congress and by the Assistant Secretary of Health to examine federal commitments to the concept of health education for the aged, both as a rightful component of health care for Medicare beneficiaries and as a means to reducing Medicare costs.

Medicaid

Title XIX of the Social Security Act, also called the Kerr-Mills medical assistance plan (Medicaid), provides medical care not only for indigents 65 years of age and older but for those of any age who were defined medically indigent. This program is a joint enterprise of the federal and state governments, which subsidize all of the costs. By 1977 every state except Arizona participated.

Like Medicare, the Medicaid "Grants to States for Medical Assistance Programs" was addressed exclusively to the problem of purchasing power and made little or no effort to deviate from "usual and customary fees" to hospitals and physicians or from the prevailing organization of delivery systems. Both programs under Public Law 89-97 were established on the assumption that the existing delivery systems would respond to the needs and demands of the population if sufficient fees for services were provided. The only thing that seems to have responded is prices. Together

the costs of the two programs rose from $5 billion in its initial year to over $38 billion in 1977. The growth and distribution of these costs are shown in Figs. 18-8 and 18-9.

The purpose of Medicaid was to provide medical assistance for the "medically indigent" families with dependent children, the aged, the blind, and the disabled. The law extended coverage to rehabilitation and other services to help such families attain independence and self-care. The distinguishing mechanism of this plan is that it authorizes appropriations on a fiscal year basis for payments to states that submit approved plans. The act requires that state plans must (1) cover the entire state, (2) contribute at least 40% of the nonfederal share, (3) provide for a fair hearing to any individual whose claim is denied or delayed, (4) provide for administration of the state program or supervision of locally administered plans, (5) designate a single state agency for administration or supervision of the plan, (6) provide reports to the Secretary of Health and Human

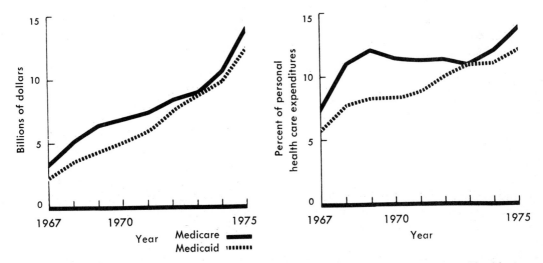

FIG. 18-8. Growth of Medicare and Medicaid funding in dollars and percent of personal health care expenditure, fiscal years 1967-1975, United States.

From Social Security Administration, Office of Research and Statistics.

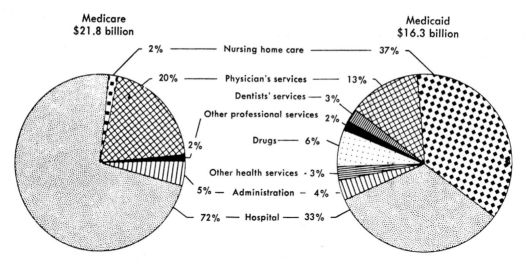

Medicare
$21.8 billion

Medicaid
$16.3 billion

2% ——————— Nursing home care ——————— 37%

20% ————— Physician's services ————— 13%

Dentists' services — 3%

Other professional services 2%

2%

Drugs —— 6%

Other health services - 3%

5% — Administration – 4%

72% — Hospital — 33%

FIG. 18-9. Medicare and Medicaid payments by type of service, 1977, United States.
From Social Security Administration, Office of Research and Statistics.

Services, (7) provide safeguards for confidentiality of records, (8) provide that all individuals wishing to make application for medical assistance under the plan have an opportunity to do so, and (9) designate an authority for establishing and maintaining standards for participating institutions.

Consider some of the implications of these nine requirements. Numbers 1 and 2 clearly distinguish Medicaid from Medicare as a *state* plan. Number 3 places emphasis on repairing damage that should be prevented by requirements 8 and 9. If number 8 is viewed from the educational perspective, it would require states to include coordinated programs to assure that all eligible beneficiaries know of their eligibility and that all applicants know of and have access to sources of assistance in maneuvering the application process. According to a survey in California, 95% of the potential beneficiaries and many of the community workers interviewed confused Medi-Cal (the California name for Medicaid) with welfare and with Medicare. (Some thought it was a soft drink.) Even among those using the program, 90% thought it was

the same as welfare. The welfare stigma was found to be highly unsettling for most users, a cause of misuse, and a clear deterent to use by potential beneficiaries (Berger, 1969).

Requirements 10 and 11 for state plans specify the relationships with welfare. Number 10 requires the state to provide medical assistance to all individuals under their existing welfare categories *plus* coverage of the "medically indigent" with services of the same scope (no less than services provided under any other state plan). Number 11 then requires cooperative arrangements with health agencies, thus allowing Welfare to be the coordinating agency but suggesting that the state health department should assume responsibility for the health aspects of the program. In view of the California study and experience in other states that have placed the Medicaid administration in welfare departments, the administration *at least* of the part of the program dealing with nonwelfare medically indigent patients should be delegated to health departments. Along with this transfer, health educators should replace welfare workers as planners of community organization, information, and education programs. Emphasis then might be placed more on prevention of illnesses and their recurrence, appropriate use of health resources, anticipation of problems in negotiating the health care system, preparing unsophisticated patients to get the most out of their brief encounters with physicians (what questions to ask, what rights to demand, etc.), and related problems that health educators could presumably deal with more adequately than welfare workers. But most important is the removal of Medicaid from identification with welfare.

These needs are underscored by the "Report of the Task force on Medicaid and Related Programs" submitted to the Secretary of Health, Education and Welfare in 1970:

Programs of health education, provided they meet adequate standards set by the Federal Government, should be considered integral components of any health care service, and therefore, included in the budget of such service. All agencies and institutions providing health services that receive Federal support must provide continuing programs of health education to their consumers.

The report continues:

State Medicaid Programs should be required to undertake educational efforts designed to: improve recipients' use of the Medicaid program; improve the health of Medicaid recipients through preventive education; improve providers' use of the program; and provide for greater participation by provider and consumer in the planning, implementation, and evaluation of the program.

In order to assist State Medicaid Programs in developing effective educational and informational programs, guidelines, materials, consultation and technical assistance should be provided by Health, Education and Welfare. "Model educational programs" should be developed in consultation with the States. The approach used should also include "outreach" education utilizing potential Medicaid beneficiaries. Efforts should be made to involve voluntary health agencies, consumer organizations and professional organizations, many of which have substantial and successful health education experience.

This last recommendation relates to the need for coordinating existing community health resources and planning for health on a more comprehensive basis. Medicare and Medicaid must be regarded as failures if they were expected to achieve this kind of coordinated and comprehensive approach to community health planning. The real potential for such an approach was intended to be provided by legislation passed the following year as Public Law 89-749.

Health planning

Comprehensive Health Planning Act of 1966. The Comprehensive Health Planning Act of 1966 (PL 89-749) declared as its purpose (1) "promoting and assuring the highest level of health attainable for every person" (2) through "an effective partnership, involving close intergovernmental collaboration, official and voluntary efforts, and participation of individuals and organizations" (3) with federal financial assistance "to support the marshalling of all health resources—national, state, and local—to assure comprehensive health services of high quality for every person," (4) "but without interference with existing patterns of private professional practice of medicine, dentistry, and related healing arts," therefore requiring (5) "comprehensive planning for health services, health manpower, and health facilities . . . at every level of government," (6) "strengthening the leadership and capacities of State health agencies," and (7) "support of health services provided people in their communities should be broadened and made more flexible."

This law has since been replaced (superceded) by the National Health Planning and Resource Development Act of 1974 (PL 93-641).

National Health Planning and Resources Development Act of 1974. The National Health Planning and Resources Development Act of 1974 combined and redirected the efforts of a number of federally supported state and local agencies that had been performing health planning and resource development activities for their communities. The Hill-Burton program, begun in 1946, assumed that the states would use health facilities construction funds in such a way as to fill unmet needs. In 1964 this concept was clarified under legislative authority, which resulted in the creation of non-profit private corporations, governed by boards of community leaders and health care providers, to plan for their whole community the development of needed hospitals and other health care facilities.

The Regional Medical Program, enacted in 1965, also had a planning component, but its primary focus was on development of resources.

The Comprehensive Health Planning program from 1966 to 1974 broadened the planning concept to include health services and manpower development as well as facilities construction, and emphasized the elimination of unnecessary duplication in facilities and equipment. The Comprehensive Health Planning program established state and areawide agencies to plan for and promote the rational and orderly development of health resources in their respective communities.

The National Health Planning and Resource Development Act of 1974 was to build on the experience of these three programs and to combine their best features into one new health planning and resource development program with the following provisions.

- Require the Department of Health and Human Services (HHS) to issue guidelines on national health planning policy
- Establish a National Council on Health Planning and Development
- Specify procedures for designating health service areas
- Create a network of Health Systems Agencies (HSAs) responsible for health planning and development

- Authorize planning grants for HSAs
- Authorize HHS to enter into agreements with State Health Planning and Development Agencies designated by the governor of each state
- Create Statewide Health Coordinating Councils
- Authorize grants for state health planning and development
- Authorize grants to six states for demonstrating effectiveness of rate regulation
- Provide technical assistance for HSAs and State Agencies
- Establish a National Health Planning Information Center
- Authorize at least five regional centers for study and development of health planning
- Revise the existing Medical Facilities Construction Program
- Provide assistance through grants, loans, and loan guarantees for projects for modernizing medical facilities; building new outpatient medical facilities; building new inpatient medical facilities in areas that have experienced recent rapid population growth

Limitations of the planning programs. The ultimate concession to the medical establishment is found in part 4 of the Comprehensive Health Planning Act. Not to interfere with "existing patterns of private professional practice" virtually nullified the community potential of the act. The main emphasis of the law became the development and support of planning capacities, especially at the state health department level (see Chapter 20). One section of the act provided for Project Grants for Areawide Health Planning.

The appointment of community planning councils was required to have consumers in a majority of the councils. How to define "consumers of health services" and how to obtain "representatives" of such consumers has been one of the most controversial aspects of the planning programs. Some communities merely relabeled selected professionals and agency representatives as "consumers." The interaction of health professionals and lay consumers working together on planning councils has been an exciting and at times difficult process. Professionals tend to be threatened by and resistant to the challenge to their traditional roles. Consumers are sometimes intimidated by their lack of technical knowledge, but because they usually are placed on these councils as representatives of special interest groups rather than as representatives-at-large or homemakers, they have usually acted as advocates for specific groups rather than as consumers in general. The successful conduct of planning meetings bringing together such diverse interests and skills calls for training and experience in group process and discussion leadership. These and other planning skills are in relatively short supply.

The availability of planners with such skills was recognized as a problem and has been addressed by manpower legislation. Unfortunately, the planning agencies and councils had to be set up before training programs could turn out skilled planners. One of the reasons that health educators in the 1960s disappeared from other programs (Medicare and community health department programs) is that their general skills in planning, community organization, training, and group process were suddenly in great demand with the enactment of Public Law 89-749 and many became reclassified as "administrators," "planners," and "directors" in Comprehensive Health Planning Agencies.

Later amendments. In early October 1979 President Jimmy Carter signed the Health Planning and Resources Development Amendments of 1979, although he expressed some disappointment at parts of the legislation he said may weaken the planning agencies' authority to check spending and unneeded facility building. Parts of the new legislation cut into the health planning system's power. Conservative forces and an antiregulatory feeling had come together to attach restrictive amendments to the bill.

The new law exempts HMOs from having to get a certificate of need (CON) for offering an inpatient service, acquisition of major equipment, or capital expenditure. It had been feared that this provision would allow almost any provider to call itself an HMO and be exempt from health planning. But final language defines HMOs as described in the HMO definition in the Public Health Service Law. In addition, the HMO must have an enrollment of 50,000 (although HMOs can combine enrollments). Its exempt services must have reasonable access for HMO members, and 75% of the patients who can be reasonably expected to receive an exempted service must be the HMO's enrollees.

The language of the law limits the planning agency in making a CON decision to criteria spelled out in the planning act, in federal regulations promulgated before these amendments were passed, or in state regulations. This amendment prohibits, for instance, a health planning agency ruling on a new wing of a hospital from taking into account such things as the facility's fulfillment of charity obligation or use of minorities.

The CON requirement is expanded to cover acquisition of major medical equipment that is not owned or located in a health care facility if the equipment will be used by inpatients of a facility. This is designed to regulate instances such as physicians buying large pieces of equipment, like CAT scans, for their offices after the local hospital has been turned down for approval. The amendments also allowed states already regulating other uses of major medical equipment outside health facilities to continue that regulation.

Representative boards. Now deleted from the 1979 planning law is language that required the board of a health systems agency (HSA) to be broadly representative of the major population groups in the health services area. Instead, the HSA boards are required to be broadly representative of the health services area and "include" representatives of the principal social, economic, linguistic, handicapped, and racial populations and of geographic areas of the service area. The congressional conference committee stated: "Several different approaches in insuring meaningful involvement in HSA decisions by all segments of society are permissible. However, it was not the intent of the Congress in enacting this provision to mandate a quota system requiring the selection of representatives of a particular category strictly proportionate to its representatives of a category of members of the class they represent."

Self-perpetuation of the governing bodies of HSAs is prohibited through a clause requiring that at least one half of those bodies be chosen by means other than selection by present governing body members. The conference report expressed concern that "these agencies, which are supposed to be open and accessible, can become closed with a self-perpetuating board providing policy direction unsupported by the general public."

Competition encouragement. The 1979 law adds to the HSAs' responsibilities the preservation and promotion of competition in health care. The agencies, says the law, should aid competition where competition allocates supply that is consistent with the agency's plan.

The new planning law also prohibits individuals on the planning agency from voting on a matter dealing with some person or entity with whom they have had "ownership, employment, medical, staff, fiduciary, contractual, creditor, or consultative relationship" in the last 12 months; requires that governing body membership include persons knowledgeable about mental health services; makes review and development of the health systems plan of each HSA a 3-year instead of 1-year process to allow more time for implementation; gives a nod to primary prevention but restricts the descrip-

tions of "healthful environment" in health plans to meaning "primarily with regard to health care equipment and to health services provided by health care institutions, health care facilities and other providers of health care and other health resources;" and establishes a new financial assistance program to help hospitals discontinue unneeded services or convert them to more appropriate services.

The Reagan administration proposes to phase HSAs out of existence over a 3-year period beginning in 1982. As with other programs previously sponsored, supported, or regulated by the federal government, HSAs are expected to be taken over by the states with a minimum of federal direction, control, or support.

SUMMARY OF EXISTING AND PROPOSED NATIONAL HEALTH POLICIES IN THE UNITED STATES

We have ranged rather superficially over personal health services and the history and current status of health legislation. We have identified some major gaps and weaknesses in these acts, especially as related to their failure to take adequately into account the knowledge, attitudes, behavior, resources, and health needs of consumers and communities and thereby to challenge the existing medical establishment to make significant changes in the structure and form of personal health care delivery systems. The tacit assumption underlying these acts is that given more resources and better coordination of existing resources, the existing system (or nonsystem) can be strengthened to meet the needs and demands of the population.

The Comprehensive Health Planning Act and the National Health Planning and Resources Development Act come closest to challenging the existing order through participation of professionals and consumers in decentralized decision making, but the financial support to implement some of the decisions still are lacking at the community level.

Proposed national medical care programs

A growing nationwide realization that the existing national program for providing medical and hospital care is not adequate has motivated groups in and out of government to propose national health care or health security programs. These proposals differ both in philosophy and in their basic forms, yet their differences are not irreconcilable. Any final program doubtless will contain elements of these various proposals. For purposes here, two types of proposals will be presented for contrast: that of the AMA, and that of Senator Edward M. Kennedy and 24 other senators.

The United States has not suddenly decided to follow the example of other countries. Although the 17 countries that rank higher than the United States in life expectancy statistics all have a national health program (either financing or providing services) and all have lower per capita costs for health care than the United States, these experiences only lend support to a movement for national health insurance in the United States that began with the 1912 presidential campaign of Theodore Roosevelt. Franklin Roosevelt's report to Congress in 1935, which formed the basis of the Social Security Act, endorsed the principle of compulsory national health insurance but made no specific program recommendation.

President Harry S. Truman also proposed a comprehensive, prepaid medical insurance plan in 1945 and again in 1947, 1949, and 1950, which led ultimately to OASI, which in turn led to the Kerr-Mills bill (Medicare) in 1965.

Numerous proposals on restructuring the health care system have been introduced recently by public and private groups recognizing the inadequacy of the Social Security Amendments on Medicare and Medicaid to provide health insurance for the elderly and the medically indigent. The major proposals now before Congress for national health insurance plans place major emphasis on insurance protection. The National Health Insurance Plan, proposed by the Committee of 100 and first introduced by Senator Edward M. Kennedy, is probably the most comprehensive of all and strongly emphasizes preventive care and manpower training. Even this relatively "liberal" proposal, however, exempts the government from managing direct care services. At the other extreme, the AMA proposal would minimize government intrusion into the financing and management of all aspects of personal health services.

All of the proposals offer protections to the pocketbooks and assets of both consumers and providers. All involve some use of federal tax devices, and at least one proposal makes further use of state taxes. The AMA proposal, of course, would interfere least with the existing organization and delivery of medical care. It involves federal income tax credits for individuals who purchase health insurance; voluntary free choice of benefit packages that include all physician services; some method of pooling of risks among insuring agencies; and control of quality, use, and efficiency by providers only. An approach that minimizes the possibility of change in the health care delivery system and the participation of consumers may fall short of national needs.

There is increasing general agreement that some form of universal coverage is essential through federal legislation. Nevertheless, there are substantial disagreements over the extent of coverage and the approach that should be taken. Principally, there is the contention that a mandate for payment for a national health insurance program would inflate the cost of medical services because of deficiencies in organization, facilities, and manpower available to furnish medical care under the uncoordinated schemes that we now operate. Medicare and Medicaid are prime examples of the inflationary results of pumping large sums of federal financial resources into the present health complex. Billions of dollars placed in the hands of health services consumers, pressing against a system incapable of providing these services on an adequate scale, would produce further inflation of the cost of medical care unless specific resources are developed and the system restructured.

Underlying the promotion of any national health insurance program is the recognition that there is little point in pouring vast federal sums into health insurance without a concomitant commitment to reorganize the delivery system, to continue developing manpower resources, to place emphasis on prevention, and to involve consumers in decisions regarding the delivery of services at the local level.

The American Medical Association (AMA). The AMA advanced what has been termed the *Medicredit* plan. The protection would be in the form of a health insurance policy from a company; membership in a prepayment plan such as Blue Cross–Blue Shield; or membership in a prepaid group practice plan. Choice of the kind of protection desired would be made by the individual or the family. Medicredit would be approved by the respective states to assure that benefits meet national standards. Medicredit would not obligate the government to pay for the care of people who can afford to provide most of the payment for their medical problems themselves.

There are two forms of protection offered under the plan: basic coverage, and catastrophic coverage. Basic coverage would provide for the payment of expenses for services such as inpatient care in a hospital or extended day facility for 60 days during a 12-month policy period, in a semiprivate room. Within the 60-day limit, 2 days in an extended care facility would count as only 1 day. Inpatient hospital coverage would include all care customarily provided in a hospital including nursing services, drugs, oxygen, blood and plasma (after the first 3 pints), biologicals, appliances, surgery, delivery or recovery room, intensive care or coronary care unit, rehabilitation unit, and other customary provisions. Extended care coverage would include all care customarily provided in an extended care facility. Outpatient emergency

care would cover diagnostic services: x-ray tests, laboratory tests, electrocardiograms, and other diagnostic tests.

Medical services—preventive, diagnostic, or therapeutic—provided or ordered by a doctor of medicine or doctor of osteopathy, wherever provided, would be covered. This includes dental or oral surgery, and ambulance service, but does not include cosmetic (plastic) surgery unless related to birth defects or burns or scars caused by injury or illness.

Catastrophic coverage would pay for an additional 30 days in a hospital or extended care facility. Since medical care services would continue without limit under basic coverage, no additional medical services would be necessary.

Who pays for what? Medicredit is designed to give maximum help to those who need it most, and minimum help to those who are best able to pay their own way. Financial condition would be determined solely by the amount of federal income tax a person or family pays whether by withholding or direct payment by individuals when they file their tax return. A person or family paying no federal income tax would have all basic and catastrophic coverage paid by the federal government. For a person or family who pays federal income tax, the federal government would pay for the catastrophic coverage. The cost of the basic plan is prorated on the basis of federal income tax paid.

What is covered? Under basic coverage in the original AMA proposal the patient would pay

1. $50 per stay in the hospital as an inpatient
2. 20% of the first $500 of expenses for outpatient or emergency care (maximum of $100) in a 12-month period
3. 20% of the first $500 of expenses for medical care services (maximum of $100) in a 12-month period

Medicredit was designed to solve the most immediate problem relating to medical and health care. Companion programs are being proposed by the AMA to solve the various problems inherent in providing medical and hospital services for all citizens.

The Health Security Act. The Health Security Act was introduced in the U.S. Senate by Senator Edward M. Kennedy as a national health insurance plan to be administered by the federal government, covering all U.S. citizens and certain aliens. It would repeal Medicare but would continue Medicaid as a supplemental program.

The plan provides for comprehensive health benefits, including physicians services, inpatient and outpatient hospital care, home health services, supporting services such as optometry, podiatry, devices, and appliances subject to the following exclusions:

1. Dental care initially limited to children under 15; covered age group is to be extended in each of the succeeding 5 years until all under age 25 are covered
2. Drug benefit limited to inpatient drugs, specified drugs necessary for chronic conditions, drugs provided through group practice systems
3. Skilled nursing home care initially limited to 120 days with provision for expansion when feasible
4. Mental hospital care limited to 45 days per year active treatment; limit of 20 consultations per year for outpatient psychiatric care if provided by solo practitioner

Benefits would be covered in full with no deductibles, coinsurance, waiting periods, maximums, or cutoffs other than as previously indicated.

Hospitals, homes with skilled nursing, and home health agencies would be paid on a schedule of reasonable costs. HMOs or professional foundations would be paid on a per capita basis or approved budget. Independent physicians and dentists may be paid on fee-for-service basis or per capita. Supplemental stipends may be paid to practitioners located in remote or deprived areas. Practitioners may be reimbursed for costs of continuing education.

Administration of the program would be by

means of a five-member Health Security Board within the Department of Health and Human Services. A National Health Security Council, representing consumers, providers of care, health organizations, and others would advise the board on program operation. Regional authorities would be given strong discretionary powers. The program would substantially supplant private health insurance.

The program would be financed by a 3.5% tax on employer's payrolls (36% of costs); 1.0% tax on employees (12% of costs); 2.5% tax on self-employed (2% of costs); and the balance (50%) from general tax revenues. The original Kennedy bill also provided $600 million for a Health Resources Development Fund to be used in 2 years preceding program operations for development of health manpower.

Some general principles under which the Kennedy-type of proposal would operate are the following:

1. The national health insurance program should be an integral part of the national social insurance system financed by employer-employee and federal tax revenues.
2. The spectrum of program benefits should include preventive, curative, and rehabilitative services.
3. Payments for the services provided as benefits should assure full financial protection for the consumers and should be fair to the providers of services.
4. There should be provisions within the program design to safeguard quantity, quality, effectiveness, continuity, and economy of the family health care services it finances.
5. Organization of auxiliary and professional health personnel into health teams should be supported, financed, and trained.
6. There should be public control of the basic policies governing the program through consumer participation and full public accountability for its financial and operational activities.
7. National development of adequate manpower, facilities, and organizations needed for effective delivery of health care services should be an integral part of the program design.

8. Although primarily directed to the development of comprehensive personal health care services, the national health insurance program should have concern for the development of effective community health and welfare programs at the national, state, regional, and local levels through comprehensive health planning.
9. There should be advocation of reform and realignment of federal agencies concerned with personal and community health programs into a coordinated entity that will provide common objectives and common action toward developing integrated health systems.

One of the most positive aspects of this bill from the point of view of political development and participation is the broad base of support and input that has been included in its formulation. The Committee for National Health Insurance or "Committee of 100" was originally formed by the late Walter Reuther in 1968. Three of the 100 members, along with 12 other senators, first sponsored the bill in August 1970. It was later merged with a similar bill sponsored by Congresswoman Martha Griffiths and the AFL-CIO. Unlike the other plans with their emphasis on the private sector, this bill convincingly proposed "a working partnership between the public and private sectors." Although the bill clearly disavowed any intention of government-owned or government-managed facilities, it did set down a variety of provisions for consumer and community participation. For example, consumer organizations would be encouraged to give health care a high priority in their overall activities and to sponsor and develop comprehensive, community-wide health care organizations. Along with comprehensive health care programs to be developed by hospitals, physician groups, and combinations of professionals, the consumer-sponsored organizations would be supported and recognized by Health Security.

Effective participation by consumers at all levels of policy formulation and program development of Health Security would be assured on the board, on the National Advisory Council assisting in its continuing public administration, and on regional and local advisory councils. There would be public control of the basic policies governing the program, and full public accountability for its financial and operational activities.

There are also major provisions for and commitments to preventive health in this bill, along with concomitant concerns for the development of health manpower and support for the location of needed health personnel in urban and rural poverty areas. Health education is specifically cited as an essential component of the program.

Appraisal. All of the porposed national health program proposals have certain merits. Doubtless any final program accepted and put into operation will incorporate certain features of each of the proposals. When such a national program will be instituted in the United States depends on a combination of circumstances. The economic recession has dramatized the need for some type of program, but it also has made the prospects of funding it less likely.

Private health insurance. The inability of private health insurance to meet the medical and other health needs of the U.S. population fully has been demonstrated. The commercial plans have taken away most of the low-risk, high-income consumers, leaving the nonprofit Blue Cross and Blue Shield plans with the necessity of raising premium rates on their poorer customers. As Senator Kennedy pointed out in his first speech introducing the Health Security Act (Congressional Record, 5.4297, August 27, 1970), private insurance in 1968 met only one third of the private costs of health care and much of that was where it was needed least:

20% of all Americans under 65 had no hospital insurance
22% had no surgical insurance
34% had no inpatient medical insurance
50% had no outpatient x-ray and laboratory insurance

57% had no insurance for office visits or home visits

61% had no insurance against the cost of prescription drugs

97% had no dental care insurance

Moreover, Kennedy continued, private health insurance is not sufficiently prevention-oriented, it is *sickness* rather than *health* insurance. It gives partial rather than comprehensive benefits. It fails to control either costs or quality. "Health insurance coverage in America today is more loophole than protection," he said.

The health insurance industry itself has acknowledged the problem and has developed a series of "new objectives" for which a program has been proposed for federal action.

1. Health care delivery systems should be *responsive and relevant* to the continuing health needs of people rather than only to their episodic medical needs. Systems should be oriented to the whole person and his needs for disease prevention and health maintenance, rather than primarily to medical treatment and management of disabling conditions.
2. Health care delivery systems should *integrate and interact* with other social and environmental systems that serve in the public interest, including employment, education, housing, transportation, communications, recreation, etc.
3. Health care delivery systems should be *reflective of consumer and professional interests,* operating not only to provide the quality of care needed and desired by the citizen-consumer, but to assure that the means of delivering services are in keeping with the professional concepts and standards of the providers of service.
4. Health care delivery systems should be adaptively structured and interrelated so as to *provide access to quality health care by all residents* regardless of such factors as geographical location, economic resources or cultural or social variables.

The personal health system for the future as envisioned by the Health Insurance Association of America would have the following characteristics:

5. Multiple and organized systems providing relatively comprehensive services and continuity of care, with the needs of the individual taking precedence over institutional requirements, and with extensive utilization of group practice and team methods of delivering personal health care services.
6. Access to personal health care reasonably near to those being served, with more care provided on an ambulatory basis, and limited inpatient care adapted to the needs of the patient and economy and effectiveness of service.
7. Emphasis on preventive services, health maintenance procedures, and health education concerning individual and family health behavior and the use of health services.
8. Active involvement of "consumers"—including those of low income, of minority and ethnic groups, and of the areas being served, as well as middle and upper income people—in planning, development, and management of services and facilities, and in determination of priorities.
9. Many different efforts separately and jointly by governments, professions, and private industry to try out new ways and means of delivering health care services and similar pluralistic approaches to financing—including strong reliance on insurance and other forms of prepayment as well as governmental subsidies (Gulick, 1970).

The United States will someday have a national health insurance program, but when and how is still a matter of conjecture. To duplicate Sweden's program would be a formidable and questionable task. What works effectively in Sweden, a nation of about 8 million people, may not fit at all for a nation of more than 26 times that population. The medical profession, with much at stake, will have its voice heard in any proposal for a nationalized program. Other professional and consumer groups less well organized will need to combine forces to be heard as clearly.

QUESTIONS AND EXERCISES

1. Why is it paradoxical that the United States does not have the highest level of health nor the greatest life expectancy?
2. Why is health education of the poor an urgent need in the United States?
3. Why does quackery tend to flourish?
4. Why has the administrator of the FDA proposed that most patent medicines be banned from sale in the United States?
5. Name some patent medicines you think should be banned from sale and indicate the reasons.
6. Why will an adult citizen wear a charm around his neck to keep sickness away?
7. What should the communications media do to protect the public from quackery?
8. Is the U.S. general and special hospital admissions rate of 168 per 1,000 population too high or too low? Why?
9. What is the ratio of physicians to population in your county, and what is your appraisal of the situation?
10. How does your country measure up to the standard of four beds per 1,000 people?
11. Why is the average length of stay in a hospital of limited value in the analysis of medical and hospital costs to citizens?
12. To what extent should nursing homes and personal care homes be increased in the next 10 years in your community?
13. Why are medical and hospital costs increasing faster than the cost of living index?
14. What is your proposal for paying for hospital and medical care for the low-income families not on welfare?
15. Why are people slow in paying their medical and hospital bills?
16. What is the case for and against the federal government totally subsidizing education in the medical, dental, and other health professions?
17. Why should the consumer of medical service have a voice in how medical service is to be paid?
18. What evidence have you that the public seeks to control medical practice?
19. Make a survey among 100 adult acquaintances under age 65 to determine the percentage carrying hospital and medical insurance and compare it with national figures.
20. Propose a National Hospital and Medical Service Program for the United States.

BIBLIOGRAPHY

Andersen, R., Anderson, O.W., and Kozak, L.J.: The status of hospital discharge data in three countries, Center for Health Administration Studies, Chicago, 1979, University of Chicago.

Anderson, D.C., editor: Health education in practice, London, 1979, Croom Helm Ltd.

Anderson, O.W.: Health care: can there be equity? The United States, Sweden, and England, New York, 1973, John Wiley & Sons, Inc.

Australian Bureau of Statistics, Queensland Office: Patients treated in hospitals, 1976, Ref. No. 4303.3, Brisbane, Austrialia, 1978.

Australian Bureau of Statistics, Tasmania Office: Hospital morbidity, 1976, Ref. No. 4301.6, Hobart, Australia, 1978.

Australian Bureau of Statistics, Western Australian Office: Hospital in-patient statistics, 1976, Ref. No. 4301.5, Perth, Australia, 1977.

Becker, M.H., editor: Personal health behavior and the health belief model, Health Educ. Monog. 2:324, 1974.

Bennett, A.E.: Communication between doctors and patients, London, 1976, Oxford University Press for the Nuffield Provincial Hospitals Trust.

Berger, J.: A study of information needs in the community on the Medi-Cal program, Berkeley, Calif., 1969, Bureau of Health Education, California State Department of Public Health.

Bernstein, B.J.: Public health—inside or outside the mainstream of the political process? Lessons from the passage of Medicaid, Am. J. Public Health 60:1690, Sept., 1970.

Blum, H.L.: Expanding health care horizons: from a general systems concept of health to a national health policy, Oakland, Calif., 1976, Third Party Associates.

Brenner, M.H.: Estimating the social costs of national economic policy, Washington, D.C., 1976, U.S. Government Printing Office.

Cambridge Research Institute: Trends affecting the U.S. health care system, Rockville, Md., Bureau of Health Planning and Resources Development, DHEW Publication No. (HRA) 76-14503, 1976.

Chapman, J.E., and Chapman, H.H.: Behavior and health care: a humanistic helping process, St. Louis, 1975, The C.V. Mosby Co.

Commonwealth Department of Health, Australia: Handbook on health manpower, Canberra, 1977, Australian Government Publishing Service.

Crowley, A., editor: Medical education in the United States, 1973-1974, J.A.M.A. Suppl., Jan., 1975.

Department of Health and Social Security: Health and personal social services statistics for England, 1977, London, 1977, Her Majesty's Stationery Office.

Department of Health and Social Security, Office of Population Censuses and Surveys, and Welsh Office: Hospital in-patient enquiry, 1975, main tables, London, 1978, Series MB4-No. 5, Her Majesty's Stationery Office.

Editors of Consumer Reports: The medicine show, Mount Vernon, N.Y., rev. ed. 1974, Consumers Union.

Federal Office of Statistics, Federal Republic of Germany: Hospitals, 1977, health care statistics, vol. 6, Stuttgart, West Germany, 1979, W. Kohlhammer.

Forward Plan for Health, FY 1978-82, Washington, D.C., 1976, Public Health Service, DHEW Pub. No. (05) 76-50046.

Fuchs, V.R.: Who shall live? Health, economics and social choice, New York, 1974, Basic Books, Inc., Publishers.

Garb, S.: Abbreviations and acronyms in medicine and nursing, New York, 1976, Springer Publishing Co., Inc.

Garfield, S.R.: The delivery of medical care, Sci. Am. **222:**15, April, 1970.

Golden, A.S.: An inventory of primary health care practice, Cambridge, Mass., 1976, Ballinger Publishing Co.

Goodrich, C.H., et al.: Welfare medical care, an experiment, Cambridge, Mass., 1970, Harvard University Press.

Gulick, M.A.: The health care crisis, The Conference Board Record **7:**50, 1970.

Haynes, R.B., Taylor, D.W., and Sackett, D.L.: Compliance in health care, Baltimore, 1979, The Johns Hopkins University Press.

Health Care Financing Administration: Health care financing trends, HCFA Pub. No. 03055, Washington, D.C., 1980, U.S. Department of Health and Human Services.

Health Insurance Commission, Australia: Third annual report, 1976-77, Canberra, Australia, 1978, Australian Government Publishing Service.

Health Resources Statistics, 1976, Rockville, Md., National Center for Health Statistics, DHEW Pub. No. (HRA) 75-1509.

Hepner, J.O., and Hepner, D.M.: The health strategy game: a challenge for reorganization and management, St. Louis, 1973, The C.V. Mosby Co.

Hiatt, H.H.: The politics of health care: nine case studies of innovative planning in New York City, New York, 1973, Praeger Publishers, Inc.

Hospital Morbidity Section of Health Division, Statistics Canada: Hospital morbidity, 1975, Ref. No. 32-206, Ottawa, June, 1978.

Information Services Division of the Common Services Agency, Scottish Health Service: Scottish hospital in-patient statistics, 1976, Edinburgh, 1978, Her Majesty's Stationery Office.

Information Services Division of the Common Services Agency, Scottish Health Service: Hospital utilization statistics, ISD(S)1 Scheme, Year Ending March 1978, Edinburgh, Jan., 1979.

Kennedy, E.M.: In critical condition: the crisis in America's health care, New York, 1972, Simon & Schuster, Inc.

Koch, J.H., Toftemark, C., and Andersen-Rosendal, P.: Health services in Denmark, Copenhagen, 1976, Association of County Councils.

Kozak, L.J., Andersen, R., and Anderson, O.W.: Short-term hospital discharge data in ten countries, a case study in data adjustment. Unpublished document, 1980.

Lalonde, M.: A new perspective on the health of Canadians: a working document, Ottawa, 1974, Ministry of National Health and Welfare, Government of Canada.

Levin, L.S.: Self-care: new initiatives in health, New York, 1976, Neale Watson Academic Publications, Inc.

Lewis, C.E., Fein, R., and Mechanic, D.: A right to health: the problem of access to primary medical care, New York, 1976, John Wiley & Sons, Inc.

McKinlay, J.B., editor: Economic aspects of health care, New York, 1973, Prodist.

Ministry of Health and Social Security, France: Reference statistics of health, 1978, Information Note No. 136, Paris, 1978, French Documentation.

Munts, R.: Bargaining for health: labor unions, health insurance and medical care, Madison, Wis., 1967, University of Wisconsin Press.

Myers, E.S.: Insurance coverage for mental illness: present status and future prospects, Am. J. Public Health **60:**1921, 1970.

National Board of Health, Finland: Health services, year book of the national board of health, 1971-77, Helsinki, 1978.

National Board of Health and Welfare, Sweden: In-patient statistics from hospitals in the Uppsala region and in the countries of Skane, 1973, Consumption of hospital care by age and sex, Patient Statistics, No. 17, Stockholm, 1976.

National Board of Health and Welfare, Sweden: Hospital service statistics for 1976, Statistical Reports, Ref. No. HS 1978:5, Stockholm, 1978, National Central Bureau of Statistics.

National Board of Health and Welfare, Sweden: Public health in Sweden, 1976, Stockholm, 1979.

National Center for Health Statistics: The nations' use of health resources, 1976 edition, Rockville, Md., 1977, Health Resources Administration, Public Health Service, DHEW Pub. No. (HRA) 77-1240.

National Center for Health Statistics: Detailed diagnoses and surgical procedures for patients discharged from short-stay hospitals, United States, 1977, DHEW Pub. No. (PHS) 79-1274, Public Health Service, Washington, D.C., 1979, U.S. Government Printing Office.

National Center for Health Statistics: Health, United States, 1980, DHEW Pub. No. (PHS) 81-1232, Public Health Service, Washington, D.C. 1980, U.S. Government Printing Office.

National Health Service, Denmark: Output statistics for the hospital system, 1977. Medical Statistics Reports, Ref. No. 1978:7, Copenhagen, 1978.

Navarro, V.: Medicine under capitalism, New York, 1976, Prodist.

Norman, J.C.: Medicine in the ghetto, New York, 1969, Appleton-Century-Crofts.

Preventive Medicine USA: Theory, practice and application of prevention in personal health services and quality control and evaluation of preventive health services, New York, 1976, Prodist.

Robert Wood Johnson Foundation: A new survey on access to medical care, Special Report No. 1, Princeton, N.J., 1978, The Foundation.

Roemer, M.I.: Organization of medical care under Social Security, Washington, D.C., 1971, International Labour Office.

Roemer, M.I.: Rural health care, St. Louis, 1976, The C.V. Mosby Co.

Shenkin, B.N.: Change in Swedish health care: what lessons for us? N. Engl. J. Med. **302**:10, Feb. 28, 1980.

Shonick, W.: Elements of planning for area-wide personal health services, St. Louis, 1976, The C.V. Mosby Co.

Squyres, W., editor: Patient education: an inquiry into the state of the art, New York, 1980, Springer Publishing Co., Inc.

State Statistical Office of Schleswig-Holstein, Federal Republic of Germany: Diseases of inpatients in Schleswig-Holstein, 1976, Kiel, West Germany, 1978.

Stimmel, B.: The Congress and health manpower: a legislative morass, N. Engl. J. Med. **293**:68, July 10, 1975.

U.S. National Center for Health Services Research: Changes in the costs of treatment of selected illnesses 1951-1964-1971, Rockville, Md., 1976, DHEW Pub. No. (HRA) 77-3161.

U.S. National Center for Health Statistics: Hospital discharges and length of stay; short-stay hospitals, United States—1972, Rockville, Md., 1976, DHEW Pub. No. (HRA) 77-1534.

Weaver, J.L.: National health policy and the underserved: ethnic minorities, women, and the elderly, St. Louis, 1976, The C.V. Mosby Co.

Welsh Office: Health and personal social services statistics for Wales, Cardiff, Wales, 1978, Her Majesty's Stationery Office.

White, K.L.: Epidemiology as a fundamental science—its uses in health services planning, administration, and evaluation, New York, 1976, Oxford University Press, Inc.

Wing, K.: The law and the public's health, St. Louis, 1976, The C.V. Mosby Co.

World Health Organization: World health statistics annual, 1978, vol. 3, Geneva, 1979, Health Personnel and Hospital Establishments.

19

COMMUNITY HEALTH SERVICES

In the final analysis, our most basic common link is that we all inhabit this small planet. We all breathe the same air. We all cherish our children's future. And we are all mortal.

John F. Kennedy

A community recognizes there are some goals in the promotion of health that individuals cannot attain by themselves and that must be pursued through collective action. There are also some things that the individual can do but that can be done better on a community or cooperative basis. In the complex society of today, no one is totally self-sufficient in dealing with all threats to health. To facilitate and supplement what the individual does in health promotion, official and voluntary health organizations have been established on local, state, provincial, national, and international levels. Operating both cooperatively and independently, these organizations protect and promote the health of the community.

COMMUNITY RESPONSIBILITY

Need, demand, custom, and gradual development have led society to accept as a community responsibility certain health services on behalf of all citizens. As the population increases and tends to concentrate in urban centers, some new health problems develop, but most of the health problems that have long been with communities become more complex and more difficult to manage. If community health problems of today are more complex, society has advanced its technology in dealing with some of them.

Most community health services directly or indirectly will be of value to all citizens but of greater value to lower income groups than to higher economic groups. As an example, community immunization services will have a greater protective impact on lower income groups but will have some value, direct or indirect, for people on all income levels.

Health services and functions accepted as responsibilities of the community include safe, ample water supply; safe milk supply; regulation of food establishments; waste disposal; control of air pollution, insects, and rats; nuisance elimination; screening and referral for detection of genetic and chronic diseases; collection and recording of vital statistics; communicable disease control; infant, maternal, child, adult, and senior citizen health promotion; mental health; nutrition education; health education; laboratory service; and other services specific for certain communities.

PROFESSIONAL PERSONNEL

In the previous chapter the supply and demand for physicians, nurses, dentists, and other providers of *personal* health services were reviewed. These personnel provide the base for community health services as well, but an additional cadre of professionally qualified community health specialists is needed to plan, organize, administer, and evaluate community health programs. Of the employed nurses in the United States, for example, only about 7% were employed in public health agencies and schools, compared with 74% in hospitals and nursing homes. Less than 5% of these nurses employed in schools and public health agencies have master's level training in public health (Hall, Jackson, and Parsons, 1980).

Table 19-1 presents the developing manpower picture for the United States in the coming decades. The "supply" includes the graduates of schools of public health as well as those receiving similar advanced degrees in community health education from schools of education, community health nursing from schools of nursing, health services administration from schools of business, and environmental health from schools of engineering. The

Milbank Memorial Fund Commission on Higher Education for Public Health (Sheps, 1976), concluded, ". . . the greatest relative increases in public health manpower requirements will occur in mental health, health education, and health services administration."

Health education manpower requirements in the United States were expected to triple because of new programs in smoking, alcohol, diabetes, hypertension, and cancer control, which depend heavily on health education as the main approach to behavioral change. Currently, 17 of the 21 accredited schools of public health have active graduate programs conferring some 180 master's degrees per year in community health education (University of Alabama, University of California at Berkeley, UCLA, Columbia University, Harvard University, University of Hawaii, University of Illinois, The Johns Hopkins University, Loma

TABLE 19-1. Projected supply of economically active public health graduates for selected categories of professional health manpower for community health, United States, selected years, 1980-2000*

Area of specialization†	Estimated no. of graduates economically active in the specialty‡		
	1980	1990	2000
Biomedical and laboratory sciences	1,066	1,673	2,164
Biostatistics	1,777	2,787	3,606
Environmental sciences	4,620	7,247	9,377
Epidemiology	3,554	5,575	7,213
Health education	2,488	3,902	5,049
Health services administration	9,951	15,609	20,196
Nutrition	1,777	2,787	3,606
Occupational safety and health	711	1,115	1,443
Public health practice and program management	4,265	6,690	8,655
Other	5,331	8,362	10,819
TOTAL	35,540	55,747	72,128

*Based on estimates and assumptions in Hall, T.L., Jackson, R.S., and Parsons, W.B.: Schools of public health, trends in graduate education, Washington, D.C., May, 1980, Division of Associated Health Professions, DHHS Pub. No. (HRA) 80-45.

†See Appendix A of this text for description of the areas of specialization with illustrative jobs and job settings.

‡Based on adjustments that eliminate (approximately) Canadian and other foreign graduates as well as the double counting that might result from persons with two or more degrees from schools of public health.

Linda University, University of Massachusetts, The University of Michigan, The University of Minnesota, The University of North Carolina, The University of South Carolina, The University of Texas, University of Puerto Rico, and Yale University). Another seven programs in other educational units have master's level programs accredited by the Council on Education for Public Health (California State University at Northridge and San Jose, Columbia Teachers College, Hunter College, University of Missouri at Columbia School of Medicine, New York University, and the University of Tennessee). An estimated 20 other programs are applying or soon will be qualified to apply for accreditation, indicating the rapid growth of this field. These programs admit graduates of nursing and other clinical programs, health education, social and biological sciences, and others with at least 1 year of community health experience.

Mental health specialists with graduate preparation in public health are in increasing demand because of the growth of community mental health centers and other programs related to mental health in community agencies. In the United States there were only 60 graduates of schools of public health with a major in mental health between 1978 and 1979, less than 2% of the 3,735 graduates during that period. Most of those receiving master's degrees in mental health from schools of public health had prior graduate degrees in medicine, psychiatric nursing, psychology, or social work.

Health services administration has seen a growth pattern similar to that of community health education, but on a larger scale. The number of new graduate programs more than doubled between 1960 and 1972, and many new programs are now applying for accreditation to add to the 750 master's level graduates per year from schools of public health. Most of the new programs have grown out of hospital administration programs in the same way that new community health education programs are

growing out of school health education programs outside schools of public health.

Another trend that may partially offset the shortages in other specialties for community health is the development of specialty tracks within graduate programs of health services and public health administration, such as mental health, emergency health services, health maintenance organizations, family planning services, long-term care, and ambulatory care services. A list of common job titles in community health is in Appendix B of this book.

SOURCES OF PUBLIC HEALTH LAW IN THE UNITED STATES

Woodrow Wilson defined law as "that portion of the established thought and habit which has gained distinct and formal recognition in the shape of uniform rules backed by the authority and power of government." A more concise definition is: law is crystallized public opinion. Public health law is that branch of jurisprudence that applies common and statutory law to the principles of hygiene.

Public health law in the United States is derived from several sources discussed in the following paragraphs. All sources of public health law have some impact on health, but the closer to a community the source of a public health law, the greater will be its acceptance by and value to the community.

Statutory authority

The U.S. Constitution. The Constitution is a grant of authority by the states to the federal government but with reservations as expressed in the Tenth Amendment. "The powers not delegated to the United States by the Constitution, nor prohibited by it to the States, are reserved to the States respectively, or to the people." The word *health* is not used in the Constitution and nowhere in the Constitution is there any reference to public health. The states did not surrender their control over health and they retain it today under the "police power." While the control of public health is primarily a state function, the Constitution contains many broad provisions that affect the control of health and spell out the general responsibilities of the federal government in promoting the public well-being. These are described in Chapter 21.

State constitution and legislation. Fundamentally, promotion of public health is the function of the state. Governments have long recognized health as a basic essential that government has an inherent obligation, right, and power to protect and promote. From colonial times, states have taken measures to safeguard and promote the health of their citizens. This authority is vested in the *police power,* which is recognized by the courts as well as by the federal government. (See Chapter 20.)

Delegated authority

County and municipal ordinances and regulations. The state legislature has the authority to delegate the police power to counties and cities to exercise within their own territorial boundaries. This is done through the delegation of "home rule" to counties and municipalities. A city thus may present a proposed city charter to the state legislature for consideration. If the legislature approves, it grants this charter and home rule to the city. In health matters, counties and cities may pass health ordinances and regulations to be effective within their own geographical boundaries. Community standards may be higher than state standards, but not lower. Generally, counties and cities adopt the same health standards and regulations found in the state sanitary code.

Common law. A heritage from Great Britain, the common law is distinguished from civil law and from ecclesiastical law. It is unwritten law and is based on custom or court decision as distinguished from statutory laws. Based on practice and experience, the common law is founded on court interpretation of a present situation in terms of court decisions of the past. Some health problems or controversies may be

adjudicated on the basis of custom or past practice. To this extent, the common law represents a source of public health law.

Police power

Police power is the authority of the people, vested in the state government, to enact laws, within constitutional limits, to promote the health, comfort, safety, order, morality, and general welfare of the people. This means the authority to promote the welfare of the public, although it may mean regulating and restraining the use of freedom and property. The police power is based on the greatest good for the greatest number and may operate to the inconvenience and even distress of certain individuals. All persons, business firms, and corporations must regulate their conduct subject to the police power.

Any *reasonable* act done under the shield of police power will tend to be upheld unless contrary to constitutional provisions. Amendments 1, 4, 6, and 14 of the Bill of Rights safeguard the personal rights of the citizen. Although the Constitution guarantees freedom of religious belief, such a guarantee does not invalidate a school board regulation requiring students to have a health examination for admission to school. Likewise, it is a valid exercise of the police power for a state law to require marriage license applicants to have a physician's statement showing they are free from venereal diseases.

Jurisdiction. Any official health department has jurisdiction over all persons and things within its boundaries. A state law may extend the jurisdiction of a county or city health department beyond the county or city boundaries. Even in the absence of such law, a local health department may take action to abate a nuisance outside of its territory if its own citizens are affected. The state health department can assume jurisdiction in a health dispute or health problem involving two or more cities or two or more counties.

Nuisance. A public health nuisance is one

detrimental to the physical or mental health of one person or a large number of people. Most nuisances are not health nuisances. Not all health nuisances are of major importance.

Health departments take all possible action to prevent nuisances by passing regulations declaring certain conditions to be a nuisance. Such action is taken by state boards of health and local boards of health. The following conditions, which are nuisances, are of importance in terms of their threat to human health: pollution of water, improper sewage disposal, air pollution, contaminated milk, contaminated food other than milk, lead paint in housing, rat infestation, stagnant water providing for insect breeding, and excessive noise (see Chapter 17). Some conditions declared to be health nuisances are actually of minor health significance. Yet the public regards these factors as threats to health. Further, even though these conditions may have a minor effect on health, they can interfere with the enjoyment of life. Such things as the following, which have been declared to be nuisances, have slight health significance—rubbish, untidy back yards, odors, pig styes, stables, dead animals, garbage, and dumps. Well-defined legislation or regulations that make it an offense to cause or maintain objectionable conditions can be the basis on which health officials can proceed to correct offensive conditions. In dealing with a nuisance, even when a condition has been defined as a nuisance by law or regulation, diplomacy and tact are still important. It is an indication of competence in health administration when undesirable conditions can be corrected without resorting to extreme measures. Education and diplomacy are sometimes not enough, and court action may be necessary. In the absence of a regulation covering the situation, the board of health may cite a person to appear before it to answer charges of maintaining a nuisance. The following recognized principles of responsibility apply to a nuisance.

1. Motive is not a consideration.
2. Time is not a consideration.
3. Possession of a license to conduct a business does not excuse a nuisance.
4. Negligence is not an excuse.
5. Lack of financial means to correct the condition is not a valid excuse.
6. Municipalities are not responsible for a nuisance in connection with a governmental function but are responsible in connection with a proprietary function.
7. A nuisance is a basis for the revocation of a license.

Courts recognize three classes of nuisances—private, public, and mixed. If the nuisance cannot be corrected by negotiation, action to abate any one of these may be taken by a private citizen or a public health official.

Private nuisance is one that affects, injures, or damages only one individual or relatively few people. Sewage from a septic tank from one house flowing on to neighboring property may be declared to be a nuisance if the offended citizen takes court action. Abatement of a private nuisance may occur following a formal complaint or may require a suit for damages.

Public nuisance is one that injures a considerable number of people. An industrial plant emitting objectionable fumes affecting a neighborhood could be considered a public nuisance. A group of citizens may themselves file court action or may request local health officials to take action in a court of equity. Plaintiffs ask the court to issue an injunction forbidding the continuance of the condition, or the court may order the defendant to reduce the degree of offensiveness.

Mixed nuisance is one that affects both an individual and a considerable number of persons. Smoke from a factory may affect one person and a whole neighborhood. Remedy could be a suit for damages or a suit in equity, asking that an injunction be issued restraining the responsible party from continuing the condition.

Immediate action is sometimes necessary, and there is not always sufficient time to resort to court action. In this event, summary abatement is the remedy. Before any action is taken, however, notice should be given to the person responsible for the condition to permit correction of the condition. If action is not taken, summary abatement is necessary. Persons correcting the nuisance must proceed with caution because they are personally liable for their acts. Courts have held that summary action must be reasonable. If the person responsible for the condition should elect to sue the individual who undertook the summary abatement, the disposition of the case would depend on whether the action taken was reasonable.

CITY HEALTH DEPARTMENTS IN THE UNITED STATES

In the early development of official health agencies in the United States, it was the city health department that was most in evidence. Baltimore established the first city health department in the United States in 1798. Virtually all cities by the mid-twentieth century had a health department of some description. In the smaller towns the department consisted of a part-time health officer, a quarantine officer, a sanitarian, and a clerk. Activities consisted largely in enforcing isolation and quarantine in communicable disease control and in the inspection of unsanitary conditions. Some small communities still have part-time health officers who are not trained in public health, who are political appointees, and who regard their health duties as a sideline to their medical practice. They have neither the time nor the inclination to carry out the many necessary health duties, and they sometimes use their official position to promote their private practice. Fortunately, this is giving way to complete, professionally staffed health departments.

Large cities maintain well-qualified health staffs with a director, nurses, sanitarians, sanitary engineers, laboratory technicians, health educators, and other highly specialized personnel, such as experts in air quality control. The Washington, D.C., health agency is equivalent to a city as well as state health department. In many situations city health departments are consolidating with county health departments. A city of 30,000 people in a county of 70,000 will usually depend on a county health department rather than have its own separate department. Yet some cities still retain their health departments, which have programs similar to those of the county departments. Baltimore still has its city health department because the surrounding county is politically separate and does not include the city. What will be said later about the program and services of county health departments applies equally to full-time, professionally staffed city health departments.

COUNTY BOARDS OF HEALTH IN THE UNITED STATES

Authority to establish a board of health and a health program in the United States is delegated by the state legislature to the legislation body of the county or parish, the county board of supervisors, county board of commissioners, or other title. State statutes may specify how the county health board is to be chosen and the number of people to be on the board. The county board of supervisors (or commissioners) usually appoints the county board of health. In some instances a county supervisor or commissioner may be appointed to the county board of health. This arrangement can provide a coordination between the board of supervisors and the board of health. In other states the members of the county board of health must be from outside the membership of the supervisors.

Organization

A county board of health may be composed of five, seven, nine, or any other number of members. Too small a membership may not provide adequate representation of the diverse public interests, and too large a number of members may create a debating assembly. Length of term of office varies from 3 to 6 years, and terms are staggered to provide for

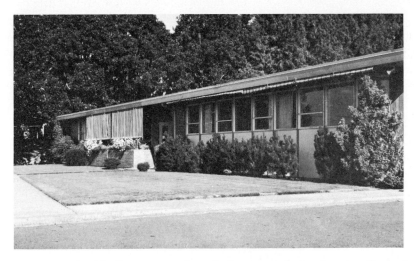

FIG. 19-1. A county health department. These facilities provide for the 60 staff members of the health department of a small county of 150,000 people.

continuity as well as replacement. Many segments of the population are represented on the board so that a cross section of the population is represented. At least one physician is usually on the board, but no one profession should dominate the membership. A chairman is elected by the board from among its own members. The county health office usually serves as an ex officio member or as executive secretary of the board.

Board responsibilities. Health authority in the county is vested in the county board of health. In many instances this authority will not extend over cities in the county that have their own full-time professional health department. The board has administrative, legislative, and quasi-judicial functions.

The board appoints a director of the county health department, a "health officer," to whom most *administrative* functions are delegated, including the recommendation of professional staff for board approval. The director is usually a medical doctor with professional preparation in public health. Increasingly, nonmedical directors are being appointed. The board also passes on the budget, as recommended by the

director, and then sends the budget to the board of supervisors for approval. The board of supervisors has responsibility for the entire county budget, including that portion relating to health.

Legislative functions of the county board of health begin with the adoption of a county sanitary code. This code is the recommendation of the professional staff and is usually the state sanitary code modified to fit the county situation. The county can have more rigid standards than the state, but not less rigid. This county code has the effect of law and will be amended by the board from time to time as conditions require.

Quasi-judicial powers of the county board of health are inherent in the authority of the board to hold hearings preliminary to granting or revoking a license. The board has the authority to summon people to appear before it in cases where health regulations have been violated. Any decision by the board may be appealed to the courts by any citizen who believes that the decision was unjust.

Staff and finances. The health program of the county is carried on by salaried professional personnel. Size of the staff depends on the territorial area of the county, the population, special health problems, resources of the county, and the public's view of the importance of the work of the health department. No rule of thumb exists, but a general guide for professional staff can be represented somewhat as follows:

One health director	per	50,000 people
One public health nurse	per	6,000 people
One psychiatrist	per	50,000 people
One psychologist	per	50,000 people
One psychiatric social worker	per	50,000 people
One public health sanitarian	per	15,000 people
One public health educator	per	50,000 people
One laboratory technician	per	40,000 people
One public health dentist	per	100,000 people

Employment of an administrative assistant is economically sound because it relieves the director of many routine, time-consuming tasks. This action would increase the number of people the director could serve from 50,000 to 75,000.

For economic reasons, a population of 50,000 is regarded as the minimum unit for which a health department should be established. Smaller counties either contract for services from the state or unite two or more sparsely populated counties into a district health unit to have a population in the order of 50,000. Using a minimum of $7 per capita per annum and a population of 50,000, a minimum staff and budget could be proposed.

Personnel	Salary	Expense
One director	$ 50,000	$ 4,000
Eight nurses	130,000	14,000
One laboratory technician	15,000	2,000
Two sanitarians	35,000	8,000
One health educator	25,000	5,000
Two clerks	20,000	
Office		18,000
Quarters		10,000
Miscellaneous		14,000
TOTAL	$350,000	

This budget represents a minimum per capita appropriation. Acceptable and adequate funding will depend on the problems of the community and the public's definition of their acceptability and their causes.

Staff functions

Direct health services to the people of the community are provided by the full-time professional staff. General and specific services vary greatly from county to county within a state and in counties from one state to another. State legislatures may require county health officials to perform certain special services. For example, one state requires county health directors to make medical investigations of deaths and to make investigations of the "battered child" cases. In many instances two county health departments will be giving the same service but under two different titles. One health department may give family health service and another health department may be giving the same service as maternal and child health service.

To cite all types of services given by county health departments would be to make an interminable list of unusual, rare, and minor services, as well as essential services. Services listed here are those that are quite generally accepted as the core of county health services. While each county health department has its own particular program, virtually all full-time county health departments carry on the following essential, highly important health services: (1) vital statistics, (2) communicable disease control, (3) promotion of maternal and child health, (4) promotion of dental health, (5) chronic disease control, (6) mental health promotion, (7) environmental health promotion, (8) laboratory service, and (9) health education.

Vital statistics. Biostatistics, public health statistics, human biometrics, and other terms are used to designate public health recordkeeping. Vital statistics consists of the application of statistical methods to the vital facts of human existence. For the health staff, vital statistics

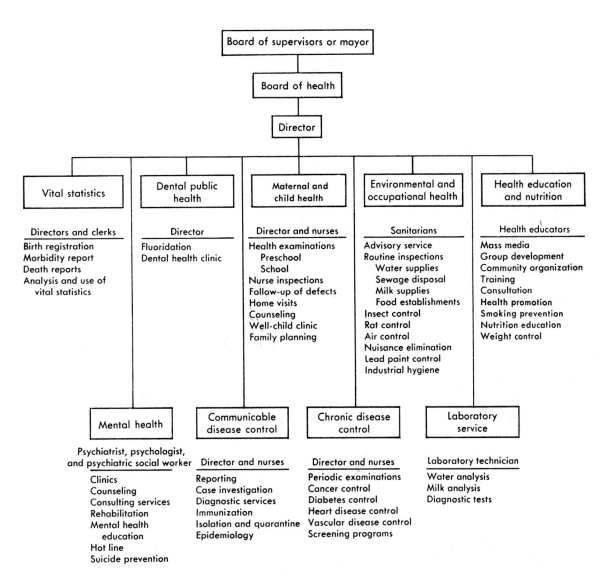

FIG. 19-2. Organization and services of a city or county health department. Many variations in health department organization exist and services vary from one health department to another, but the services listed in this chart represent the core of local health department activities.

point out the health needs of the city or county as well as the strengths and weaknesses of the health program. Health data are obtained by registration and enumeration.

Registration of certain health information is required by law and health regulations. Physicians must report to the health department cases of certain communicable diseases. To make reporting easy, health departments provide all physicians with a simple form on which the physician can quickly record pertinent data and mail postage-free to the health department. Birth and death records usually come to the county health department from the county clerk.

Enumeration of health data usually requires that the health staff actually collect information. Health examinations, dental examinations, and water samples provide important information. Special surveys and studies also provide information regarded as important by the health staff.

Health statistics are not an end in themselves but are a means to an end. They can picture health conditions, health levels, health needs, and health problems. Certain rates per year are of particular health significance.

1. Birthrate is the number of live births per 1,000 of the population in a year.

$$\frac{\text{Number of live births}}{\text{Population}} \times 1{,}000 = \text{Birthrate}$$

2. General, or crude, death rate is the number of deaths per 1,000 of the population.

$$\frac{\text{Number of deaths}}{\text{Population}} \times 1{,}000 = \text{Death rate}$$

3. Infant mortality rate is the number of deaths under 1 year of age per 1,000 live births in the same year.

$$\frac{\text{Number of deaths under 1 year}}{\text{Number of live births}} \times 1{,}000$$
$$= \text{Infant mortality rate}$$

4. Maternal mortality rate is the number of deaths of mothers from childbirth per 10,000 live births in the same year.

$$\frac{\text{Number of deaths of mothers (from childbirth)}}{\text{Number of live births}}$$
$$\times 10{,}000 = \text{Maternal mortality rate}$$

5. Specific mortality rate is the number of deaths for a specific cause (or age group) per 100,000 population.

$$\frac{\text{Number of deaths (specific cause)}}{\text{Population}} \times 100{,}000$$
$$= \text{Specific mortality rate}$$

6. Case fatality rate is the number of deaths from a specific cause to the number of cases and is always expressed as a percent.

$$\frac{\text{Number of deaths from a specific cause}}{\text{Number of cases of the cause}} \times 100$$
$$= \text{Case fatality rate (\%)}$$

Other rates are also calculated to obtain an accurate picture of vital facts of health significance, such as marriage rates and divorce rates. Net and gross reproduction rates can be meaningful in terms of population directions. Within populations, rates for selected factors and for specific age, sex, and racial groups may have significance.

Rates will be affected by many variables that must be considered in interpreting the significance of a particular rate. For example, a particular "retirement" county in Florida had a low birthrate and a high death rate, understandable when one studies the age distribution of the population and finds a disproportionate concentration of older age people.

Communicable disease control. Constant vigilance is necessary to hold communicable diseases to a minimum. Programs can be planned and effectively administered so that epidemics do not occur and the number of outbreaks of communicable disease is held to a minimum. Such a program requires certain preventive measures: (1) immunization, (2) public health education, (3) protection of water, milk, and other food supplies, (4) promotion of sanitation, and (5) control of carriers. Control measures must concentrate on infected persons and their environment: (1) recognition of the disease, (2) prompt reporting of all cases, (3) isolation procedures, (4) quarantine when warranted, and (5) decontamination. Most city and county health departments provide immunization service. Others at least provide biologicals to be administered by private practitioners.

Promotion of maternal and child health. A public health nurse is a family health counselor. In some community health departments the nurse is given this title. The public health nurse does no bedside or hospital nursing except as a demonstration for the instruction of some member of the family or in an emergency. The health nurse is the key person in maternal and infant health.

In maternal health promotion, certain *direct* means are taken in behalf of the health of expectant mothers, the fetus, and the expected infant.

1. Promotion of prenatal care through early medical examination, prevention and correction of impairments, proper rest, proper nutrition, moderate exercise, sunshine, and avoidance of fatigue, alcohol, smoking, drugs, and infection
2. Adequate delivery facilities in a hospital or home
3. Obstetrical and nurse-midwifery services
4. Postnatal care

Similarly, there are certain *indirect* means for promoting maternal health.

1. Public education and health education for other family members
2. Laws governing employment of women
3. Medical and hospital insurance with maternity benefits
4. Improvement of socioeconomic and environmental conditions

Infant health must begin with the education of the parents in the importance of considering all factors affecting infant well-being. In addition, the public health nurse must assist parents in understanding the particular health needs and health problems of the infant, encourage the parents to have the infant examined at regular intervals by a physician, help

secure medical diagnosis and treatment for the infant when such needs are indicated, and teach the mother care of the infant, including good nutrition, feeding, and parenting practices. The public health nurse can serve as a liaison between the family and the pediatrician or well-child clinic of the health department.

Many agencies, including the school, contribute to child health, and the county health department has an obligation to cooperate with all recognized agencies contributing to child health. This is in the best interests of the child. The health department contributes more directly to child health through the following activities of the public health nurse:

1. Counseling parents on health matters relating to children
2. Assisting parents in understanding the health needs and conditions of their children
3. Urging parents to have children receive a health examination at regular intervals and to complete their immunization series
4. Helping parents in securing medical services for diagnosis and treatment of illness in the family
5. Helping families to carry out essential sanitary and other health measures
6. Teaching home nursing and parenting skills to members of the family
7. Supervising family members who care for the ill children in the home
8. Assisting in improving social conditions that affect health
9. Recognizing and reporting signs of child abuse

Family planning. As an example of guidelines for a specific, high-priority program area, the recommendations of the Planned Parenthood Federation for family planning programs are more generally instructive:

1. Expand family planning services— through hospitals, health departments, private physicians, welfare agencies, Planned Parenthood and other voluntary

agencies, and antipoverty groups—to reach seven out of eight poor American women still denied these services.

2. Direct priority attention to incorporating effective services in existing big city health facilities and adding satellite clinics to serve outlying neighborhoods. Programs should also be initiated to deliver services in rural areas.

3. Priority should be given to development of convenient, familiar, and accessible services in or near officially designated "poverty" neighborhoods.

4. Services should not be directed exclusively to any ethnic or racial group. Emphasis on services for blacks alone, for example, will fail to reach the bulk of the population in need and may feed the suspicion that family planning advocates seek to reduce their numbers rather than to meet essential health needs.

5. Welfare referral and reimbursement programs and even Medicaid programs can meet only a small proportion of the need. Overemphasis on such programs diverts attention from needed changes in the health system to make family planning available to all of the poor.

6. Family planning clinics should be open evenings and weekends to serve working women. Adequate transportation and baby-sitting are needed for mothers who must remain home to care for young children.

7. Some of the women in need can be reached through newspapers, magazines, television, radio, and other traditional media, with information on the safety, effectiveness, and convenience of modern contraception, and where they can get help. More personalized educational methods must be emphasized for some.

8. Humiliating marital status restrictions on provision of services will fail to meet the needs of a significant number of women who are separated, widowed, divorced, or single.

9. Good follow-up procedures are feasible and will have long-term benefits for the families in need of help.

10. Family planning programs should emphasize child spacing. By delaying and spacing pregnancies, couples will have a better chance to get more education and increase family income as well as to enjoy better health. Thus family planning services should seek to reach poor couples in their early twenties or even their teens.

Some of these recommendations illustrate the general approach to preventive health delivery that should characterize all components of community health services. Similar recommendations would apply to other programs such as mental health, diabetes, hypertension, maternal and infant care, and sexually transmitted disease control.

Chronic disease control. Many if not most of the organic diseases of the late years had their genesis in middle age. Accordingly, adult health promotion gives emphasis to the middle years of life as well as to the elderly years. Indeed, preventive efforts directed toward the younger years of age can yield the most productive dividends. A constructive adult health promotional program concentrates on the following three factors:

1. Periodic screening and examination
2. Correction of all remediable disorders
3. Health education that emphasizes moderation in living, avoiding infection, diagnosing and treating infection and other symptoms immediately when they occur, exercise, proper diet, avoiding undue stress, and checking with a physician when any abnormal condition persists

Community organization on the part of the health department is called for in getting adults examined. This is particularly true in getting

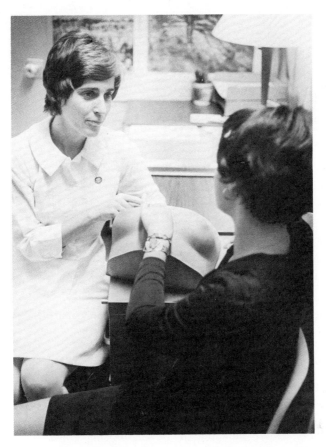

FIG. 19-3. Breast self-examination is a major strategy of the American Cancer Society and local health departments to detect early signs of breast cancer and to reduce delay in treatment. Breast self-examination is taught in clinics, classes, and women's self-help groups.

Courtesy Johns Hopkins Medical Institutions.

men examined and assuring proper follow-up of those screened. Cooperation with the medical society, industry, labor unions, and service organizations backed by a good promotional program through various media is required.

Mental health promotion. Major emphasis in mental health promotion is placed on the mental health of the normal individual. The modern mental health program offers counseling, seminars, institutes, hot lines, demonstrations, lectures, and other services. Psychiatric, psychological, and social work services are available to normal individuals, people with minor disturbances, delinquents, people with serious emotional problems, the disordered, people in the process of rehabilitation, and to groups. The mere fact that the city or county health department provides a mental health center where a person may go for consultation is extremely significant for citizens in the community. It takes experience with this service before the public uses it effectively. It will take a few more years before mental health service is accepted as a phase of community health the way immunization has been accepted as an inherent service of the health department.

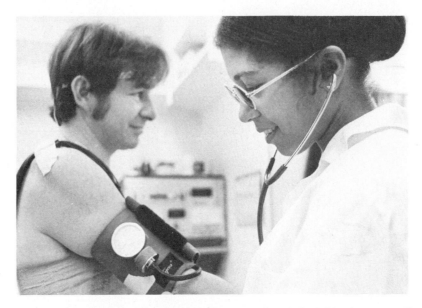

FIG. 19-4. Hypertension screening programs attempt to identify high blood pressure through special clinics and readings taken at fairs, work sites, and home visits. Only about 50% of the detected cases are followed up adequately in treatment.

Courtesy Johns Hopkins Medical Institutions.

Environmental health promotion. Sanitarians are primarily occupied with public sanitation but provide consulting services when requested by householders. Home sanitation is encouraged through continuous educational measures. Most of the sanitarian's time and attention is directed to the inspection and appraisal of public water supplies, milk and milk products, sewage disposal, public buildings, swimming pools, insect infestation, industrial operations, and nuisances. Preventing disease is the primary goal of the sanitation program, but promotion of an esthetic environment is usually a secondary benefit.

Laboratory service. Most health departments in low-census counties do not have their own laboratories but depend on the centralized laboratory of the state health department or a local laboratory in a hospital or a clinic. Water plant operators are usually competent to run bacteriological examinations of water. Even without its own laboratory a county health department can improvise sufficiently to provide limited laboratory service.

Having a county health department laboratory has many advantages in convenience and reduced time for running laboratory tests. Communicable disease control by means of laboratory tests requires promptness. Diagnostic tests, water and milk examinations, and food contamination tests can be done promptly in the county health department laboratory. When the health department supplies immunizations, the laboratory technicians keep the biologicals in stock and assume responsibility for dispensing them.

Health education. The base of the pyramid called community health is public health education, and the breadth and stability of the base largely determines the height to which the pyramid can rise. Health education is effective to the extent that it constructively affects people's health knowledge, health attitudes, and health practices. To be effective, public health educa-

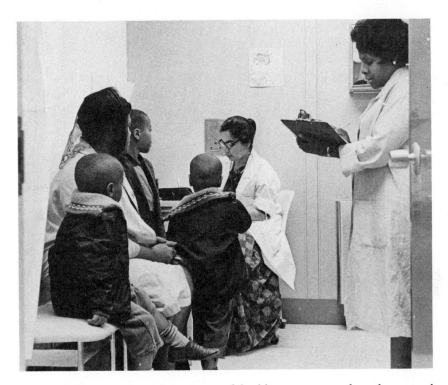

FIG. 19-5. Ambulatory care, primary care, and health maintenance through maternal and child health, children and youth, family health, and related clinical services are central to community health.

Courtesy Johns Hopkins Medical Institutions.

tion must get public *acceptance* of a program or practice, arouse a *desire* in people to benefit by it, and obtain *involvement* of the people.

Effective public health education is directed to different segments of the population for different purposes. Communications directly with those whose health behavior places them at risk are designed to inform and gain their acceptance of a program or practice and to increase their motivation to benefit by it. Communications indirectly through parents, teachers, officials, employers, and peers are designed to provide a supportive social environment and reinforcement for the behavior. Communications directed to organizations, such as parent-teacher associations, service clubs, church groups, labor unions, health

agencies, insurance companies, child study organizations, parent groups, and neighborhood organizations are designed to enable and facilitate the behavior by organizing community resources required for the health behavior to occur.

Public health education is beset with many obstacles, particularly false advertising, quackery, cultism, attitude toward health, superstition, professional indifference, and the human tendency to seek the easiest solution to every health problem. Yet a well-organized and effectively administered community health education program can be highly effective and can have a substantial influence on the community's health.

The head of the community health education

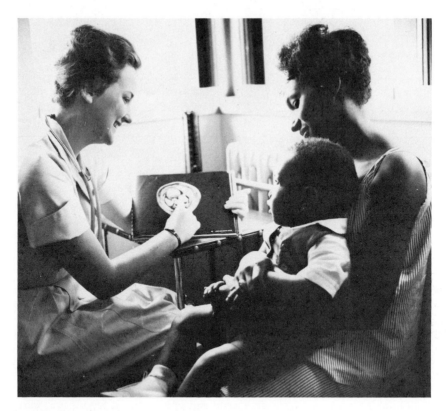

FIG. 19-6. Health education in prenatal care and other clinical services complements the home visits of public health nurses and the community organization and mass communications efforts coordinated by the community health educator.

Courtesy Johns Hopkins Medical Institutions.

program is a professionally prepared community health educator. This person supervises a number of organized units and individuals who have contributions to make. All members of the local health department staff properly are engaged in health education as part of their professional activities. The health educator coordinates the educational efforts of the staff, provides consultation, and initiates action that will involve other staff members of the department as well as other agencies in the community.

In addition to the health department, the voluntary health agencies, child health councils, schools, medical society, dental society, and a number of other organizations in the city or county have contributions to make to health education. It requires imaginative, sensitive, and persistent leadership to get all of these organizations and individuals contributing in a coordinated way so that the health education program is effective and consistent.

Numerous services and materials constitute the methods used in community health education. Each medium makes its own contribution, but it is the composite effect of a coordinated program that achieves the goal of a health-educated public.

Services

Speaker's bureau (including others in addition to
   the health department staff)
Demonstrations
Seminars
Conferences
Health councils
Exhibits and health fairs
In-service education for teachers and others
Community organization
Consultation to health practitioners
Self-care discussion groups
Telephone hot lines and "dial-a-message" services
Smoking cessation groups
Weight control groups
Prenatal and parenting groups

Materials

Bulletins
Pamphlets
Newsletters
Health hazard appraisals
Self-tests
Minicomputers
Films
Individual letters
Newspaper articles
Radio programs
Television interviews
Special reports for the media
Annual reports

Not indiscriminate use of every conceivable gimmick or device, but the considered use of the most effective means for obtaining specific health objectives is the scientific and professional discipline of health education.

Health education of the public is a continuous process. While some circumstances occasion a justifiable "blitz" program, these are of value only as they are part of the overall, year-round, continuing public health education program.

   Other county health department services. Either through legislative requirement, local pressure, custom, or even coincidence, a county health department may be engaged in one or more unique services not included in the usual list of responsibilities. Some county health departments are responsible for the medical investigation of deaths of unknown cause. "Battered child" cases may be referred to the health department. Inspection of foster care homes is an activity of some county health departments. Speech therapy, occupational and physical therapy, rehabilitation, and medical questions relating to commitment to mental hospitals are but some of the unique activities of different county health departments. Someone must perform these services, but if these activities interfere with the effective performance of the basic public health functions of the department, the public may lose more in health protection than it gains in social services.

Community health council

   On the county level, health councils have been valuable in coordinating the health services of various agencies and individuals. Health councils are usually not official organizations but are voluntary and composed of representatives from various organizations and groups having special health interests or needs. Councils may vary from 10 to 30 in membership, with representatives from such groups as voluntary health agencies, medical profession, dental profession, parent-teacher organizations, labor unions, chambers of commerce, women's clubs, church groups, social agencies, and various other groups. The council usually represents a cross-section of the population and can make known the health needs of the people. It can make recommendations to the county health department and can be called on to support certain activities of the department.

   A community health council can provide a valuable community service so long as it considers the overall health needs of the county and strives to assist, support, and supplement the health department. It serves as a health-promoting force in the community and provides for citizen involvement in public health.

U.S. FEDERAL SUPPORT FOR COMMUNITY HEALTH SERVICES

Most countries subsidize local health services from state or national revenues. In the United States the early stage was federal grants-in-aid to states for maternal and child health programs and to state and local governments for the establishment and development of health departments (Titles V and VI of the 1935 Social Security Act). Then came the Hill-Burton Hospital Survey and Construction Act of 1946, which assisted more than 3,800 communities to build hospitals, extended-care and rehabilitation facilities, and public health centers. The National Institutes of Health was also developed during this postwar period of federal investment, contributing over $14 billion toward the development and support of biomedical and health-related research. Support for health manpower development also began during this period, providing traineeships for public health specialists, most of whom were already employed in community health agencies but without formal training in public health.

The "years of ferment"

By the early 1960s there was considerable disillusionment with the results of these massive investments in the three major areas of national health resources—facilities, knowledge, and manpower. The United States had reached the highest level of per capita expenditures for health in the world, but American health services and health statistics rated poorly among developed nations—thirteenth among industrial countries in death of infants during the first year of life; seventh in the percentage of mothers who died in childbirth; eighteenth in the life expectancy of males and eleventh for females; and sixteenth in the death rate of males in their middle years.

It was apparent that the investment period had succeeded in building a massive health and medical care complex, but this complex had failed to adjust its structure appropriately to trends in the distribution of illness, demands for services, specialization of practitioners and medical equipment, and demands among office and hospital personnel for competitive wages. Physicians and hospitals clung tenaciously to traditions of individualism, endeavoring to be all things to their patients despite the obvious need to pool specialized facilities and services. Rural areas most notably were still without community health services. By the mid-1960s the United States had entered what Kissick (1970) called the "years of ferment" in the evolution of national health policy. Particular emphasis was placed on community health services and consumer participation in health planning.

Community mental health centers. In 1963 President Kennedy signed the Community Mental Health Centers Act. This act differed from earlier construction assistance acts in that it required centers to provide comprehensive services including outpatient care, consultation, and education. Approximately 400 community mental health centers had been established by 1970, which was significantly behind schedule for the original target of 2,000 by 1975, but the comprehensive approach required and the consequent innovations in delivery systems marked a new departure in organizational arrangements with a community education orientation. Community mental health centers form a network of comprehensive services and continuity of care for patients discharged from state psychiatric facilities, as well as preventive services for the general population.

This act provided specifically for "a State advisory council which shall include representatives of non-government organizations or groups, and of State agencies, concerned with planning, operation, or utilization of community mental health centers or other mental health facilities, *including representatives of consumers* of the services. . . ." This clause was the forerunner of more sweeping provisions for consumer participation in the Economic Opportunity Act and later legislation.

The Community Mental Health Centers Act authorized grants to public or nonprofit private agencies to assist "in the establishment and initial operation of community mental health centers providing all or part of a *comprehensive* community mental health program. . . ." Approximately 10% of staff time is spent in consultation, education, and other indirect services. By 1973 nearly 28% of all outpatient mental health episodes were seen at community mental health centers.

MCH, Mental Retardation, and Economic Opportunity Acts of 1963-1964. Also in 1963, the Maternal and Child Health and Mental Retardation Amendments provided for similarly comprehensive, community-based approaches to prenatal and postnatal services for high-risk, low-income groups. Maternity and Infant Care Projects have been funded by grants to many state and local health departments.

The most salient legislation marking the "years of ferment" was the Economic Opportunity Act of 1964. Support for research, demonstration, and training for Neighborhood Health Centers resulted in widespread experimentation with health care teams, indigenous community workers, or community health aides and—most significantly from an educational perspective—serious attention to participation of the poor in the planning and evaluation of services. By mid-1969 about 50 projects had been funded, a drop in the bucket in relation to needs and legitimate demands of the poor, but again significant in terms of the concepts demonstrated. Federal support for Neighborhood Health Centers declined in the 1970s.

Regional Medical Programs. The purposes of this 1965 law were (1) to provide federal grants to establish regional cooperative arrangements among medical schools, research institutions, and hospitals for research and training (including continuing education) and for related demonstrations of prevention and patient care in the fields of heart disease, cancer, and stroke; (2) to afford the medical profession the opportunity of making available to patients the latest advances in diagnosis and treatment; and (3) by these means to improve generally the health manpower and facilities available in the nation, ". . . without interfering with the patterns, or the methods of financing, of patient care or professional practice, or with the administration of hospitals, and in cooperation with practicing physicians, medical center officials, hospital administrators, and representatives from appropriate voluntary health agencies."

Note particularly the hesitation in this legislation to offend or challenge the medical establishment. There was no mention of official (state or local) health agencies and no mention of health professionals or paraprofessionals other than those of the hospital "establishment." The Regional Medical Programs were phased out of existence in 1976 with the development of regional Health Systems Agencies (HSAs).

Consumer participation in community health planning

Community Action Programs (CAP). The Economic Opportunity Act of 1964 moved consumer participation from a matter of voluntary action to a matter of public policy. Community action was suddenly defined in legal terms, which carried both opportunities and new obligations for the poor. "Maximum feasible participation" was further legislated in Public Law 89-749 in 1965 (authorizing the establishment of Comprehensive Health Planning Agencies) and in the Model Cities Demonstration Act of 1966. The concept has survived a variety of setbacks and assaults (Green, 1975; Partridge, 1973; Wang, et al., 1975).

For all of the good intentions behind the

consumer participation movement, its legislated implementation was misunderstood or mistrusted by many professionals and consumers. The "Maximum feasible misunderstanding" created by the law was summarized by Moynihan (1969, p. 11):

> Community action was originally seen as a means of shaping unorganized and even disorganized city dwellers into a coherent and self-conscious group, if necessary by techniques of protest and opposition to established authority. Somehow, however, the higher civil service came to see it as a means for coordinating at the community level the array of conflicting and overlapping departmental programs that proceeded from Washington. . . .

The co-optation of consumer participants in managerial functions undermined the intent of the legislation and left many volunteer participants feeling exploited and suspicious of governmental purposes. If other consumer initiatives in health become similarly enmeshed in governmental relations with health care providers and agencies, they are likely to take a different form, or at least a different flavor for the consumer, than they now take. This caution has special meaning in relation to activities in which voluntary participation of consumers becomes qualitatively a different experience when it is required by law.

The lesson from governmental implementation of maximum feasible participation laws is not necessarily that governmental support should not be offered to voluntary programs but that it should be offered with carefully designed safeguards for the voluntary character of the programs.

National Health Planning and Resources Development Act of 1974. Under a later federal health planning program, consumers participated in local and state efforts to correct many deficiencies and inequities in the delivery of health care. Public Law 93-641, the National Health Planning and Resources Development Act of 1974, provided for a majority of consumers (51% to 60%) to serve on two major planning bodies—the more than 200 HSAs and the Statewide Health Coordinating Councils. These bodies, together with the State Health Planning and Development Agencies, have broad authority over the allocation and development of health resources, including manpower, facilities, and services.

Virtually everyone is a "consumer" of health care—if not of personal medical services, then certainly of those preventive services that help one stay healthy. As used here, "consumer" refers to an individual who has not been a provider of health services for the preceding 12 months. Such a person is eligible to serve as a consumer on the governing bodies of HSAs and on Statewide Health Coordinating Councils.

If the health-planning program survives the proposed phaseout of HSAs by the Reagan Administration, consumers will be contributing to decisions that help produce a more rational, responsive, effective, and equitable health care system. Good planning can, for example, help change the emphasis in health care from crisis intervention for the cure of sick patients to a well-thought-out program of prevention and health maintenance. Consumers can help restrain hospitals in acquiring expensive equipment—the community may not need all the available technology. Other problems also can be alleviated through more effective planning for the production and use of community health resources and services. Consider, for example, the following facts concerning the present U.S. system of health care.

- In general, inner-city areas and remote rural sections are served by too few physicians.
- Primary care is often available only after long waits in crowded waiting rooms or after driving long distances to see a physician.
- The affluent areas of cities may be building more hospitals than needed.
- The costs of medical care have been rising rapidly. Part of this rise in health care costs is attributable to the poor location of health

care facilities and the costs of staffing and equipping these facilities.

Aside from correcting some of the more gross deficiencies in the health care system, such as these, an active consumer leadership in health planning can help produce a more immediate and tangible impact on patients through improved service and staffing patterns, more equitable fees, a mechanism to respond to patient grievances, improved physical facilities, and, above all, care that protects the dignity and well-being of the individual patient.

Moreover, for the individual consumer participating in health planning, there are also benefits beyond promoting improvements in the health care system. Many consumers who have served on planning boards in the past report a deep sense of personal involvement that has enriched their lives. Others found they had increased their effectiveness in other community activities.

Individuals who report dissatisfaction with consumer participation usually mention the difficulty of finding the time and acquiring the training necessary to do a good job. Consumers, for example, have reported that being a representative took more time, effort, and knowledge than they expected.

In one respect, health planning is an educational process for the community. It is a way of making citizens and public officials as well as providers of health care aware of better ways of allocating health resources. By adding a non-provider perspective, consumers can help create a climate in which community interests take precedence over special interests.

Some idea of the complexity of the planning process nationwide can be seen from the following description of the major components established under the National Health Planning and Resources Development Act of 1974. Familiarity with the broad outlines of this program is necessary before one can even begin to think constructively about participation.

Health Systems Agency (HSA). The HSA is the local or regional planning agency under Public Law 93-641. One HSA is designated for each of more than 200 health service areas throughout the United States. A health service area is a geographic region appropriate for the effective planning and development of health services, designated by the state governor on the basis of such factors as population and the availability of resources to provide necessary health services for residents in the area.

Each HSA gathers and analyzes health data and prepares a Health Systems Plan or detailed statement of goals for improving the health of its residents and increasing the accessibility, continuity, and quality of health services, while restraining costs. In addition, it must develop an annual implementation plan, setting forth its objectives for attaining those goals and priorities among those objectives.

The HSA must review the appropriateness of services provided by hospitals, nursing homes, and other health institutions within the area. It also recommends approval or disapproval of applications for new health service or medical facilities projects. The HSA also reviews and approves or disapproves proposed projects within the health service area under several federal health programs. It is this last function, the approval and disapproval of new or expanded facilities and programs, that makes the HSAs a target for termination in the plans of the anti-regulatory Reagan Administration.

VOLUNTARY HEALTH AGENCIES IN THE UNITED STATES

Non-tax-supported, voluntary health agencies provide opportunities for people to fulfill their needs beyond what official agencies provide. These voluntary health organizations have pioneered in promoting health programs and in demonstrating what can be done. Frequently, when a voluntary health organization demonstrates what can be done, the official health agencies then enter the field and supplement what the voluntary health organization does.

Two types of voluntary health agencies—

professional health organizations and health foundations—will be discussed in Chapter 21 because these have relatively fewer local affiliates to provide direct support to community health programs.

Background

In the late nineteenth and early twentieth centuries, governmental agencies were slow to recognize existing health problems and the need to use available means for dealing with these problems and to develop new measures for disease prevention and control. Voluntary agencies were organized in response to the recognized need to take action dealing with the problems of disease, to use all available means for solving problems of disease prevention and control, and to develop new measures. Many such organizations have been formed, several of which will be discussed as representative of the types of voluntary health agencies that have served the public over the past half century or more at both national and community levels.

Examples

The American Lung Association. Founded in 1904 as the National Tuberculosis and Respiratory Disease Association, the American Lung Association was the first voluntary agency of the educational, promotional type. From the outset, education has been the foundation of this association's program, based on the premise that, while it is essential to extend knowledge through scientific research, such knowledge is of little value unless it is available to the public, medical practitioners, health personnel, and patients.

With the tuberculosis problem largely under control, the American Lung Association is directing much of its attention and efforts to the problem of emphysema and other disorders of the chest. Some state associations have a subsidiary Thoracic Society composed of physicians who are specialists in thoracic diseases.

From the outset, the association's program has operated primarily on the community level. In part this has been responsible for much of the success of the program. The state association or chapter has supervision over the local units. Financing of the association's program has been through Christmas seal campaigns, and more people have contributed to this program than to any similar philanthropical enterprise. At no time has the association paid medical or hospital costs for patients with tuberculosis, emphysema, or other chronic lung diseases. The American Lung Association has had an intensive and extensive research program. This research is not limited to tuberculosis but includes research in various diseases of the chest.

The March of Dimes Birth Defects Foundation. Formerly known as the National Foundation for Infantile Paralysis, the March of Dimes Birth Defects Foundation was founded in 1938. President Franklin D. Roosevelt, stricken by poliomyelitis, gave his personal support to the foundation and thereby gave great impetus to the organization. From its start, the foundation has been financed through the March of Dimes Program. Several state chapters and more than 900 local chapters reach into virtually every county in the United States with programs now concentrated on birth defects.

In 1958 the organization shortened its name to the National Foundation and its objectives were expanded to become "an organized force for medical research, patient care and professional education, flexible enough to meet new health problems as they arise." The present program includes investigation into birth defects (congenital defects) and genetic and nutritional disorders associated with birth.

Local chapters that are branches of the national organization give direct medical assistance and raise funds to maintain national and local activities. A considerable part of the funds raised locally remains in the community to promote the local program.

Financial assistance from the March of Dimes was instrumental in demonstrating the effectiveness of the Salk vaccine in the 1954

Poliomyelitis Vaccine Field Trial. This resulted in the shortest elapsed time between the discovery of a preventive measure and its widespread use.

The American Cancer Society, Inc. The American Cancer Society, Inc. was founded in 1913 "to disseminate knowledge concerning the symptoms, diagnosis, treatment, and prevention of cancer; to investigate the conditions under which cancer is found; and to compile statistics in regard thereto." The society was established largely through the efforts of medical persons, although the work of the organization has been carried on largely by laypeople.

The leadoff educational program was designed to acquaint the public with the fact that early cancer can be cured, that early diagnosis is of primary importance, and that prompt, scientific treatment is the acknowledged method of cure. The educational campaign used an impersonal approach in the effort to avoid arousing fear of cancer.

In addition to public health education, the society encouraged health departments to expand their cancer programs, stimulated medical schools to extend their work in cancer, helped to organize a National Advisory Cancer Council, and influenced the passage of the National Cancer Act and the creation of the National Cancer Institute as a part of the U.S. Public Health Service.

The state organization is called a division and, as an example, is titled American Cancer Society, Inc., Michigan Division. Operation of the program is basically on the county level and is controlled and supervised by the local medical profession. The women's auxiliary group enlists the active participation of laypeople in a program of health education.

Income of the American Cancer Society, Inc., is derived from donations, dues, endowments, and legacies. In many instances citizens losing a family member because of cancer assign life insurance benefits to the society. The official publication of the society is *CA—A Bulletin of Cancer Progress*. This is a publica-

tion for members of the professions dealing with cancer.

The American Heart Association. Originally formed as a scientific and professional organization of physicians interested in heart disease, the American Heart Association in 1948 was reorganized as a voluntary health agency with thousands of nonprofessional members. The objective of the association is to prevent and control heart disease through research, professional education, public education, and community service.

Each state has a state heart association and county heart councils. A large corps of volunteers composed of physicians and laymen work together to plan and execute the association's programs. The state heart association has a professional staff, which provides consultation services and works with the volunteers in planning and implementing both the education and fund-raising aspects of the program.

Through community service, the association provides training of volunteers in blood pressure measurement. It provides rheumatic fever control programs to prevent secondary attacks in individuals who have had a first attack. It also provides smoking cessation, nutrition, and weight control programs; a Speaker's Bureau; a school health program; and a work simplification program, which demonstrates methods to help housekeepers to organize their work in a manner that will prevent unnecessary fatigue. The association also maintains an information and referral service, which is a directory of cardiac services. Throughout, the American Heart Association works through and with physicians by making services available to the physician and to the patient as the physician requests.

Funds are raised by state drives and come from voluntary contributions, endowments, and legacies. At times people losing a family member because of heart disease will turn insurance benefits over to the state heart association. Most of the American Heart Association funds go into heart research or an allied activity.

The Red Cross. The American Red Cross has a quasi-governmental status because it is incorporated under a charter granted by Congress. The President of the United States is president of the American Red Cross, which is an affiliate of the international organization.

The Red Cross was founded in 1881 in accordance with the Geneva Treaty of 1864, which was ratified by the United States in 1882. The Red Cross provides relief services during wartime and other disasters. In times of peace the American affiliate has established health centers, helped to conduct public health surveys, sponsored health demonstration projects and first aid and water safety programs, and provided public health nursing service for rural areas that were otherwise not served. In 1981 the American Red Cross adopted a new set of priorities emphasizing health promotion and disease prevention.

It is an established policy of the Red Cross to work closely with private and governmental agencies at all levels—national, state, and community. County chapters are formed but operate under the supervision of the national office, which establishes policies and must approve all local projects.

National Urban League. Health has been a core program activity of the National Urban League since 1910. The 70-year experience of the "health program" has fluctuated between being a separate division for health with its own specially funded projects and at other times an adjunct of the Social Welfare Division. During the early years the National Urban League published a monthly health education bulletin and for more than 20 years stimulated local efforts such as dental clinics, immunization programs, tuberculosis screening, well-baby clinics, and a variety of convalescent care programs through its Annual Health Education Week.

Frustrated in its attempt to remove discrimination in employment in the health profession and in health facilities, the National Urban League, led by Dr. Montague Cobb, joined forces with the National Medical Association, the NAACP, and the Medico-Chirurgical Society. This coalition became known as Imhotep and spearheaded a vigorous attack on hospital discrimination between the late 1950s and the mid-1960s. In 1965 the National Urban League Health Committee published *Health Care in the Negro Population*, reporting its findings of this period and its recommendations for the future.

In 1962, based on initial experience in family planning and sex education, the National Urban League Board of Trustees adopted a policy statement supportive of family planning in the interest of strengthening family life and reducing individual and family dependency. This was a courageous move at a time when family planning was viewed by some black activists as genocide.

The league has administered a number of federally funded research and demonstration programs in the health field. These projects have included an evaluation of consumer health education and training programs, a study of health manpower resources and facilities in 30 cities, a National Urban League Poison Control Project, the development of allied health careers curriculum in the traditionally black colleges, dental services for preschool children, and a sickle-cell education and screening program.

The National Urban League is firmly on record in support of comprehensive-universal national health insurance, the Child Health Assurance Program, and improving health services in local communities. The league continues to address these crucial programs through public testimony and participation in organized, broad-based coalitions.

The issue most disturbing and threatening to the health of black and poor people, however, is the national strategy to reduce health care cost by closing down public general hospitals in inner-city communities. Increased efforts to inform and assist affiliates to respond to local initiatives in this direction and to rally support for new legislation to address the special needs of inner-city public general hospitals have been recent priorities of the National Urban League.

The Preparing Adolescents for Responsible Parenthood Project has been the centerpiece to the national office's concern with the increase of pregnancies among black and other minority teenagers. Its importance has been increased by the Supreme Court's ruling that neither the Medicaid statute nor the Constitution require the federal government or states to provide funding for all medically necessary abortion services. It has been estimated that 35% of women receiving Aid to Families with Dependent Children (AFDC) who would have had abortions financed by Medicaid will now go full term with their pregnancies. Many of these will be young teenagers, ages 12 to 16, who are least capable emotionally, physically, or economically to be parents. The National Urban League project seeks to increase the quality and quantity of information and services, both preventive and supportive, available to minority youth.

Health promotion and health education directed at disease prevention and early detection will represent a major programmatic direction of the National Urban League in the 1980s. This move is entirely consistent with the current national strategy toward improved personal health management. It does not, however, minimize the reality that the poor health status of black Americans requires increased medical services and programs for health restoration. Rather, the National Urban League health promotion plan is an attempt to ensure that black communities benefit from a total range and mixture of health approaches. It further seeks to identify appropriate roles for nonmedical community-based organizations in the provision of community health care.

To accomplish this, the National Urban League has identified health promotion and disease prevention as the area in which nonmedical community-based organizations can plan a significant and strategic role in im-

proving the health status of black Americans. Organized programs in local affiliates and at the national office that are centered on health advocacy and health promotion activities are realistic for National Urban League affiliates with limited health personnel and financial resources. Toward these ends the national office has been attempting to ensure that new health legislation and special federal initiatives addressing community health education and disease prevention provide for the participation of nonmedical community-based organizations. Thus future health programs such as high blood pressure education, cancer education and screening, physical fitness, and nutrition all provide for local outreach information and education activity. Community-based organizations such as National Urban League affiliates can qualify to operate funded programs in these areas. Funding, for the most part, must be obtained at the state level. This makes it particularly important for local affiliates of such organizations to stay abreast of comprehensive statewide planning and the allocation of health funds through block grants at the state level.

SCHOOL HEALTH PROGRAM

The school health program properly should be considered as part of the public health program and thus be integrated with it. Not only the health of the children, but also the health of the home and the health of the community should be the concern of the school, because the school can contribute to all three.

Scope of a school health program. Six basic policies point up the role of a school health program.

1. To provide for healthful school living through standards for safety and sanitation, adequate food service, maintenance of teacher's health, and promotion of mental and emotional health of teachers and pupils

2. To provide health instruction in the entire curriculum, especially in courses designed for the elementary, junior, and se-

nior high schools, and through school participation in community health education

3. To provide services for health protection and improvement through first aid for emergencies, prevention and control of communicable disease, and health appraisal, guidance, and assistance

4. To emphasize the fitness and hygienic aspects of physical education, to seek to adapt programs to individual needs, to secure adequate activity programs, and to develop health safeguards in athletics

5. To designate the education and care of handicapped persons through identification of the need, adjustment of programs, adjustment of individuals, special classes, and properly prepared teachers

6. To denote the needed qualifications of health education personnel

These policies are usually translated into a school health program of health services, health instruction, and healthful living.

Health services deal with the present health of the school youngster and have three aspects. The first is health *appraisal,* consisting of health examinations, teacher health assessment, vision screening, hearing testing, height and weight determinations, health guidance and supervision, and teacher health. The second is *preventive* aspects, which consist of communicable disease control, safety, emergency care, and first aid. The third is *remedial* aspects, consisting of the follow-up services, correction of remediable defects, practitioner services, and school remedial functions.

Health instruction includes planned instruction, correlated instruction, integrated learning, and incidental instruction. Health education through all possible experiences is the objective of health instruction.

Healthful environment includes a sanitary and safe physical environment but also incorporates consideration of the mental health of students and teachers. It is represented in practices that promote the highest level of physical and mental health.

An effective school health program requires elementary school teachers who have preparation in health services, health instruction, and healthful environment; certified secondary school health teachers who have specialized in health; and a school health director who has a master's degree in health education. Above all, to have an effective health program a school must have administrators who understand health and provide leadership, counsel, and encouragement for all people involved in the school health program. This properly means everyone in the school.

APPRAISAL OF COMMUNITY HEALTH SERVICES

It is difficult to measure the effectiveness or value of a community health program in terms of lives saved, illnesses prevented, and health improved. There are inferential means of appraising a health program based on the assumption that, if certain activities or services are provided by a health staff, it can be inferred that certain health benefits accrue to the public. This inference is based on independent studies, which have shown that certain services and activities produced certain public health results. This approach to appraisal is simply an accounting of services rendered. A considerable segment of the public health profession prefers to specify the services a health department should provide and contends that appraisal *should* be based on the proficiency with which the health staff performs these services. This approach to evaluation is called quality assurance or quality control.

Full-time county health departments provide a direct health service available to all citizens within the respective county. It provides the various means for reducing the incidence of disease, lowering the death rate, reducing invalidism and dependency, preventing disabilities, correcting remediable defects, decreasing wage losses, reducing hospital and medical costs, and reducing hazards to health and life. Some agencies attempt to get periodic measures of these outcomes to appraise their programs.

In the final analysis the evaluation of community health services is severely compounded by the relationship of health outcomes with aspects of poverty, culture, and the environment over which community health agencies have little control. These relationships were acknowledged in some of the recommendations of the American Health Assembly (1970), which help to cast this chapter in perspective:

It must be recognized that illness produces poverty; and that in turn poverty breeds health problems. Health services will not alone overcome the disadvantages of poverty itself nor be able to correct the disabling impact of inferior nutrition, housing, recreation, and education. As the level of health services rises, a point of diminishing returns from such services may be reached as compared with investment in the quality of the living environment.

Poverty itself involves a variety of handicapping conditions that can result in irreversible health problems. The tragic fact of malnutrition among millions of poor and near poor is a national shame. The economic base of malnutrition should be promptly eliminated by expansion of nutritional support programs.

Because of the vulnerability of infants and young children to the environment of poverty, programs of high quality such as day care and early childhood education should be directed to these age groups.

Special problems of health care delivery exist in poverty areas: urban ghettos and barrios and many rural sections of the country. Until a comprehensive financing system is implemented, we vigorously oppose the curtailment, and instead favor all possible expansion, of existing programs providing health care for the poor or other low-income people.

Consumers have an obviously deep and primary interest in community health services. The health professions alone cannot be the sufficient guardians of that interest. Consumers must have effective representation—wherever possible a majority—in the policy-making processes of major health facilities and organizations. This representation must reflect all aspects of the community, including cultural, racial, and linguistic diversities. Special emphasis should be placed on meaningful representation of the poor.

QUESTIONS AND EXERCISES

1. In a republic such as the United States, what individuals or groups are most nearly self-sufficient in dealing with all health matters?
2. About one third of the counties (and parishes) in the United States are without full-time professional health service. What is the explanation?
3. If you lived in a county or parish without a full-time health department, what measures would you take to obtain full-time public health service?
4. Why do people in the low-income groups benefit most from the county health department program?
5. Is it just or unjust that some people get more service than others from the county health department?
6. Which health department in the United States—federal, state, or county—is most likely to give service to the individual citizen? Cite examples to illustrate.
7. What are some nonhealth regulations the state has established through the exercise of the police power in the United States?
8. Why not pass laws and regulations identifying as nuisances all conditions and practices that might cause hurt, injury, damage, or inconvenience to people?
9. If a county health department refuses to take court action to stop a condition that citizens regard as a nuisance, what action can the citizens take?
10. A dog in public was thought to have rabies. Rather than risk being bitten, a deputy sheriff shot the dog. What are the possible legal implications?
11. Why not have only medical doctors on the county board of health?
12. Why should decisions by the county board of health be subject to appeal to a court?
13. What justification can you make for the expenditure of $5 per person per year for a county health department?
14. What was the national birthrate and death rate for a recent year?
15. Why was mental health promotion not included in the U.S. county health department program until recently?
16. Why is it not logical to say that one position on the county health staff is more important to the public than is another?
17. Why should public health education employ a variety of media and methods of communication?
18. If an HSA was to be formed in your county, what organizations should be represented?
19. Why should the school be concerned with more than health education in the school?

20. What evidence can you present that people in the United States have better health today than those who lived there at the turn of the century, and what has been the contribution of official and voluntary health agencies?
21. What are some respects in which voluntary health agencies differ from official health agencies?
22. Which voluntary promotional health agency in the United States do you regard as being most important? Why?
23. Does the medical profession in the United States exercise too great an influence or even control of the voluntary promotional health agencies? What is your line of reasoning?

BIBLIOGRAPHY

Accredited U.S. schools of public health and graduate public health programs, 1979-80, Am. J. Public Health **70:**329, 1980.

Aday, L.A., Andesen, R., and Fleming, G.V.: Health care in the U.S.: equitable for whom? Beverly Hills, 1980, Sage Publications.

American Health Assembly: The health of Americans, New York, 1970, Columbia University Press.

American Public Health Association: Health is a community affair, Cambridge, Mass., 1970, Harvard University Press.

Anderson, C.L., and Creswell, W.H.: School health practice, ed. 7, St. Louis, 1980, The C.V. Mosby Co.

Bartlett, E.E.: The contribution of school health education to community health promotion: what can we reasonably expect? Am. J. Public Health **71:**1384, 1981.

Cornacchia, H.J., and Staton, W.M.: Health in elementary schools, ed. 5, St. Louis, 1979, The C.V. Mosby Co.

Curran, W.J.: Public health and the law, Am. J. Public Health **60:**2208, 1970.

Division of Associated Health Professions: Preparation and practice of community, patient, and school health educators, Washington, D.C., 1978, Bureau of Health Professions, DHHS Pub. No. (HRA)78-71.

Division of Associated Health Professions: Initial role delineation for health education, final report, Washington, D.C., 1980, Bureau of Health Professions, DHHS Pub. No. (HRA)80-44.

Eisner, V., and Callan, L.B.: Dimensions of school health, Springfield, Ill., 1974, Charles C Thomas, Publisher.

Enthoven, A.C.: Health plan, Reading, Mass., 1980, Addison-Wesley Publishing Co.

Freeman, R.: Community health nursing, ed. 2, Philadelphia, 1970. W.B. Saunders Co.

Freeman, R.: The expanding role of nursing, some implications, Int. Nurs. Rev. **19:**351, April, 1972.

Ginsberg, E.: Urban health services: the case of New York City, New York, 1970, The Columbia University Press.

Green, L.W.: Constructive consumerism, Health Educ. **2:**3, 1975.

Hall, T.L., Jackson, R.S., and Parsons, W.B.: Schools of public health, trends in graduate education, Washington, D.C., May, 1980, Division of Associated Health Professions, DHHS Pub. No. (HRA)80-45.

Health Resources Administration: A report on public and community health personnel, Washington, D.C., 1980, Bureau of Health Professions, DHHS Pub. No. (HRA)80-43.

Iverson, D.C., editor: Promoting health through the schools: a challenge for the 80s. Special issue of Health Education Quar. **8:**5, Spring 1981.

Kissick, W.: Health policy directions for the 1970's, N. Engl. J. Med. **282:**1343, June 11, 1970.

Kosa, J., and Zola, I.K.: Poverty and health, a sociological analysis, Cambridge, Mass., 1975, Harvard University Press.

Maxcy, K.F., and Startwell, P.E.: Preventive medicine and public health, ed. 10, New York, 1976, Appleton-Century-Crofts.

Mayshark, C., Shaw, D.D., and Best, W.H.: Administration of school health programs: its theory and practice, ed. 2, St. Louis, 1977, The C.V. Mosby Co.

Mico, P.R., and Ross, H.S.: Health education and behavioral science, Oakland, Calif., 1975, Third-Party Associates.

Miller, C.A., Brooks, E.F., DeFriese, G.H., et al.: A survey of local health departments and their directors, Am. J. Public Health **67:**931, 1977.

Moynihan, D.P., editor: Maximum feasible misunderstanding, community action in the War on Poverty, New York, 1969, The Free Press.

Partridge, K.B.: Community and professional participation in decision making at a health center, Health Serv. Rep. **88:**527, 1973.

Richardson, A.H.: Report of the fiscal scheme for the Association of Schools of Public Health (Bureau of Health Manpower Contract NIH 71-4159), Baltimore, 1973, The Johns Hopkins University Press.

Sheps, C.G., chairman: Higher education for public health, a report of the Milbank Memorial Fund Commission, New York, 1976, Prodist.

Smith, B.C.: Community health: an epidemiological approach, New York, 1979, Macmillan Publishing Co., Inc.

Wang, V.L., et al.: An approach to consumer-patient activation in health maintenance, Public Health Rep. **90:**449, 1975.

White, K.L., and Henderson, M.M.: Epidemiology as a fundamental science: its uses in health services planning, administration, and evaluation, New York, 1976, Oxford University Press, Inc.

World Health Organization: Postgraduate education and training in public health, Geneva, 1973, Technical Report Series No. 533.

20

STATE OR PROVINCIAL HEALTH ORGANIZATIONS AND SERVICES

The final end of government is not to exert restraint but to do good.

Rufus Choate

In most countries health planning and resources are coordinated at some level between the local community and the national or federal agencies responsible for public health. In the United States this intermediate layer is the state health agency (SHA), usually referred to as the State Department of Public Health, which is provided by the state constitution with broad functions. The state constitution permits or directs the state legislature to pass supplemental statutory provisions. Canada, Australia, and most European countries have provincial health agencies with varying degrees of autonomy and independence from their national ministries of health. In small countries, such as Ireland, the county is the equivalent of a state or province.

The function of state and provincial health agencies is to assure a long-range, equitable, comprehensive, and balanced approach to the several needs of many individual communities, rather than allowing each community complete autonomy in addressing short-range health concerns of local interest groups who may be the most affluent or the most politically powerful.

State and provincial agencies are a backup of the community health department, providing the services of experts when requested or needed for an emergency or for an important

health problem. The SHAs also provide local health departments with laboratory services and with equipment and facilities for special surveys and other purposes. Mobile x-ray units and devices for measuring air pollution and other equipment are made available by the state to local authorities for the promotion of community health.

The SHA acts as the link between the federal health agencies and the local health departments. Federal health funds are channeled through the SHA to the local health agency. Through the SHA, community health departments are able to obtain the services of national or federal health experts to solve unique or difficult health problems or to deal with an emergency when summary action is required.

HEALTH AUTHORITY

Sovereignty, or ultimate authority, in matters of health rests with the people, and this authority is vested in local and state or provincial governments to pass such legislation and take such action as may be necessary to promote the health and general welfare of the people. The state in the United States has virtually unlimited authority to do what is necessary to promote the greatest good for the greatest number. There is but one limitation on the state's power to legislate in health matters—a statute may not be contrary to nor violate the provisions of the U.S. Constitution. In the exercise of power to act in matters of health, the act or performance under the state's police power must be *reasonable* and *constitutional*.

The people of a state or province approve a constitution that may merely provide that the legislature is charged with the responsibility to set up health agencies and make such other provisions as are necessary for the protection and promotion of the health of the public. In some states in the United States the constitution delineates in some detail what the state health organization and services shall be. Most public health authorities agree that the state constitution should contain broad, general provisions granting to the state legislature authority to establish the necessary health agencies, their responsibilities, and their authority. This provides for changes through legislation as future circumstances develop.

Most legislatures choose to delegate their health authority to a state or provincial board of health to pass health regulations, standards, and requirements, but the health board must restrict itself to health matters. In effect, the state or provincial board of health acts as a quasi-legislative body. The legislature also charges the health board with the responsibility for the enforcement of these regulations, which have the force of law.

In summary, health authority is exercised through the state or provincial constitution, legislation, and health board regulations. Custom and reasonable action may also enter into matters of health authority and action so long as it is reasonable and constitutional.

Health agencies in the state or province

Each state or province has both official health agencies and voluntary health agencies. Official health agencies and services are those supported by tax funds and recognized as a governmental agency or service. Official health agencies have staffs appointed by some official governmental body, and the staff members are government employees and may be classified as officials.

Voluntary health agencies are those supported entirely or primarily by financial contributions from citizens and private organizations. Services of voluntary health agencies are carried on by full-time, salaried, professional personnel. Most of the recognized voluntary health agencies in the United States have a national organization with state divisions and local chapters. The effective, principal sphere of operation of most voluntary agencies is at the state level where funds are raised, programs are planned, and services are developed. A small part of the state-raised funds are contributed to the national office, and some of the funds may be channeled to the local chapters.

Official health agencies

In every state or province the official health department is the principal health agency. Yet each state or province has many other agencies that are also engaged in health promotion. For most of these agencies, health is a secondary service or even an incidental activity. In some instances many health benefits are somewhat in the nature of a by-product of the primary activities of the agency. Yet the composite health contributions of these agencies are significant. In some instances more than one agency may carry on the same health function. At times this duplication is justifiable, but too often the duplication is without merit and is the result of empire building, long-established custom or priority, and political protectionism. On the state or provincial level as well as the local and national levels, agencies multiply and often outgrow their original purpose, so they create new activities to justify their continuing existence. Too often, tax funds diverted to unnecessary agencies and outmoded services are desperately needed by other essential and worthy services and agencies.

To record all state or provincial agencies that are involved in health in some form would mean an almost interminable list. Some of these agencies found in virtually all states will indicate how extensive the spectrum is. In many cases the title of the agency gives some indication of the nature of its health function.

Department of Agriculture
Department of Education
Department of Labor and Industry
Department of Welfare
Department of Conservation
Department of Mines and Minerals
Department of Motor Vehicles
Department of Public Safety
Department of Civil Service and Registration
Department of State Institutions
Department of Parks and Recreation
University
College
Experiment Station
Commissions
  Blood pressure
  Cancer
  Crippled children's
  Blind
  Mental health
  Dairy and food
  Hotel
  Workmen's compensation
  Hospital
Boards
  Industrial accident
  Water resources
  Examining and licensing
    Medicine
    Osteopathy
    Dentistry
    Nursing
    Medical laboratory
    Podiatry
  Livestock sanitation
Independent Offices
  Toxicologist
  Veterinarian

All of the health services given by these agencies are important, but the administrative need for combining agencies and for coordinating services is apparent. Such reorganization could result in a reduction in costs and in an improvement in services but in large states sometimes creates overly complex and confusing bureaucracies. A neglected criterion of organization is public familiarity with agency structures and procedures.

Department of health

An executive agency or department responsible for the activities necessary to protect and promote health is found in most every state or province.

In four states in the United States the state constitution names the department and specifies its functions. In the remaining states the state constitution delegates this authority to the state legislature. Massachusetts established the first state health board in the United States in 1869. Local official health agencies had been in operation for more than a century prior to the creation of the Massachusetts State Board of Health. No two states have precisely the same structure for their health programs, but, generally, state health authority is vested in a council or board that appoints a full-time health commissioner who administers the health program and agency.

The usual practice is to appoint a board of about nine members. Board members are appointed by the governor—subject to legislature approval—and serve without pay but are reimbursed for personal expenses in connection with their duties, such as attending meetings and participating in special functions. Board members usually are appointed for terms of 6 years, with terms staggered to provide for changes in board membership but with desirable continuity as well. The board is not composed of health specialists but ideally is made up of a cross-section of the population of the state or province and is representative of various interests, geographical areas, and backgrounds. The board's role is to reflect the viewpoints, interpretations, desires, and needs of the public. There could be no objection to having one medical physician on the board, but to have the medical profession dominate would defeat the very purpose for which the board is created. Just as education policies are left to nonexperts in education rather than professional academicians, so too general health policies are decided by lay citizens with the viewpoint and judgment of the general public. Services of experts are provided to the board by the professional staff of the health department.

Powers of the board of health. The state or provincial board of health has such powers and functions as have been granted to it by the state or provincial constitution and the legislature. There are seven acknowledged powers of any board of health—code making, quasi-judicial powers, administration, investigation, supervision and consultation, education, and coordination with other health agencies.

Code-making power of the board is a quasi-legislative function that gives the board the authority to make necessary rules and regulations to carry out the authority and functions granted to it by the legislature. The professional health staff recommends certain health rules and regulations, which are assembled into a sanitary code. This code has the effect of law when approved by the board of health. Courts have upheld the power of the board to enact binding rules and regulations, providing these rules and regulations do not go outside of health matters.

Quasi-judicial powers are exercised by the board in its authority to summon before it anyone alleged to have violated state or provincial health regulations. The board has the further recognized authority to summon witnesses. Hearings may be held by the board before granting or revoking a license. In all cases the citizen concerned has the right to contest any adverse action of the board by filing an appeal in court.

Administrative functions of the state or provincial board of health are delegated to the full-time staff of health specialists. In Australia, Canada, and many Asian, African, South American, and European countries, the chief provincial officer is called the Minister of Health. In most states of the United States the chief administrator is called the health commissioner, although "health officer," "health director," "secretary of health," and other titles are used. In some states of the United States the board elects the commissioner and in other states the governor appoints the commissioner. State health commissioners usually are medical physicians with preparation and experience in public health. The commissioner has certain recognized responsibilities: (1) general administration, (2) recommendation of health legislation, rules and regulations for consideration by the board, (3) appointment of personnel, (4) preparation of the budget, (5) supervision of divisions or bureaus, (6) enforcement of health rules and regulations, and (7) relationship with official agencies, organizations, and the public.

Department organization. The structure of the health department or organization varies. At the top of the administrative pyramid is the health commissioner, officer, or Minister of Health. At the next level are the primary administrative units usually called *divisions*, which in turn are divided into bureaus or sections. There may be further subdivisions, but this would be necessary only in departments in the heavily populated states or provinces. A large state or provincial health department may have 10 divisions, and a small state or provincial health department may have but five administrative divisions. Each division has a director or chief, and each bureau or section has a head as administrator.

In most instances, the title of the division or bureau, as shown in Fig. 20-1, indicates the function or areas of health service. For present purposes, the distribution of program effort can

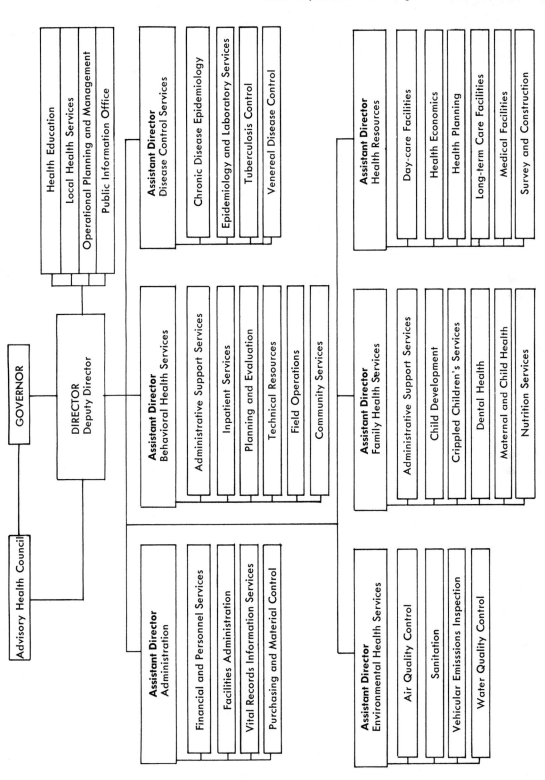

FIG. 20-1. State or provincial health organization and services. In states or provinces of less than average population, the organization of health services is kept as simple and unified as possible.

be illustrated best by reviewing recent expenditures of state health departments in various program areas in the United States.

Programs of state health agencies (SHAs) in the United States

The 50 states, the District of Columbia, and the six territories (Guam, Puerto Rico, the Virgin Islands, American Samoa, the Northern Mariana Islands, and the Trust Territory of the Pacific Islands) all participated in 1980 and 1981 surveys of the programs and expenditures of SHAs,* which were made by the National Public Health Program Reporting System of the Association of State and Territorial Health Officials (1980).

Differences among the SHAs arise primarily from size of population, the wealth of the state, the extent to which local health department expenditures are included, and the wide variance in the responsibility only for traditional public health programs such as maternal and child health, communicable disease control, and for more specialized chronic disease programs. At the other extreme are states whose health agencies have responsibility for the same traditional areas; for institutional care programs; for environmental health services; for health resources planning, development, and regulation; for Medicaid (Title XIX) programs; and for added social services.

There has been a considerable movement among the states to delegate certain health programs to agencies other than the SHA and to establish "super agencies" or "umbrella agencies" that provide a wide (but not a consistent) variety of services that have been traditionally considered as public health, medical care, environmental health, welfare, and educational

*Defined as the agency or department headed by the state or territorial health official. Puerto Rico did not report on its fiscal year 1979 expenditures. Selected data for fiscal year 1980 were provided by the Association of State and Territorial Health Officials prior to their publication in 1981.

services. Therefore the programs of the SHAs cannot be understood without an awareness of the changing patterns of assignment of function within the larger agency.

The 57 official SHAs or departments spent a total of $4.5 billion in 1980 for all of their public health programs. These programs provided general services for protection of the health and well-being of the entire population in addition to direct personal health services to an estimated 72 million persons. Seven of the SHAs were also the single state agencies responsible for administering the Medicaid program. These seven SHAs reported an additional $5.3 billion in Medicaid expenditures in 1979.

The public health programs of SHAs are generally classified into six program areas: personal health, environmental health, health resources, laboratory, general administration, and funds to local health departments (LHDs) not allocated to program areas. The personal health, environmental health, health resources, and laboratory program areas can be divided into program categories. Although the expenditures and sources of funds reported by the 57 state agencies in 1980 are exclusively those of SHAs, the persons served and types of services offered include not only those served directly by the SHA, but also, in many instances, those served by LHDs with the support of state health departments.

Public health expenditures. The largest expenditures (79%) of SHAs for fiscal years 1975 to 1980 were for personal health programs (including 21% for SHA-operated institution programs). Expenditures and trends for the other program areas were as shown in Fig. 20-2. Approximately 6% was used for general administration. About 3% was also reported as "funds to local health departments not allocated to program areas."

Sources of funds. State funds accounted for about 54% of the total expenditures of SHAs during 1975 to 1980 (Fig. 20-3). Direct federal grants and contracts provided 36%, and funds

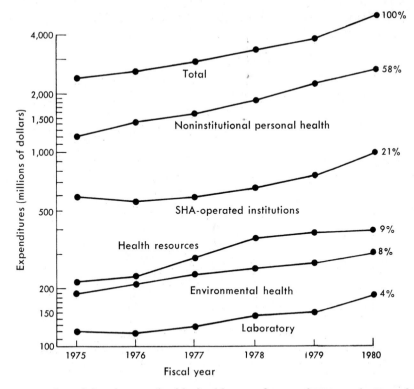

FIG. 20-2. Trends and distribution of public health expenditures of SHAs in the United States for fiscal years 1975-1980.

From Association of State and Territorial Health Officials, National Public Health Program Reporting System, 1980 and 1981.

from local sources, fees and reimbursements, and other sources accounted for the remaining 11%.

Expenditures from the U.S. Department of Health and Human Services sources included $246 million from the Maternal and Child Health portion of Title V of the Social Security Act; $74 million from the Crippled Children's portion of Title V; $64 million in comprehensive public health services formula grants (Section 314[d] [7] [A] of the Public Health Service Act); and $71 million in family planning grants under Title X of the Public Health Service Act. The largest federal funding source was the Supplemental Food Program for Women, Infants, and Children (WIC), which is administered by the Department of Agriculture. The

SHAs spent $649 million from these funds in 1980.

Preventive services. The portions of the total SHA expenditures for 1979 attributed to treatment and "preventive" health services as part of personal health services are shown in Fig. 20-4. More than two fifths of the total public health expenditures were spent for services that were primarily preventive, but this varies widely from more than 90% of immunization and health education to less than 10% of institutional and home health care.

Local health departments (LHDs). There are multiple variations in the relationships between SHAs and LHDs. These range from strong SHA control over the budgets and activities of the LHDs in those states in which

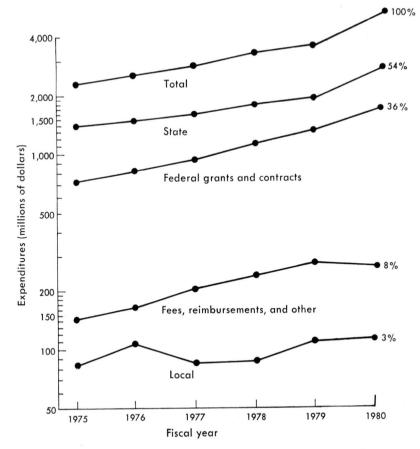

FIG. 20-3. Trends in the source of funds for public health expenditures by SHAs in the United States for fiscal years 1975-1980.

From Association of State and Territorial Health Officials, National Public Health Program Reporting System, 1980 and 1981.

LHD staff members are SHA employees, to complete autonomy of LHDs. In states where SHA programs are carried out jointly by SHAs and LHDs, or by LHDs under the direction of SHAs, the services reported include both direct services of SHAs and direct services of LHDs. In other states the services provided by LHDs are underreported or omitted.

Forty-seven states and Puerto Rico reported a combined total of 3,134 LHDs in their states in 1980. The District of Columbia and the territories (except Puerto Rico) do not have LHDs. About 76% of funds granted by SHAs

to LHDs was spent for personal health services, and 13% for environmental health, as shown in Fig. 20-5, *A*. For each dollar the SHAs granted to LHDs, the LHDs spent an additional $2.90, which they received from other sources, including local governments, fees, and direct federal or state grants, as seen in Fig. 20-5, *B*.

Personal health. Personal health programs of SHAs include maternal and child health, handicapped children's services, communicable disease control, dental health, chronic disease, mental health and related programs, op-

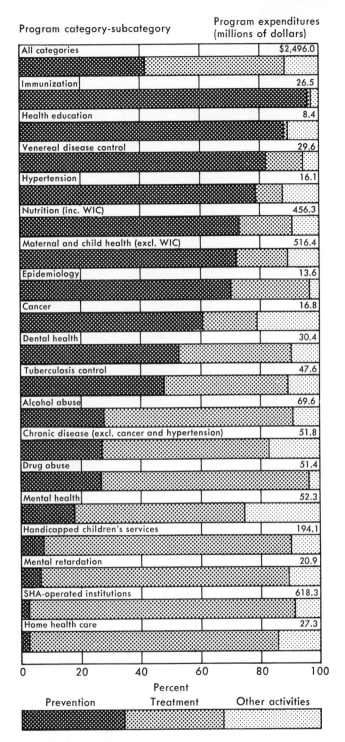

FIG. 20-4. Total SHA expenditures in 18 categories of personal health programs and the proportion of each of these devoted to prevention, treatment, and other activities in fiscal year 1979.

From Association of State and Territorial Health Officials, National Public Health Program Reporting System, 1980.

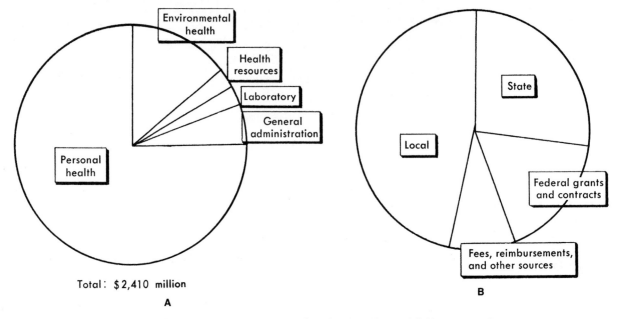

Total: $2,410 million

A

B

FIG. 20-5. Expenditures **(A)** and sources **(B)** of funds (in millions of dollars) granted to LHDs in the United States in fiscal year 1980.

From Association of State and Territorial Health Officials, National Public Health Program Reporting System, 1981.

eration of hospitals and other health care institutions, and other personal health programs such as financial assistance, accident prevention, and general services to special population groups such as agricultural migrants. Of the $2.5 billion spent for personal health programs in 1979, the largest amounts were for maternal and child health programs and for SHA-operated institutions, as seen in Fig. 20-4.

In addition to providing inpatient care through SHA-operated institution programs, many other personal health programs purchased inpatient hospital services, amounting to almost one third of all personal health expenditures.

An estimated 72 million people were served directly by the personal health programs of the SHAs. The services provided to the greatest number of people were health screening, immunizations, and dental services. The programs that provided direct services to the

greatest number of persons were communicable disease control and maternal and child health.

Environmental health. Environmental health programs have been classified into seven categories: consumer protection and sanitation, water quality, air quality, waste management, occupational health and safety and related areas, radiation control, and general and combined environmental health. The largest SHA program expenditures for environmental health programs in 1980 were for consumer protection and sanitation and water quality, as shown in Fig. 20-6.

Certain activities are common to most SHAs in their efforts to prevent or intervene in environmental health hazards. All of the 54 SHAs with environmental health programs had standard-setting or enforcement responsibilities. They made 3.9 million field inspections and took almost 179,000 enforcement actions. In

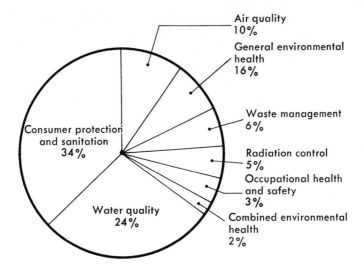

Total: $299 million for 56 SHAs

FIG. 20-6. Environmental health program expenditures (in millions of dollars) of 54 SHAs, fiscal year 1980.

From Association of State and Territorial Health Officials, National Public Health Program Reporting System, 1981.

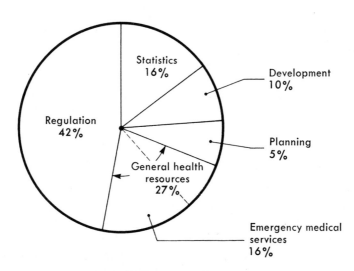

Total: $358 million for 57 SHAs

FIG. 20-7. Health resources program expenditures (in millions of dollars) of 54 SHAs, fiscal year 1980.

From Association of State and Territorial Health Officials, National Public Health Program Reporting System, 1981.

addition, these SHAs trained a total of 226,000 individuals, including 2,300 emergency response team members. They also licensed or certified 270,000 persons through environmental health programs and issued 1.3 million licenses, registrations, and permits. Finally, SHAs made design reviews and reviewed environmental impact statements.

Health resources. In 1979 states performed one or more of the following functions in developing health resources: health planning; the development and regulation of health services, facilities, and manpower, including the development and regulation of emergency medical services; or the collection, analysis, and publication of health statistics. The distribution of such activities for health resources programs is shown in Fig. 20-7.

Laboratory. Laboratory services offered by SHAs in 1980 included analytical services (clinical, environmental, toxicological, forensic, and related), production of biologics, research and development, laboratory improvement (including quality control, regulation, licensing or certification, consultation, and training), reference services, and professional consultation.

Most of the laboratory programs provided services in support of other SHA programs or activities. Those laboratory programs able to allocate their expenditures to other public health services reported that about 43% of their expenditures were in support of communicable disease control services, 38% for environmental health services, and 19% for personal health services other than communicable disease.

General administration. The SHAs together spent a total of $201 million for general administrative and support services in 1979. These expenditures, which accounted for 6% of all of their public health expenditures, were spent at the central level for general agency management. The expenditures for administration of specific programs are usually reported with program expenditures in the appropriate program area.

Appraisal of official state health services in the United States

The expenditures reported by the Association of State and Territorial Health Officials (1980) have been presented here to provide the student with a sense of the relative magnitude of different state health services and programs. The figures should not be memorized because their exact meaning is transitory, but they should provide a more realistic picture of the current areas of responsibility and emphasis in state health departments than the organization chart in Fig. 20-1. Organization charts can be deceptive because the boxes are all approximately the same size, giving the illusion that the programs and services are of similar scope. The examination of budgets or expenditure figures casts each program or service into perspective.

As a support service to many programs, it is assumed that health education funds are set aside within the program budgets. This often is not the case, even though the programs require health education services. Hence certain basic functions such as health education sometimes end up with no budget and their expenditures are from leftover funds. The Association of State and Territorial Health Officials (1980) could identify only $8.4 million expended for health education, less than one half of 1% of the expenditures on personal health services. The Report of the President's Committee on Health Education (1973) could identify only 0.5% of state health expenditures devoted to health education. The relative position of health education had not changed. In 1980, however, a new grant program from the U.S. government began to channel "Health Education–Risk Reduction" funds through the state health departments, resulting in at least a doubling of expenditures for health education, all of it in prevention.

No instrument is available to make a precise appraisal of the value and significance of the official state health services. Yet there is ample empirical evidence that, as state health services have expanded and technology has advanced, the health of the public has been advanced, diseases have been prevented, and deaths have been postponed. Many of the state health services do not deal with life and death matters but contribute to the enjoyment and effectiveness of living. These services serve as a backup for the local health services, medical care, hospital care, and other services related to human well-being. The state health department also serves as the agent of the state in dealings with the federal health agencies and those of other states.

In matters of state public health three cardinal needs exist. The first is the need for more funds to do adequately what is needed in state health promotion. A second need is to relieve the state health department of functions and services that are not strictly the province of the public health department. A third need is to integrate the health functions of all state agencies that provide health services in some form. The state health department, agriculture department, labor department, and other state agencies that have health functions must work closely together to allocate responsibility for overlapping health services. This would result in some agencies transferring certain health activities to other agencies where these functions more logically belong. Only when the public demands such coordination and shifting of functions will this actually take place.

HEALTH PLANNING IN THE UNITED STATES

The Federal Comprehensive Planning Act of 1966 (PL 89-749) and the Partnership for Health Amendments of 1967 (PL 90-174) were enacted in the United States to establish comprehensive planning for health services, health manpower, and health facilities essential at every level of government; to strengthen the leadership and capabilities of SHAs; and to broaden and make more feasible and relevant federal support of health services provided people in their communities. This legislation was superceded by the National Health Planning and Resources Development Act of 1974.

Health Systems Agencies (HSAs)

The National Health Planning and Resources Development Act of 1974 (PL 93-641) created a network of HSAs responsible for health planning and development throughout the United States. In creating such a network, the governors of the states were asked to designate throughout the U.S. health service areas for planning and development purposes that meet the requirements specified in the legislation. These requirements were as follows:

1. There must be a geographic region appropriate for the effective planning and development of health services, determined on the basis of factors including population and the availability of resources to provide all necessary health services for residents of the area.
2. To the extent practicable, the area must include at least one center for the provision of highly specialized health services, such as a University hospital or major teaching hospital.
3. Each area must have a population of not less than 500,000 or more than three million, except that an area may be less than 500,000 if the area comprises an entire state with a population of less than 500,000 or more than three million if the area includes a standard metropolitan statistical area with a greater population.
4. The area boundaries, to the maximum extent feasible, must be appropriately coordinated with those of Professional Standards Review Organizations, existing regional planning areas, and State planning and administrative areas.
5. The boundaries are also to be established so that, in the planning and development of health services to be offered within the health service area, any economic or geographic barrier to the receipt of such services in nonmetropolitan areas is taken into account. Determination of boundaries is to reflect the differ-

ences in health planning and health services development needs between nonmetropolitan and metropolitan areas.

6. Each standard metropolitan statistical area (SMSA) must be entirely within the boundaries of a single health service area. This requirement may be waived if a governor determines, with the approval of the Secretary,* that in order to meet the above-mentioned requirements, a health service area may contain only part of the SMSA.

The act also provided that no areas need be designated for states that have no county or municipal public health institution or department and that have maintained a health planning system that complies with the purposes of this title.

Health plans

In each health service area, the Department of Health and Human Services, after consulting with the governor of the appropriate state, then designated either a private nonprofit corporation or a public entity as the HSA responsible for health planning and development in that area. An HSA may not be or operate an educational institution. The legislation specifies minimum criteria for the legal structure, staff, governing body, and functioning of the HSAs. They are generally responsible for preparing and implementing plans designed to improve the health of the residents of their health service area; to increase the accessibility, acceptability, continuity, and quality of health services in the area; to restrain increases in the cost of providing health services; and to prevent unnecessary duplication of health resources. In performing these responsibilities, the HSAs were required to

1. Gather and analyze suitable data
2. Establish health systems plans (goals) and annual implementation plans (objectives and priorities)

3. Provide either technical and/or limited financial assistance to people seeking to implement provisions of the plans
4. Coordinate activities with PSROs* and other appropriate planning and regulatory entities
5. Review and approve or disapprove applications for federal funds for health programs within the area
6. Assist states in the performance of capital expenditures reviews
7. Assist states in making findings as to the need for new institutional health services proposed to be offered in the area
8. Assist states in reviewing existing institutional health services offered with respect to the appropriateness of such services
9. Annually recommend to states projects for the modernization, construction, and conversion of medical facilities in the area

State agency

An agency of state government was chosen by the governor in each state to serve as the state health planning and development agency (state agency). To be designated, the state agency was to prepare and submit to the Secretary of the Department of Health and Human Services for approval an administrative program for carrying out its functions. The state agency was then to be advised by a Statewide Health Coordinating Council whose composition and responsibilities are specified in the legislation, including requirements that the council

1. Have 60% of its members appointed by the governor from the state's health systems agencies and have a consumer majority
2. Review annually and coordinate the health systems plans and annual implementation plans of the state's health systems agencies and make comments to the Secretary
3. Prepare a state health plan made up of the health systems plans of the health systems agencies, taking into account the preliminary plan developed by the State Agency

---

*Secretary of the U.S. Department of Health and Human Services.

*Professional Standards Review Organizations.

4. Review for the Secretary budgets and applications for assistance of health systems agencies
5. Advise the State Agency on the performance of its functions
6. Review and approve or disapprove state plans and applications for health-type formula grants to the state

The required functions of the state agency were specified by the act to include

1. Conducting the state's health planning activities and implementing the parts of the state health plan and plans of health systems agencies which relate to the government of the state
2. Preparing a preliminary state plan for approval or disapproval by the Council
3. Assisting the Council in the review of the state medical facilities plan and in the performance of its functions
4. Reviewing new institutional health services proposed and making findings as to the need for such services
5. Reviewing existing institutional health services offered with respect to the appropriateness of such services and making public its findings

Any of the functions described above may be performed by another agency of state government on the request of the governor under an agreement with the state agency satisfactory to the Secretary of the Department of Health and Human Services.

The state facilities plan includes a list of the projects for which assistance will be sought and the priorities for the funding of these projects. For each project an application must be submitted to the Secretary for approval, which must set forth a number of assurances including one that services in assisted facilities will be made available to all persons residing or employed in the areas served by the facilities and that a reasonable volume of services will be available to persons unable to pay.

Allotments to the states are made on the basis of population, financial need, and the need for medical facilities. Not more than 20% of a

state's allotment may be used for projects for construction of new inpatient facilities in areas that have experienced recent rapid population growth, and less than 25% may be used for projects for outpatient facilities that will serve medically underserved populations, half of which must be expended in rural medically underserved areas. The intent to replace expensive inpatient care with less expensive outpatient care is evident here. In the case of a project to be assisted under an allotment, the federal share may not exceed two thirds of the costs, except that a project in a rural or urban poverty area may receive 100% federal funding.

The National Health Planning and Resources Development Act of 1974 also revised the Hill-Burton medical facilities construction program and related their activities more closely to the planning programs. Development funds for each HSA will enable the agency to establish and maintain an Area Health Services Development Fund. This fund, together with grants, loans, loan guarantees, and interest subsidies, will support

1. Modernization of medical facilities
2. Construction of new outpatient medical facilities
3. Construction of new inpatient medical facilities in areas which have experienced recent rapid population growth
4. Conversion of existing medical facilities for the provision of new health services

It is also the purpose to provide grant assistance for construction and modernization projects designed to eliminate or prevent safety hazards or avoid noncompliance with licensure or accreditation standards.

When the HSA has determined what health problems are being taken care of adequately and who is dealing with them, the state coordination council's role is to determine whether all concerned agencies are coordinating their efforts to deal efficiently and effectively with these problems. It then follows that areas of health not being adequately provided for is where the planning committees must devote their major attention. This means recruiting the services of all persons and agencies having possible contributions. It means obtaining necessary grants and other funding required for a solution to a particular health problem. A continuing program conceivably could attain the goal of no health problems unrecognized, no problems neglected, and an organized citizenry using its full resources in the protection and promotion of the health of all the people. This was the objective of the health planning legislation in the United States.

QUESTIONS AND EXERCISES

1. To what extent are SHAs the "middleman" of health organization?
2. Is the state's authority over the health of the people in the United States too great or not great enough? Why?
3. What check does the public have to prevent health authorities from being too powerful and arrogant?
4. Why should citizens always have the right to appeal to a court when they believe that they have been unjustly dealt with by health officials?
5. What health functions does your state or provincial department of agriculture engage in?
6. How do you explain that local health departments were formed long before state health departments were established?
7. How frequently does your state or provincial board of health meet?
8. Present the case for and against having the state or provincial board of health composed entirely of medical physicians.
9. Obtain a copy of your state or provincial sanitary code and report your reactions.
10. Who is your health commissioner or Minister of Health, what has been his or her professional preparation, experience, and for how many years has he or she been in the position?
11. When was the last time you or any member of your family received direct service from personnel of your state or provincial health department?
12. What are some health problems in your area on which the state or provincial health department should be conducting research?
13. What service now required of or otherwise carried on by your state or provincial health department should not be a part of the department's activities?
14. What consolidation of official health services have taken place in your state or province in the last 10 years?
15. Evaluate comprehensive health planning as it affects the health of your community.
16. Why has the U.S. Congress enacted laws to regulate health planning in states and regions?

BIBLIOGRAPHY

Association of State and Territorial Health Officials: Services, expenditures and programs of state and territorial health agencies, Washington, D.C., 1980 and 1981, U.S. Government Printing Office.

Christmas, J.J.: The challenge of change, the 1980 presidential address, Am. J. Public Health 71:235, 1981.

DeFriese, G.H., Hetherington, J.S., Brooks, E.F., et al.: The program implications of administrative relationships between local health departments and state and local government, Am. J. Public Health 71:1109, 1981.

Dye, T.R.: Politics in states and communities, ed. 3, Englewood Cliffs, N.J., 1977, Prentice-Hall, Inc.

Felman, Y.M.: Repeal of mandated premarital tests for syphilis: a survey of state health officers, Am. J. Public Health 71:155, 1981.

Hamilton, J.A., editor: The impact of centralization on the administration of health care services, Minneapolis, 1967, University of Minnesota Press.

Hanlon, J.J., and Pickett, G.E.: Public health: administration and practice, ed. 7, St. Louis, 1979, The C.V. Mosby Co.

Jain, S.C.: Role of state and local governments in relation to personal health services, Suppl. to Am. J. Public Health 71:5, 1981.

Krause, E.A., editor: Power and illness: the political sociology of health and medical care, New York, 1977, Elsevier North-Holland, Inc.

Last, J.M.: Public health and preventive medicine, ed. 11, New York, 1980, Appleton-Century-Crofts.

National Governor's Association Center for Policy Research: Fiscal survey of the states, 1979-1980, Washington, D.C., 1980, The Center.

Pickett, G.E.: The future of health departments: the governmental presence. In Breslow, L., editor: Annual review of public health, vol. 1, Palo Alto, Calif., 1980, Annual Reviews, Inc.

Report of the President's Committee on Health Education, 1973, Rockville, Md., Department of Health, Education, and Welfare, Health Services and Mental Health Administration.

Rocheleau, B., and Warren, S.: Health planners and local public finance: the case for revenue sharing, Public Health Rep. 95:313, 1980.

21

NATIONAL AND INTERNATIONAL
HEALTH SERVICES

Our true nationality is mankind.

H.G. Wells

The authority of national governments in matters of health varies from country to country, depending on the constitutional, imperial, or martial law. At one extreme, constitutions that create a republic, federation, or commonwealth of disparate states will tend to reserve most powers for the states and grant only essential authorities for the *common* good to the central government. At the other extreme, small countries, some monarchies, most socialist countries, and any country existing under martial law tend to centralize power at the national level and depend on state or local governmental bodies merely to carry out central plans and directives. Most countries swing between these extremes during their history.

The Constitution founding the United States, for example, acknowledged that the authority to promote public health rests with the states. Yet the U.S. federal government has provided many indispensable health services, as outlined in this chapter. The Constitution grants the federal government no direct authority to engage in public health activities, but authority to promote health is derived from general clauses concerning federal responsibilities.

SOURCES OF U.S. FEDERAL AUTHORITY IN HEALTH

As a result of the broad, general clauses in the U.S. Constitution, the federal government carries on many health functions.

1. Regulation of *interstate commerce* gives Congress the right to pass Pure Food and Drug Acts controlling the interstate shipment of foods and drugs. This power enables Congress to pass legislation governing the movement of people and livestock on interstate carriers. Control of insects, air pollution, stream pollution, and other threats to health become federal functions under the authority to regulate interstate commerce.

2. *Taxing power* is vested in Congress and is used to control narcotics by requiring a tax for a permit to possess and sell narcotics and a tax on each transaction. Oddly, courts have held that these are measures primarily for revenue purposes and not for regulatory reasons.

3. *Postal power* of the national government permits the passage of legislation prohibiting the use of the mails in any frauds, including health frauds. Misbranded or fraudulent drugs, patent medicines, and foods cannot be shipped through the mails, nor can any promotional material relating to fraudulent drugs or foods.

4. *Patent authority* enables the national government to require that any newly developed drug or medicine that is to be distributed to the public must be registered or patented.

5. *Treaty-making power* enables the federal government to enter into agreements with other nations on the control of communicable diseases, regulation of sanitary conditions, exchange of health information, and other health

matters that are international in nature.

6. *National war power* grants to the national government the authority to protect and maintain the health of all personnel in the Armed Services.

7. Authority to govern the District of Columbia carries an implied responsibility for the health of residents of the District.

8. Power to appropriate money for the general welfare, together with the right to create agencies, forms the great umbrella under which most federal health activities operate. Appropriating money for health agencies of the national, state, and local governments, for the construction of hospitals, for research, for health personnel training, for stream pollution control, and for other health projects has been the major contribution of the national government to health.

9. Power to create agencies for the general welfare has enabled the federal government to set up agencies to deal with each health problem that arises. Within each of the federal executive departments there exist bureaus, divisions, or branches directly or indirectly concerned with some aspect of health.

OFFICIAL U.S. HEALTH AGENCIES

In the United States more than 50 federal departments, bureaus, and other agencies are engaged in some sphere of health work. In most cases health is a minor or subordinate function of the agency. No particular overall organizational relationship exists between these agencies. When cooperation does occur, it is the result of the judgment and action of the administrators involved or occasionally by legislative requirement for joint action.

Often health functions are assigned to agencies less logically structured for the function than some other agency. This has resulted when a special interest group has succeeded in having a certain health program assigned to a particular agency. Once the program has been lodged with a certain agency, the special interests will guard the agency's prerogative.

Most of the federal agencies with health functions are concerned with special problems or serve special groups. The U.S. Public Health Service is the only federal agency that truly deals with general health promotion. All others contribute one or more of the health services of the jigsaw puzzle referred to as the federal health program.

EXECUTIVE DEPARTMENTS WITH HEALTH SERVICES

Every executive department of the U.S. government has one or more branches directly or indirectly involved in health work. In almost every instance, health is a minor concern of the agency. For the purpose of the present discussion, only a limited number of agencies in each executive department will be identified and their health activity indicated. Agencies give direct health services, regulatory services, advisory services, and grants-in-aid, and they loan personnel, conduct special studies, disseminate information, and conduct research, as well as provide other services related to their primary mission.

Department of Agriculture. Except for the Department of Health and Human Services (HHS) with its U.S. Public Health Service, the Department of Agriculture contributes more community health service to the United States than any other executive department. Some of its health services are the following.

Agricultural and industrial chemistry—study of food, feed, and drugs of importance to health

Animal industry—study of the cause, prevention, control, and treatment of diseases affecting humans and lower animals

Dairy industry—sanitary methods for handling milk and milk products

Entomology and plant quarantine—control of vectors affecting the health and well-being of humans

Extension service—promotion of rural health and environmental sanitation

Human nutrition and home economics—wholesomeness and sanitation of meat or food products

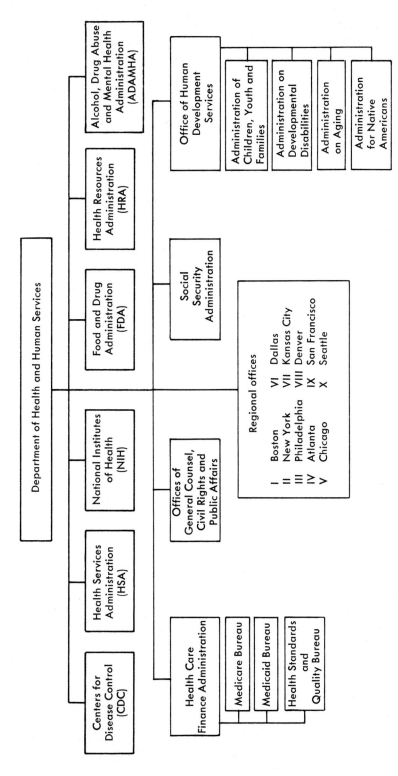

FIG. 21-1. Organizational plan of the U.S. Department of Health and Human Services. The six units on the second row make up the Public Health Service.

Department of Commerce. Responsibilities in health would appear to be misplaced in the Department of Commerce, but two health functions carried out by this department are of significance and are not too illogically placed.

Bureau of Census—collection and publication of statistics relating to the population, which is of value in planning health programs

Maritime Administration—medical and dental services for members of the Merchant Marine Cadet Corps and operation of the health program at merchant marine training stations

Department of Defense. As the title indicates, the health responsibilities of the Department of Defense would be that of providing health and medical care programs for military personnel and their dependents. This includes the provision of healthful environmental conditions and the training of personnel for duties in the field of health. The department cooperates with other federal agencies on health and medical problems.

Department of Health and Human Services (HHS). HHS is continually restructuring its operating divisions, all of which are involved in matters of health in one form or another.

The six units of the Public Health Service contain numerous offices, bureaus, centers, institutes, and divisions that change their names, locations, or functions to some degree with every major health bill passed by Congress. They grow, shrink, split, or disappear with each year's appropriations. Of the 62 units of HHS that were listed in the 1973 edition of this book, only a few still exist under the same administrative division and with the same name in 1981, and it is expected that President Ronald Reagan will make major bureaucratic changes as promised in his campaign. Fig. 21-1 outlines the current units by their bureaucratic names, which are sure to change. Table 21-1 presents the major program or service areas of the six units of the Public Health Service and the Office of the Assistant Secretary for Health. Most of the budgeted areas shown

are identified organizationally with a bureau, center, office, institute, or division containing the name (for example, the $5.3 million requested for health promotion would be the entire budget of the Office of Health Information and Health Promotion).

The 1982 budget included a block grant system with $1.4 billion to provide states with greater control of resources to deliver health services and conduct health promotion and disease prevention activities previously financed through 26 categorical grant programs. Of the funds included in the budget, $1,139 million would be allocated to the states for health services and $260 million for preventive health through two separate block grants.

This consolidation of the current array of categorical project and formula grants is expected to promote efficiency and responsiveness, allow states and localities to decide on the allocation of resources, and eliminate unnecessary restrictions on the exercise of state responsibility. The only limitations on the states are that funds may not be used for cash payments, for construction, or for the purchase of land and facilities. Performance standards are required only in the area of immunization of children against preventable diseases. As this book goes to press, Congress has voted on the Reagan Administration's proposal for block grants, and has created four rather than two block grants. The Omnibus Budget Reconciliation Act of 1981 (H.R. 3982) creates health block grants to states for preventive health, primary care, health services, and maternal and child health. All four are authorized for three years until the 1984-1985 fiscal year.

Under the Reagan Administration's proposal, a state would be allocated under the block grant the same proportion as the proportion received in 1981 of federal health services and prevention funds by the state and entities within the state. Savings realized through the elimination of duplication in activities and administration and reductions achieved in unnecessary administrative requirements are expected to make possible significant cost savings. Therefore the budget proposed for the block grants is 75% of the previous services level for the programs that would be replaced. Programs Reagan proposed to consolidate into each of the two block grants included the following.

Health services block grant	Preventive health block grant
Primary health care centers	High blood pressure control
Primary care research and demonstrations	Health incentive grants
Black lung services	Risk reduction and health education
Migrant health	Venereal disease
Home health services	Immunization
Maternal and child health	Fluoridation
Hemophilia	Rat control
Sudden infant death syndrome	Lead-based paint poisoning prevention
Emergency medical services	Genetic diseases
Mental health services	Family planning services
Drug abuse project grants and contracts	Adolescent health services
Drug abuse grants to states	
Alcoholism project grants and grants to states	

For administration closer to the grass roots, the HHS has 10 regional offices. (See the list on this page.) All divisions of the HHS will have offices and personnel complements in these regional headquarters. This is especially true as it relates to the Public Health Service. The organization and functions of this unit and the National Institutes of Health (NIH) will be presented in more detail following a brief account of some of the health activities of other departments of the executive branch of the federal government.

Region	Area	Office location
I	Connecticut, Maine, Massachusetts, New Hampshire, Rhode Island, Vermont	Boston, Mass.
II	New Jersey, New York, Puerto Rico, Virgin Islands	New York, N.Y.
III	Delaware, Maryland, Pennsylvania, Virginia, West Virginia, District of Columbia	Philadelphia, Pa.
IV	Alabama, Florida, Georgia, Kentucky, Mississippi, North Carolina, South Carolina, Tennessee	Atlanta, Ga.
V	Illinois, Indiana, Michigan, Minnesota, Ohio, Wisconsin	Chicago, Ill.
VI	Arkansas, Louisiana, New Mexico, Oklahoma, Texas	Dallas, Tex.
VII	Iowa, Kansas, Missouri, Nebraska	Kansas City, Mo.
VIII	Colorado, Montana, North Dakota, South Dakota, Utah, Wyoming	Denver, Colo.
IX	Arizona, California, Hawaii, Nevada, American Samoa, Guam, Trust Territory of the Pacific	San Francisco, Calif.
X	Alaska, Idaho, Oregon, Washington	Seattle, Wash.

Department of the Interior. Many highly significant health problems are the responsibility of the Department of the Interior. These responsibilities are adjuncts of the primary purpose of the department and are an essential service.

Bureau of Mines—inspection of mines, investigation of mine accidents, and training personnel in mine rescue work

Text continued on p. 550.

TABLE 21-1. Appropriations for the U.S. Public Health Service: actual 1980 level compared with 1981 budget request of the Carter Administration, the congressional action on the 1981 budget, and the 1982 budget requests of the Reagan Administration

Program	Millions of dollars			
		1981		1982
	1980 actual	Carter request	House action	Reagan request
Health Services Administration				
A. Community health services				
1. Community health center (CHC) primary care centers	320.0	353.1	325.0	*
2. CHC research and demonstration centers	10.0	—	7.0	*
3. CHC black lung services	4.5	4.5	4.5	*
4. Home health services	5.0	—	4.0	*
5. Hypertension	20.0	20.0	20.0	*
6. Maternal and child health (MCH) grants to states	345.5	357.4	357.4	*
7. MCH sudden infant death syndrome	2.8	2.8	2.8	*
8. MCH research and training	30.8	24.0	30.0	*
9. Genetic services	14.6	14.9	16.4	*
10. Family planning	162.0	162.0	166.0	*
11. Migrant health	39.7	44.7	43.4	*
12. National Health Service Corps (unauthorized)	(74.1)	(87.2)	—	95.0
13. Program support	33.9	38.7	36.0	*
B. Health care services and systems				
1. Public Health Service hospitals and clinics	171.2	164.0	164.0	73.0
2. Federal employees health program	0.8	0.8	0.8	1.0
3. Payments to Hawaii	1.8	1.8	1.8	2.0
4. Emergency medical services	32.1	21.1	30.0	*
5. Program support	10.0	10.0	10.0	10.0
6. Indian Health Service	620.0	682.0	682.0	635.0
C. Refugee assistance	36.0	—	—	*
D. Buildings and facilities	3.0	4.8	4.8	} 27.0
E. Program management	7.7	7.8	7.8	

Food and Drug Administration	325.0	355.0	355.0	336.0
Centers for Disease Control				
A. Disease control				
1. Health incentive grants to states	68.0	—	36.0	*
2. Risk reduction and health education	13.5	13.7	13.7	*
3. Venereal diseases	47.3	47.6	47.6	7.0*
4. Immunizations	30.1	30.4	30.4	7.0*
5. Fluoridation	6.8	6.8	6.8	2.0*
6. Chronic diseases	17.7	19.3	19.3	19.0
7. Urban rat control	14.5	13.5	13.5	*
8. Lead-based paint poisoning prevention	11.8	10.8	10.8	*
9. Other environmental hazards	3.7	5.2	5.2	4.0
B. Occupational safety and health				
1. Research	61.5	62.4	62.4	59.0
2. Training	13.9	14.3	14.3	
3. Program support	4.2	4.5	4.5	
C. Epidemic services	27.0	29.2	29.2	33.0
D. Technology development and application	24.9	26.8	26.8	26.0
E. Buildings and facilities	11.4	5.0	5.0	2.0
F. Program management	3.7	3.9	3.9	2.0
National Institutes of Health				
A. National Cancer Institute	1,000.0	965.1	1,001.3	1,026.0
B. National Heart, Lung, and Blood Institute	527.5	532.8	560.3	580.0
C. National Institute of Dental Research	68.3	70.0	71.2	75.0
D. National Institute of Arthritis, Metabolism, and Digestive Disorders	341.2	361.2	372.;	380.0
E. National Institute of Neu. and Comm. Disorders and Stroke	242.0	246.8	253.8	276.0
F. National Institute of Allergy and Infectious Diseases	215.4	226.4	232.4	244.0
G. National Institute of General Medical Sciences	312.5	328.1	335.7	341.0
H. National Institute of Child Health and Human Development	209.0	215.0	223.6	231.0
I. National Eye Institute	113.0	115.6	120.3	132.0
J. National Institute of Environmental Health Sciences	83.9	93.8	97.3	110.0
K. National Institute on Aging	70.0	74.3	76.1	84.0

*Most of the 1982 budget lines with no figure have been placed in block grants to states and reduced by 25% from 1981 levels. See text.   *Continued.*

TABLE 21-1. Appropriations for the U.S. Public Health Service: actual 1980 level compared with 1981 budget request of the Carter Administration, the congressional action on the 1981 budget, and the 1982 budget requests of the Reagan Administration—cont'd

Program	Millions of dollars			
	1980 actual	1981 Carter request	1981 House action	1982 Reagan request
National Institutes of Health—cont'd				
L. Research resources	169.2	173.9	184.4	
M. John E. Fogarty Center	9.0	9.1	9.1	
N. National Library of Medicine	44.0	44.4	44.7	283.0
O. Buildings and facilities	3.3	11.8	11.8	
P. Office of the Director	21.1	22.2	22.5	
Alcohol, Drug Abuse, and Mental Health Administration				
A. General mental health				
1. Research	141.2	156.5	147.0	
2. Rape (unauthorized)	(4.1)	(5.7)	—	
3. Training	90.4	90.4	93.9	
4. Community mental health centers (continuations)	235.4	257.3	253.0	235.0*
5. Community demonstrations	7.6	47.1	20.0	
6. Other (unauthorized)	(50.9)	(63.4)	—	
7. Program support	34.9	38.1	37.0	
B. Drug abuse				
1. Research	46.0	50.2	46.0	
2. Training	8.7	7.6	7.6	
3. Project grants and contracts	161.0	161.0	161.0	65.0*
4. Grants to states	38.0	—	30.0	
5. Program support	18.5	19.4	19.4	
C. Alcoholism				
1. Research	22.3	25.1	22.3	
2. Training	7.2	5.8	5.8	
3. Project grants and contracts	78.7	108.3	73.0	38.0*
4. Grants to states	54.8	—	50.0	
5. Program support	10.2	10.8	10.2	

D. Buildings and facilities	—	5.4	5.4	6.0
E. Program management	9.8	10.9	10.9	
Health Resources Administration				
A. Health planning and resource development				58.0
1. Local planning	124.7	101.7	86.7	
2. State planning and regulation	32.0	32.0	32.0	
3. Technical assistance	1.0	1.7	1.7	
4. Program support	9.2	9.7	9.7	
B. Health facility financing and conversion				5.0
1. Health teaching facilities	5.3	4.3	4.3	
2. Program support	4.2	4.8	4.8	
C. Health professions education	325.0	140.0	140.0	120.0
D. Program management	12.4	14.1	14.3	10.0
E. Medical facilities guarantee and loan fund	45.0	—	—	35.0
Assistant Secretary for Health	(1,492.0)	—	(1,405.0)	1,139.0
A. Health services and preventive health block grants to states (unauthorized)	43.1	38.7	38.7	39.0
B. Health statistics	29.7	30.9	34.5	20.0
C. Health services research	3.3	4.0	4.8	
D. Health care technology	0.7	0.7	0.7	20.0
E. Program management (A-D above)	54.4	55.3	62.4	8.0
F. Health maintenance organizations	7.5	10.0	8.7	*
G. Adolescent health	12.5	13.0	13.0	3.0
H. Smoking and health	1.7	3.3	5.3	
I. Health promotion	0.7	0.8	0.8	1.0
J. International health	0.9	0.9	0.9	2.0
K. Physical fitness and sports				18.0
L. Public Health Service management	21.6	22.2	22.9	

Fish and Wildlife Service—research on sanitary processing of fishery products, elimination of hazards of stream pollution, and the destruction of wildlife that jeopardize the health and life of humans

National Park Service—provision of environmental sanitation measures in national parks

Department of Justice. At first glance one would be inclined to disbelieve that the Department of Justice could have any health responsibilities. Yet the duties of the Justice Department encompass certain social responsibilities that logically incorporate health.

Bureau of Prisons—With the assistance of the Public Health Service, provision of medical and dental services to inmates in federal correctional institutions and prisons

Immigration and Naturalization Service—With assistance from the Public Health Service, provision of medical examinations and medical care of immigrants

Department of Labor. Responsibility for the welfare of the worker includes responsibility for health and health conditions. Indeed, health of workers is a primary consideration of the department.

Bureau of Employment Security—health and medical services for migrant farm workers en route from one contractor to another and at reception centers

Bureau of Labor Standards—promotion of health in industry of all descriptions and magnitude

Bureau of Labor Statistics—collection, analysis, and application of data relating to significant health conditions in industry

Women's Bureau—studies on health and working conditions of women in industry and the promotion of the health and welfare of working women

Other agencies. A considerable number of somewhat independent federal agencies provide health services to a significant degree. From a long list, a few of these agencies are identified as examples.

Federal Trade Commission—control of deceptive advertising of foods, drugs, cosmetics, and devices shipped in interstate commerce

Interstate Commerce Commission—enforcement and promotion of health standards in the operation of interstate carriers

National Science Foundation—development of fundamental research in biological, physical, medical, and health sciences

Veterans Administration—providing health and medical services, including hospitalization and rehabilitation to Armed Forces veterans; training of personnel in health work

It is thus apparent that scores of federal agencies are engaged in health work. In each case the service is significant and in some essential. Yet the principal health organization in the federal government, the one that carries on virtually all health functions to an extended degree, is the U.S. Public Health Service. In terms of classic public health, this is perhaps the largest, most formidable, and most effective health organization in the world.

U.S. PUBLIC HEALTH SERVICE

What began in 1798 as the Marine Hospital Service in the Treasury Department evolved into the Public Health and Marine Hospital Service in 1902. In 1912 the name was changed to the U.S. Public Health Service. The responsibilities of the agency continued to be increased. In 1917 the Public Health Service was charged with responsibility for the physical and mental examinations of all aliens entering the country. In the same year a national leprosarium was opened in Carville, Louisiana, and the Public Health Service was designated as the operating agency. In 1929 the medical care of federal prisoners and narcotic addicts became a responsibility of the Public Health Service. In the same year a program in mental hygiene was launched. The Social Security Act of 1935 extended the responsibilities of the Public Health Service. All grants-in-aid to states to strengthen local and state health departments were administered by the Public Health Service.

In subsequent years a series of congressional acts increased the functions of the Public Health Service. In 1937 the National Cancer Act was passed, followed by the Venereal Disease Control Act a year later. In 1939 the U.S. Public Health Service was moved from the Treasury Department to the Federal Security Agencies. Health agencies of other departments were also affected by this action.

The Public Health Law enacted in 1944 was a landmark in the development of the Public Health Service, because this act provided for an expansion, reorganization, and consolidation of the Public Health Service and a revision of laws relating to public health. When the Department of Health, Education, and Welfare (now the HHS) was established in 1953, the Public Health Service became a part of the new department.

In the reorganization of the Department of Health, Education, and Welfare in 1968, Health Services and Mental Health Administration became the designation of what had largely been the U.S. Public Health Service. In the same reorganization, the National Institutes of Health (NIH) became independent of the Health Services and Mental Health Administration as a division of the Department of Health, Education, and Welfare. The Food and Drug Administration (FDA) became the third major division along with the Health Services and Health Institutes. Today, the Assistant Secretary for Health is the administrative head of the six divisions of the Public Health Service (see Table 21-1).

The Environmental Health Service is no longer operational. Its pollution control programs—National Pollution Control Administration, Bureau of Solid Wastes Managements, Bureau of Water Hygiene, and elements of the Bureau of Radiological Health—were trans-

ferred to the Environmental Protection Agency (EPA). In 1971 Community Environmental Management and the Bureau of Occupational Safety and Health became the National Institute of Occupational Safety and Health.

On May 4, 1980, the Department of Education was created, and the Department of Health, Education, and Welfare was renamed the Department of Health and Human Services (HHS).

National Institutes of Health (NIH). In 1887 the Marine Hospital Service founded a research laboratory at the Marine Hospital, Staten Island, New York. In 1891 the name was changed to Hygienic Laboratory, and the unit was moved to Washington, D.C. In 1930 the Hygienic Laboratory became the NIH and moved to Bethesda, Maryland, on land donated by Mr. and Mrs. Luke I. Wilson of Bethesda.

The mission of the NIH is the discovery of knowledge for the prevention and control of disease and the extension of life. A broad, complex program is designed to meet the needs in biomedical science. Scientists in the laboratories and clinical center of the NIH carry on part of the program of research. Most of the research is done outside of the NIH through grants administered by the NIH. About 90% of the institute's appropriation of more than $3 billion yearly goes to the extramural program of grants to scientists and research institutions throughout the nation.

The grants program is planned to provide a continuous supply of competent scientists in biomedical disciplines. In addition to the training grants, fellowships, and traineeships, the program also provides facilities, equipment, and other resources, including computers and primate centers. Basic research now cuts across several of the traditional areas. Special attention is given to national trends and to neglected research areas.

The NIH has an international research program, which seeks to make use of the abilities of qualified scientists the world over. Grants have been made to scientists in various health disciplines in many countries. The NIH has also provided opportunities for promising young American scientists to work abroad as members of the established research groups. No foreign grants are made unless they are of a high value and are related to health objectives of value to the United States. Nobel Prize awards in medicine and physiology have been made to foreign investigators who were working under grants from the NIH.

The NIH makes contracts with foreign institutions to conduct research and provides fellowships to American scientists to study at foreign centers of excellence. NIH also promotes a visiting program that brings distinguished scientists to the United States to work in the NIH laboratories or the John E. Fogarty International Center.

The NIH expends some $3 billion to finance research in hospitals, medical schools, and nonprofit research centers. Altogether, it underwrites about 40% of all the biomedical research done in the United States. (The reader can obtain more information by writing National Institutes of Health, Office of Public Affairs, Room 309, Building 1, 9000 Rockville Pike, Bethesda, MD 20014.)

Food and Drug Administration (FDA). The FDA regulates products that account for 20 cents of every dollar spent by consumers. Its responsibilities range from making sure that the radiation emission levels of color television sets are safe, to inspecting cosmetics to assure that they are free from harmful bacteria, and from requiring nutrition information on food packages, to assuring the safety and effectiveness of medicines. The work of the FDA's scientists—physicians, chemists, nutritionists, microbiologists, pharmacologists—forms the basis of its regulatory activities. (For more information, write Food and Drug Administra-

tion, Office of Public Affairs, Room 15B-42, 5600 Fishers Lane, Rockville, MD 20857.)

Centers for Disease Control. Based in Atlanta, the Centers for Disease Control are well known for their efforts to combat communicable diseases. They also work in occupational safety and health, diabetes control, nutrition, health education, and family planning. They train state and local health officials in epidemic control and in operating local disease prevention programs. (For more information, write Centers for Disease Control, Office of Information, Atlanta, GA 30333.)

Health Resources Administration. The Health Resources Administration works with the people who provide health care, the schools that train them, and the facilities in which they work—all with an eye toward assuring that the nation's health resources are adequate. It also supports and works with the nationwide network of state and local health planning agencies to improve the availability and adequacy of medical services in all parts of the country, while constraining the rising costs of such services. The administration has recently been severely reduced by budget cuts. (For more information, write Health Resources Administration, Office of Communications, Room 10-44, Center Building, 3700 East-West Highway, Hyattsville, MD 20782.)

Health Services Administration. Most of the programs of the Health Services Administration will be rolled into the health services and maternal and child health block grants under the Omnibus Budget Reconciliation Act of 1981 passed by Congress. More than 600 community health centers have been funded, bringing health care to thousands of inner-city and isolated rural residents. The administration's migrant health program focuses on meeting the health needs of migrant workers and their families. Migrant health care represents a good example of justified federal intervention because of the interstate migration patterns and con-

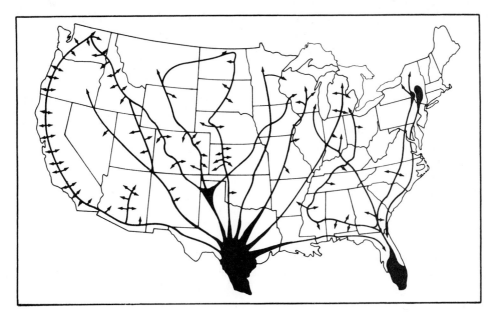

FIG. 21-2. Schematic diagram of travel patterns of migrant agricultural workers.
From Office of Migrant Health, U.S. Public Health Service.

comitant spread of communicable diseases (Fig. 21-2).

The Health Services Administration also operates the National Health Service Corps, recruiting medical professionals and placing them in both rural and urban medically underserved areas, and the Indian Health Service, providing direct care to nearly $1/2$ million American Indians and Alaska natives through a network of 51 hospitals, 86 care centers, and 300 field clinics.

In 1979 the Health Services Administration also treated more than 2 million people in its eight hospitals, 27 clinics, and the National Hansen's Disease Center in Louisiana. (For more information, write Health Services Administration, Office of Communications and Public Affairs, Room 14A-55, Parklawn Building, 5600 Fishers Lane, Rockville, MD 20857.)

Alcohol, Drug Abuse, and Mental Health Administration. The Alcohol, Drug Abuse, and Mental Health Administration spearheads the federal effort to prevent and treat problems related to alcohol and drug misuse and mental and emotional illnesses. Through its three institutes—the National Institute of Alcohol Abuse and Alcoholism, the National Institute on Drug Abuse, and the National Institute of Mental Health—it funds research, supports local treatment offices, and finances nationwide campaigns aimed at the prevention of drug and alcohol misuse and the promotion of mental health. Most of its programs will be placed in block grants, and most of its behavioral research will be terminated by the Reagan Administration. (For more information, write Alcohol, Drug Abuse, and Mental Health Administration, Office of Communications and Public Affairs, 5600 Fishers Lane, Rockville, MD 20857.)

• • •

As the HHS enters the 1980s, it is conducting major initiatives focusing on the prevention of disease and illness and the promotion of health. These include protecting millions of youngsters from crippling and sometimes lethal illnesses through early and regular childhood immunization; assuring early identification and treatment of health problems that would otherwise be undetected among the nation's 10 million lower-income children; and improving the health of all Americans by encouraging them to lead life-styles that will greatly reduce their risk of developing chronic diseases. (For more information about the disease prevention and health promotion initiatives of the Public Health Service, write Public Health Service, Office of Health Information, Health Promotion, and Physical Fitness and Sports Medicine, 721B Hubert Humphrey Building, 200 Independence Avenue, S.W., Washington, D.C. 20201.)

OTHER COMPONENTS OF THE DEPARTMENT OF HEALTH AND HUMAN SERVICES (HHS)
Health Care Finance Administration

The creation of Medicare and Medicaid culminated a quarter century of legislative efforts to assure that no elderly, disabled, or poor American need forego basic health care because of cost. Within HHS, Medicare and Medicaid are managed by the Health Care Finance Administration.

Medicare provides low-cost health insurance for aged and disabled Social Security and railroad retirement beneficiaries. In 1979 27.6 million aged or disabled Americans were eligible for Medicare benefits, which in that year totaled more than $28 billion.

Medicaid, jointly funded by federal and state governments, provides virtually free health insurance coverage for those unable to afford any other kind of insurance or health care. In 1979 the national Medicaid bill totaled more than $20 billion for health care provided to nearly 23 million people.

The Health Care Finance Administration also develops and enforces standards to assure high quality health care and to guarantee the safety and quality of all health services financed by federal funds. (For more information, write Health Care Finance Administration, Office of Information, Room 5218, Switzer Building, 330 C Street, S.W., Washington, D.C. 20201.)

Office of Human Development Services

For millions of Americans, dignity and hope would be beyond reach without the broad range of human services provided by HHS. Generating hope for a better life are programs of HHS's Office of Human Development Services that serve millions of children, youth, American Indians, Alaska natives, native Hawaiians, families in need, the aged, and the disabled. These programs enable families to remain together, provide permanent care for homeless children, serve victims of spouse or child abuse, and help developmentally disabled people live in their own homes and communities instead of institutions. Few of these services existed 2 decades ago. Most of the programs of the Office of Human Development Services will be included in a single social services block grant to states under the Reagan Administration's proposal.

Under Title XX of the Social Security Act, the Office of Human Development Services supports and helps to coordinate a comprehensive range of in-home and community-based social services including day-care, homemaker-chore services; training and employment; protective services; foster care; counseling; and family planning. It provides funding directly to states and gives technical assistance to governmental units that administer the aid. The social services and training funds under Title XX are slated by the Reagan Administration to be included in the social services block grants.

The Office of Human Development Services also supports the Work Incentive Program (WIN), which provides training, employment, and social services designed to shift families from welfare dependency to self-sufficiency. The program is administered jointly by HHS and the Department of Labor.

The principal goal of the Office of Human Development Services, in addition to assuring proper and efficient management of the programs it oversees, is to improve the quality of all human service programs throughout the United States. A more cohesive social service network would not only improve cost-effectiveness, but also assure assistance for people who need it. (For more information, write Office of Human Development Services, Office of Public Affairs, Room 329-D, Hubert Humphrey Building, 200 Independence Avenue, S.W., Washington, D.C. 20201.)

The following are the major program components of the Office of Human Development Services.

Administration for Children, Youth, and Families. Programs for children, from infancy through adolescence, and their families bring healing and protection for abused children, provide services for battered women and their families, reach out to runaway or homeless youths, support quality day-care services to meet the needs of working parents, and give society's vulnerable children a "head start." The Head Start budget will increase under the Reagan Administration and will not be included in the social services block grants. (For more information, write Administration for Children, Youth, and Families, Office of Public Information, Room 3853, Donohoe Building, 400 6th Street, S.W., Washington, D.C. 20201.)

Administration for Native Americans. The Administration for Native Americans provides a departmental focus for the special concerns (other than health) of American Indians, Alaska natives, and native Hawaiians. Financial assistance is provided through grants to promote economic and social self-sufficiency, thereby reinforcing the programs of the Indian Health Service. (For more information, write Admin-

istration for Native Americans, Room 329-D, Hubert Humphrey Building, 200 Independence Avenue, S.W., Washington, D.C. 20201.)

Administration on Aging. The Administration on Aging was established to provide a focal point in government for the concerns and needs of older people and to coordinate federal policies that affect them. It supports community-based nutrition and companionship programs, transportation services, legal aid, homemaker and home health service, residential repair, and recreational activities for older people. A primary goal of all programs for the elderly is to provide supportive services in the community that will enable older people to lead fully independent lives, avoid unnecessary institutionalization, and be a part of the community. (For more information, see Chapter 7 or write Administration on Aging, Office of Public Information, Room 4553, North Building, 330 Independence Avenue, S.W., Washington, D.C. 20201.)

Administration on Developmental Disabilities. The Administration on Developmental Disabilities is responsible for overall program advocacy and leadership within the Office of Human Development Services for the needs of disabled people. The unit works through state agencies to improve services to people with developmental disabilities or severe mental or physical impairments that are manifested before age 22. (For more information, write Administration on Developmental Disabilities, Room 3070, Switzer Building, 330 C Street, S.W., Washington, D.C. 20201.)

In addition, the President's Committee on Mental Retardation, located within the Office of Human Development Services, advises the President and works with government agencies to prevent mental retardation.

Social Security Administration

Through its Social Security Administration, HHS operates the world's largest social insurance program. Each month some 35 million Americans receive Social Security benefits. These benefits total more than $117 billion annually. Most beneficiaries are retired workers. Some are disabled workers and their family members. Others are young children or eligible spouses of workers who have died. Through payroll taxes, 115 million Americans are making cash contributions to a Social Security system that guarantees direct benefits to them or their dependents in the event of retirement, death, or disability.

In addition, more than 4 million aged, blind, and disabled Americans—all with little or no resources—receive monthly cash benefits from the separate Supplemental Security Income Program administered by the Social Security Administration.

Another program administered by the Social Security Administration is Aid to Families with Dependent Children. This program provides cash welfare payments to more than 10 million individuals, mostly mothers and children, who have little or no other source of income. The cost of the program is shared by the states and, in a few cases, the cities.

Information about Social Security or Supplemental Security Income can be obtained by contacting the nearest of more than 1,300 Social Security Administration offices throughout the United States. All are listed in local telephone books under Social Security Administration. Information about Aid to Families with Dependent Children can be obtained by contacting county welfare, social service, or human resources offices.

Office of the Inspector General

The Office of the Inspector General (General Counsel) is charged by law with preventing misuse of HHS's funds and promoting economy and efficiency in HHS operations. Created by Congress in 1976, the office is the auditing and investigating arm of HHS. Each year it conducts about 8,000 audits of departmental grantees, contractors, and state agencies that receive federal funds.

The Office of the Inspector General is continually acting to detect any fraud or abuse through such activities as

- Analyzing Medicaid and Medicare program billings by physicians, dentists, and other medical practitioners and agencies
- Conducting special studies of operations of nursing homes, home health care agencies, and hopsitals that derive some support from Medicaid and Medicare
- Making computer comparisons of welfare rolls of various states

The Office of the Inspector General also evaluates the operation of departmental systems and programs and seeks ways of improving their performance for the people they serve. The Office of the Inspector General is the intradepartmental "watchdog agency," whose job is to see that HHS's programs operate honestly, efficiently, and effectively. (For more information, write HHS/Office of the Inspector General, Room 5250, North Building, 330 Independence Avenue, S.W., Washington, D.C. 20201.)

Office for Civil Rights

The Office for Civil Rights spearheads the effort to guarantee the civil rights of people participating in HHS programs. The office monitors and enforces those laws barring federal financial assistance to programs or institutions that discriminate on the basis of race, color, national origin, age, or physical and mental handicap.

In cases of alleged discrimination, the Office for Civil Rights attempts to help organizations or institutions comply with the law through mediation and negotiation. When such attempts fail, the Office for Civil Rights is required to initiate legal proceedings to achieve compliance.

The Office for Civil Rights was created in response to the national determination in the 1960s to end discrimination against members of ethnic and racial minority groups. The Civil Rights Act of 1964 gave the office authority to terminate federal funding when voluntary action to end proven discrimination failed. Additional legislation in the 1970s gave the office strong new legal tools to protect the rights of the aged and of physically and mentally handicapped people.

Some individuals may be reluctant to file complaints, fearing retaliation, and others simply may not know of their rights and how to ensure them. Thus the Office for Civil Rights has recently given increased emphasis to what it calls "compliance reviews." In such a review the office will look at an entire institution—a university, a welfare agency, a hospital, a nursing home, a mental health center, a program for the aged—to see whether its practices are nondiscriminatory. (For more information, write HHS/Office for Civil Rights, Room 5400, North Building, 330 Independence Avenue, S.W., Washington, D.C. 20201.)

Office of Refugee Resettlement

The Office of Refugee Resettlement administers a series of refugee assistance programs authorized by the Refugee Assistance Act of 1980. The programs include 100% reimbursement to states for their cost of providing cash assistance, medical assistance, and social services to persons forced to flee their homelands because of persecution on religious, political, or ethnic grounds. In addition, the office directly funds grants to state and local social service organizations. The Reagan Administration's 1982 budget assumes that 173,500 refugees will be admitted to the United States in 1982, including 144,000 Indo-Chinese and 29,500 refugees from other parts of the world. Continued assistance is projected for the 168,000 Cuban and Haitian refugees admitted

in 1981. Polish refugees were not anticipated before the budget was approved. (For more information, write Office of Refugee Resettlement, Room 1229 Switzer Building, 330 C Street, S.W., Washington, D.C. 20201.)

PROFESSIONAL HEALTH ORGANIZATIONS

Professional societies or associations are formed by people who have completed a prescribed curriculum and training and have met standards of certification. These people of common purpose organize to uphold professional standards and to serve society better through their organized efforts. While the primary purpose of a professional society is to promote the interests of the profession and its members, its image and prestige depend on its service to humankind, and members of these professional societies are fully aware of this fact. What best serves the public should be in the best interests of the professional organization.

American Medical Association (AMA). The AMA was founded in 1847. Its constitution states that "the object of the Association is to promote the art of medicine and the betterment of public health." Primarily, the AMA serves the interests of private medical practitioners, but its activities are planned to protect and serve the interests of the public and particularly to provide the best possible medical service.

The AMA is a federation of state societies, and these in turn are made up of county societies, which means that the national organization is an association of state societies rather than of individual practitioners. The AMA strives to improve the quality of medical service by informing members of advancements in medicine and related fields. It has three different agencies investigating possible quackery in drugs, nostrums, foods, cosmetics, and other possible health frauds that might jeopardize the health of the public. The AMA participates in the accreditation of hospital standards.

The *Journal of the American Medical Association* is a weekly publication and is generally regarded as a leading journal in its field. The AMA also publishes much pamphlet material for distribution.

American Dental Association. The American Dental Association was formed in 1860 to advance the dental profession by raising the quality of dental education and dental practice. The association is the profession's agency for keeping practitioners informed of new developments in equipment, procedures, and techniques.

In its early years the American Dental Association was an organization of individual dental practitioners; later it became an association of state societies, which in turn are composed of representatives from county societies. The American Dental Association publishes the *Journal of the American Dental Association* and a yearly index of periodical dental literature. The association also publishes pamphlets for distribution to patients.

American Public Health Association. The American Public Health Association was established in September 1872 and rapidly expanded from a limited interest in sanitation to a broad public health program to encompass all factors affecting the health of the people.

The American Public Health Association carries on a wide variety of activities through 25 sections including laboratory, health administration, community health planning, statistics, environment, radiological health, food and nutrition, injury control, international health, maternal and child health, public health education, gerontological health, veterinary public health, social work, population, public health nursing, epidemiology, school health education and services, dental health, mental health, occupational health, vision care, and medical care. The association has developed standards that have been widely accepted and adopted. These include methods for the examination of water, milk, and sewage, the operation of swimming pools, diagnostic reagents and procedures, the appraisal of local health work, a model health code for cities, the accreditation of public health training, and many other standards, procedures, and guides. The association conducts surveys and other studies, which it initiates and carries out at the request of organizations or of individuals. Its publication, *American Journal of Public Health,* is issued each month. In addition, the association publishes *The Nation's Health,* a monthly newsletter, pamphlets, special reports, and other material.

National League for Nursing. The National League for Nursing was formed in 1952 when three national nursing organizations and four national committees combined their resources and programs—the National League of Nursing Education (founded in 1893), the National Organization for Public Health Nursing (1912), the Association of Collegiate Schools of Nursing (1933), the Joint Committee on Practical Nurses and Auxiliary workers in Nursing Services (1945), the Joint Committee on Careers in Nursing (1948), the National Committee for the Improvement of Nursing Services (1949), and the National Nursing Accrediting Service (1949).

The principal purpose of the National League for Nursing is simply stated, "That the nursing needs of the people may be met." The Department of Public Health Nursing continues the practices and objectives of the previous National Organization for Public Health Nursing. The following are the objectives of the Department of Public Health Nursing:

1. To stimulate responsibility for the health of the community by establishing and extending public health nursing
2. To bring about cooperation among nurses, physicians, and all others interested in public health
3. To develop standards of public health nursing
4. To maintain a central bureau of informa-

tion and assistance in such services

5. To publish periodicals and bulletins

The league has both professional and non-professional members including both public health nurses and friends of public health nurses. The official periodical of the National League for Nursing is *Nursing Outlook*. The league is also the sponsor of *Nursing Research*.

Society of Public Health Education. The Society of Public Health Education was formed in 1958 as the Society of Public Health Educators. Its change in name reflects its commitment to promotion of health education of the public more than the interests of its professional members. With a membership of less than 1,500, the society has been remarkably effective in influencing national policy related to health education, including the Health Information and Promotion Act of 1976 (PL 94-317). The society publishes *Health Education Quarterly* and meets annually in conjunction with the American Public Health Association.

American Alliance for Health, Physical Education, Recreation and Dance. The American Alliance for Health, Physical Education, Recreation and Dance began in 1885 as the American Association for the Advancement of Physical Education and became a department of the National Education Association in 1937. "Alliance" refers to its several constituent organizations, including the Association for the Advancement of Health Education. Several areas of alliance activity are related to health, such as school nursing, school medical service, health teaching, nutrition education, dental health, mental health, and recreation. The alliance recommends program standards for communities. The alliance publishes the monthly *Health Education* and the *Research Quarterly*.

HEALTH FOUNDATIONS

The United States is blessed with a considerable number of philanthropical foundations, many of which are engaged in public health programs. Some foundations have broad programs and operate in a variety of fields. Others are specific in their activities and tend to concentrate on relatively few projects. Five foundations will be described as examples of the different types that engage in health projects.

Rockefeller Foundation. The Rockefeller Foundation was chartered in 1913 under the laws of the state of New York for the purpose of "promoting the well-being of mankind throughout the world." In part, the charter states:

It shall be within the purposes of said corporation to use as means to that end research, publications, the establishment and maintenance of charitable, benevolent, religious, missionary, and public education activities, agencies, and institutions already established and any other means and agencies which from time to time shall seem expedient to its members or trustees.

In its organization the foundation consists of five divisions: (1) International Health, (2) Medical Sciences, (3) Natural Sciences, (4) Social Sciences, and (5) Humanities.

The International Health Division is an operating agency with its own laboratories and staff of scientists. Three phases of work have been pursued: (1) control of specific diseases such as yellow fever, tuberculosis, and influenza, (2) aid to health departments, and (3) health demonstrations, aid to selected schools, public health education, and grants of postgraduate fellowships in public health. Out of the research laboratories of the foundation have come many significant contributions in the treatment of yellow fever, typhus, influenza, and malaria.

The other divisions support university, laboratory, and other research groups. Fellowships for postdoctoral work are also granted. These divisions support a wide range of activities through various grants and appropriations.

Milbank Memorial Fund. The Milbank Memorial Fund was established in 1905 with the objective "to improve the physical, mental, and moral condition of humanity and generally to advance charitable and benevolent objects." Its activities for the most part have been in preventive medicine. Objectives of the organization have been attained through grants and fellowships. Contributions of the fund have been to the fields of public health, medicine, social welfare, research, and education. The fund has sponsored population studies, demonstrations, projects, a recent study of schools of public health, and the measurement of various aspects of public health services. The organization has extended its activities to mental hygiene, school lunches, food research, defective vision, dental studies, prenatal and postnatal instruction, and public health demonstrations.

Commonwealth Fund. The Commonwealth Fund was founded in 1918 with a simple but meaningful objective: "To do something for the welfare of mankind." Activities have included health, medical education and research, education, and mental hygiene. The fund has been instrumental in advancing public health practices and procedures through research, improved teaching in medical schools, extension of public health services to rural communities, provision and improvement of hospital facilities, and strengthening mental health services in the United States and in Great Britain.

W.K. Kellogg Foundation. The W.K. Kellogg Foundation was established in 1930 for "the promotion of health, education, and the welfare of mankind, but principally of children and youth, directly or indirectly, without regard to sex, race, creed, or nationality." The 19 points listed in the Children's Charter of the White House Conference on Child Health and Protection in 1930 have been accepted as goals. A functional problem-solving approach has been used rather than one of research or relief. The foundation's program begins in the home by teaching people to help themselves. Grants have been made to various counties to establish county health departments. A recent priority is health education programs to link the school and community in health promotion.

Robert Wood Johnson Foundation. The Robert Wood Johnson Foundation received the bulk of General Johnson's estate and began its work on the national scene in 1972. With offices just outside Princeton, New Jersey, the foundation made grants totaling more than $400 million by 1980, with a primary emphasis on improving access to general medical and dental care. The statistics on access improved considerably during this period, so two new priorities have been added since 1980: (1) support for research programs to make health care arrangements more effective and care more affordable and (2) support for research, development, and demonstration projects that show promise of helping large numbers of people avoid disabilities and maintain or regain maximum attainable function in their everyday lives.

Cooperation and coordination. Voluntary health agencies have made a significant contribution to the health of the United States and the world. Each agency is free to choose its own course of action and is sufficiently flexible to adjust to changing conditions and needs. These agencies tend to specialize and demonstrate what can be done in a specific field of health. In theory, when this has been accomplished, the task or field is taken over by an official health agency and the need for the voluntary agency no longer exists. In practice, few voluntary agencies are ever dissolved.

Overlapping of programs exists to some degree. The need for cooperation and coordination has long existed, and in 1921 the National Health Council was organized with about 50 voluntary national groups represented. The U.S. Public Health Service served as an advisory member. At the outset the council was well financed and well staffed. Within 5 years after its inception, the council had become ineffective and had abandoned many of its projects. Some revitalization has occurred in recent years through the organization of National Health Forums, the inauguration of Community Health Week, the creation of working committees, and various publications. The council recently assisted in the establishment of a National Center for Health Education based in San Francisco and cosponsored a series of Regional Health Promotion Forums with the U.S. Office of Health Information and Health Promotion.

Voluntary health agencies perform a unique and important role in the promotion of health in every state and in most nations. No health program is complete in the sense that it serves every individual who could benefit from the program. Thus these agencies have a need to expand and intensify their services. Further, there are areas of health needs that receive little attention and less service. Perhaps the National Foundation for Infantile Paralysis (now the March of Dimes Birth Defects Foundation) charted the course that all existing voluntary as well as official agencies might consider. When the agency's original goal is virtually achieved, the agency directs its attention and energies to other health problems in need of solution rather than returning to the public with requests for funds to do more of the same.

OFFICIAL INTERNATIONAL HEALTH ORGANIZATIONS

For more than a century, health scientists of the world have worked cooperatively and harmoniously in promoting the health of all people. National interests have given way to world interests. Exchange of health knowledge, loan of the services of experts, and united efforts in preventing the spread of disease have characterized the international activities of public health personnel the world over. In the early years of international health activities, virtually all attention was directed to the control of communicable diseases, but programs have expanded to encompass the entire spectrum of health promotion.

International congresses on hygiene and epidemiology have been held at irregular intervals since 1852, when the first congress met in Brussels. After a series of such meetings, the International Office of Public Health was created on December 9, 1907, by agreement among 40 nations. Until the formation of the Health Section in the Secretariat of the League of Nations, the International Office of Public Health served as the medium for the international exchange of health knowledge and for cooperation on health matters. In 1950 the International Office of Public Health was absorbed by the World Health Organization (WHO).

Pan American Health Organization. Creation of the Pan American Sanitary Bureau was authorized by the Second International Conference of the American States, which met in Mexico City in 1901. It was formally organized as the International Sanitary Office at the First Inter-American Sanitary Conference, held in Washington, D.C., in 1902. The Fifth Conference, which met in Santiago, Chile, in 1911, changed the name to Pan American Sanitary Bureau.

From its inception the Pan American Sanitary Bureau has devoted its attention primarily to the control of communicable diseases. This has been done through cooperation between the participating nations by exchanging vital statistics reports, exchanging health information on travellers, reporting new advances in disease control, exchanging knowledge on advances in sanitation procedures, training health personnel, and making technical experts available to other nations on a consulting basis. The Pan American Sanitary Bureau is now known as the Pan American Health Organization and is an independent health organization, but at present is essentially an agency integrated with WHO as one of its regional offices.

League of Nations Health Section. In September 1923, under Article 23 of the covenant of the League of Nations, participating nations established a Health Section in the Secretariat of the League of Nations. The Health Section developed a moderately effective program. In cooperation with the International Office of Public Health, the Health Section took steps to control epidemics, improved the worldwide epidemiological reporting system, initiated research in the control of communicable diseases, established standards for biological products, began studies on the underlying foundations of health, and assisted governments in improving their public health services.

With the formation of the United Nations and the creation of WHO, the League of Nations Health Section was duly dissolved. WHO took over all functions of the League of Nations Health Section and of the International Office of Public Health. The Pan American Health Organization became a regional office of WHO.

WORLD HEALTH ORGANIZATION (WHO)

The International Health Conference that convened in New York City on June 19, 1946, ushered in a new era in health cooperation. The conference was attended by representatives from all of the member states of the United Nations and by observers from 13 countries that were not members. At the closing session on June 22, the final instruments were approved and signed by the conference. This included a protocol providing for the absorption by WHO of the International Office of Health and the League of Nations Health Section. The constitution provided for the eventual integration of the Pan American Sanitary Bureau with WHO. By April 7, 1948, the required 26 countries that were members of the United Nations had confirmed their approval of the constitution and their membership in WHO.

The founding principles of WHO and a widely quoted definition of health are set forth in the preamble of its consititution

Health is a state of complete physical, mental, and social wellbeing and not merely the absence of disease or infirmity.
The enjoyment of the highest attainable standard of health is one of the fundamental rights of every human being without distinction of race, religion, political belief, or economic or social conditions.

The health of all peoples is fundamental to the attainment of peace and security and is dependent upon the fullest cooperation of individuals and states.
The achievement of any state in the promotion and protection of health is of value to all.
Unequal development in different countries in the promotion of health and control of disease, especially communicable disease, is a common danger.
Healthy development of the child is of basic importance; the ability to live harmoniously in a changing total environment is essential to such development.
The extension to all peoples of the benefits of medical, psychologic, and related knowledge is essential to the fullest attainment of health.
Informed opinion and active cooperation on the part of the public are of the utmost importance in the improvement of the health of the people.
Governments have a responsibility for the health of their peoples that can be fulfilled only by the provision of adequate health and social measures.

Financing. The WHO budget is raised by assessments of Member States according to a formula, with a limitation that no nation shall pay more than $33^{1}/_{3}\%$ of the total assessment. In addition, the organization receives funds from various other sources—Pan American Health Organization and voluntary contributions from governments, institutions, and individuals.

Organization. The democratic nature of WHO is reflected in its organization, where legislation, administration, and services are under the direction of the Member States. A great deal of the services of participants are contributed without any cost to the organization.

World Health Assembly is the legislative branch of WHO. Delegates of the Member States and Associate Members meet annually in Geneva, Switzerland. The World Health Assembly establishes policy and decides on the program and budget for the next year.

Executive Board is the board of directors of

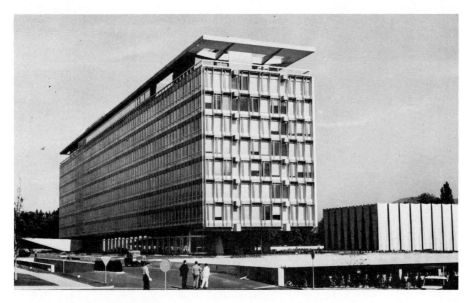

FIG. 21-3. WHO headquarters in Geneva is a monument to people's concern for one another and a symbol of cooperation in a world of conflict.

Courtesy WHO.

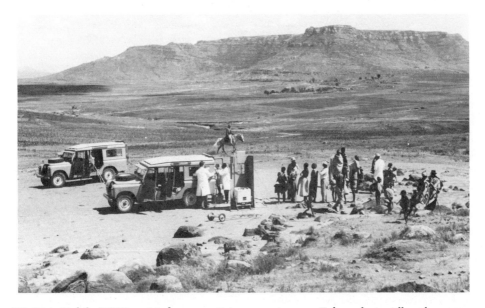

FIG. 21-4. Mobile WHO-assisted x-ray unit in a remote area. Tuberculosis still ranks among the world's greatest scourges. WHO is helping to develop large-scale programs in diagnosis and control.

Courtesy WHO.

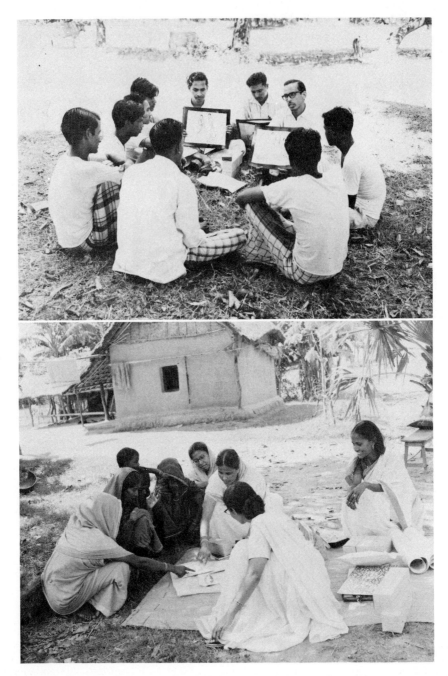

FIG. 21-5. Family planning education for villages in Bangladesh. Cultural factors require local adaptations of media and channels of communication in traditional societies.

Courtesy Public Health Education Research Project, University of California, Berkeley.

the organization. The board is composed of 24 persons qualified in health matters. It meets at least twice a year to advise and act for the assembly. Each year the assembly elects eight governments to designate members to serve for 3 years and to replace eight retiring members.

Secretariat designates the professional management of WHO at headquarters in Geneva and in 140 countries of the world. The Director-General is the chief executive, and in organization the Secretariat is composed of three departments—advisory services, central technical services, and administration and finance. Each department is composed of divisions that in turn are made up of sections.

Regions are used for effectiveness in organization and operation. For WHO purposes, the world is divided into six regions, each with its own organization consisting of a regional committee composed of delegates from governments in the region, and a regional office that administers WHO-aided projects and supervises the staff in the various projects. Regional offices of WHO are logically distributed.

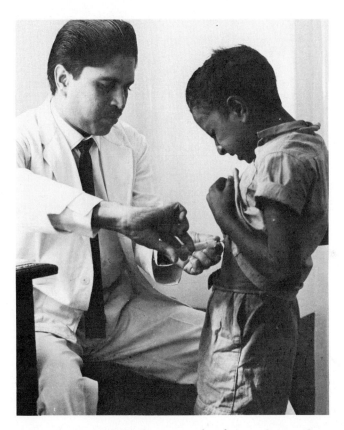

FIG. 21-6. Rabies immunization, WHO International Reference Centre, Coonoor, India. The long incubation period provides the victim the chance to be immunized before the virus reaches the brain. Rabies must be eliminated in lower animals if rabies is to be eradicated in humans.

Courtesy WHO.

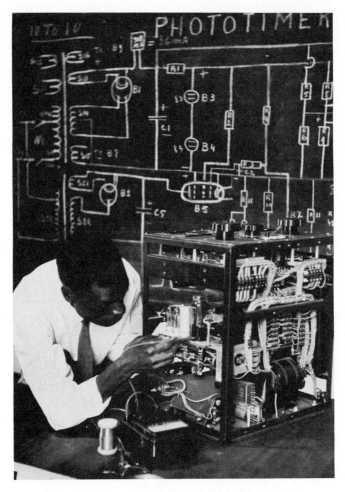

FIG. 21-7. Training of health personnel. WHO helps to build up national and regional teaching and training institutions. At the Tuberculosis Chemotherapy Laboratory in Nairobi, Kenya, trainees learn to repair x-ray equipment.

Courtesy WHO.

Region	Regional office
Southeast Asia	New Delhi
Eastern Mediterranean	Alexandria
The Americas (Pan American Health Organization)	Washington, D.C.
Western Pacific	Manila
Africa	Brazzaville
Europe	Copenhagen

Each regional office has its own staff and method of operation.

Advisory panels consist of more than 12,000 scientists, health administrators, and educators from many nations. These 44 panels provide expert advice in their respective fields. Committees of experts are chosen from these panels to provide the necessary expertise to deal with particular health problems.

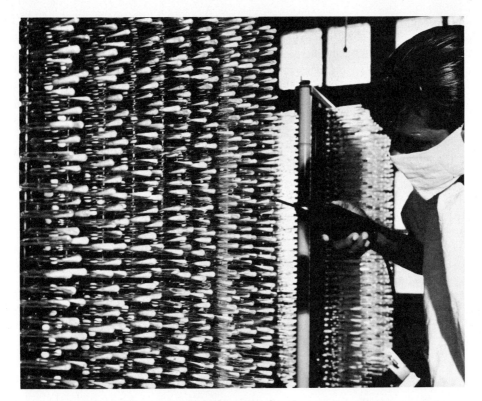

FIG. 21-8. Smallpox eradication. Modern freeze-dried and tropical stable vaccine production in India. In a massive 10-year assault (1967-1977), WHO has worked together with all the countries of the world to defeat one of the greatest killers of all times. In 1979 smallpox became a fear of the past.

Courtesy WHO.

Functions of WHO. To meet the objectives of its charter, WHO recognizes specific functions that are its responsibilities.

1. International health—to act as the directing and coordinating authority on world health
2. International conventions—to propose conventions, agreements, and regulations and make recommendations concerning international health matters
3. International standards—to develop, establish, and promote international standards for food, biologic, pharmaceutical, and similar products
4. Nongovernmental organizations—to promote cooperation among scientific and professional groups that contribute to the advancement of science
5. Research—to promote and conduct research in health
6. Public health—to study and report on public health and medical care from preventive and curative points of view, including hospital services and social security
7. Health services—to assist governments, upon request, in strengthening health services
8. Maternal and child health—to promote maternal and child health and welfare and to foster the ability to live harmoniously in a changing environment
9. Diseases—to stimulate and advance work to

eradicate epidemic, endemic, and other disease

10. Diagnosis—to standardize diagnostic procedures as necessary

11. Living conditions—to promote the improvement of nutrition, housing, sanitation, recreation, economic, or working conditions, and other aspects of environmental hygiene

12. Accidents—to promote the prevention of accidental injuries

13. Mental health—to foster activities in mental health, especially those affecting human relations

14. Education—to promote improved standards of teaching and training in health, medical, and related professions

WHO is helping many nations to solve many health problems. In helping a nation, it is always the objective of WHO to build up the nation's potential and train its personnel so that eventually outside help will not be needed. In some instances the services of WHO are merely advisory, but in many instances WHO personnel are on the scene to do the job that is necessary. WHO also takes part in the United Nations Expanded Programme of Technical Assistance for economic development of underdeveloped countries. WHO operates closely with the United Nations Children's Fund, the United Nations Specialized Agencies, especially the Food and Agriculture Organization, and the United Nations Educational, Scientific and Cultural Organization, the Technical Assistance Board, and the International Labor Organization.

It is significant that public health people

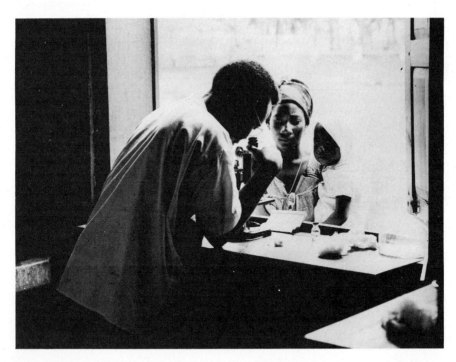

FIG. 21-9. Rural health services. Well-organized rural health services are essential to improve health conditions of the areas concerned and to help in the consolidation and integration phases of eradication campaigns against communicable diseases.

Courtesy WHO.

from all over the world can work together harmoniously and cooperatively. This is possible in a profession guided by the idea of service to humanity. Professional public health people are motivated to improve the health and general well-being and to extend the life expectancy of all people.

QUESTIONS AND EXERCISES

1. In your judgment, which of the eight broad general clauses of the Constitution of the United States provides the federal government with the best means for the promotion of health, and what is your reasoning?
2. Give some examples of how the U.S. government has used the taxing power in matters of health.
3. Evaluate this statement: "One price paid for democracy is inefficiency and illogical organization."
4. Recall any time that you or any member of your family received a direct health service from a U.S. federal agency. Why is such service rare for a student?
5. Identify one health service in a U.S. federal agency, other than the U.S. Public Health Service, which should be assigned to the Public Health Service, and explain your reasons.
6. What reasons can you give for and against lodging the function of stream pollution prevention and control in the U.S. Department of the Interior?
7. What are your reasons for or against establishing the U.S. Public Health Service as an independent agency?
8. What is your reaction to the U.S. Public Health Service having a semimilitary character?
9. What is the significance of the fact that 95% of the professional public health people in the United States are nonmedical people?
10. Evaluate this statement: "Appropriations for the U.S. Public Health Service represent investments rather than expenditures."
11. Justify the grants for Public Health Traineeships. Present a case for extending these grants to other traineeship programs.
12. What justification is there for the NIH subsidizing the research of scientists in other countries?
13. Why should the federal government concern itself with research in the health sciences?
14. In your judgment, what specific health problem is most in need of more extensive and intensive research?
15. What voice does a local medical practitioner have in the policies of the AMA?
16. Which of the professional health organizations do you regard as most public spirited and least self-interested? Why?
17. Some Western nations give far more to WHO than they receive. What is your comment?
18. Why does WHO place so much emphasis on communicable disease control in view of all the recent technological advances in this field?
19. Why is it so important that WHO place primary emphasis on helping nations to help themselves?
20. What do you regard as the number one health problem in the world today and why?

BIBLIOGRAPHY

Allagrante, J.P., and Green, L.W.: When health policy becomes victim blaming, New Eng. J. Med. **305:**1528, December 17, 1981.

Altman, S.H., and Sapolsky, H.M.: Federal health programs, Lexington, Mass., 1981, Lexington Books.

Bryant, J.: Health and the developing world, Ithaca, N.Y., 1969, Cornell University Press.

Epstein S., and Epstein, B.: First book of the World Health Organization, New York, 1964, Franklin Watts, Inc.

Green, L.W.: Determining the impact and effectiveness of health education as it relates to federal policy, Health Educ. Monogr. **6:**28 (Suppl. 1), 1978.

Green, L.W.: Toward national policy for health education. In Blane, H., and Chafetz, M.E., editors: Alcohol, youth, and social policy, New York, 1979, Plenum Publishers.

Green, L.W.: Health promotion policy and the placement of responsibility for personal health care, Family and Community Health **2:**51, 1979.

Green, L.W.: National policy in the promotion of health, Int. J. Health Educ. **22:**161, 1979.

McNerney, W.J., editor: Working for a healthier America, Cambridge, Mass., 1980, Ballinger Publishing Co.

National Nutrition Policy Study—1974: hearings before the Select Committee on Nutrition and Human Needs, United States Senate, 93rd Congress, Part I: Famine and the world situation, Washington, D.C., 1974, U.S. Government Printing Office.

Pflanz, M., and Schach, E., editors: Cross-national sociomedical research: concepts, methods, practice, Stuttgart, 1976, Georg Thieme Publishers.

Profiles in health caring: A report on the voluntary health agency members of the National Health Council, New York, 1980, National Health Council.

Promoting Health, Preventing Disease: Objectives for the nation, Washington, D.C., 1980, Public Health Service, U.S. Department of Health and Human Services.

Sivin, I.: Contraception and fertility change in the international postpartum program, New York, 1974, The Population Council.

Smoking and health programs around the world, Bethesda, 1973, DHEW Publication No. 74-8707, National Clearinghouse for Smoking and Health, Center for Smoking and Health, Centers for Disease Control.

UNESCO: World of promise, Dobbs Ferry, N.Y., 1965, Oceana Publications, Inc.

World Health Organization, what it is, what it does, how it works, Irvington-on-Hudson, N.Y., 1965, Columbia University Press.

PUBLICATIONS OF WHO

The following publications of WHO may be obtained from Q Corporation, 49 Sheridan Avenue, Albany, N.Y. 12210 (variably priced).

Technical report series

No. 548—Planning and organization of geriatric services. Report of a WHO expert Committee, 1974, 46 pages.

No. 553—Ecology and control of rodents of public health importance. Report of a WHO Scientific Group, 1974, 42 pages.

No. 554—Health aspects of environmental pollution control: planning and implementation of national programmes. Report of a WHO Expert Committee, 1974, 57 pages.

No. 558—Community health nursing. Report of a WHO Expert Committee, 1974, 28 pages.

No. 559—New approaches in health statistics. Report of the Second International Conference of National Committees on Vital and Health Statistics, 1974, 40 pages.

No. 562—Services for cardiovascular emergencies. Report of a WHO Expert Committee, 1975, 129 pages.

No. 564—Organization of mental health services in developing countries. Sixteenth Report of the WHO Expert Committee on Mental Health, 1975, 41 pages.

No. 569—Evaluation of family planning in health services. Report of a WHO Expert Committee, 1975, 67 pages.

No. 571—Early detection of health impairment in occupational exposure to health hazards. Report of a WHO Study Group, 1975, 80 pages.

No. 573—Veterinary contribution to public health practice. Report of a joint FAO/WHO Committee, 1975, 79 pages.

No. 584—Food and nutrition strategies in national development. Ninth report of the Joint FAO/WHO Expert Committee on Nutrition, 1976, 64 pages.

No. 586—Health hazards from new environment pollutants. Report of a WHO Study Group, 1976, 96 pages.

No. 589—Planning and evaluation of public dental health services. Report of a WHO Expert Committee, 1976, 35 pages.

Public health papers

No. 57—The teaching of human sexuality in schools for health professionals, 1974, 47 pages.

No. 58—Suicide and attempted suicide, 1974, 127 pages.

No. 59—Administration of environmental health programs. A systems view, 1974, 242 pages.

No. 61—Educational strategies for the health professions, 1974, 106 pages.

Appendixes

AREAS OF COMMUNITY HEALTH SPECIALIZATION IN THE UNITED STATES*

Area of specialization	Differentiating characteristics (pertaining to the area of specialization and illustrative ways it contributes to improved health)	Illustrative jobs and job settings (for graduates of the area of specialization)
Biostatistics *The application of statistical procedures, techniques, and methodology to characterize or investigate health problems and programs.*	Biostatistics is concerned with such activities as the collection, organization, retrieval, and analysis of data; design of experiments; and application of techniques of inference and probability to the examination of biologic, social, and environmental data. Biostatistics closely interacts with the field of epidemiology, while also extending into the congruent areas of vital statistics and demography, computer systems, programming and analysis, and program planning and evaluation. The specialty helps to anticipate needs and improve decision making with regard to health problems, programs, and technologies through (1) the development and operation of ongoing statistical information systems concerned with vital events, health status, and program operations and (2) the proper design and conduct of studies, and the analysis and interpretation of data obtained from such studies.	In local and state agencies employment includes the collection, tabulation, and analysis of statistics bearing on all aspects of health problems and programs. In state, federal, and academic settings employment includes providing assistance to investigators in the design, conduct, and data analysis of research on health problems and programs. In academic institutions employment includes training health workers in the use and interpretation of statistics and carrying out research to discover improved ways of using statistical measures and procedures.

*Based on Hall, T.L., Jackson, R.S., and Parsons, W.B.: Schools of public health, trends in graduate education, Washington, D.C., May, 1980, Division of Associated Health Professions, Public Health Service, DHHS Pub. No. (HRA) 80–45.

Area of specialization	Differentiating characteristics (pertaining to the area of specialization and illustrative ways it contributes to improved health)	Illustrative jobs and job settings (for graduates of the area of specialization)
Epidemiology *The science devoted to the systematic study of the distribution and determinants of disease or disability.*	Epidemiology determines disease frequencies and trends in populations, and those factors that augment or reduce disease and disability. Epidemiology has both a descriptive and analytic role. In the former, and in conjunction with the field of biostatistics, it makes use of the statistical methods to determine morbidity, mortality, prevalence, incidence and case fatality rates, and estimates of risk of developing specific diseases in a given population. In its analytic role, epidemiology uses a variety of techniques to examine and evaluate data that seek to identify predisposing, precipitating, and prolonging factors bearing on disease and disability. By developing new or improved information on the distribution and determinants of disease, epidemiology helps the health system design better ways to prevent, detect, and treat disease and disability.	In health agencies at all levels epidemiologists are employed in the design and execution of studies or information systems concerned with determining the distribution and determinants of disease or disability. In academic settings epidemiologists teach, do research, and assist clinical investigators in the study of disease and in the evaluation of new or improved measures for disease prevention, therapy, and rehabilitation.

Area of specialization	Differentiating characteristics (pertaining to the area of specialization and illustrative ways it contributes to improved health)	Illustrative jobs and job settings (for graduates of the area of specialization)
Health services administration *Concerned with the application and skills in resource management to accomplish the effective and efficient delivery of health services.*	Areas of expertise relevant to this specialization include those of planning, organizing, directing, controlling, policy formulation and analysis, financial management, economics, accounting, and operations research. Faculties of health services administration programs tend to be specialists in one of the administrative knowledge base areas, either as a basic discipline or from later specialization and research. While persons with prior professional degrees are not uncommon, students in specialized programs of health services administration tend to have recent bachelor's degrees or have been practicing administrators without other advanced training. Health services administrators seek to ensure that the resources available for the promotion, protection, and restoration of health are applied as effectively and efficiently as possible, consistent with the scientific knowledge base that exists about health and disease.	Health services administrators are employed at all levels of government and in the private sector to plan, implement, manage, coordinate, and evaluate programs for the delivery of health care and to design administrative systems appropriate for the needs of the population being served.

Area of specialization	Differentiating characteristics (pertaining to the area of specialization and illustrative ways it contributes to improved health)	Illustrative jobs and job settings (for graduates of the area of specialization)
Public health practice and program management *The application of specialized knowledge and skills to the planning, implementation, management, and evaluation of activities carried out relevant to selected types of health professional disciplines and health problems or target populations.*	This area of specialization encompasses many of the identifiable public health programs and activities, some of which are organized according to the demographical characteristics of the target population (maternal and child health, gerontology), others according to a health problem or organ system (mental health, dental public health), and still others according to professional discipline (nursing, social work). Specialists in each of these programmatic areas usually have a prior professional degree in one or more health disciplines in addition to speciality training relevant to their field of choice. They seek to integrate the body of knowledge of the basic discipline (medicine, nursing, etc.) with skills relevant to public health practice (planning, program development, etc.) to design and implement programs appropriate to specific health needs.	Employed at all levels of government and in the private and educational sectors, these specialists assume leadership roles in community-based health care programs and systems; apply technical expertise to planning, implementation, and evaluation of technical programs within a defined organizational framework; and carry out training and research activities.
Health education *Concerned with the process of influencing health-related social and behavioral change in human populations by predisposing, enabling, and reinforcing voluntary decisions conducive to health.*	Health education specialists use specific methods, skills, and program strategies to help people change to healthier life-styles, to make more efficient use of health services, to adopt self-care practices wherever possible, and to participate actively in the design and implementation of programs that affect their health. Skills in the social and behavioral sciences, communication dynamics, educational theory, and community organization as well as other fields are all relevant to this specialization.	Employment is available in many different types of agencies in both the public and private sectors to identify social and health needs of population groups, adapt the health care delivery system to the needs of individuals and communities, develop and implement patient education in health care and community settings, and use the media effectively as a means of achieving the above. Health education and health promotion programs in schools, worksites, and clinical and other community settings employ health educators.

Area of specialization	Differentiating characteristics (pertaining to the area of specialization and illustrative ways it contributes to improved health)	Illustrative jobs and job settings (for graduates of the area of specialization)
Environmental sciences *Those specialties concerned with the identification and control of factors in the natural environment that affect health.*	Environmental sciences specialists are concerned with the relationships between the characteristics of the natural environment (air, water, soil, chemicals, etc.) and mental and physical health. This information is used to establish limits on pollutants that the environment can absorb without detrimental effects, to develop control technology, and to implement controls as necessary for the benefit of human and animal populations. The educational background of most environmental scientists usually includes disciplinary training in one or more of the natural sciences plus advanced courses in those aspects of environmental health relevant to their primary discipline.	Employment is available at all levels of government, public and private organizations, and industry to provide technical knowledge and methods in the investigation, planning, controlling, and regulation of matters pertaining to environmental health hazards. In addition, employees carry out basic and operational environmental research procedures and provide training to community workers and interest groups in methods and techniques of environmental protection.
Occupational safety and health *Concerned with the identification of health and safety hazards related to work and the work environment, and with their prevention and control.*	In collaboration with many disciplines such as medicine, nursing, statistics, engineering, psychology, this area of specialization seeks to minimize ill health, injury, and maladjustments to work that may arise as a result of a person's association with work and the work environment.	In industry occupational safety and health specialists are concerned with establishing the causes and effects of industrial health problems and the implementation of acceptable control methods. In government they are involved with monitoring morbidity and mortality associated with the work environment, formulating and enforcing safety standards, investigating specific health and safety problems, and planning and implementing appropriate health programs. Those employed by academic institutions are involved with the training of specialists in this field and with research.

Area of specialization	Differentiating characteristics (pertaining to the area of specialization and illustrative ways it contributes to improved health)	Illustrative jobs and job settings (for graduates of the area of specialization)
Nutrition *Concerned with the study of the interaction between nutrients, nutrition, and health, and with the application of sound nutritional principles and maintenance of good health.*	One specialization in nutrition is concerned primarily with the scientific study in laboratory and clinical settings of the effects of nutrients or their lack of growth, development, and health; and the other with the application of specialized nutrition knowledge and skills to improve or maintain the health of target population groups. In the former category are found persons with basic preparation in biochemistry, medicine, and related sciences; while in the latter are persons with training in dietetics, clinical nutrition, and related fields.	Employment opportunities for specialists in nutrition exist at all levels of government and in private agencies, institutions, and industry. Examples of typical job activities include the assessment of nutritional problems in individuals and population groups, development and implementation of programs to change patterns of food consumption, and fundamental research into human and animal nutrition.
Biomedical and laboratory practice *Encompasses various specialty disciplines that use laboratory techniques for the diagnosis and treatment of disease, and for the investigation of conditions affecting health status.*	The two main defining characteristics of this broad area of specialization are (1) the type of facilities and equipment used and (2) the fact that it is concerned with the scientific investigation in individuals of biological and biochemical processes that affect or reflect health status. Specialists working in this area may be primarily concerned with developing new knowledge or with the application of existing laboratory-based techniques for the maintenance of health and for the prevention, early detection, and treatment of disease, both in individuals and in mass screening and prevention programs.	Those trained in this specialization are employed at all levels of government, in medical and academic institutions, and in public and private laboratories. Illustrative job opportunities include laboratory research for the detection and treatment of disease and the planning and operation of training programs concerned both with the basic training of laboratory personnel as well as their needs for continuing education.

Area of specialization	Differentiating characteristics (pertaining to the area of specialization and illustrative ways it contributes to improved health)	Illustrative jobs and job settings (for graduates of the area of specialization)
Other *A diverse group of specialties, although not fitting within any of the preceding, nevertheless make important contributions to community health. These specialties are defined in different ways, such as by disciplinary background (e.g., behavioral and social sciences) or by the kinds of phenomena under consideration (e.g., the study and treatment of health problems in an international setting).*		Employment opportunities exist primarily at the federal and state levels, in academic institutions, and in some private agencies and foundations. Skills of particular relevance to this broad area of specialization include the collection and analysis of data pertinent to the health status of defined populations, and the planning, development, and operation or evaluation of programs designed to deal with particular health needs.

COMMON JOB TITLES— PUBLIC AND COMMUNITY HEALTH

Administrator
Director (of a specific service or program)
Health administrator
Health care administrator
Health officer
Health services administrator
Hospital administrator
Nursing home administrator

Analyst
Computer specialist
Demographer
Epidemiologist
Systems analyst

Dentist
Public health dentist

Engineer
Air pollution engineer
Environmental engineer
Product safety engineer
Sanitary engineer
Waterworks engineer

Health Educator
Community health educator
Health promotion specialist
Public health educator
School health educator

Hygienist
Dental hygienist
Industrial hygienist

Inspector
Food and drug inspector
Hospital inspector
Milk and food inspector
Nursing home inspector

Laboratory Technician/ Technologist
Biochemical technologist
Food technologist
Laboratory technician
Microbiology technologist
Radiologic technologist
Veterinary lab technician

Nurse
Industrial health nurse
Mental health nurse
Nurse practitioner
Occupational health nurse
Public health nurse
School nurse
Visiting nurse

Nutritionist
Community nutritionist
Public health nutritionist
School nutritionist

Physician
Industrial health physician
Occupational health physician
Public health physician
School health physician

Planner
Facilities planner
Health planner
Manpower planner
Services planner
Program planner

Sanitarian
Environmental technician
Sanitarian

Scientist
Anthropologist
Bacteriologist
Behavioral scientist
Biologist
Chemist
Dairy scientist
Ecologist
Entomologist
Microbiologist
Parasitologist
Psychologist
Social scientist
Sociologist
Soil scientist
Zoologist

Social Worker
Medical social worker
Mental health counselor
Public health social worker
Psychiatric social worker

Statistician
Analyst
Biometrician
Biostatistician
Survey statistician
Vital statistician

Therapist
Occupational therapist
Physical rehabilitation therapist
Physical therapist
Recreation therapist
Speech therapist
Vocational rehabilitation therapist

Veterinarian
Public health veterinarian
Vector control technician

INDEX

Morbidity—cont'd
  of diabetes, 155
  new, 117-118
Morphine, 330-332, 334
Mortality
  accidents and, 291
  air pollution and, 424
  alcohol-related, 314
  barbiturates and, 339-340, 347
  burns and fires and, 294
  cancer and, 142, 148, 150
  causes of, 141, 142
    projected distribution and, 321
  children and, 119, 120, 121
    school, 305
  cigarette smoking and, 317
  communicable diseases and, 256
  drug-related, reduction of, 347
  farms and, 301, 302
  fetal, 110
  heroin overdose and, 335
  home injuries and, 297
  infant; see Infant mortality
  maternal, 107-109, 504
    causes of, 108
    reduction of, 121
    reporting of, 127
  neonatal, 111, 112
    reduction of, 121
  occupational illnesses and, 413
  perinatal, 110
    reduction of, 121
  postneonatal, 111-112
  rate of, 504
    age-adjusted, 139, 141
    by age and sex, 140, 141
    evaluation and, 76
    specific, 504
    vital index and, 60
  recreational accidents and, 305, 306
  reproductive, 110-111
  residential fires and, 300
  seasonal variations in, 58, 59
  violent deaths and, 294-295
Mosaic law, 4
Mosquito control, 442-443
Motivation, 23, 24
Motor vehicles
  air pollution and, 425

Motor vehicles—cont'd
  injuries and, 291-293, 296-297, 307-308
    personality and, 213
Motorcycle safety, 293, 297
Mottling of teeth, 367
Multiple methods principle, 86
Multiple targets principle, 85
Multipurpose Arthritis Centers, 155-156
Mumps, 284
Municipal ordinances and regulations, 498; *see also* City health departments; Local health departments
Myocardial infarction, 143

N

NAACP, 518
Narcotics, tax for, 539; *see also* Drug misuse
National Academy of Sciences, 430, 434
National Advisory Cancer Council, 517
National Aeronautic and Space Administration, 245
National Ambient Air Quality Standards, 432
National Association for Mental Health, 206, 213
National Association of Registered Nursing Homes, 191
National Basketball Association, 115
National Cancer Act, 517
National Cancer Institute, 517
National Catholic Youth Council, 244
National Center for Health Education, 559
National Center for Health Statistics, 77
National Clearinghouse for Alcohol Information, 160
National Clearinghouse for Family Planning Information, 160
National Commission on Air Quality, 428
National Commission on Marihuana and Drug Abuse, 334, 351
National Committee on Radiation, 434
National Community Water Supply Study of 1970, 369
National Council on Environmental Quality, 386
National Council on Health Planning and Development, 484
National Council of Negro Women, 115
National Council of Senior Citizens, 181
National Drinking Water Advisory Council, 370
National environmental data registry, 412
National Fire Protection Association, 300
National Football League, 115
National forest systems, 222, 223